# ORAL AN
# HISTOLOGY and
# EMBRYOLOGY

*Commissioning Editor:* Alison Taylor
*Development Editor:* Lulu Stader
*Project Manager:* Jane Dingwall
*Designers:* Sarah Russell/Kirsteen Wright
*Illustrator:* Marion Tasker (new figures)
*Illustration Manager:* Merlyn Harvey

Fourth Edition

# ORAL ANATOMY, HISTOLOGY and EMBRYOLOGY

**B. K. B. Berkovitz** BDS, MSc, PhD, FDS (Eng)

*Emeritus Reader, Anatomy and Human Sciences, Biomedical and Health Sciences, King's College, London, UK*

**G. R. Holland** BSc, BDS, PhD, CERT ENDO

*Professor, Department of Cariology, Restorative Sciences and Endodontics, School of Dentistry and Department of Cell and Developmental Biology, University of Michigan, Ann Arbor, USA*

**B. J. Moxham** BSc, BDS, PhD

*Professor of Anatomy, Cardiff School of Biosciences, Cardiff University, Cardiff, UK*

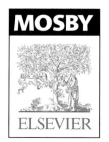

MOSBY

ELSEVIER

EDINBURGH  LONDON  NEW YORK  OXFORD  PHILADELPHIA  ST LOUIS  SYDNEY  TORONTO  2009

# MOSBY
### ELSEVIER

First edition 1992
Second edition 2002
Third edition 2005
Fourth edition 2009

ISBN 9780723434115
International ISBN 9780723435518

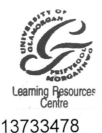

**British Library Cataloguing in Publication Data**

A catalogue record for this book is available from the British Library

**Library of Congress Cataloging in Publication Data**

A catalog record for this book is available from the Library of Congress

**Notice**

Neither the Publisher nor the Authors assume any responsibility for any loss or injury and/or damage to persons or property arising out of or related to any use of the material contained in this book. It is the responsibility of the treating practitioner, relying on independent expertise and knowledge of the patient, to determine the best treatment and method of application for the patient.

**The Publisher**

**ELSEVIER** your source for books,
journals and multimedia
in the health sciences

**www.elsevierhealth.com**

Working together to grow
libraries in developing countries

www.elsevier.com | www.bookaid.org | www.sabre.org

ELSEVIER    BOOK AID International    Sabre Foundation

The publisher's policy is to use paper manufactured from sustainable forests

Printed in China

# Contents

# Preface

This, the fourth edition of our book, follows the form and principles we established in the earlier third edition. Thus, although in that third edition we changed the format of the book from a textbook and atlas to a textbook, we retained the considerable number of illustrations, believing strongly that anatomical and histological textbooks must present information in a visual format. This fourth edition maintains this principle and we have expanded the book considerably to incorporate nearly 1100 illustrations (over twenty percent of the illustrations being new). This time, the expansion of the book has been accomplished without removing any of the topics covered in the previous edition. On the contrary, we have added a chapter on ageing of orodental tissues, because of the increased longevity of humans and the consequences of this to the types of patient seeking dental treatment. This chapter also includes some information concerning forensic dentistry and dental archaeological material. As for the earlier editions of our book, we have preferred, wherever possible, to use photographs and photomicrographs for our illustrations rather than diagrams or drawings, however expertly and artistically presented, as we wish to encourage students to look at 'real' material, warts and all!

As for the previous edition, we are adamant that dental students should not just learn basic ('core') material for oral anatomy, histology and embryology. These are important subjects that provide essential scientific material that should be appreciated by all dental surgeons who wish to consider themselves professionals (in all senses of the term). Indeed, it seems to us that a book such as this that attempts to be encyclopaedic in scope is increasingly necessary where there is a shortage of experienced teachers for the subjects covered! Furthermore, because of the increasing shortage of teachers with clinical backgrounds in dentistry, we have expanded the 'clinical considerations' section in most chapters of our book.

It is, unfortunately, increasingly difficult to obtain funding for basic dental research that involves significant amounts of morphological investigation. And yet, such research does continue and considerable advances in our knowledge of the microscopic anatomy and development of orodental tissues have occurred in recent times. All chapters have been reviewed. In some (e.g. enamel integuments), only minor changes were deemed necessary whereas in others (e.g. alveolar bone and the salivary glands) we have made significant additions. We have also taken the opportunity to improve some of the illustrations where no changes in the text were required. For example, all of the photographs relating to tooth morphology are new. Finally, we are, as ever, grateful to those readers who have provided comments and criticisms. We do not pretend to be infallible and would ask for indulgence if we have strayed from scientific rectitude!

2008
B. K. B. Berkovitz
G. R. Holland
B. J. Moxham

# Acknowledgements

We are most grateful to the numerous colleagues who generously provided photographic material for our book and these have been acknowledged in the text. In addition, we owe a debt of thanks to the following researchers for their constructive criticisms of draft chapters: Dr T. Arnett, Dr A. E. Barrett, Dr J. H. Bennett, Dr S. R. Berkovitz, Dr R. Brooks, Dr M. Cobourne, Dr R. J. Cook, Professor M. C. Dean, Dr A. Grigoriadis, Dr J. D. Harrison, Dr M. Ide, Professor R. W. A. Linden, Dr H. Liversidge, Professor F. McDonald, Dr T. A. Mitsiadis, Professor P. R. Morgan, Dr I. Needleman, Professor R. G. Oliver, Dr C. Orr, Professor R. M. Palmer, Professor T. Pitt-Ford, Dr G. D. Procter, Professor P. T. Sharpe, Dr A. Thexton, Professor T. J. Watson.

We are grateful to Ms K. Kirwan for much photographic help and for producing a number of the new line diagrams. We also acknowledge photographic help from Mr G. Fox.

# In vivo appearance of the oral cavity

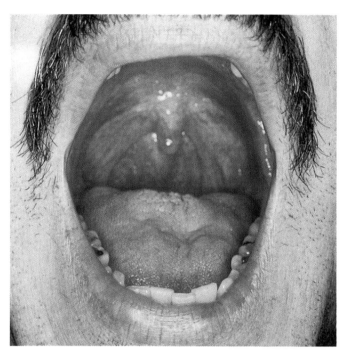

**Fig. 1.1** The oral cavity.

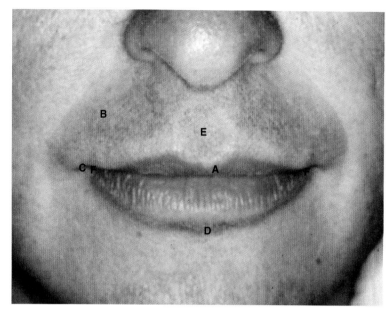

**Fig. 1.2** The lips. A = tubercle; B = nasolabial groove; C = labiomarginal sulci; D = labiomental groove; E = philtrum; F = labial commissure.

The oral cavity (Fig. 1.1) extends from the lips and cheeks externally to the pillars of the fauces internally, where it continues into the oropharynx. It is subdivided into the vestibule external to the teeth and the oral cavity proper internal to the teeth. The palate forms the roof of the mouth and separates the oral and nasal cavities. The floor of the oral cavity consists of mucous membrane covering the mylohyoid muscle and is occupied mainly by the tongue. The lateral walls of the oral cavity are defined by the cheeks and retromolar regions. The primary functions of the mouth are concerned with the ingestion (and selection) of food, and with mastication and swallowing. Secondary functions include speech and ventilation (breathing).

## LIPS

The lips (Fig. 1.2) are composed of a muscular skeleton (the orbicularis oris muscle) and connective tissue, and are covered externally by skin and internally by mucous membrane. The red portion of the lip (the vermilion) is a feature characteristic of humans. The sharp junction of the vermilion and the skin is termed the vermilion border. In the upper lip the vermilion protrudes in the midline to form the tubercle. The lower lip shows a slight depression in the midline corresponding to the tubercle. From the midline to the corners of the mouth the lips widen and then narrow. Laterally, the upper lip is separated from the cheeks by nasolabial grooves. Similar grooves appear with age at the corners of the mouth to delineate the lower lip from the cheeks (the labiomarginal sulci). The labiomental groove separates the lower lip from the chin. In the midline of the upper lip runs the philtrum. The corners of the lips (the labial commissures) are usually located adjacent to the maxillary canine and mandibular first premolar teeth. The lips exhibit sexual dimorphism; as a general rule, the skin of the male is thicker, firmer, less mobile and hirsute. The lips illustrated are lightly closed at rest and are described as being 'competent'.

Incompetent lips (Fig. 1.3) describe a situation where, at rest and with the facial muscles relaxed, a lip seal is not produced. It is of some importance that this is distinguished from conditions where the lips are merely held apart habitually (as often occurs with 'mouth breathers'). The lip posture illustrated in Figure 1.3 can be described as being 'potentially competent', as the lips would be capable of producing a seal at rest if there were no interference caused by the protruding incisors. Where the lips are incompetent, the pattern of swallowing is often modified to produce an

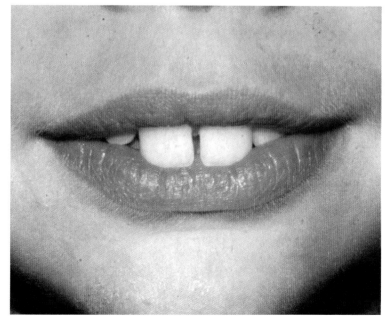

**Fig. 1.3** Incompetent lips.

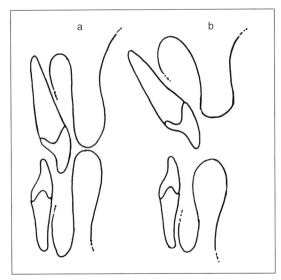

**Fig. 1.4** (a) Competent lips maintaining normal inclination of the incisors. (b) Incompetent lips resulting in proclination of the upper incisors.

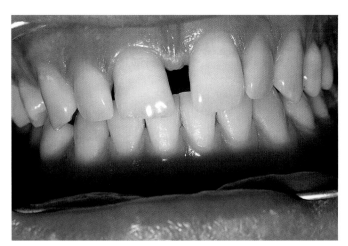

**Fig. 1.6** Midline diastema between upper central incisor teeth, produced by an enlarged labial frenum.

anterior oral seal. Accordingly, an oral seal may be formed by contact between the lower lip (or the tongue) and the palatal mucosa, and there may even be a forcible tongue thrust. It has been estimated that in the UK and the USA about 50% of children at the age of 11 years have some degree of lip incompetence.

The position and activity of the lips are important in controlling the degree of protrusion of the incisors. With competent lips (Fig. 1.4a) the tips of the maxillary incisors lie below the upper border of the lower lip, this arrangement helping to maintain the 'normal' inclination of the incisors. With incompetent lips (Fig. 1.4b) the maxillary incisors may not be so controlled and the lower lip may even lie behind them, thus producing an exaggerated proclination of these teeth. If there is tongue thrusting to provide an anterior oral seal, further forces that tend to protrude the incisors are generated. A tight, or overactive, lip musculature may be associated with retroclined incisors.

## ORAL VESTIBULE

The oral vestibule (Fig. 1.5) is a slit-like space between the lips and cheeks, and the teeth and alveolus. At rest, or with the mouth open, the vestibule and oral cavity proper directly communicate between the

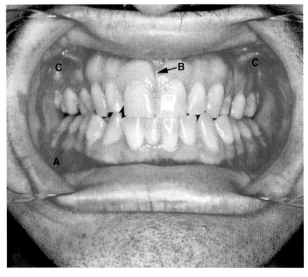

**Fig. 1.5** The oral vestibule. A = vestibular fornix; B = upper labial frenum; C = frenum in the region of the upper premolar teeth.

teeth. When the teeth occlude, the vestibule is a closed space that communicates with the oral cavity proper only behind the last molars (the retromolar regions). This provides a pathway for the administration of nutrients in a patient whose jaws have been wired together following a fracture.

The mucosa covering the alveolus is reflected on to the lips and cheeks, forming a trough or sulcus called the vestibular fornix. In some regions of the sulcus, the mucosa may show distinct sickle-shaped folds running from the cheeks and lips to the alveolus. The upper and lower labial frena or frenula are such folds in the midline. Other folds of variable dimensions may traverse the sulcus in the region of the canines or premolars. Such frena are said to be more pronounced in the lower sulcus. All folds contain loose connective tissue and are neither muscle attachments nor sites of large blood vessels.

The upper labial frenum should be attached well below the alveolar crest. A large frenum with an attachment near this crest may be associated with a midline diastema between the maxillary first incisors (Fig. 1.6). Prominent frena may also influence the stability of dentures.

## GINGIVA

The gums or gingivae, the oral mucosa covering the alveolar bone (which supports the roots of the teeth) and the necks (cervical region) of the teeth, are divided into two main components (Fig. 1.7). The portion lining the lower part of the alveolus is loosely attached to the periosteum via a diffuse submucosa and is termed the alveolar mucosa. It is delineated from the gingiva (which covers the upper part of the alveolar bone and the necks of the teeth) by a well defined junction, the mucogingival junction. The alveolar mucosa appears red, the gingiva pale pink. These colour differences relate to differences in the type of keratinization and the proximity to the surface of underlying blood vessels. Indeed, small blood vessels may readily be seen coursing beneath the alveolar mucosa (Fig. 1.7b). The gingiva may be further subdivided into the attached gingiva and the free gingiva. The attached gingiva is firmly bound to the periosteum of the alveolus and to the teeth, and the free gingiva lies unattached around the cervical region of the tooth. A groove (the free gingival groove) may be seen between the free and attached gingiva. This groove corresponds roughly to the floor of the gingival sulcus that separates the inner surface of the attached gingiva from the enamel itself (see Fig. 14.36). The interdental papilla is that part of the gingiva that fills the space between adjacent teeth. A feature of the attached gingiva is its surface stippling. The degree of stippling varies from individual to individual and according to age, sex and the health of the gingiva. Unlike the attached gingiva, the free gingiva is not stippled. On the lingual surface of the lower

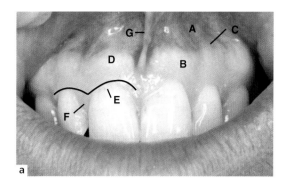 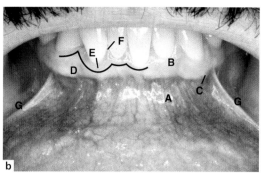

**Fig. 1.7** Upper (a) and lower (b) gingivae. A = alveolar mucosa; B = gingiva; C = mucogingival junction, D = attached gingiva; E = free gingiva; F = interdental papilla; G = labial frenum.

jaw the attached gingiva is sharply differentiated from the alveolar mucosa towards the floor of the mouth by a mucogingival line. On the palate, however, there is no obvious division between the attached gingiva and the rest of the palatal mucosa as this whole surface is keratinized masticatory mucosa.

## CHEEKS

The cheeks extend intra-orally from the labial commissures anteriorly to the ridge of mucosa overlying the ascending ramus of the mandible posteriorly. They are bounded superiorly and inferiorly by the upper and lower vestibular fornices (Fig. 1.5). The mucosa is non-keratinized and, being tightly adherent to the buccinator muscle, is stretched when the mouth is opened and wrinkled when closed. Ectopic sebaceous glands without any associated hair follicles may be evident in the mucosa and are called Fordyce spots (Fig. 1.8). They are seen as small, yellowish-white spots,

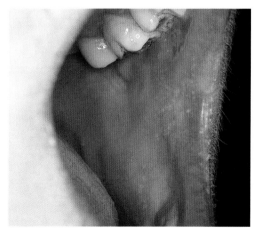

**Fig. 1.8** Inner surface of the cheek, showing Fordyce spots as yellowish patches.

occurring singly or in clusters on the margin of the lips or the mucosa of the cheeks (and other sites such as genital skin). They can be seen in the majority of patients and are said to increase with age.

Few structural landmarks are visible in the cheeks. The parotid duct drains into the cheek opposite the maxillary second molar tooth and its opening may be covered by a small fold of mucosa termed the parotid papilla (see Fig. 1.25). In the retromolar region, in front of the pillars of the fauces, a fold of mucosa containing the pterygomandibular raphe extends from the upper to the lower alveolus (Fig. 1.9). The pterygomandibular space, in which the lingual and inferior alveolar nerves run, lies lateral to this fold and medial to a ridge produced by the mandibular ramus. The groove lying between the ridges produced by the raphe and the ramus of the mandible is an important landmark for insertion of a needle for local anaesthesia of the lingual and inferior alveolar nerves (see page 88).

## PALATE

The palate forms the roof of the mouth and separates the oral and nasal cavities. It is divided into the immovable hard palate anteriorly and the movable soft palate posteriorly. As their names imply, the skeleton of the hard palate is bony while that of the soft palate is fibrous.

The hard palate is covered by a masticatory, keratinized mucosa that is firmly bound down to underlying bone and also contains some taste buds. It shows a distinct prominence immediately behind the maxillary central incisors, the incisive papilla (Fig. 1.10). This papilla overlies the incisive fossa through which the nasopalatine nerves enter on to the palate. Extending posteriorly in the midline from the papilla runs a ridge termed the palatine raphe. Here, the oral mucosa is attached directly to bone without the presence of a submucous layer of tissue. Palatine rugae are elevated ridges in the anterior part of the hard palate that radiate somewhat transversely from the incisive papilla and the anterior part of the palatine raphe. Their pattern is unique to the individual and, like fingerprints, can be used for forensic purposes to help identify individuals. At the junction of the

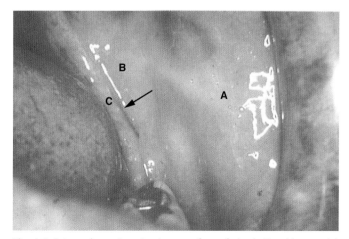

**Fig. 1.9** Retromolar region. A = inner surface of cheek; B = ridge overlying ramus of mandible; C = ridge overlying the pterygomandibular raphe. The arrow indicates a landmark for the insertion of needle for local anaesthesia of the lingual and inferior alveolar nerves.

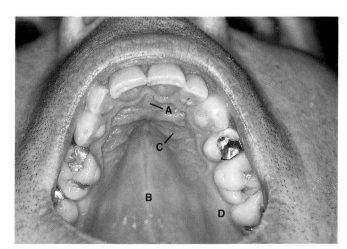

**Fig. 1.10** The hard palate. A = incisive papilla; B = palatine raphe; C = palatine rugae; D = alveolus.

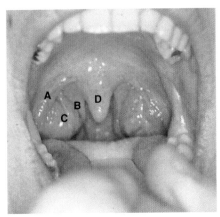

**Fig. 1.11** The soft palate and oropharyngeal isthmus. A = palatoglossal fold; B = palatopharyngeal fold; C = palatine tonsil; D = uvula.

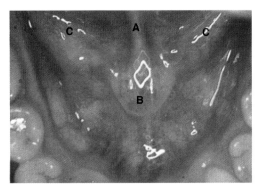

**Fig. 1.13** Floor of the mouth. A = lingual frenum; B = sublingual papilla; C = sublingual folds.

## FLOOR OF THE MOUTH

The moveable floor of the mouth is a small, horseshoe-shaped region above the mylohyoid muscle and beneath the movable part of the tongue (Fig. 1.13). It is covered by a lining of non-keratinized mucosa. In the midline, near the base of the tongue, a fold of tissue called the lingual frenum extends on to the inferior surface of the tongue. The sublingual papilla, on to which the submandibular salivary ducts open into the mouth, is a large centrally positioned protuberance at the base of the tongue. On either side of this papilla are the sublingual folds, beneath which lie the submandibular ducts and sublingual salivary glands.

## TONGUE

The tongue is a muscular organ with its base attached to the floor of the mouth. It is attached to the inner surface of the mandible near the midline and gains support below from the hyoid bone. It functions in mastication, swallowing and speech and carries out important sensory functions, particularly those of taste. The lymphoid material contained in its posterior third has a protective role.

The inferior (ventral) surface of the tongue, related to the floor of the mouth, is covered by a thin lining of non-keratinized mucosa that is tightly bound down to the underlying muscles. In the midline, extending on to the floor of the mouth, lies the lingual frenum (Fig. 1.14). Rarely, this extends across the floor of the mouth to be attached to the mandibular alveolus. Such an overdeveloped lingual frenum (ankyloglossia) may restrict movements of the tongue. Lateral to the frenum lie irregular, fringed folds: the fimbriated folds. Also visible through the mucosa are the deep lingual veins.

The upper (dorsal) surface of the tongue may be subdivided into an anterior two-thirds (palatal part) and a posterior one-third (pharyngeal part). The junction of the palatal and pharyngeal parts is marked by a

palate and the alveolus lies a mass of soft tissue (submucosa) in which run the greater palatine nerves and vessels. The shape and size of the dome of the palate varies considerably, being relatively shallow in some cases and having considerable depth in others.

The boundary between the soft palate and the hard palate is readily palpable and may be distinguished by a change in colour, the soft palate having a yellowish tint. Extending laterally from the free border of the soft palate on each side are the palatoglossal and palatopharyngeal folds (pillars of the fauces), the palatoglossal fold being more anterior (Fig. 1.11). These folds cover the palatoglossus and palatopharyngeus muscles and between them lies the tonsillar fossa that, in children, houses the palatine tonsil. The palatine tonsil is a collection of lymphoid material of variable size that is likely to atrophy in the adult. It exhibits several slit-like invaginations (the tonsillar crypts), one of which is particularly deep and named the intratonsillar cleft. The free edge of the soft palate in the midline is termed the palatal uvula. The oropharyngeal isthmus is where the oral cavity and the oropharynx meet. It is delineated by the palatoglossal folds.

Knowledge of the anatomy of the palate has clinical relevance when siting the posterior border (postdam) of an upper denture. The denture needs to bed into the tissues at the anterior border of the soft palate (at a location sometimes referred to as the 'vibrating line' because the soft palate can be seen to move here on asking a patient to say 'ah'). In most individuals two small pits, the fovea palatini, may be seen (Fig. 1.12) on either side of the midline; these represent the orifices of ducts from some of the minor mucous glands of the palate. The fovea palatini can also be seen on impressions of the palate and a postdam may usually be safely placed a couple of millimetres behind the pits.

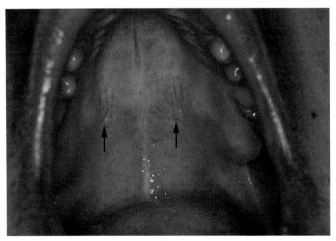

**Fig. 1.12** Oral surface of the soft palate showing the fovea palatini (arrows).

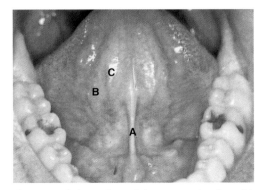

**Fig. 1.14** Inferior surface of the tongue. A = lingual frenum; B = fimbriated fold; C = deep lingual vein.

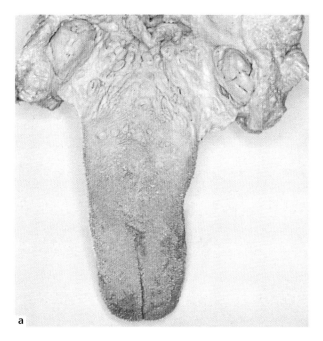

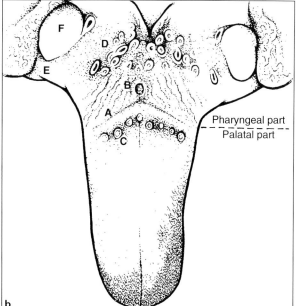

**Fig. 1.15** Dorsum of the tongue.
A = sulcus terminalis
B = foramen caecum
C = circumvallate papillae
D = lingual follicles
E = palatoglossal arches
F = palatine tonsil.

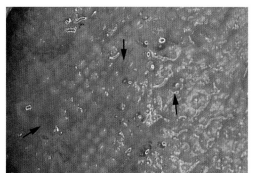

**Fig. 1.16** Dorsum of the tongue, showing filiform and fungiform (arrows) papillae.

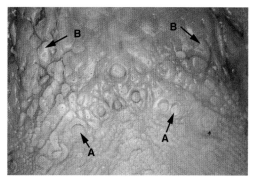

**Fig. 1.17** Dorsum of the tongue, showing circumvallate papillae (A). B = lingual follicles.

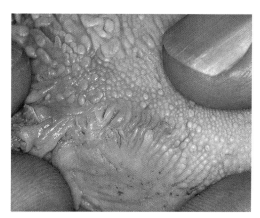

**Fig. 1.18** Side of the tongue, showing slit-like appearance of foliate papillae.

shallow V-shaped groove, the sulcus terminalis (Fig. 1.15). The angle (or 'V') of the sulcus terminalis is directed posteriorly. In the midline, near the angle, may be seen a small pit called the foramen caecum. This is the primordial site of development of the thyroid gland.

The mucosa of the palatal part of the dorsum of the tongue is mainly keratinized and is characterized by an abundance of projections (papillae). The most numerous are the filiform papillae appearing as whitish, conical elevations (Fig. 1.16). Interspersed between the filiform papillae and readily seen at the tip of the tongue are isolated reddish prominences, the fungiform papillae. The largest papillae on the palatal surface of the tongue are the circumvallate papillae, which lie immediately in front of the sulcus terminalis. There are about 10–15 circumvallate papillae (Fig. 1.17). They do not project beyond the surface of the tongue and are surrounded by a circular 'trench'. Foliate papillae (Fig. 1.18) appear as a series of parallel, slit-like folds of mucosa on each lateral border of the tongue, near the attachment of the palatoglossal fold. The foliate papillae are of variable length in humans and are the vestige of large papillae found in many other mammals. Apart from the filiform papillae, the papillae are the site of taste buds.

The pharyngeal surface of the dorsum of the tongue is non-keratinized and is covered with large rounded nodules termed the lingual follicles. These follicles are composed of lymphatic tissue, collectively forming the lingual tonsil. The posterior part of the tongue slopes towards the epiglottis, where three folds of mucous membrane are seen: the median and lateral glossoepiglottic folds. The anterior pillars of the fauces (the palatoglossal

arches) extend from the soft palate to the sides of the tongue near the circumvallate papillae.

## CLINICAL CONSIDERATIONS

There are a number of conditions in the mouth that can be inspected in the non-clinical environment. They provide examples of 1) normal variation, 2) common benign disorders and 3) disorders that may highlight normal features, which may be otherwise inconspicuous.

As examples of normal variation, we can consider pigmentation, Fordyce spots and black hairy tongue. In dark-skinned patients, patches of melanin pigment may be seen in the mouth, particularly in the gingiva (Fig. 1.19). This pigmentation is due to the extra melanosome granules present within the oral epithelium (see Fig. 14.22). Such pigmentation needs to be distinguished from other forms of mucosal pigmentation and from increased melanin pigmentation associated with a range of inflammatory conditions, such as lichen planus where melanin pigment is held within macrophages in the lamina propria (Figs 1.20, 1.21). Fordyce spots are seen in varying degrees as small, yellowish-white spots, occurring singly or in clusters on the margin of the lips (Fig. 1.22) or in the mucosa of the cheeks (Fig. 1.8) (and other sites such as genital skin). They can be seen in the majority of patients and are said to increase with age. They represent collections of sebaceous glands (Fig. 1.23) without any associated hair follicles. The range of variation in the filiform papillae on the dorsum of the tongue is

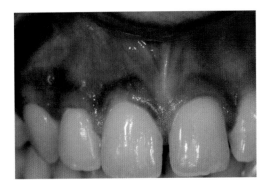

**Fig. 1.19** Patches of dark melanin pigment appearing in the region of the attached gingiva. Courtesy of Professor P.R. Morgan.

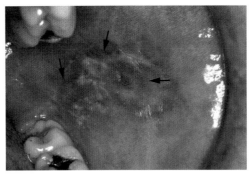

**Fig. 1.20** Area of increased pigmentation (arrowed) associated with whitish patches due to lichen planus. Courtesy of Professor P.R. Morgan.

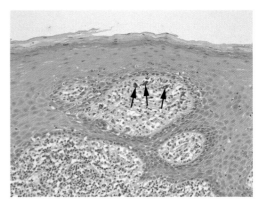

**Fig. 1.21** Micrograph of biopsy taken from pigmented area seen in Fig. 1.20, showing melanin pigment within macrophages (arrows) lying within the lamina propria. The epithelium is parakeratinized, giving the whitish patches (H & E; ×100). Courtesy of Professor P.R. Morgan.

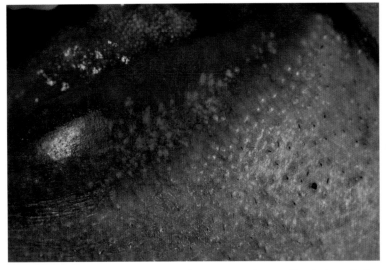

**Fig. 1.22** Fordyce spots appearing as yellow spots on the vermilion (red zone) of the lip. The black spots below represent hair follicles on the surface of the adjacent skin of the chin. Courtesy of Professor P.R. Morgan.

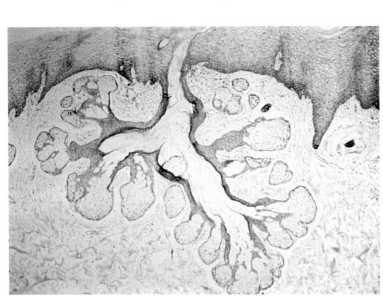

**Fig. 1.23** Micrograph of a Fordyce spot, showing it to be a sebaceous gland (H & E;. ×50). Courtesy of Professor P.R. Morgan.

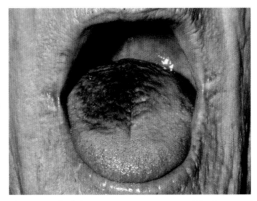

**Fig. 1.24** Black hairy tongue. Courtesy of Professor P.R. Morgan.

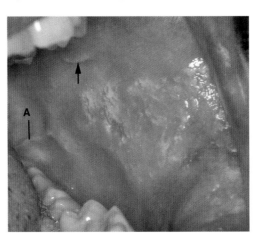

**Fig. 1.25** View of buccal mucosa showing a linea alba adjacent to the molar teeth (A) at the level of the occlusal plane. In front of this line, the white patches on the cheek represent more diverse cheek chewing. Arrow shows the parotid papilla. Courtesy of Professor P.R. Morgan.

well illustrated by black hairy tongue (lingua villosa nigra), a benign condition in which there is hypertrophy of these papillae (Fig. 1.24). Instead of being about 1 mm in length, the filiform papillae may reach up to 15 mm, giving the dorsum an appearance of being covered in fine hairs. This provides a suitable environment for bacteria (and sometimes fungi)

to accumulate and, together with retained pigments of dietary or microbial origin, may colour the surface of the tongue black. The condition may be associated with the administration of antibiotics or mouthwashes that may alter the normal bacterial population. It has a frequency of about 5% of the population.

Examples of common benign disorders are linea alba and tori. On the inside of the cheek and level with the occlusal plane, a linear, slightly raised whitish ridge may be seen, the linea alba (Fig. 1.25). It is commonly the result of low-grade, intermittent trauma due to folds of cheek mucosa being trapped between the teeth. More active trauma associated with cheek chewing produces a much larger, irregular white patch (Fig. 1.25). The

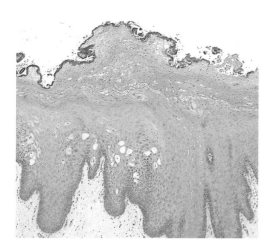

**Fig. 1.26** Section of buccal mucosa showing the linea alba to be parakeratinized compared with the normal non-keratinized state of the buccal mucosa (H & E; ×50). Courtesy of Professor P.R. Morgan.

**Fig. 1.27** Upper jaw showing a relatively small torus palatinus as an overgrowth of bone along the midline of the palate. Courtesy of Dr C. Dunlap.

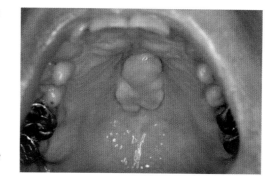

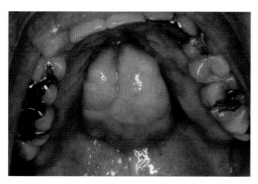

**Fig. 1.28** Upper jaw showing a large torus palatinus as an overgrowth of bone along the midline of the palate. Courtesy of Dr C. Dunlap.

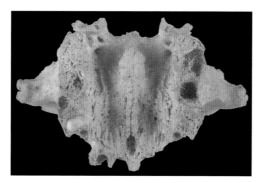

**Fig. 1.29** Isolated palate showing torus palatinus as an overgrowth of bone along the midline. Courtesy of the Royal College of Surgeons of England.

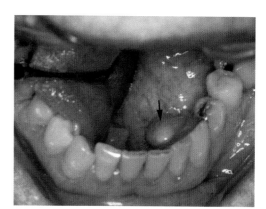

**Fig. 1.30** Unilateral torus mandibularis (arrow) on the lingual surface of the mandible. Courtesy of Professor P.R. Morgan.

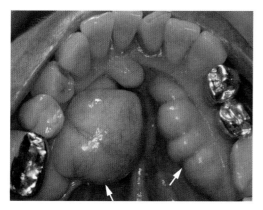

**Fig. 1.31** Bilateral torus mandibularis (arrows) on the lingual surface of the mandible. Courtesy of Dr C. Dunlap.

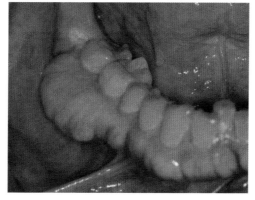

**Fig. 1.32** Torus mandibularis on the buccal surface of the mandible. Courtesy of Dr C. Dunlap.

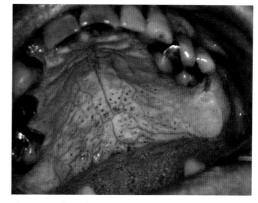

**Fig. 1.33** The palate of a heavy smoker presenting with an overall whitish appearance to the mucosa that highlights the orifices of the mucous glands as red spots. Courtesy of Professor P.R. Morgan.

constant irritation converts the surface epithelium from its normal non-keratinized state into a parakeratinized layer (Fig. 1.26).

Individual variation in the shape of the jaws is recognized by anatomists and pathologists. Such variations blend with benign conditions. As an example, tori are benign localized overgrowths of bone found in both the upper (torus palatinus) and lower (torus mandibularis) jaws, resulting in an increased radiopacity in the region. In the upper jaw, the enlargement is typically seen in the midline (Figs 1.27–1.29), while in the lower jaw it is usually on the lingual aspect in the canine/premolar region and may be unilateral (Fig. 1.30) or bilateral (Fig. 1.31). However, a torus mandibularis may also affect the buccal surface of the mandible (Fig. 1.32). Torus palatinus is more common in females, while torus mandibularis is slightly more common in males. Tori vary in size from small to very large and there is a tendency for them to increase in size

with age. Tori may be related to functional adaptations, as there is some evidence that their incidence is decreased in association with fewer teeth being present in the jaws. They require no treatment unless they interfere with the construction of satisfactory removable dentures. Their incidence varies from about 0.5% to over 65%, being less frequent in Caucasians and more frequent in Eskimos, Mongoloids and other Asian groups.

As an example of a disorder that highlights normal features that may be otherwise inconspicuous, one can inspect the palate of a patient who smokes heavily, revealing a whitish appearance that highlights numerous reddish spots (Fig. 1.33). The white appearance is the result of a pronounced orthokeratinized layer being present due to chronic irritation and this highlights the orifices of the ducts (as red spots) associated with the numerous mucous salivary glands present.

# Dento-osseous structures

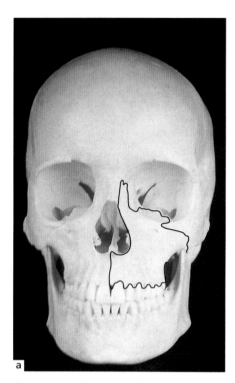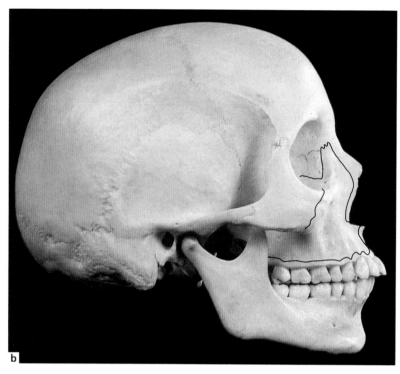

**Fig. 2.1** Front (a) and side (b) views of the skull, showing the relationship between the jaws and the remainder of the skull. The black line describes the boundaries of a maxillary bone.

## JAWS

The jaws are the tooth-bearing bones. They comprise three bones. The two maxillary bones form the upper jaw. The lower jaw is a single bone, the mandible (Fig. 2.1).

The skull is the most complex osseous structure in the body. It protects the brain, the organs of special sense and the cranial parts of the respiratory and digestive systems. The skull is divided into the neurocranium (which houses and protects the brain and the organs of special sense) and the viscerocranium (which surrounds the upper parts of the respiratory and digestive tracts). The jaws contribute the major part of the viscerocranium, comprising about 25% of the skull. The jaws have evolved from the gill arch elements of early agnathan vertebrates. It is probable that one or two anterior gill arches gradually disappeared with the expansion of the mouth cavity, so that the gill arch that developed phylogenetically into the jaws of ancestral gnathostomes was not the first of the series. Note that the upper jaw not only contains teeth but also contributes to the skeleton of the nose, orbit, cheek and palate.

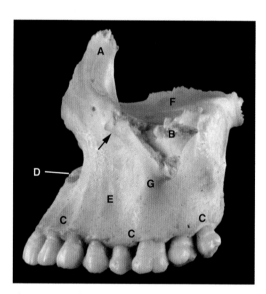

**Fig. 2.2** Lateral aspect of the maxilla. A = frontal process; B = zygomatic process; C = alveolar process; D = site of anterior nasal spine; E = canine fossa; F = orbital plate; G = jugal crest. The infra-orbital foramen is arrowed.

## MAXILLA

The maxilla consists of a body and four processes: the frontal, zygomatic, alveolar and palatine processes. Only the palatine process cannot be seen from the lateral aspect of the maxilla (Fig. 2.2). The anterolateral surface of the maxilla (the malar surface) forms the skeleton of the anterior part of the cheek. In the midline, the alveolar processes of the two maxillae meet at the intermaxillary suture whence they diverge laterally to form the opening into the nasal fossae (the piriform aperture). At the lower border of the piriform aperture, in the midline, lies the bony projection termed the anterior nasal spine. The malar surface of the body of the maxilla is concave, forming the canine fossa. Superiorly, the malar surface is continuous with the orbital plate of the maxilla and forms the floor of the orbit.

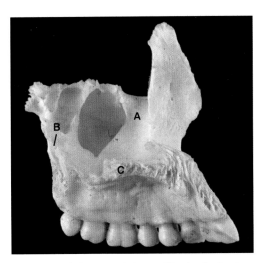

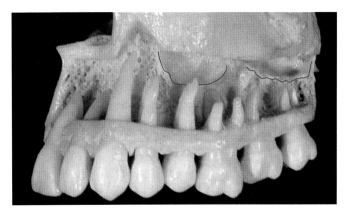

**Fig. 2.5** Lateral view of the maxilla, showing close relationship of roots of the cheek teeth to the floor of the maxillary sinus (red outline).

**Fig. 2.3** Medial aspect of the maxilla. A = lacrimal groove; B = palatine groove; C = palatine process of maxilla. Note the large opening into the maxillary sinus.

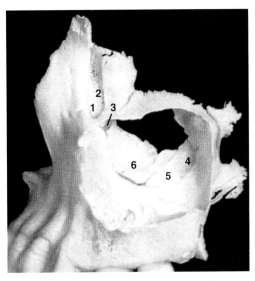

**Fig. 2.4** Osteology of the maxillary air sinus showing adjacent bones reducing the size of the ostium. 1 = lacrimal groove of maxilla; 2 = lacrimal groove; 3 = lacrimal bone; 4 = ethmoid bone; 5 = palatine bone; 6 = inferior nasal concha. Courtesy of Professor R.M.H. McMinn.

Anterior to the orbital plate, the frontal process extends above the piriform aperture to meet the nasal and frontal bones. Below the infra-orbital rim lies the infra-orbital foramen through which the infra-orbital branch of the maxillary nerve and the infra-orbital artery from the maxillary artery emerge on to the face. The posterolateral surface of the maxilla (the infratemporal surface) forms the anterior wall of the infratemporal fossa. The malar and infratemporal surfaces meet at a bony ridge extending from the zygomatic process to the alveolus adjacent to the first molar tooth. This ridge is called the zygomatico-alveolar, or jugal, crest. The posterior convexity of the infratemporal surface is termed the maxillary tuberosity and presents several small foramina associated with the posterior superior alveolar nerves (which supply the posterior maxillary teeth). The zygomatic process extends from both the malar and the infratemporal surfaces of the maxilla. From the entire lower surface of the body arises the alveolar process, which supports the maxillary teeth.

The medial aspect of the maxilla is illustrated in Figure 2.3. This part of the maxilla forms the lateral wall of the nose. In the specimen illustrated, the central hollow of the body of the maxilla (the maxillary air sinus or antrum) is divided by a bony septum. In front of the antrum lies a deep vertical groove called the lacrimal groove. This groove meets the lower edge of the lacrimal bone to form the nasolacrimal canal. Behind the antrum lies the palatine groove, which is converted into a canal carrying the greater palatine nerve and artery by the perpendicular plate of the palatine bone. The maxillary palatine process extends horizontally from the medial surface of the maxilla where the body meets the alveolar process.

The lateral wall of the nasal fossa consists mainly of the medial surface of the maxilla. This surface of the isolated bone is occupied mainly by the large maxillary hiatus (Fig. 2.3). To reduce the size of this space in vivo, the hiatus is overlapped by the lacrimal bone and the ethmoid bone above, the palatine bone behind and the inferior concha below (Fig. 2.4).

## Maxillary sinus

The maxillary sinus (antrum) is the largest of the paranasal sinuses and is situated in the body of the maxilla. It is pyramidal in shape. The base (medial wall) forms part of the lateral wall of the nose. The apex extends into the zygomatic process of the maxilla. The roof of the sinus is part of the floor of the orbit and the floor of the sinus is formed by the alveolar process and part of the palatine process of the maxilla. The anterior wall of the sinus is the facial surface of the maxilla and the posterior wall is the infratemporal surface of the maxilla. Running in the roof of the sinus is the infra-orbital nerve and vessels. The anterior superior alveolar nerve and vessels run in the anterior wall of the sinus. The posterior superior alveolar nerve and vessels pass through canals in the posterior surface of the sinus. The medial wall of the maxillary sinus contains the opening (ostium) of the sinus that leads into the middle meatus of the nose. As this opening lies well above the floor of the sinus, its position is unfavourable for drainage (see Fig. 5.4a). Infections of the maxillary sinus may therefore require surgical intervention, creating a more favourable drainage channel closer to the floor of the sinus.

The roots of the cheek teeth are related to the floor of the maxillary sinus (Fig. 2.5). The most closely related are the roots of the second permanent maxillary molar, especially the apex of its palatal root; the roots of the first and third molars and the second premolar are only slightly further away. Sometimes, only mucosa separates the roots from the sinus. Care must be taken (particularly when extracting fractured roots in this region) to avoid creating an oro-antral fistula, when an epithelium-lined channel exists between the oral cavity and maxillary sinus.

The maxillary air sinus is lined by respiratory epithelium (a ciliated columnar epithelium), with numerous goblet cells. The sinus is innervated by the infra-orbital nerve and superior alveolar branches of the maxillary nerve.

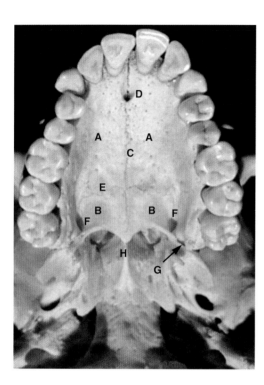

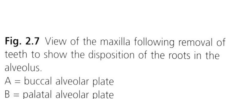

**Fig. 2.6** Oral surface of the hard palate.
A = palatine processes of maxillae
B = horizontal plates of the palatine bones
C = median palatine suture
D = incisive fossa
E = transverse palatine suture
F = greater palatine foramina
G = lesser palatine foramen
H = posterior nasal spine.

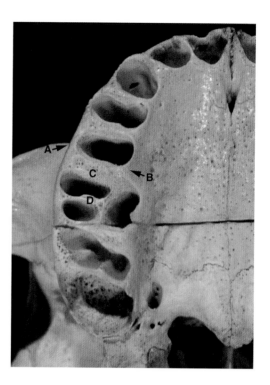

**Fig. 2.7** View of the maxilla following removal of teeth to show the disposition of the roots in the alveolus.
A = buccal alveolar plate
B = palatal alveolar plate
C = interdental bony septa between the second premolar and first permanent molar
D = interradicular septum between the buccal roots of first permanent molar.

An inferior view of the maxillae shows their important contributions to the hard palate (Fig. 2.6). The four major bones contributing to the hard palate are the palatine processes of the maxillae and the horizontal plates of the palatine bones. The maxillary palatine processes arise as horizontal plates at the junction of the bodies and alveolar processes of the maxillae. The boundary between the palatine and alveolar processes is well defined in its posterior aspect only; anteriorly, the angle between the two is less well defined. The junction between the palatine processes in the midline is termed the median palatine suture. Anteriorly, behind the central incisors, this junction is incomplete, thus forming the incisive fossa, through which pass the nasopalatine nerves. Unlike the nasal surface, the oral surface of the palatine process is rough and irregular. The posterior edges of the palatine processes articulate with the horizontal plates of the two palatine bones to form the transverse palatine suture. Laterally, this junction is incomplete, forming the greater palatine foramina, through which pass the greater palatine nerves and vessels. Behind the greater palatine foramina lie the lesser palatine foramina, through which pass the lesser palatine nerves and vessels. The junction of the two palatine bones in the midline completes the median palatine suture. The posterior borders of the horizontal palatine plates are concave and, in the midline, form a sharp ridge of bone called the posterior nasal spine. To the posterior edge of the hard palate is attached the fibrous palatine aponeurosis of the soft palate, which is formed by the tendons of the tensor veli palatini muscles.

## MAXILLARY ALVEOLUS

The maxillary alveolar processes extend inferiorly from the bodies of the maxillae and support the teeth within bony sockets (Fig. 2.7). Each maxilla can contain a full quadrant of eight permanent teeth or five deciduous teeth. The form of the alveolus is related to the functional demands put upon the teeth. When the teeth are lost the alveolus resorbs.

Essentially, the alveolar process consists of two parallel plates of cortical bone, the buccal and palatal alveolar plates, between which lie the sockets of individual teeth. Between each socket lie interalveolar or interdental septa. The floor of the socket has been termed the fundus, its rim the alveolar crest. The form and depth of each socket is defined by the form and length of the root it supports, and thus shows considerable variation. In multirooted teeth, the sockets are divided by interradicular septa.

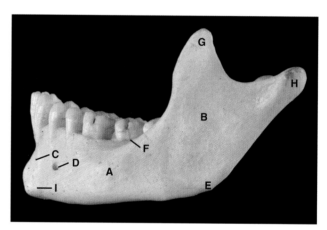

**Fig. 2.8** Lateral aspect of the mandible. A = Body; B = ramus; C = incisive fossa; D = mental foramen; E = angle; F = external oblique line; G = coronoid process; H = condyle; I = mental protuberance.

The apical regions of the sockets of anterior teeth are closely related to the nasal fossae, while those of posterior teeth are closely related to the maxillary air sinuses. The positions of the sockets in relation to the buccal and palatal alveolar plates are shown in Figure 2.12.

## MANDIBLE

The mandible consists of a horizontal, horseshoe-shaped component, the body of the mandible, and two vertical components, the rami. The rami join the body posteriorly at obtuse angles. The body of the mandible carries the mandibular teeth and their associated alveolar processes. Before birth, the body consists of two lateral halves that meet in the midline at a symphysis. As viewed laterally (Fig. 2.8), on either side of the midline, close to the inferior margin of the body lies a distinct prominence called the mental tubercle. These tubercles constitute the mental protuberance or chin. Above the mental protuberance lies a shallow depression termed the incisive fossa. Behind this fossa, the canine eminence overlies the root of the mandibular canine. Midway in the height of the body of the mandible, related to the premolar teeth, is the mental foramen. The mental branches

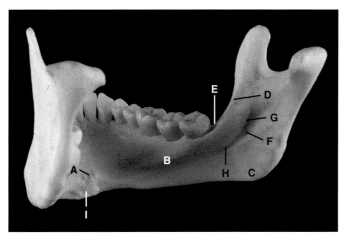

**Fig. 2.9** Inner (medial) surface of the mandible. A = genial spines (tubercles); B = internal oblique ridge (mylohyoid ridge); C = attachment area for medial pterygoid muscle; D = temporal crest; E = retromolar triangle; F = mandibular foramen; G = lingula; H = mylohyoid groove; I = digastric fossa.

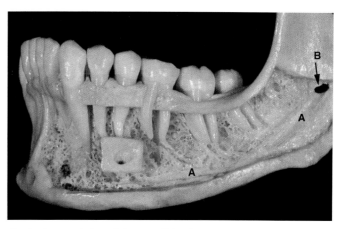

**Fig. 2.10** Lateral view of the mandible, showing the roots of the teeth and the relationship to the mandibular canal (A). B = mandibular foramen.

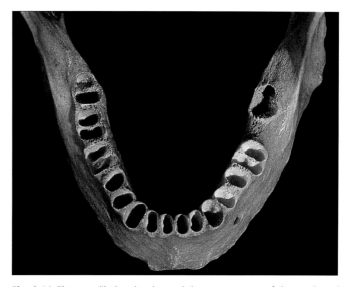

**Fig. 2.11** The mandibular alveolus and the arrangement of the tooth sockets. Note that the left second permanent mandibular molar has previously been extracted and the socket has healed.

of the inferior alveolar nerve and artery pass on to the face through this foramen. The most common position for the mental foramen is on a vertical line passing through the mandibular second premolar. During the first and second years of life, as the prominence of the chin develops, the direction of the opening of the mental foramen alters from facing forwards to facing upwards and backwards. Rarely, there may be multiple mental foramina. The inferior margin of the mandibular body meets the posterior margin of the ramus at the angle of the mandible. This area is irregular, being the site of insertion of the masseter muscle and stylomandibular ligament. The alveolus forms the superior margin of the mandibular body. The junction of the alveolus and ramus is demarcated by a ridge of bone, the external oblique line, which continues downwards and forwards across the body of the mandible to terminate below the mental foramen. As this line progresses upwards, it becomes the anterior margin of the ramus and ends as the tip of the coronoid process. The coronoid and condylar processes form the two processes of the superior border of the ramus. The coronoid process provides attachment for the temporalis muscle. The condylar process has a neck supporting an articular surface, which fits into the mandibular fossa of the temporal bone to form a moveable synovial joint (the temporomandibular joint). The concavity between the coronoid and condylar processes is called the mandibular notch.

Several important features are seen on the internal (medial) surface of the mandible (Fig. 2.9). Close to the midline, on the inferior surface of the mandibular body, lie two shallow depressions called the digastric fossae, into which are inserted the anterior bellies of the digastric muscles. Above the fossae, in the midline, are the genial spines or tubercles. There are generally two inferior and two superior spines, which serve as attachments for the geniohyoid muscles and the genioglossus muscles, respectively. Passing upwards and backwards across the medial surface of the body of the mandible is a prominent ridge. This is termed the mylohyoid or internal oblique ridge. From this ridge, the mylohyoid muscle takes origin. The mylohyoid ridge arises between the genial spines and digastric fossa and increases in prominence as it passes backwards to end on the anterior surface of the ramus. Because the mylohyoid muscle forms the floor of the mouth, the bone above the mylohyoid ridge forms the anterior wall of the oral cavity proper, while that below the ridge forms the lateral wall of the submandibular space (see page 78). The following features may be seen on the medial surface of the ramus. Around the angle of the mandible, the bone is roughened for the attachment of the medial pterygoid muscle. Commencing at the tip of the coronoid process, a ridge

of bone called the temporal crest runs down the anterior surface of the ramus to end behind the mandibular molars at the retromolar triangle. In the centre of the medial surface of the ramus lies the mandibular foramen, through which the inferior alveolar nerve and artery pass into the mandibular canal. A bony process, the lingula, extends from the anterosuperior surface of the foramen. The lingula is the site of attachment of the sphenomandibular ligament (see page 64). The mylohyoid groove may be seen running down from the posteroinferior surface of the foramen.

The mandibular canal, that transmits the inferior alveolar nerve, artery and veins, begins at the mandibular foramen and extends to the region of the premolar teeth, where it bifurcates into the mental and incisive canals (Fig. 2.10). The course of the mandibular canal and its relationship with the teeth is variable; this variation is illustrated in connection with the course of the inferior alveolar nerve (Fig. 4.6).

## MANDIBULAR ALVEOLUS

As for the maxilla, the mandibular alveolus consists of buccal and lingual alveolar plates joined by interdental and interradicular septa (Fig. 2.11). In the region of the second and third molars, the external oblique line is superimposed upon the buccal alveolar plate. The form and depth of the tooth sockets are related to the morphology of the roots of the mandibular teeth and the functional demands placed upon them.

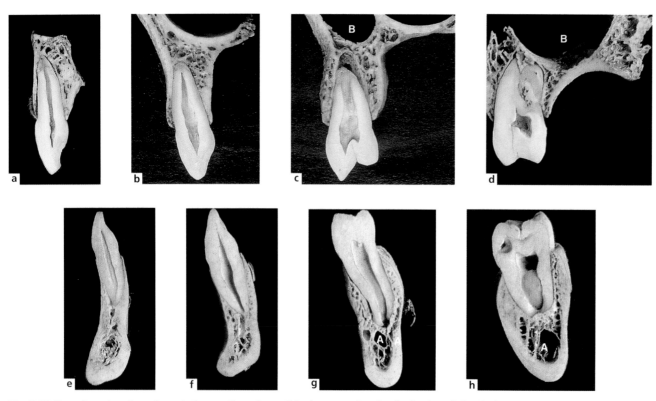

**Fig. 2.12** Buccolingual sections through the maxilla and mandible demonstrating the distribution of alveolar bone in relation to the roots of the teeth. (a) Maxillary incisor region. (b) Maxillary canine region. (c) Maxillary premolar region. (d) Maxillary molar region. (e) Mandibular incisor region. (f) Mandibular canine region. (g) Mandibular premolar region. (h) Mandibular molar region. Note the relationship of the mandibular cheek teeth to the mandibular canal (A) and of the maxillary cheek teeth to the maxillary sinus (B). Courtesy of the Royal College of Surgeons of England.

Figure 2.12 illustrates buccolingual sections through the teeth and jaws, demonstrating the directional axes and bony relationships of the teeth and their alveoli and the relative thickness of the buccal and lingual alveolar plates. The relationships of the mandibular teeth to the mandibular canal, and the maxillary teeth to the maxillary sinus have clinical significance. Thus, the thickness of bone may determine the direction in which teeth are levered during extractions and explain why local infiltration techniques can be used for anaesthetizing anterior mandibular teeth but not mandibular molar teeth. Care must be taken when exploring for fractured roots in the maxillary region in order to avoid an oro-antral fistula, due to the presence of the maxillary sinus in close relationship to the maxillary molar teeth, while the presence of the inferior alveolar nerve and its branches requires care when placing dental implants in the mandibular region.

## TOOTH MORPHOLOGY

Humans have two generations of teeth: the deciduous (or primary) dentition and the permanent (or secondary) dentition. No teeth are erupted into the mouth at birth but, by the age of 3 years, all the deciduous teeth have erupted. By 6 years, the first permanent teeth appear and thence the deciduous teeth are exfoliated one by one to be replaced by their permanent successors. A complete permanent dentition is present at or around the age of 18 years. Thus, given the average life of 75 years, the functional lifespan of the deciduous dentition is only 5% of this total while, with care and luck, that of the permanent dentition can be over 90%. In the complete deciduous dentition there are 20 teeth – 10 in each jaw; in the complete permanent dentition there are 32 teeth – 16 in each jaw.

In both dentitions, there are three basic tooth forms: incisiform, caniniform and molariform. Incisiform teeth (incisors) are cutting teeth, with thin, blade-like crowns. Caniniform teeth (canines) are piercing or tearing teeth, having a single, stout, pointed, cone-shaped crown. Molariform teeth

(molars and premolars) are grinding teeth possessing a number of cusps on an otherwise flattened biting surface. Premolars are bicuspid teeth; they are peculiar to the permanent dentition and replace the deciduous molars. Table 2.1 gives definitions of terms used for the descriptions of tooth form.

## DENTAL NOTATION

The types and numbers of teeth in any mammalian dentition can be expressed using dental formulae. The type of tooth is represented by its initial letter – I for incisors, C for canines, P for premolars, M for molars. The deciduous dentition is indicated by the letter D. The formula for the deciduous human dentition is $DI_2^2 DC_1^1 DM_2^2 = 10$, and for the permanent dentition $I_2^2 C_1^1 PM_2^2 M_3^3 = 16$, where the numbers following each letter refer to the number of teeth of each type in the upper and lower jaws on one side only. Identification of teeth is made not only according to the dentition to which they belong and basic tooth form but also according to their anatomical location within the jaws. The tooth-bearing region of the jaws can be divided into four quadrants: the right and left maxillary and mandibular quadrants. A tooth may thus be identified according to the quadrant in which it is located – e.g. a right maxillary deciduous incisor or a left mandibular permanent molar. In both the permanent and deciduous dentitions, the incisors may be distinguished according to their relationship to the midline. Thus, the incisor nearest the midline is the central (or first) incisor and the more laterally positioned incisor the lateral (or second) incisor. The permanent premolars and the permanent and deciduous molars can also be distinguished according to their mesiodistal relationships (see Fig. 2.13). The molar most mesially positioned is designated the first molar, the one behind it being the second molar. In the permanent dentition, the tooth most distally positioned is the third molar. The mesial premolar is the first premolar, the premolar behind it being the second premolar.

**Table 2.1** *Some terms used for the description of tooth form*

| | |
|---|---|
| Crown | Clinical crown – that portion of a tooth visible in the oral cavity<br>Anatomical crown – that portion of a tooth covered with enamel |
| Root | Clinical root – that portion of a tooth which lies within the alveolus<br>Anatomical root – that portion of a tooth covered by cementum |
| Cervical margin | The junction of the anatomical crown and the anatomical root |
| Occlusal surface | The biting surface of a posterior tooth (molar or premolar) |
| Cusp | A pronounced elevation on the occlusal surface of a tooth |
| Incisal margin | The cutting edge of anterior teeth, analogous to the occlusal surface of the posterior teeth |
| Tubercle | A small elevation on the crown |
| Cingulum | A bulbous convexity near the cervical region of a tooth |
| Ridge | A linear elevation on the surface of a tooth |
| Marginal ridge | A ridge at the mesial or distal edge of the occlusal surface of posterior teeth. Some anterior teeth have equivalent ridges |
| Fissure | A long cleft between cusps or ridges |
| Fossa | A rounded depression in a surface of a tooth |
| Buccal | Towards, or adjacent to, the cheek. The term buccal surface is reserved for that surface of a premolar or molar which is positioned immediately adjacent to the cheek |
| Labial | Towards, or adjacent to, the lips. The term labial surface is reserved for that surface of an incisor or canine which is positioned immediately adjacent to the lips |
| Palatal | Towards, or adjacent to, the palate. The term palatal surface is reserved for that surface of a maxillary tooth which is positioned immediately adjacent to the palate |
| Lingual | Towards, or adjacent to, the tongue. The term lingual surface is reserved for that surface of a mandibular tooth which lies immediately adjacent to the tongue |
| Mesial | Towards the median. The mesial surface is that surface which faces towards the median line following the curve of the dental arch |
| Distal | Away from the median. The distal surface is that surface which faces away from the median line following the curve of the dental arch |

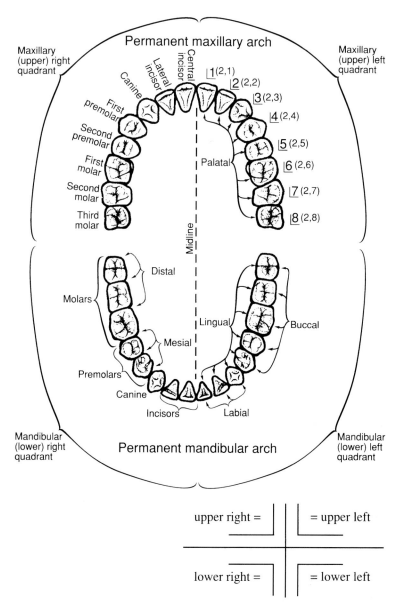

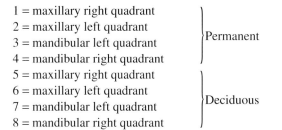

**Fig. 2.13** Terminology employed for the identification of teeth according to their location in the jaws.

A dental shorthand may be used in the clinic to simplify tooth identification. The permanent teeth in each quadrant are numbered 1–8 and the deciduous teeth in each quadrant are lettered A–E. The symbols for the quadrants are derived from an imaginary cross, with the horizontal bar placed between the upper and lower jaws and the vertical bar running between the upper and lower central incisors. Thus, the maxillary right first permanent molar is allocated the symbol $\underline{6|}$ and the mandibular left deciduous canine $\overline{|c}$. This system of dental shorthand is termed the Zsigmondy system. An alternative scheme has been devised by the Federation Dentaire Internationale, in which the quadrant is represented by a number:

1 = maxillary right quadrant ⎫
2 = maxillary left quadrant ⎪
3 = mandibular left quadrant ⎬ Permanent
4 = mandibular right quadrant ⎪
⎭
5 = maxillary right quadrant ⎫
6 = maxillary left quadrant ⎪
7 = mandibular left quadrant ⎬ Deciduous
8 = mandibular right quadrant ⎭

In this system, the quadrant number prefixes a tooth number. Thus, the maxillary right first permanent molar is symbolized as 1,6 and the mandibular left deciduous canine as 7,3.

Figure 2.13 summarizes some of the terminology employed for the identification of teeth according to their location in the jaws.

## DIFFERENCES BETWEEN TEETH OF THE DECIDUOUS AND PERMANENT DENTITIONS

1. The dental formula for the deciduous dentition is:
   $DI\frac{2}{2} DC\frac{1}{1} DM\frac{2}{2} = 10$
   That of the permanent dentition is:
   $I\frac{2}{2} C\frac{1}{1} PM\frac{2}{2} M\frac{3}{3} = 16$.
2. The deciduous teeth are smaller than their corresponding permanent successors although the mesiodistal dimensions of the permanent premolars are generally less than those for the deciduous molars.
3. Deciduous teeth have a greater constancy of shape than permanent teeth.
4. The crowns of deciduous teeth appear bulbous, often having pronounced labial or buccal cingula.
5. The cervical margins of deciduous teeth are more sharply demarcated and pronounced than those of the permanent teeth, the enamel bulging at the cervical margins rather than gently tapering.

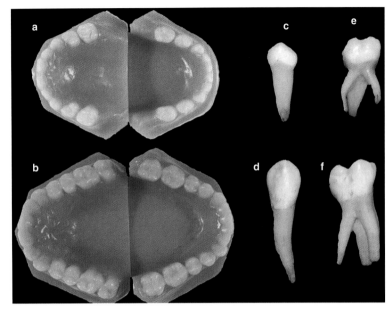

**Fig. 2.14** Models of deciduous (a) and permanent (b) dental arches and some examples of deciduous and permanent teeth. (c) Deciduous canine. (d) Permanent canine. (e) Deciduous second molar. (f) Permanent first molar.

**Table 2.2** *Average dimensions of the permanent teeth*

| Tooth | Crown height (mm) | Length of root (mm) | Mediodistal crown diameter (mm) | Labiolingual crown diameter (mm) |
|---|---|---|---|---|
| **Maxillary** | | | | |
| 1 | 10.5 | 13.0 | 8.5 | 7.0 |
| 2 | 9.0 | 13.0 | 6.5 | 6.0 |
| 3 | 10.0 | 17.0 | 7.5 | 8.0 |
| 4 | 8.5 | 14.5 | 7.0 | 9.0 |
| 5 | 8.5 | 14.0 | 7.0 | 9.0 |
| 6 | 7.5 | 12.5 | 10.5 | 11.0 |
| 7 | 7.0 | 11.5 | 9.5 | 11.0 |
| 8 | 6.5 | 11.0 | 8.5 | 10.0 |
| **Mandibular** | | | | |
| 1 | 9.0 | 12.5 | 5.0 | 6.0 |
| 2 | 9.5 | 14.0 | 5.5 | 6.5 |
| 3 | 11.0 | 15.5 | 7.0 | 7.5 |
| 4 | 8.5 | 14.0 | 7.0 | 7.5 |
| 5 | 8.0 | 14.5 | 7.0 | 8.0 |
| 6 | 7.5 | 14.0 | 11.0 | 10.0 |
| 7 | 7.0 | 12.0 | 10.5 | 10.0 |
| 8 | 7.0 | 11.0 | 10.0 | 9.5 |

**Table 2.3** *Average dimensions of the deciduous teeth*

| Tooth | Crown height (mm) | Length of root (mm) | Mediodistal crown diameter (mm) | Labiolingual crown diameter (mm) |
|---|---|---|---|---|
| **Maxillary** | | | | |
| A | 6.0 | 10.0 | 6.5 | 5.0 |
| B | 5.6 | 10.2 | 5.2 | 4.0 |
| C | 6.5 | 13.0 | 6.8 | 7.0 |
| D | 5.1 | 10.0 | 7.1 | 8.5 |
| E | 5.7 | 11.7 | 8.4 | 10.0 |
| **Mandibular** | | | | |
| A | 5.0 | 9.0 | 4.0 | 4.0 |
| B | 5.2 | 9.8 | 4.5 | 4.0 |
| C | 6.0 | 11.2 | 5.5 | 4.9 |
| D | 6.0 | 9.8 | 7.7 | 7.0 |
| E | 5.5 | 12.5 | 9.7 | 8.7 |

6. The cusps of newly erupted deciduous teeth are more pointed than those of the corresponding permanent teeth.
7. The crowns of deciduous teeth have a thinner covering of enamel (average width 0.5–1.0 mm) than the crowns of permanent teeth (average width 2.5 mm).
8. The enamel of deciduous teeth, being more opaque than that of permanent teeth, gives the crown a whiter appearance.
9. The enamel of deciduous teeth is softer than that of permanent teeth and is more easily worn.
10. Enamel of deciduous teeth is more permeable than that of permanent teeth.
11. The aprismatic layer of surface enamel (see pages 111–112) is wider in deciduous teeth.
12. The enamel and dentine of all deciduous teeth exhibit neonatal lines (see pages 115, 142).
13. The roots of deciduous teeth are shorter and less robust than those of permanent teeth.
14. The roots of deciduous incisors and canines are longer in proportion to the crown than those of their permanent counterparts.
15. The roots of deciduous molars are widely divergent, extending beyond the dimensions of the crown.
16. The pulp chambers of deciduous teeth are proportionally larger in relation to the crowns than those of the permanent teeth. The pulp horns in deciduous teeth are more prominent.
17. The root canals of deciduous teeth are extremely fine.
18. The dental arches for the deciduous dentition are smaller.

Some of these differences are illustrated in Figure 2.14.

The following descriptions of individual teeth will be considered according to tooth class (incisors, canines, premolars and molars) rather than by membership of the permanent or deciduous dentition. For each class, the permanent teeth will be described before the deciduous teeth. This arrangement allows emphasis of the basic features common to each class to be made.

To help visualize the tooth as a three-dimensional object, the illustrations of each tooth are arranged according to the 'third angle projection technique', which aligns each side of a tooth to its occlusal or incisal aspect. The morphology of the pulp is treated independently of the morphology of the external surfaces of the teeth on pages 28–33. For the chronology of the developing dentitions see page 365, for the average dimensions of the teeth see Tables 2.2 and 2.3, and for ethnic variations in tooth morphology see pages 24–28.

## INCISORS

Human incisors have thin, blade-like crowns that are adapted for the cutting and shearing of food preparatory to grinding. Viewed mesially or distally, the crowns of the incisors are roughly triangular in shape, with the apex of the triangle at the incisal margin of the tooth (Fig. 2.15). This shape is thought to facilitate the penetration and cutting of food. Viewed buccally or lingually, the incisors are trapezoidal, the shortest of the uneven sides being the base of the crown cervically.

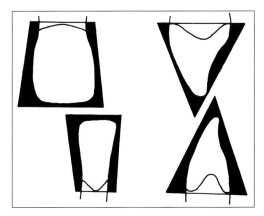

**Fig. 2.15** Schematic drawings of incisor crown form, illustrating the relationship between the anatomical and geometrical forms. Redrawn after Dr R.C. Wheeler.

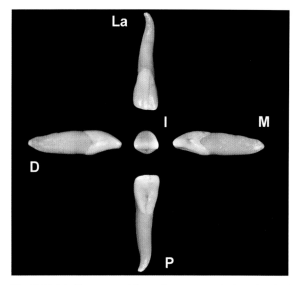

**Fig. 2.17** Maxillary second (lateral) permanent incisor. A = incisal surface; B = labial surface; C = palatal surface; D = mesial surface; E = distal surface.

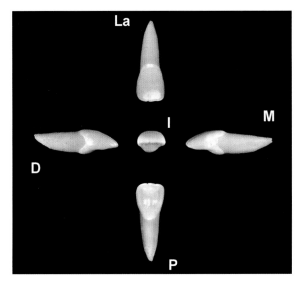

**Fig. 2.16** Maxillary first (central) permanent incisor. A = incisal surface; B = labial surface; C = palatal surface; D = mesial surface; E = distal surface.

## Maxillary first (central) permanent incisor

This tooth (Fig. 2.16) is the widest mesiodistally of all the permanent incisors and canines, the crown being almost as wide as it is long. Like all incisors, it is basically wedge- or chisel-shaped and has a single conical root.

From the incisal view, the crown and incisal margin are centrally positioned over the root of the tooth. The incisal margin presents as a narrow, flattened ridge rather than as a fine, sharp edge. The incisal margin may be grooved by two troughs, the labial lobe grooves, which correspond to the divisions between three developmental lobes (or mamelons) seen on newly erupted incisors. The mamelons are lost by attrition soon after eruption. From the incisal aspect, the crown outline is bilaterally symmetrical, being triangular. However, the mesial profile may appear slightly larger than the distal profile. From the labial view, the crown length can be seen to be almost as great as the root length. The crown has a smooth, convex labial surface. It may be marked by two faint grooves that run vertically towards the cervical margin and are extensions of the labial lobe grooves. The convexity of the labial surface is especially marked cervically, the labial surface sometimes being flat at its middle and incisal regions. The mesial surface is straight and approximately at right angles to the incisal margin. The distoincisal angle, however, is more rounded and the distal outline more convex. A line drawn through the axial centre of the tooth lies roughly parallel to the mesial outline of the crown and root. Viewed palatally, the crown is more irregular, its middle and incisal regions being concave, giving a slightly shovel-shaped appearance to the incisor. The palatal surface of the crown is bordered by mesial and distal marginal ridges. Near the cervical margin lies a prominent cingulum. The cingulum may be single, divided or replaced by prominent portions of the marginal ridges. Occasionally, a slight ridge of enamel may run towards the incisal margin, dividing the palatal surface into two shallow depressions. The mesial and distal views of the crown illustrate the fundamental wedge-shaped or triangular crown form of the incisor.

The sinuous cervical margin is concave towards the crown on the palatal and labial surfaces and convex towards the crown on the mesial and distal surfaces, the curvature on the mesial surface being the most pronounced of any tooth in the dentition. The single root of the first incisor tapers towards the apex. The root is conical in cross-section and appears narrower from the palatal than from the labial aspect.

## Maxillary second (lateral) permanent incisor

Shown in Figure 2.17, this is one of the most variable teeth in the dentition, although generally it is morphologically a diminutive form of the maxillary central incisor with slight modifications. The crown is much narrower and shorter than that of the first incisor, although the crown : root length ratio is considerably decreased.

From the incisal aspect, the crown has a more rounded outline than the adjacent first incisor. Viewed labially, the mesioincisal and distoincisal angles and the mesial and distal crown margins are more rounded than those of the first incisor. The palatal aspect of the crown is similar to that of the first incisor, although the marginal ridges and cingulum are often more pronounced. Consequently, the palatal concavity appears deeper. Lying in front of the cingulum is a pit (foramen caecum) that may extend some way into the root. The mesial and distal aspects of the second incisor differ little from those of the first incisor. A common morphological variation is the so-called 'peg-shaped' lateral incisor, which has a thin root surmounted by a small conical crown (see Fig. 2.47).

The course of the cervical margin and the shape of the root are similar to those of the first incisor. However, the root is often slightly compressed and grooved on the mesial and distal surfaces.

The mandibular incisors have the smallest mesiodistal dimensions of any teeth in the permanent dentition. They can be distinguished from the maxillary incisors not only by their size but also by the marked lingual inclination of the crowns over the roots, the mesiodistal compression of their roots and the poor development of the marginal ridges and cingula.

## Mandibular first (central) permanent incisor

Viewed incisally, this tooth has a bilaterally symmetrical triangular shape (Fig. 2.18). The incisal margin in the specimen shown in the figure has been worn and appears flat, although the newly erupted tooth has three mamelons. The incisal margin is at right angles to a line bisecting the tooth labiolingually. Viewed labially, the crown of the incisor is almost twice as long as it is wide. The unworn incisal margin is straight and approximately at right angles to the long axis of the tooth. The mesioincisal and distoincisal angles are sharp and the mesial and distal surfaces are approximately at right angles to the incisal margin. The profiles of the mesial and distal surfaces appear very similar, being convex in their incisal thirds and relatively flattened in the middle and cervical thirds. The lingual surface is smooth and slightly concave, the lingual cingulum and mesial and distal marginal ridges appearing less distinct than those of the maxillary incisors. The mesial and distal views show the characteristic wedge shape of the incisor and the inclination of the crown lingually over the root.

The cervical margins on the labial and lingual surfaces show their maximum convexities midway between the mesial and distal borders of the root. The cervical margin on the distal surface is said to be less curved than that on the mesial surface. The root is narrow and conical, although flattened mesiodistally. It is frequently grooved on the mesial and distal surfaces, the distal groove being more marked and deeper.

## Mandibular second (lateral) permanent incisor

The mandibular second incisor (Fig. 2.19) closely resembles the mandibular first incisor. However, it is slightly wider mesiodistally and is more asymmetrical in shape. The distal surface diverges at a greater angle from the long axis of the tooth, giving it a fan-shaped appearance, and the distoincisal angle is more acute and rounded. Another distinguishing characteristic is the angulation of the incisal margin relative to the labiolingual axis of the root: in the first incisor the incisal margin forms a right angle with the labiolingual axis, whereas that of the second incisor is 'twisted' distally in a lingual direction.

## Maxillary first (central) deciduous incisor

This is similar morphologically to the corresponding permanent tooth (Fig. 2.20). However, because the width of the crown of the deciduous incisor nearly equals the length it appears plumper than its permanent successor.

From the incisal view, the straight incisal margin appears to be centred over the bulk of the crown. Unlike the permanent teeth, no mamelons are seen on the incisal margin of the newly erupted deciduous incisor. The labial surface is slightly convex in all planes and unmarked by grooves, lobes or depressions. The mesioincisal angle is sharp and acute, while the distoincisal angle is more rounded and obtuse. On the palatal surface, the cingulum is a very prominent bulge that extends some way up the crown (sometimes to the incisal margin to form a ridge). Unlike those of its permanent successor, the marginal ridges are poorly defined and the concavity of the palatal surface is shallow. Mesial and distal views show the typical incisal form of the crown. There is a low, rounded cingulum at the margin of the labial surface.

As with all deciduous teeth, the cervical margins are more pronounced but less sinuous than those of their permanent successors. The fully formed root is conical in shape, tapering apically to a rather blunt apex. Compared with the corresponding permanent tooth, the root is longer in proportion to the crown.

## Maxillary second (lateral) deciduous incisor

This is similar in shape to the maxillary first deciduous incisor, although smaller (Fig. 2.21). One obvious difference is the more acute mesioincisal angle and the more rounded distoincisal angle. The palatal surface is more concave and the marginal ridges more pronounced. Viewed incisally, the crown appears almost circular (in contrast to the first incisor, which appears diamond-shaped). As with the first deciduous incisor, there is a rounded labial cingulum cervically. The palatal cingulum is generally lower than that of the first deciduous incisor.

The course of the cervical margin and the shape of the root are similar to those of the first deciduous incisor.

## Mandibular first (central) deciduous incisor

The mandibular first incisor (Fig. 2.22) is morphologically similar to its permanent successor. However, it is much shorter and has a low labial cingulum. The mesioincisal and distoincisal angles are sharp right angles and the incisal margin is straight in the horizontal plane. The lingual cingulum and the marginal ridges are poorly defined.

The single root is more rounded than that of the corresponding permanent tooth and, when complete, tapers and tends to incline distally.

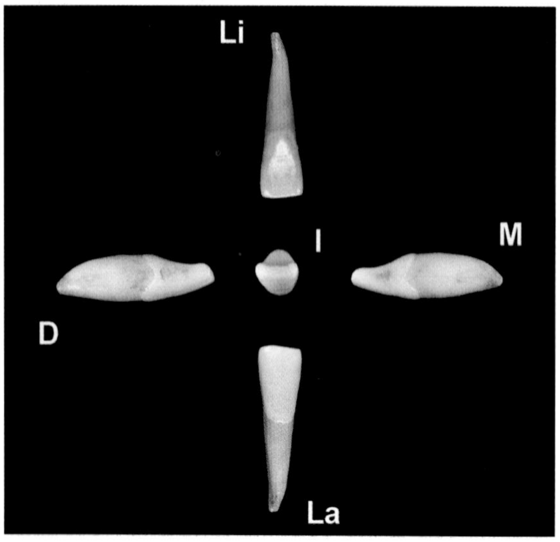

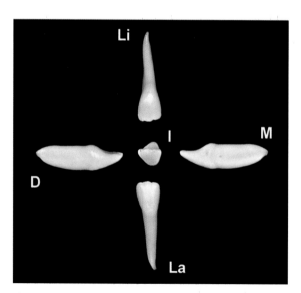

**Fig. 2.18** Mandibular first (central) right permanent incisor. A = incisal surface; B = labial surface; C = lingual surface; D = mesial surface; E = distal surface.

**Fig. 2.19** Mandibular second (lateral) right permanent incisor. A = incisal surface; B = labial surface; C = lingual surface; D = mesial surface; E = distal surface.

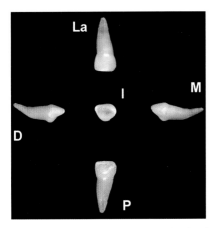

**Fig. 2.20** Maxillary first (central) right deciduous incisor. A = incisal surface; B = labial surface; C = palatal surface; D = mesial surface; E = distal surface.

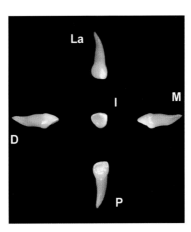

**Fig. 2.21** Maxillary second (lateral) right deciduous incisor. A = incisal surface; B = labial surface; C = palatal surface; D = mesial surface; E = distal surface.

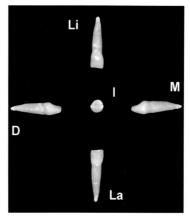

**Fig. 2.22** Mandibular first (central) right deciduous incisor. A = incisal surface; B = labial surface; C = lingual surface; D = mesial surface; E = distal surface.

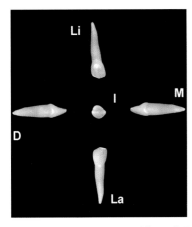

**Fig. 2.23** Mandibular second (lateral) right deciduous incisor. A = incisal surface; B = labial surface; C = lingual surface; D = mesial surface; E = distal surface.

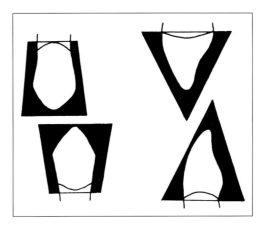

**Fig. 2.24** Schematic drawings of canine crown form, illustrating the relationship between the anatomical and geometrical forms. Redrawn after Dr R.C. Wheeler.

## Mandibular second (lateral) deciduous incisor

This is a bulbous tooth (Fig. 2.23) that resembles its permanent successor. It is wider than the mandibular first deciduous incisor and is asymmetrical. The mesioincisal angle is more obtuse and rounded than that of the mandibular first deciduous incisor and the incisal margin slopes downwards distally. Should the distoincisal angle be markedly rounded, the tooth may be difficult to distinguish from a maxillary second deciduous incisor.

Unlike the permanent tooth, the root is rounded. When complete, it is longer than the root of the mandibular first deciduous incisor.

## CANINES

Canines are the only teeth in the dentition with a single cusp. Morphologically, they can be considered transitional between incisors and premolars. As for the incisors, the crowns of canines are essentially triangular in shape when viewed mesially or distally and trapezoidal buccally and lingually (Fig. 2.24).

### Maxillary permanent canine

This is a stout tooth (Fig. 2.25) with a well developed cingulum and the longest root of any tooth. Viewed from its incisal aspect, it appears asymmetrical. If a plane is envisaged passing through the apex of the cusp to the cingulum on the palatal surface then the distal portion of the crown

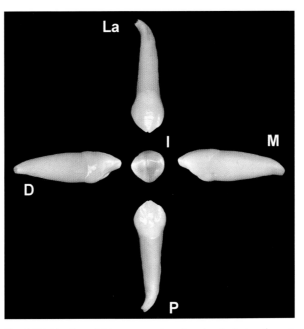

**Fig. 2.25** Maxillary right permanent canine. A = incisal surface; B = labial surface; C = palatal surface; D = mesial surface; E = distal surface.

is much wider than the mesial portion. It is thought that the pointed shape of the canine tooth is related to an increase in size of a central mamelon at the expense of mesial and distal mamelons. Prominent longitudinal ridges pass from the cusp tip down both the labial and the palatal surfaces. A relatively frequent variation in the morphology of the incisal ridge is the development of an accessory cusp on its distal arm. The labial surface of the canine is marked by the longitudinal ridge, which extends from the cusp towards the cervical margin. The incisal part of the crown occupies at least one-third of the crown height. Note that, from this view, the mesial arm of the incisal margin is shorter than the distal arm and the distoincisal angle is more rounded than the mesioincisal angle. The profiles of the mesial and distal surfaces converge markedly towards the cervix of the tooth. The mesial profile is slightly convex, the distal profile markedly convex. The mesial surface of the crown forms a straight line with the root, the distal surface meets the root at an obtuse angle. The palatal surface shows distinct mesial and distal marginal ridges and a well defined cingulum. The longitudinal ridge from the tip of the cusp meets the cingulum and is separated from the marginal ridges on either side by distinct grooves or fossae. Viewed mesially or distally, the distinctive feature is the stout character of the crown and the great width of the cervical third of both the crown and the root.

The cervical margin of this tooth follows a course similar to that of the incisors but the curves are less pronounced. The curvature of the cervical margin on the distal surface is less marked than that on the mesial surface. The root is the largest and stoutest in the dentition and is triangular in cross-section (its labial surface being wider than its palatal surface). The mesial and distal surfaces of the root are often grooved longitudinally.

### Mandibular permanent canine

This is similar to the maxillary canine but smaller, more slender and more symmetrical (Fig. 2.26). The cusp is generally less well developed: indeed, with attrition, the low cusp may be lost and the tooth may resemble a maxillary second permanent incisor.

From the incisal aspect, there are no distinct longitudinal ridges from the tip of the cusp on to the labial and lingual surfaces. Viewed labially, the incisal margin occupies only one-fifth of the crown height and the cusp is less pointed. The crown is narrower mesiodistally than that of the maxillary canine so it appears longer, narrower and more slender. The mesial and distal profiles tend to be parallel or only slightly convergent towards the cervix. The labial and mesial surfaces are clearly defined, being inclined

acutely to each other, whereas the labial surface merges gradually into the distal surface. On the lingual surface, the cingulum, marginal ridges and fossae are indistinct. The lingual surface is flatter than the corresponding palatal surface of the maxillary permanent canine and simulates the lingual surface of the mandibular incisors. Viewed mesially and distally, the wedge-shaped appearance of the canine is clear. These proximal surfaces are longer than those of the maxillary canine. The labiolingual diameter of the crown near the cervix is less than the corresponding labiopalatal diameter of the maxillary canine.

The cervical margin of this tooth follows a course similar to that of the incisors. The crownward convexity on the mesial surface is generally more marked than that on the distal surface. The root is normally single, though occasionally it may bifurcate. In cross-section, the root is oval, being flattened mesially and distally. The root is grooved longitudinally on both its mesial and its distal surfaces.

### Maxillary deciduous canine

This tooth has a fang-like appearance and is similar morphologically to its permanent successor, though more bulbous (Fig. 2.27). It is generally symmetrical but, where there is asymmetry, it is usual for the mesial slope of the cusp to be longer than the distal slope. Bulging of the tooth gives the crown a diamond-shaped appearance when viewed labially or palatally, with the crown margins overhanging the root profiles. The width of the crown is greater than its length. On the labial surface, there is a low cingulum cervically, from which runs a longitudinal ridge up to the tip of the cusp. A similar longitudinal ridge also runs on the palatal surface. This ridge extends from the cusp apex to the palatal cingulum and divides the palatal surface into two shallow pits. The marginal ridges on the palatal surface are low and indistinct.

The root is long compared with the crown height and is triangular in cross-section.

### Mandibular deciduous canine

This is more slender than the maxillary deciduous canine (Fig. 2.28). The crown is asymmetrical and the cusp tip displaced mesially. Consequently, the mesial arm is shorter and more vertical than the distal arm. On the labial surface, there is a low, labial cingulum. On the lingual surface, the cingulum and marginal ridges are less pronounced than the corresponding structures on the palatal surface of the maxillary deciduous canine. The

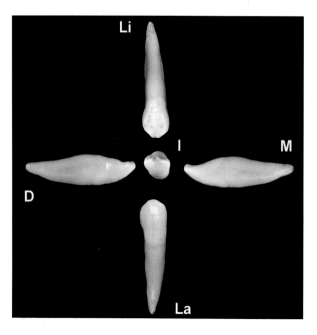

**Fig. 2.26** Mandibular right permanent canine.
A = incisal view
B = labial surface
C = lingual surface
D = mesial surface
E = distal surface.

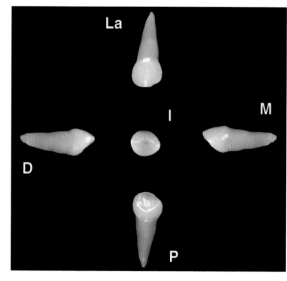

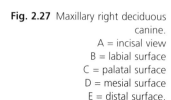

**Fig. 2.27** Maxillary right deciduous canine.
A = incisal view
B = labial surface
C = palatal surface
D = mesial surface
E = distal surface.

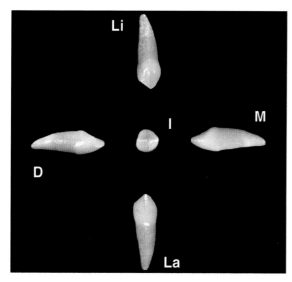

**Fig. 2.28** Mandibular right deciduous canine. A = incisal view; B = labial surface; C = lingual surface; D = mesial surface; E = distal surface.

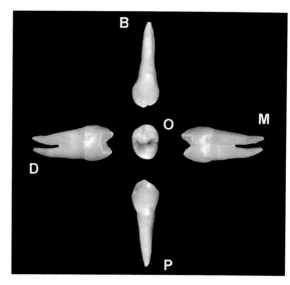

**Fig. 2.30** Maxillary first right premolar. A = occlusal surface; B = buccal surface; C = palatal surface; D = mesial surface; E = distal surface.

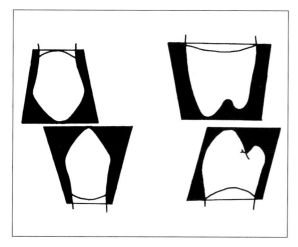

**Fig. 2.29** Schematic drawings of premolar crown form, illustrating the relationship between the anatomical and geometrical forms. Redrawn after Dr R.C. Wheeler.

longitudinal ridges on both the labial and the lingual surfaces are poorly developed. The width of the crown is less than the length.

The root is single and tends to be triangular in cross-section.

## PREMOLARS

Premolars are unique to the permanent dentition. They are sometimes referred to as 'bicuspids' because they have two main cusps – a buccal and a palatal (or lingual) cusp – separated by a mesiodistal occlusal fissure. The buccal surface of the buccal cusp is similar in shape to the cusp of a canine, to which it may be considered analogous, while the palatal or lingual cusp corresponds developmentally to the cingulum of the anterior teeth. Thus, premolars are considered to be transitional between canines and molars.

Viewed mesially or distally, the maxillary premolars are trapezoidal in shape, the longest side of the trapezoid being the base of the crown at the cervical margin (Fig. 2.29). It is thought that, because the occlusal surface is not as wide as the base of the crown, the tooth can penetrate the food more easily while minimizing the occlusal forces. The mandibular premo-

lars, however, are roughly rhomboidal in shape. The rhomboidal outline is inclined lingually, thus allowing correct intercuspal contact with the maxillary antagonists. Viewed buccally or lingually, all the premolars are trapezoidal, the shortest of the uneven sides being the bases of the crowns cervically.

### Maxillary first premolar

When viewed occlusally, this tooth has a crown that appears ovoid, being broader buccally than palatally (Fig. 2.30). Thus, the profiles of the mesial and distal surfaces converge palatally. The mesiobuccal and distobuccal corners are less rounded than the mesiopalatal and distopalatal corners. The mesial and distal borders of the occlusal surface are marked by distinct ridges, the mesial and distal marginal ridges. The buccal and palatal cusps are separated by a central occlusal fissure that runs in a mesiodistal direction. The occlusal fissure crosses the mesial marginal ridge on to the mesial surface. On the distal side, the fissure terminates in a fossa before the distal marginal ridge. Supplementary grooves from the central fissure are rare.

Viewed buccally, the first premolar bears a distinct resemblance to the adjacent canine. A longitudinal ridge may be seen passing down the buccal cusp. The mesial and distal ridges of the buccal cusp each form a 30° slope and the mesio- and disto-occlusal angles are prominent, giving the crown a 'bulging-shouldered' ovoid appearance. The mesial slope is generally longer than the distal slope.

Viewed palatally, the buccal part of the crown appears larger in all dimensions than the palatal part so that the entire buccal profile of the crown is visible from the palatal aspect. The palatal cusp is lower and its tip lies more mesially than the tip of the buccal cusp.

From the mesial aspect, the unequal height of the cusps is clearly seen. Note the canine groove extending across the marginal ridge from the occlusal surface. The cervical third of the mesial surface is marked by a distinct concavity, the canine fossa.

The distal aspect of the crown differs from the mesial aspect in that it lacks a canine groove and a canine fossa.

The cervical margin follows a fairly level course around the crown, deviating slightly towards the root on the buccal and palatal surfaces and away from the root on the mesial and distal surfaces. There are usually two roots, a buccal and palatal root, although sometimes there is only a single root. However, even a single root is deeply grooved on its mesial and distal surfaces.

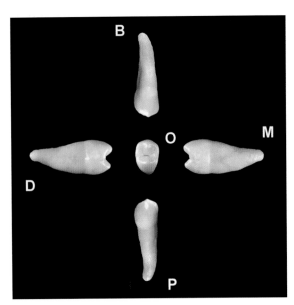

**Fig. 2.31** Maxillary second right premolar. A = occlusal surface; B = buccal surface; C = palatal surface; D = mesial surface; E = distal surface.

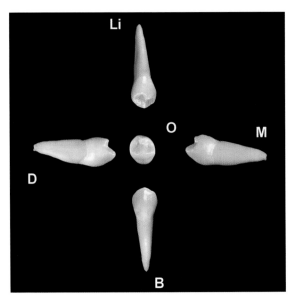

**Fig. 2.32** Mandibular first right premolar. A = occlusal surface; B = buccal surface; C = lingual surface; D = mesial surface; E = distal surface.

## Maxillary second premolar

This tooth (Fig. 2.31) is similar in shape to the maxillary first premolar, except for the following features. Viewed occlusally, the mesiobuccal and distobuccal corners are more rounded and the mesial and distal profiles do not converge lingually, being nearly parallel. The occlusal surface appears more compressed, the mesiodistal dimension of the crown being smaller. The central fissure appears shorter and does not cross the mesial marginal ridge. From the buccal aspect, the mesio- and disto-occlusal angles are less prominent. These features give the crown a 'narrow-shouldered' appearance. The two cusps are smaller and more equal in size than those of the first premolar. The height of the buccal cusp is one-quarter of the height of the crown measured from the base of the occlusal fissure, while the height of the buccal cusp of the first premolar is up to one-half the height of the crown. Viewed palatally, less of the buccal profile is visible. Mesially and distally, the tooth appears similar to the first premolar but there is no canine fossa or canine groove on the mesial surface.

The cervical margin appears similar to that of the maxillary first premolar but is slightly less undulating. The root is single.

The mandibular premolars differ from the maxillary premolars in that occlusally the crowns appear rounder and the cusps are of unequal size, the buccal cusp being the most prominent. Furthermore, the first and second premolars differ more markedly from each other than do the maxillary premolars.

## Mandibular first premolar

This is the smallest premolar (Fig. 2.32). As it comprises a dominant buccal cusp and a very small lingual cusp that appears not unlike a cingulum, some consider it to be a modified canine. From the occlusal aspect, more than two-thirds of the buccal surface is visible, although only a small portion of the lingual surface can be seen. The occlusal outline is diamond-shaped and the occlusal table, outlined by the cusps and marginal ridges, is triangular. The buccal cusp is broad with its apex approximately overlying the midpoint of the crown. The lingual cusp is less than half the size of the buccal cusp. The buccal and lingual cusps are connected by a blunt, transverse ridge that divides the poorly developed mesiodistal occlusal fissure into mesial and distal fossae. The mesial fossa is generally smaller than the distal fossa. A canine groove often extends from the mesial fossa over the mesial marginal ridge on to the mesiolingual surface of the crown. Viewed buccally, the crown is nearly symmetrical, although the mesial

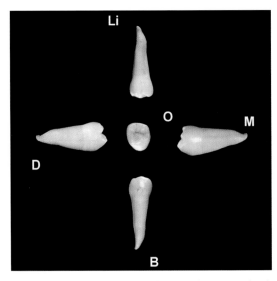

**Fig. 2.33** Mandibular second right premolar. A = occlusal surface; B = buccal surface; C = lingual surface; D = mesial surface; E = distal surface.

profile is more curved than the distal. The buccal surface is markedly convex in all planes. From the lingual aspect, the entire buccal profile and the occlusal surface are visible. Thus, the mandibular first premolar differs from other premolars in that the occlusal plane does not lie perpendicular to the long axis of the tooth but is inclined lingually. The tilt of the occlusal plane can also be appreciated from the mesial and distal aspects.

The cervical line follows an almost level course around the tooth. The root is single, conical, and oval to nearly round in cross-section. The root is grooved longitudinally both mesially and distally, the mesial groove being the more prominent.

## Mandibular second premolar

The mandibular second premolar (Fig. 2.33) differs from the mandibular first premolar in a number of respects. Its crown is generally larger. The lingual cusp is better developed, although it is not quite as large as the buccal cusp. From the occlusal aspect, its outline appears round or square, the mesial and distal profiles being straight and parallel. The mesiodistal occlusal fissure between the cusps is well defined. However, like the first premolar, the fissure ends in mesial and distal fossae, the distal fossa being generally larger than the mesial. Unlike the first premolar, a transverse ridge does not usually join the apices of the cusps. Accessory cusplets are common on both buccal and lingual cusps. The lingual cusp is usually

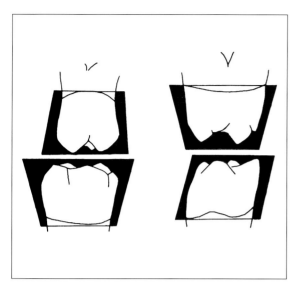

**Fig. 2.34** Schematic drawings of molar crown form, illustrating the relationship between the anatomical and geometrical forms. Redrawn after Dr R.C. Wheeler.

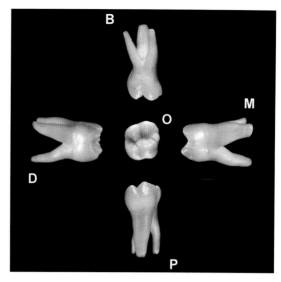

**Fig. 2.35** Maxillary first right permanent molar. A = occlusal surface; B = buccal surface; C = palatal surface, D = mesial surface; E = distal surface.

subdivided into mesiolingual and distolingual cusps, the mesiolingual cusp being wider and higher than the distolingual. The groove separating the mesiolingual and distolingual cusps lies opposite the tip of the buccal cusp. From the buccal aspect, the crown of the second premolar is symmetrical. From this view, the buccal cusp generally appears shorter and more rounded than that of the mandibular first premolar. Lingually, little if any of the occlusal surface and buccal profile is visible. From the mesial and distal aspects, the occlusal surface appears horizontal to the long axis of the tooth, unlike the mandibular first premolar. The crown is wider buccolingually than that of the first premolar and the buccal cusp does not incline as far over the root. The mesial marginal ridge is higher than the distal marginal ridge.

The cervical margin follows an almost level course around the tooth. The root is single, conical, and nearly round in cross-section.

## MOLARS

Molars present the largest occlusal surfaces of all teeth. They have three to five major cusps (although the maxillary first deciduous molar has only two). Molars are the only teeth that have more than one buccal cusp. Generally, the lower molars have two roots while the upper have three. The permanent molars do not have deciduous predecessors.

As for the premolars, the maxillary molars are approximately trapezoidal when viewed mesially and distally, while the mandibular molars are rhomboidal. Viewed buccally or lingually, the molars are trapezoidal (Fig. 2.34).

### Maxillary first permanent molar

This is usually the largest molar in each quadrant (Fig. 2.35). Viewed occlusally, the crown is rhomboid in outline. The mesiopalatal and disto-buccal angles are obtuse. The longest diameter of the crown runs from the mesiobuccal to the distopalatal corners. It has four major cusps separated by an irregular H-shaped occlusal fissure. The occlusal table may be divided into two distinct components (the trigone and talon) by an oblique ridge, which passes diagonally across the occlusal table from the mesio-palatal cusp to the distobuccal cusp. The trigone bears the mesiobuccal, mesiopalatal and distobuccal cusps and the talon bears the distopalatal cusp. The trigone is characteristically triangular in shape, the apex of the triangle being directed palatally. The mesiopalatal cusp is the largest, the buccal cusps being smaller and of approximately equal size. The buccal cusps form the base of the trigone. The mesial marginal ridge forms the mesial side of the trigone and its distal side is formed by the oblique ridge.

An accessory cusplet of variable size may be seen on the palatal surface of the mesiopalatal cusp. This cusplet is termed the tubercle of Carabelli and is found on about 60% of maxillary first permanent molars. The trigone has a central fossa from which a fissure extends mesially to terminate in a mesial pit before the mesial marginal ridge. Another fissure extends buccally from the central fossa to pass on to the buccal surface of the crown between the two buccal cusps. The distopalatal cusp of the talon is generally the smallest cusp of the tooth and is separated from the mesiopalatal cusp by a distopalatal fissure, which curves distally to end in a distal pit before the distal marginal ridge. The oblique ridge may be crossed by a shallow fissure, which connects the central fossa of the trigone with the distopalatal fissure and distal pit of the talon, completing the H-shaped fissure pattern. That the tips of the palatal cusps are situated nearer the mid-mesiodistal diameter of the crown than those of the buccal cusps is characteristic of maxillary molars.

From the buccal aspect, the buccal cusps are seen to be approximately equal in height, although the mesiobuccal cusp is wider than the distobuccal cusp. The buccal surface is convex in its cervical third but relatively flat in its middle and occlusal thirds. The buccal groove extends from the occlusal table, passing between the cusps to end about halfway up the buccal surface. The mesial profile is convex in its occlusal and middle thirds but flat, or even concave, in the cervical third. The distal profile, on the other hand, is convex in all regions.

Viewed palatally, the disproportion in size between the mesiopalatal and distopalatal cusps is most evident. The mesiopalatal cusp is blunt and occupies approximately three-fifths of the mesiodistal width of the palatal surface. The palatal surface is more or less uniformly convex in all regions. A palatal groove extends from the distal pit on to the occlusal surface between the palatal cusps to terminate approximately halfway up the palatal surface.

From the mesial and distal aspects, the maximum buccopalatal dimension is at the cervical margin, from which the buccal and palatal profiles converge occlusally. The mesial marginal ridge is more prominent than the distal ridge and may have a number of distinct tubercles, although such tubercles are rare on the distal marginal ridge.

The cervical margin follows a fairly even contour around the tooth. There are three roots, two buccal and one palatal, arising from a common root stalk. The palatal root is the longest and strongest and is circular in cross-section. The buccal roots are more slender and are flattened mesiodistally; the mesiobuccal root is usually the larger and wider of the two. At the root stalk, the palatal root is more commonly related to the distobuccal root than to the mesiobuccal root.

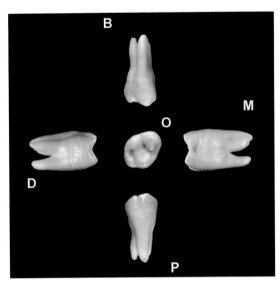

**Fig. 2.36** Maxillary second right permanent molar. A = occlusal surface; B = buccal surface; C = palatal surface; D = mesial surface; E = distal surface.

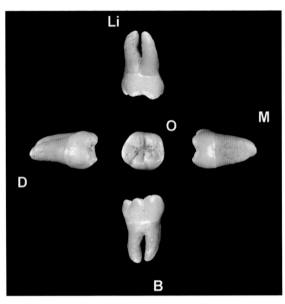

**Fig. 2.37** Mandibular first right permanent molar. A = occlusal surface; B = buccal surface; C = lingual surface; D = mesial surface; E = distal surface.

## Maxillary second permanent molar

This closely resembles the maxillary first permanent molar but shows some reduction in size and slightly different cusp relationships (Fig. 2.36). Viewed occlusally, the rhomboid form is more pronounced than in the first molar and the oblique ridge is smaller. The talon (distopalatal fissure cusp) is considerably reduced. The occlusal fissure pattern is similar to that of the first molar but is more variable, and supplemental grooves are more numerous. Two features of the buccal surface differentiate the second molar: the smaller size of the crown and the distobuccal cusp. From the palatal view, the reduction in size of the distopalatal cusp is more visible. A tubercle of Carabelli is not usually found on the mesiopalatal cusp. The mesial and distal surfaces differ little from those of the first molar, except that the tubercles on the mesial marginal ridge are less numerous and less pronounced.

As for the maxillary first molar, the second molar has three roots, two buccal and one palatal. However, they are shorter and less divergent than those of the first molar and may be partly fused. The apex of the mesiobuccal root is generally in line with the centre of the crown, unlike that of the first molar, which generally lies in line with the tip of the mesiobuccal cusp.

Variations in morphology of the maxillary second permanent molar are quite common. Total reduction of the distopalatal cusp such that only the trigone remains is frequent. Less frequently, the crown may appear compressed because of fusion of the mesiopalatal and distobuccal cusps, resulting in an oval crown possessing three cusps in a straight line.

## Maxillary third permanent molar

Being the most variable in the dentition, this tooth is not illustrated. Its morphology may range from that characteristic of the adjacent maxillary permanent molars to a rounded, triangular crown with a deep central fossa from which numerous irregular fissures radiate outwards. Most commonly, the crown is triangular in shape, having the three cusps of the trigone but no talon. The roots are often fused and irregular in form. Third permanent molars are the teeth most often absent congenitally.

## Differences between maxillary and mandibular molars

The mandibular molars differ from the maxillary molars in the following respects.

1. The mandibular molars have two roots, one mesial and one distal.
2. They are considered to be derived from a five-cusped form.

3. The crowns of the lower molars are oblong, being broader mesiodistally than buccolingually.
4. The fissure pattern is cross-shaped.
5. The lingual cusps are of more equal size.
6. The tips of the buccal cusps are shifted lingually so that, from the occlusal view, the whole of the buccal surface is visible.

## Mandibular first permanent molar

The crown of this tooth, when viewed occlusally, is somewhat pentagonal in outline (Fig. 2.37). It is broader mesiodistally than buccolingually. The occlusal surface is divided into buccal and lingual parts by a mesiodistal occlusal fissure, which arises from a deep central fossa. The buccal side of the occlusal table has three distinct cusps: mesiobuccal, distobuccal and distal. Each cusp is separated by a groove, which joins the mesiodistal fissure. On the lingual side are two cusps: mesiolingual and distolingual. The fissure separating the lingual cusps joins the mesiodistal fissure in the region of the central fossa. The lingual cusps tend to be larger and more pointed, although they are not disproportionately larger than the mesiobuccal and distobuccal cusps. The tips of the buccal cusps are displaced lingually, are rounded, and are lower than the lingual cusps. The smallest cusp is the distal cusp, which is displaced slightly towards the buccal surface. In 90% of cases, the mesiolingual cusp is joined to the distobuccal cusp across the floor of the central fossa. This feature, and the five-cusped pattern, is termed the *Dryopithecus* pattern. This 'primitive' pattern is characteristic of all the lower molars of the anthropoid apes and their early ancestors, the dryopithecines. Because of the resulting Y-shaped fissure pattern and the five cusps, the *Dryopithecus* pattern is sometimes referred to as a 'Y5' pattern. In the 10% of cases where the mesiobuccal and distolingual cusps meet, a more cruciate system of fissures is produced: this is sometimes referred to as a '+5' pattern.

From the buccal aspect, three cusps are seen, the distal cusp being the smallest. The fissure separating the mesiobuccal and distobuccal cusps arises from the central fossa on the occlusal surface and terminates halfway up the buccal surface in a buccal pit. The buccal surface appears markedly convex, especially at the cervical third of the crown. This convexity is associated with the characteristic lingual inclination of the buccal cusps.

From the lingual aspect, although the two lingual cusps are nearly equal in size, the mesiolingual cusp appears slightly larger. The fissure between the lingual cusps arises from the central fossa on the occlusal surface but

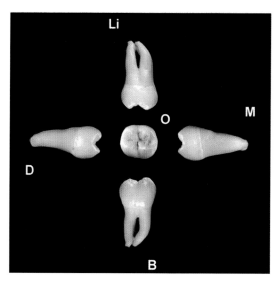

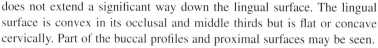

**Fig. 2.38** Mandibular second right permanent molar. A = occlusal surface; B = buccal surface; C = lingual surface; D = mesial surface; E = distal surface.

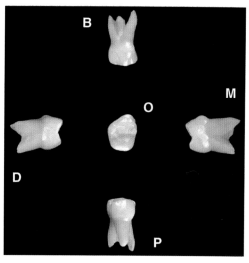

**Fig. 2.39** Maxillary first right deciduous molar. A = occlusal surface; B = buccal surface; C = palatal surface; D = mesial surface; E = distal surface.

does not extend a significant way down the lingual surface. The lingual surface is convex in its occlusal and middle thirds but is flat or concave cervically. Part of the buccal profiles and proximal surfaces may be seen.

Viewed mesially, the mesial marginal ridge joining the mesiobuccal and mesiolingual cusps is V-shaped, being notched at its midpoint. The mesial surface is flat or concave cervically and convex in its middle and occlusal thirds.

From the distal aspect, the distal marginal ridge joining the distal and distolingual cusps also appears V-shaped. The cervical third of the distal surface is relatively flat, the middle and occlusal thirds highly convex. Thus, the distal surface is more convex than the mesial surface because of the distal cusp. The proximal views of the illustration highlight the greater convex slope of the buccal surface compared with the lingual surface.

The cervical margin follows a uniform contour around the tooth. The two roots, one mesial and one distal, arise from a common root stalk. They are both markedly flattened mesiodistally and the mesial root is usually deeply grooved. Both roots curve distally.

## Mandibular second permanent molar

When viewed occlusally, the crown exhibits a regular, rectangular shape (Fig. 2.38); the buccal profile is thus nearly equal in length to the lingual profile, unlike the mandibular first permanent molar. There are four cusps, the mesiobuccal and mesiolingual cusps being slightly larger than the distobuccal and distolingual cusps. The cusps are separated by a cross-shaped occlusal fissure pattern, which may be complicated by numerous supplemental grooves. From the buccal aspect, the crown appears smaller than that of the first molar. A fissure extends between the buccal cusps from the occlusal surface and terminates approximately halfway up the buccal surface. Like that of the mandibular first molar, the buccal surface is highly convex. From the lingual aspect the buccal profiles and proximal surfaces are not visible and the crown is noticeably shorter than the first molar. The mesial and distal aspects of the second molar resemble those of the first molar although, because there is no distal cusp, the proximal surfaces are more equal in terms of their convexity. The mesial and distal marginal ridges do not converge and are not as markedly notched at their midpoint.

The mesial and distal roots are flattened mesiodistally and are smaller and less divergent than those of the first molar. They may be partly fused. The mesial root is not as broad as that of the first molar and the distal inclination of the roots is usually more marked.

## Mandibular third permanent molar

This has a variable morphology, although not as variable as that of the maxillary third permanent molar. Its clinical significance lies in the fact that it is commonly impacted. It is the smallest of the mandibular molars but can be as large as the mandibular first molar. The crown usually has four or five cusps. In shape, it is normally a rounded rectangle or circular. Its occlusal fissure pattern is generally very irregular. As a rule, the roots are greatly reduced in size and are fused. They show a marked distal inclination.

## Maxillary first deciduous molar

This is the most atypical of all molars, deciduous or permanent (Fig. 2.39). In form it appears intermediate between a premolar and a molar. It is the smallest molar.

Viewed occlusally, the crown is an irregular quadrilateral with the buccal and palatal surfaces lying parallel to one another. However, the mesiobuccal corner is extended to produce a prominent bulge, the molar tubercle. If crowns are to be fitted, this bulge may have to be smoothed over because of the undercut. The mesiopalatal angle is markedly obtuse. The tooth is generally bicuspid; the buccal (more pronounced) and palatal cusps are separated by an occlusal fissure that runs mesiodistally. A shallow buccal fissure may extend from the central mesiodistal fissure to divide the buccal cusp into two, the mesial part being the larger. The lingual cusp also may be subdivided into two. The tips of the cusps converge towards the midline, reducing the occlusal surface of the tooth. From the buccal aspect, the crown appears squat, its height being less than its width. On the mesial side lies the buccal cingulum, which extends to the molar tubercle. From the palatal aspect, the palatal surface appears shorter mesiodistally than the buccal surface, the profile of which can be seen from this view. The mesial and distal views show the cervical bulbosity of the buccal and palatal surfaces. Note the prominent molar tubercle mesially. Marginal ridges link the buccal and palatal cusps. No fissure crosses the marginal ridges.

The tooth has three roots (two buccal and one palatal), which arise from a common root stalk. The mesiobuccal root is flattened mesiodistally, the distobuccal root is smaller and more circular, and the palatal root is the largest and is round in cross-section. The distobuccal and palatal roots may be partly fused.

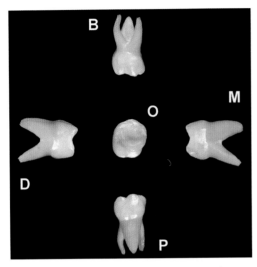

**Fig. 2.40** Maxillary second right deciduous molar. A = occlusal surface; B = buccal surface; C = palatal surface; D = mesial surface; E = distal surface.

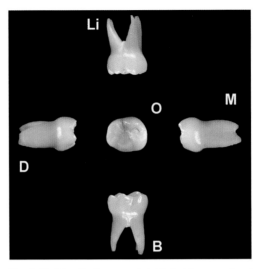

**Fig. 2.42** Mandibular second right deciduous molar. A = occlusal surface; B = buccal surface; C = lingual surface; D = mesial surface; E = distal surface.

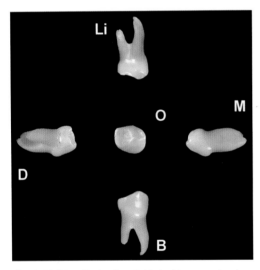

**Fig. 2.41** Mandibular first right deciduous molar. A = occlusal surface; B = buccal surface; C = lingual surface; D = mesial surface; E = distal surface.

## Maxillary second deciduous molar

The maxillary second deciduous molar (Fig. 2.40) closely resembles the maxillary first permanent molar (see Fig. 2.35), although its size, whiteness, widely diverging roots and low buccal cingulum ought to distinguish it. A tubercle of Carabelli on the mesiopalatal cusp is often well developed.

## Mandibular first deciduous molar

Unlike the maxillary first deciduous molar, this is molariform but has a number of unique features (Fig. 2.41). From the occlusal aspect the crown appears elongated mesiodistally and is an irregular quadrilateral with parallel buccal and lingual surfaces. The mesiobuccal corner is extended, forming a molar tubercle, and the mesiolingual angle markedly obtuse. The occlusal table can be divided into buccal and lingual parts by a mesiodistal fissure. The buccal part consists of two cusps, the mesiobuccal cusp being larger than the distobuccal cusp. The lingual part of the tooth is narrower than the buccal part and has two cusps separated by a lingual fissure, the mesiolingual cusp being larger than the distolingual cusp. The buccal cusps are larger than the lingual cusps. A transverse ridge may connect the mesial cusps, dividing the mesiodistal fissure into a distal fissure and a mesial pit. Often a distal pit is found just mesial to the distal marginal ridge. A supplemental groove from the mesial pit may extend over the mesial marginal ridge. From the buccal aspect, the mesiobuccal

cusp occupies at least two-thirds of the crown area and projects higher occlusally than the distobuccal cusp. The distal slopes of the buccal cusps are longer than the mesial. The profile of the mesial surface appears flat, whereas that of the distal surface is convex. The molar tubercle on the mesial corner of the buccal surface can be seen in this view. From the lingual aspect, the cusps are conical in shape. The distolingual cusp appears only as a bulging protuberance on the distal margin. Mesially and distally, the buccal and lingual aspects converge towards the midline of the crown. The mesial marginal ridge is more prominent than the distal marginal ridge. Note the bulge associated with the buccal cingulum near the cervical margin of the mesiobuccal cusp.

The mandibular first deciduous molar has two divergent roots, mesial and distal, which are flattened mesiodistally. The mesial root is often grooved.

## Mandibular second deciduous molar

This is a smaller version of the mandibular first permanent molar (see Fig. 2.37), although it is narrower, whiter and has widely diverging roots (Fig. 2.42). Other distinguishing features are the cingulum on the mesiobuccal corner of the crown, the greater convexity of the mesial and distal surfaces and the more extensive central fossa on the occlusal surface. The mesiolingual and distobuccal cusps are not usually joined to give the *Dryopithecus* pattern.

The average dimensions of the permanent and deciduous teeth are listed in Tables 2.2 and 2.3.

## SOME ASPECTS OF DENTAL ANTHROPOLOGY

Dental anthropology relates to the study of teeth and how such information can shed light on human development and relationships of both past and present populations. This topic involves detailed descriptions of the normal development and morphology of the crowns and their roots and of the type of variation found. Additional important information may be gleaned about living conditions from features such as the presence of dental mutilations (altering tooth form for cultural purposes), the nature of tooth wear (both attrition and abrasion) and the types and degrees of pathologies such as periodontal disease and dental caries. Even more specialized information relating to diet and climate can further be gleaned by the nature of radioisotopes in the enamel and dentine (see pages 381, 382).

A particular aim of dental anthropology is to use the morphology of teeth as a means of determining the relationships between populations. Thus, if the same highly heritable dental variants occur with a similar frequency in two populations, then the populations are likely to have a

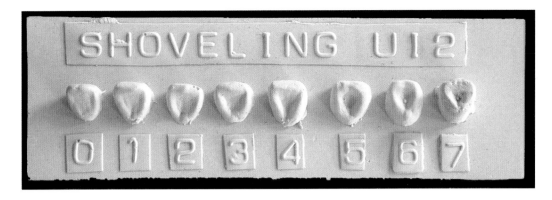

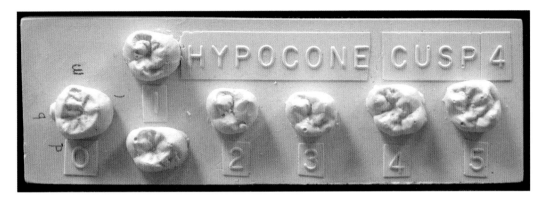

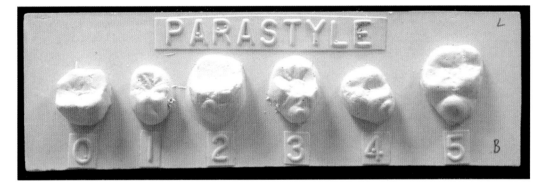

**Fig. 2.43** Arizona State University reference plaque detailing scoring system for shovelling on the maxillary second incisor. 0 = *None*: Lingual surface is essentially flat. 1 = *Faint*: Very slight elevations of mesial and distal aspects of lingual surface can be seen and palpated. 2 = *Trace*: Elevations are easily seen. 3 = *Semishovel*: Stronger ridging is present and there is a tendency for ridge convergence at the cingulum. 4 = *Semishovel*: Convergence and ridging are stronger than in grade 3. 5 = *Shovel*: Strong development of ridges, which almost contact at the cingulum. 6 = *Marked shovel*: Strongest development. Mesial and distal lingual ridges are sometimes in contact at the cingulum. 7 = (maxillary first and second incisors only) *Barrel*: Expression exceeds grade 6. Turner CG II, Nichol CR, Scott GR 1991 Scoring procedures for key morphological traits of the permanent dentition: The Arizona State University dental anthropology system. In: Kelley MA, Larsen CS (eds) *Advances in dental anthropology*. Wiley–Liss, New York, pp 13–31. Courtesy of Drs D. Hawksey and S. Haddow.

**Fig. 2.44** Arizona State University reference plaque detailing scoring system for the distolingual cusp (hypocone) in maxillary molars. 0 = No hypocone. Site is smooth. 1 = Faint ridging present at the site. 2 = Faint cuspule present. 3 = Small cusp present but not shown. 3.5 = Moderate sized cusp present. 4 = Large cusp present. 5 = Very large cusp present. Turner CG II, Nichol CR, Scott GR 1991 Scoring procedures for key morphological traits of the permanent dentition: The Arizona State University dental anthropology system. In: Kelley MA, Larsen CS (eds) *Advances in dental anthropology*. Wiley–Liss, New York, pp 13–31. Courtesy of Drs D. Hawksey and S. Haddow.

**Fig. 2.45** Arizona State University reference plaque detailing scoring system for the parastyle, most commonly appearing on the buccal surface of the mesiobuccal cusp (the paracone) of the maxillary third molar. 0 = The buccal surfaces of the buccal cusps are smooth. 1 = A pit is present in or near the buccal groove between the buccal cusps. 2 = A small cusp with an attached apex is present. 3 = A medium sized cusp with a free apex is present. 4 = A large cusp with a free apex is present. 5 = A very large cusp with a free apex is present. This form usually involves the buccal surface of both buccal cusps. 6 = An effectively free, peg-shaped crown attached to the root of the third molar is present. This condition is extremely rare, and is not shown on the plaque. Turner CG II, Nichol CR, Scott GR 1991 Scoring procedures for key morphological traits of the permanent dentition: The Arizona State University dental anthropology system. In: Kelley MA, Larsen CS (eds) *Advances in dental anthropology*. Wiley–Liss, New York, pp 13–31. Courtesy of Drs D. Hawksey and S. Haddow.

high degree of affinity. These anthropological studies generally utilize complex statistical analyses on groups of traits, rather than a single feature. Where frequencies of the features are low, a large sample size is necessary. This is particularly relevant when considering the evolution of early humans, when teeth may be the only physical traces that are preserved. Very few of the dental features to be discussed have a simple mendelian type of inheritance (i.e. autosomal dominant, autosomal recessive, sex-linked conditions). Therefore, their inheritance depends on a number of genes (polygenic) but varies minimally in response to environmental factors. As an introduction to the topic, the following section will deal with aspects of tooth morphology.

Two broad divisions of dental features can be considered. **Metric features** are those considered to be readily amenable to direct quantification, such as crown length, breadth and height. Such measurements are uncomplicated in newly erupted and unworn teeth. However, when the teeth have been functioning in the mouth, allowance must be made for any loss of dental tissues due to attrition and abrasion. The overall size of teeth in males is slightly greater (2–6%) than in females. This feature, especially in the case of lower canines, can be used in some circumstances to help separate dentitions according to sex. The teeth of females also erupt slightly earlier than their male counterparts. Using multivariate analysis, the size of teeth is also valuable in helping to distinguish different geographical populations, the largest crowns in living populations being found in Aboriginal Australians and the smallest among Asians and Europeans.

The preceding description of the morphology of teeth is, of necessity, only generalized and is related to that found in western Eurasia. However, superimposed on the basic shapes of teeth described are a number of other morphological variations affecting both deciduous and permanent teeth. In any population, these may be absent or present and display a varying degree of penetrance ranging from barely perceptible to very prominent. Because of the present difficulty in accurately quantifying such features within a reasonable period of time, these traits are considered to be **non-metric features**. However, to allow research scientists to attain some common agreement as to the degree of penetrance, a series of casts (plaques) for each feature with wide international acceptance has been produced by Arizona State University and disseminated to researchers in the field, three of which are illustrated in Figures 2.43–2.45.

Over 100 secondary dental traits have been described in the literature, but only the more common are indicated below.

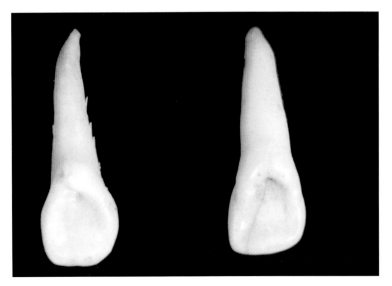

**Fig. 2.46** Shovel-shaped maxillary permanent lateral incisors. Courtesy of the Royal College of Surgeons of England.

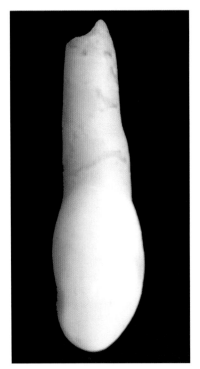

**Fig. 2.47** Peg-shaped maxillary permanent second incisor.

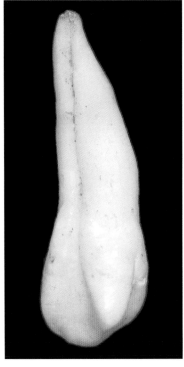

**Fig. 2.48** Maxillary permanent second incisor exhibiting a prominent palatal tubercle and a deeply grooved root. Courtesy of the Royal College of Surgeons of England.

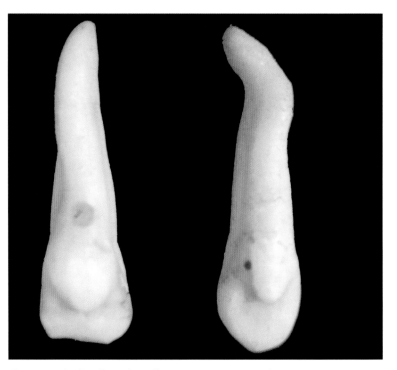

**Fig. 2.49** Palatal surface of maxillary permanent canines showing prominent tubercles. Courtesy of the Royal College of Surgeons of England.

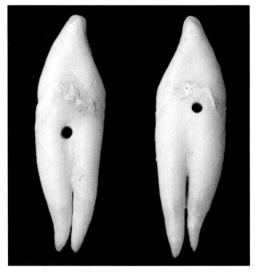

**Fig. 2.50** Two-rooted mandibular permanent canines. Courtesy of the Royal College of Surgeons of England.

## Traits found in incisors and canine teeth

***Shovel-shaped incisors.*** Exaggerated and extensive mesial and distal marginal ridges combine to result in an exaggerated palatal concavity. This gives the crown a shovel shape (Fig. 2.46). The ridging may extend on to the labial surface, giving rise to a 'double-shovelled' appearance. While it may be present on all the anterior teeth, shovelling is predominantly found in the maxillary incisors.

***Maxillary second incisor traits.*** This tooth has the most variable form in the dentition (apart from third molars), one common variant being 'peg-shaped' (Fig. 2.47).

***Cingulum traits.*** These are found on the palatal surface of the maxillary teeth and are reflected as variations in the nature of the cingulum and associate ridges, fossa and grooves (e.g. interruption grooves), especially in relation to the second incisor and canine (Figs 2.48, 2.49).

***Canine ridges.*** This trait relates to extra ridging occurring on the mesial (Bushman canine) or distal slope of the cusp of the maxillary canine.

***Winging of maxillary first incisors.*** Although not related to any variation in form, this trait concerns variation in the orientation of the teeth. Instead of the first incisors being straight and arranged along the dental arch, they are inclined mesially and their incisal edges form a V shape.

***Root variation.*** Whereas the root in all anterior teeth is usually single, that of the mandibular canine in some populations may show evidence of bifurcation at the apex in 5–10% of cases (Fig. 2.50).

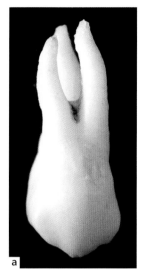
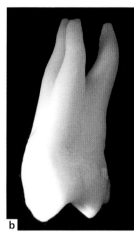

**Fig. 2.51** Three rooted maxillary first premolar: (a) View from front; (b) Viewed from side.

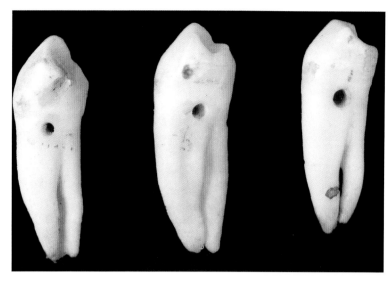

**Fig. 2.52** Two-rooted mandibular first premolars. Courtesy of the Royal College of Surgeons of England.

## Traits found in premolar teeth

***Accessory marginal tubercles.*** These tubercles are associated with the distal marginal ridge of maxillary premolars.

***Odontome.*** This rare trait is a tubercle that can occur on the inner surface of the buccal cusp of premolars. It overlies a pulp horn in about half the cases.

***Accessory buccal ridges.*** These lie within the normal mesial and distal marginal ridges associated with the buccal cusp and are more common in the maxillary premolars than the mandibular.

***Disto-sagittal ridge (Uto-Aztecan premolar).*** This trait, found in the maxillary first premolar of Native Americans, is characterized by distal displacement of the buccal cusp, associated with which is a distal fossa.

***Additional lingual cusps.*** Instead of the typical single lingual cusp present in mandibular second premolars, this trait relates to the presence of up to three cusps (cusplets).

***Root traits.*** Instead of the normal two roots (very rarely one), the first maxillary premolar tooth may have one or three roots (Fig. 2.51). Similarly, the normal single-rooted mandibular first premolar may present with two roots instead of one (Fig. 2.52).

## Traits found in molar teeth

### Maxillary molars

***Cusplet (tubercle) of Carabelli.*** This cusplet is situated on the palatal surface of the mesiopalatal cusp and is primarily considered with respect to the first molar tooth. It may be absent or show varying degrees of penetrance (see page 21).

***Distopalatal cusp.*** While this cusp is invariably present on the first molar, it may show variable degrees of reduction in the second molar tooth.

***Accessory tubercles on the marginal ridge.*** This trait can occur on both the mesial and the distal marginal ridges, primarily involving the first molar. Generally single on the distal marginal ridge (where it has been referred to as cusp 5), it may be multiple on the mesial marginal ridge.

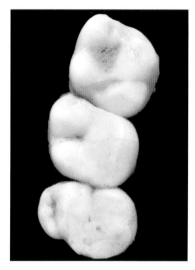
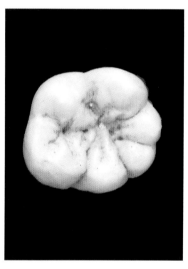

**Fig. 2.53** Maxillary right permanent third molar exhibiting a parastyle. Courtesy of the Royal College of Surgeons of England.

**Fig. 2.54** Six-cusped mandibular permanent molar. Courtesy of the Royal College of Surgeons of England.

***Paramolar tubercle (parastyle).*** This trait is represented by the presence of a tubercle on the buccal side of the mesiobuccal cusp (Fig. 2.53).

***Enamel extensions.*** Thin extensions of enamel in the region of the root bifurcation, especially on the buccal surface, may occur in maxillary and mandibular molar teeth (as well as premolars).

***Root traits.*** The typical number of three roots generally present on the first molar may be reduced to one or two in the second molar.

### Mandibular molars

***Four cusp form.*** While the first molar generally has five cusps, the second molar may be reduced to a four cusp form because of loss of the distal cusp.

***Six or seven cusp forms.*** An additional cusp (cusp 6) may occur on the first molar between the distolingual and distal cusps (Fig. 2.54). A further cusp (cusp 7) may occur between the mesiolingual and distolingual cusps.

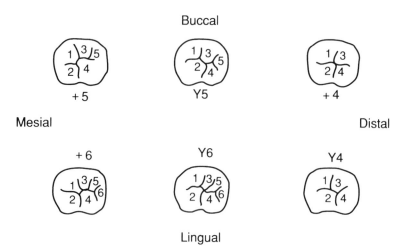

Fig. 2.55 Mandibular molars showing variation in fissure pattern and number of cusps.

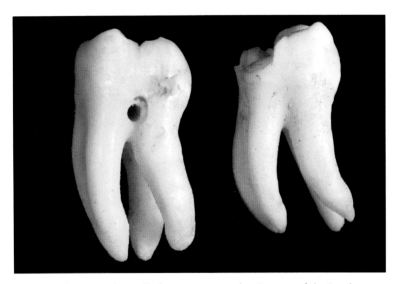

**Fig. 2.56** Three-rooted mandibular permanent molar. Courtesy of the Royal College of Surgeons of England.

*Paramolar tubercle (protostylid).* As with the maxillary teeth, the mandibular molars may exhibit the presence of a tubercle on the buccal side of the mesiobuccal cusp.

*Fissure pattern.* The classification of the fissure pattern is primarily dependent on the type of contact between the cusps in the central fossa region. If the mesiolingual and distobuccal cusps contact to intervene between the mesiobuccal and distolingual cusps, then the fissure pattern is said to have a 'Y' configuration. If the reverse is the case, the configuration is said to be an 'X' pattern. If the four cusps meet equally at the base of the fissure, the pattern is described as a '+' (Fig. 2.55).

*Ridges on the first molar.* The presence of an accessory ridge parallelling the mesial marginal ridge isolates an anterior fossa (fovea or precuspidal fossa). Another ridge may connect the two mesial cusps (distal trigonid crest). The crest passing from the mesiolingual cusp to the central fossa may be angulated (deflecting wrinkle).

*Root traits.* Whereas the mandibular molars normally have two roots, three roots may be present (Fig. 2.56), a trait associated particularly with first molars. The second molar may possess only a single root.

Two additional features are often incorporated into anthropological investigations of dental variation, even though they are not strictly morphological features. These are hypodontia (the frequency of missing teeth) and hyperdontia (the frequency of supernumerary teeth).

## Geographical variation in dentitions

It is possible to distinguish the dentitions of different geographical populations according to the distribution of the dental traits described above. Although individual dental traits may occur at high frequencies in selective populations, it is necessary to catalogue the distribution of many dental traits in helping to identify the population with more certainty. A population may be categorized by some traits occurring at high frequencies, some traits at low frequencies and others at intermediate frequencies. For example, shovel-shaped incisors have a mean frequency of about 3% in eastern Europeans and about 85% in Native Americans. Six-cusped lower first molars have a mean frequency of about 4% in European populations compared with over 50% in Aboriginal Australians. From detailed examination of the dentition, it is possible to construct a complex of dental traits that helps distinguish one geographical human population from another, allowing for the possibility of separating human populations into related groups.

A major classification of the geographical subdivisions of humanity considers it capable of being divided into five major groupings.

**Western Eurasia/Caucasoids *(to include western Europe, northern Europe and North Africa).*** The dental traits that occur with the highest frequencies compared to other groups are two-rooted mandibular canines and four-cusped first and second mandibular molars. In many other respects dental traits occur with an intermediate frequency, indicating that the group is defined more by a comparative absence of traits rather than by their presence.

**Sub-Saharan Africa *(to include West and South Africa).*** Among the traits that occur with high frequency in this group are the presence of a mesial canine ridge on the maxillary canine, a cusp 7 on mandibular first molars and a 'Y' fissure pattern on the mandibular second molar. There is a low degree of root traits and four-cusped mandibular second molars.

**Sinu-Americas *(to include China–Mongolia, Japan, North and South America, Siberia and the Eskimo–Aleuts of the American Arctic).*** This group is generally most easily recognized by the high frequency of many dental traits, such as shovelling of incisors, winging, enamel extensions, odontomes in premolars, and the low frequency of two-rooted maxillary first premolars and three-rooted maxillary second molars.

**Sunda–Pacific *(to include Southeast Asia, Polynesia and Micronesia).*** This group seems to have no characteristic dental trait occurring with a high frequency that might help characterize the group, but shows intermediate frequency of many traits (e.g. shovelling, winging, odontomes) that help to characterize their dentitions.

**Sahul–Pacific *(to include Australia, New Guinea and Melanesia).*** This group, like the Sunda–Pacific population, has few dental traits occurring at high frequency; the dentition is more characterized by a low frequency of many traits.

## PULP MORPHOLOGY

The dental pulp occupies the pulp chamber in the crown of the tooth and the root canal(s) in the root(s). The pulp chamber conforms, in basic shape, to the external form of the crown (Fig. 2.57). Root canal anatomy varies with tooth type and root morphology. At the apex of the root, the root canal becomes continuous with the periapical periodontal tissues through an apical foramen. Knowledge of the morphology of the pulp chamber and root canal is clinically significant: for example, when removing caries and

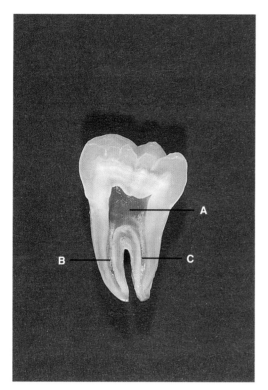

**Fig. 2.57** Ground section of a molar tooth showing the pulp chamber (A) and root canals (B, C).

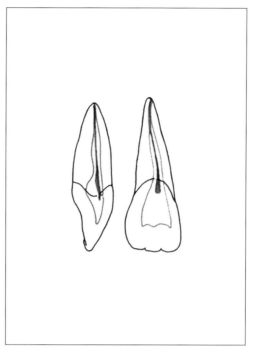

**Fig. 2.58** Schematic representation of the pulp morphology of the maxillary first permanent incisor.

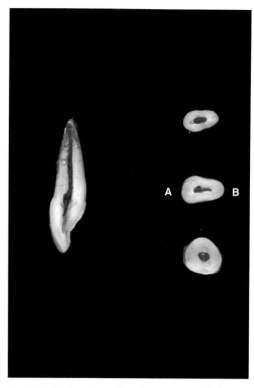

**Fig. 2.59** Sectioned maxillary first permanent incisor demonstrating pulp morphology. A = labial; B = palatal.

restoring teeth, it is important to avoid exposing the pulp. Furthermore, when the pulp is diseased and must be removed and replaced with a filling material (root canal therapy), it is essential to remove and replace all the pulp tissue and avoid injuring the periapical supporting tissues.

In the general descriptions of the pulp morphology in teeth of the permanent dentition that follow, each tooth is illustrated from the labial (buccal) and distal surfaces. The red outline shows the pulp cavity in the young tooth, the blue outline shows the pulp in the old tooth. In anterior teeth, the pulp chambers merge almost imperceptibly into the root canals. In the premolar and molar teeth, the pulp chambers and root canals are distinct. Pulp horns (or cornua) extend from the pulp chambers to the mesial and distal angles of the incisor tooth crowns and towards the cusps of posterior teeth. Each root most often contains one root canal, but two are not unusual (mandibular molars, for example, commonly have two root canals in their mesial roots). When roots are fused, the tooth still maintains the usual number of root canals. The size of the pulp chamber and the diameter of the root canals decrease significantly with age and in response to caries, attrition or other external stimuli due to the deposition of secondary (and sometimes tertiary) dentine (see pages 143–145). When the tooth first erupts into the oral cavity, root development is incomplete and the apical foramen is wide (see Fig. 25.2). The apical foramen narrows with subsequent development of the root and a constriction formed with cementum develops. This constriction marks the boundary between pulpal and periapical tissue (see Fig. 26.9).

## INCISORS

### Maxillary first (central) permanent incisor

Viewed from the labial aspect, the pulp chamber of the maxillary first permanent incisor (Figs 2.58, 2.59) follows the outline of the crown, being widest towards the incisal edge. In a young tooth, the pulp chamber has three pulp horns that correspond to the mamelons present during develop-

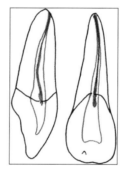

**Fig. 2.60** Schematic representation of the pulp morphology of the maxillary second permanent incisor.

ment. Viewed distally, the pulp tapers towards the incisal edge and widens cervically. A constriction (the cervical bulge) separates the single and centrally placed root canal from the pulp chamber. The root canal tapers towards the apical foramen, where it may curve slightly either distally or labially. In cross-section, the root canal is ovoid for much of its extent but, in common with canals in other teeth, becomes round as it nears the apex. With age, the dimensions of the pulp chamber and root canal are reduced as secondary dentine is laid down. The pulp chamber recedes and may disappear completely. In conducting root canal therapy on older teeth, locating the root canal in the absence of a pulp chamber may be the major clinical challenge.

### Maxillary second (lateral) permanent incisor

The pulp chamber of this incisor (Fig. 2.60) is similar to, but smaller than, that of the maxillary central incisor. The root canal is single, slightly ovoid and commonly curves both distally and palatally.

### Mandibular first (central) permanent incisor

The pulp chamber of the mandibular first permanent incisor (Figs 2.61, 2.62) is similar to that described for the maxillary first incisor although, being in a much smaller tooth, it is smaller. The pulp chamber is oval in cross-section, being wider labiolingually than mesiodistally, and is constricted at the cervical margin. The root canal is ovoid, becoming round in the apical third. As many as 30% of mandibular first incisors have two root canals, although most of these fuse near the apex and exit by a single foramen.

### Mandibular second (lateral) permanent incisor

Both tooth and root canal systems are larger than those of the mandibular first incisor (Fig. 2.63). Two root canals are somewhat more common (43%). Most of these root canals exit by separate foramina.

## CANINES

### Maxillary permanent canine

The pulp chamber of the maxillary permanent canine (Figs 2.64, 2.65) is narrow, with a single pulp horn that points cuspally. Both the pulp chamber and the single root canal are wider labiopalatally than mesiodistally. The root canal does not constrict markedly until the apical third of the root is reached. The root canal, which is always single, is oval or triangular in cross-section except in its apical third, where it is round.

### Mandibular permanent canine

The pulp cavity of the mandibular permanent canine (Figs 2.66, 2.67) resembles that of the maxillary permanent canine, although it is smaller in all dimensions. The root canal is oval in cross-section, being wider buccopalatally, but becomes round apically. About 6% of these teeth have two root canals, usually with separate foramina.

## PREMOLARS

### Maxillary first premolar

The maxillary first premolar (Figs 2.68, 2.69) usually has two roots (85% of cases), although they are sometimes fused. The two canals generally exit by separate foramina. A single root and single canal is present in less than 10% of cases. A small number (5%) have three canals (sometimes in three roots). The pulp chamber is wide buccopalatally with two distinct

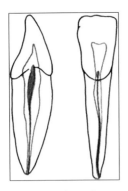

**Fig. 2.61** Schematic representation of the pulp morphology of the mandibular first permanent incisor.

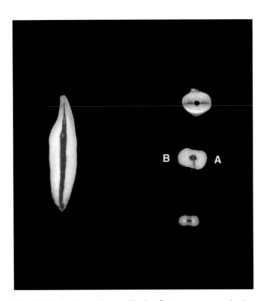

**Fig. 2.62** Sectioned mandibular first permanent incisor demonstrating pulp morphology. A = labial; B = lingual.

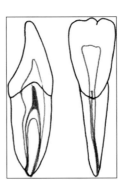

**Fig. 2.63** Schematic representation of the pulp morphology of the mandibular second permanent incisor.

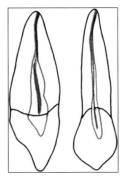

**Fig. 2.64** Schematic representation of the pulp morphology of the maxillary permanent canine.

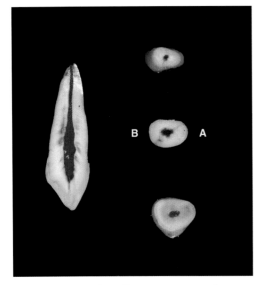

**Fig. 2.65** Sectioned maxillary permanent canine demonstrating pulp morphology. A = labial; B = palatal.

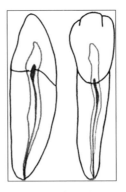

**Fig. 2.66** Schematic representation of the pulp morphology of the mandibular permanent canine.

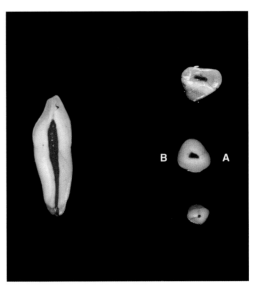

**Fig. 2.67** Sectioned mandibular permanent canine tooth demonstrating pulp morphology. A = labial; B = lingual.

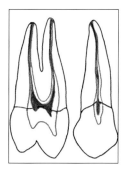

**Fig. 2.68** Schematic representation of the pulp morphology of the maxillary first premolar.

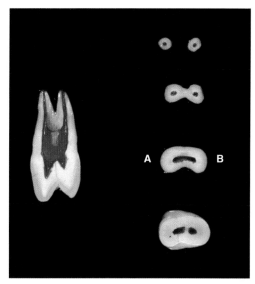

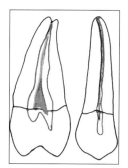

**Fig. 2.70** Schematic representation of the pulp morphology of the maxillary second premolar.

**Fig. 2.69** Sectioned maxillary first premolar demonstrating pulp morphology. A = buccal; B = palatal.

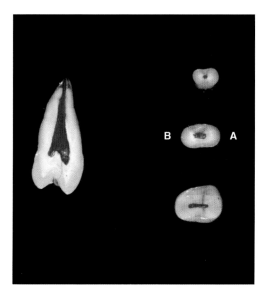

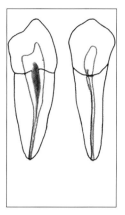

**Fig. 2.72** Schematic representation of the pulp morphology of the mandibular first premolar.

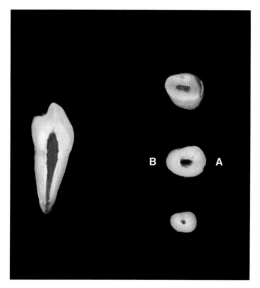

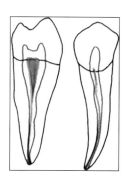

**Fig. 2.74** Schematic representation of the pulp morphology of the mandibular second premolar.

**Fig. 2.71** Sectioned maxillary second premolar demonstrating pulp morphology. A = buccal; B = palatal.

**Fig. 2.73** Sectioned mandibular first premolar demonstrating pulp morphology. A = buccal; B = lingual.

pulp horns pointing towards the cusps. From the buccal view, the pulp chamber is much narrower. The floor of the pulp chamber is rounded with the highest point in the centre. It usually lies within the root just apical to the cervix. Where the root canals arise from the pulp chamber, the orifices are funnel-shaped. The pulp chamber is closest to the surface mesially, where the shape of the crown is indented by the canine fossa. The dental pulp may be exposed in this area by caries or restorative cavities that are extended interproximally. The root canals diverge but are usually straight individually and taper evenly from their origin to the apical foramina. In cross-section, the root canals are generally round. With age, the general shape of the pulp cavity remains the same but its dimensions, particularly the height of the pulp chamber, are reduced.

## Maxillary second premolar

The maxillary second premolar (Figs 2.70, 2.71) has in most instances (75%) a single root with a single root canal. Its pulp chamber extends apically well below the cervical margin. The appearance of the pulp cavity viewed from the buccal aspect is similar to that in the first premolar. When two canals are present, they most commonly have separate apical foramina.

In cross-section the root canal is oval until the apical third of the root, where it becomes round.

## Mandibular first premolar

The pulp chamber in the mandibular first premolar (Figs 2.72, 2.73), like that of the maxillary premolars, is wider buccolingually than mesiodistally. Unlike the maxillary premolars, there is usually only one pulp horn, which extends into the buccal cusp. Occasionally, a small pulp horn may pass to the reduced lingual cusp. There is usually a single root canal (in 75% of cases) that becomes constricted towards the middle third of the root. Most teeth that have two canals have two apical foramina.

## Mandibular second premolar

The pulp morphology of the mandibular second premolar (Fig. 2.74) differs little from that described for the mandibular first premolar, although a higher proportion (85%) have single canals and there are usually two well developed pulp horns projecting towards its cusps.

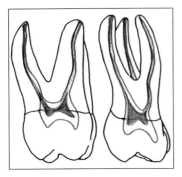

**Fig. 2.75** Schematic representation of the pulp morphology of the maxillary first permanent molar.

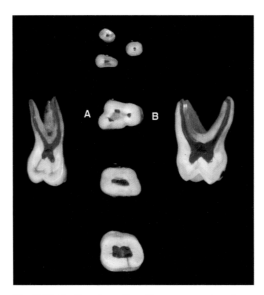

**Fig. 2.76** Sectioned maxillary first permanent molar demonstrating pulp morphology. The tooth on the left shows the root canals of the mesiobuccal and palatal roots, while that on the right shows the two buccal root canals. A = buccal; B = palatal.

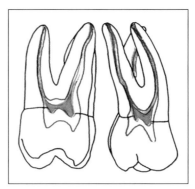

**Fig. 2.77** Schematic representation of the pulp morphology of the maxillary second permanent molar.

## MOLARS

### Maxillary first permanent molar

The pulp chamber of the maxillary first permanent molar (Figs 2.75, 2.76) is rhomboidal in shape, being wider buccopalatally than mesiodistally. Four pulp horns arise from the roof, one to each of the major cusps. The pulp horn to the mesiobuccal cusp is the longest. The floor of the pulp chamber generally lies below the cervical margin. Three root canals are present (or four in 60% of cases), their orifices being funnel-shaped. The root canal of the mesiobuccal root leaves the pulp chamber in a mesial direction and is often significantly curved. In cross-section, it appears as a narrow slit, being wider buccopalatally. Its anatomy may be complicated by irregular branching or bifurcation near the apical foramen. When a fourth canal is present, it is in the mesiobuccal root. Two-thirds of the fourth canals rejoin the main canal of the mesiobuccal root near the root apex. The palatal root canal is the widest and longest of the three root canals. The floor of the pulp chamber is marked by a series of developmental grooves that join the orifices of the root canals.

### Maxillary second permanent molar

The pulp cavity of the maxillary second permanent molar (Fig. 2.77) is similar to that of the first molar, but smaller with the rhomboidal shape more compressed. The roots of this tooth are more convergent, bringing the root canal orifices closer together on the pulpal floor. The roots are commonly fused. A second mesiobuccal canal is less common than in the first molar (40% of cases).

### Mandibular first permanent molar

The pulp chamber in the mandibular first permanent molar (Figs 2.78, 2.79) is wider mesiodistally than buccolingually. It is also wider mesially than distally. There are five pulp horns projecting to the cusps, the lingual pulp horns being longer and more pointed. The floor of the pulp chamber lies at, or just below, the level of the cervical margin. The root canals leave the pulp chamber through funnel-shaped orifices, of which the mesial are finer than the distal. The mesial root has two root canals, mesiobuccal and mesiolingual. The mesiobuccal root canal follows a curved path, the

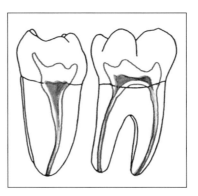

**Fig. 2.78** Schematic representation of the pulp morphology of the mandibular first permanent molar.

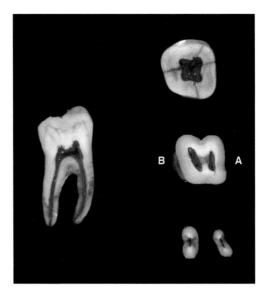

**Fig. 2.79** Sectioned mandibular first permanent molar demonstrating pulp morphology. A = buccal; B = lingual.

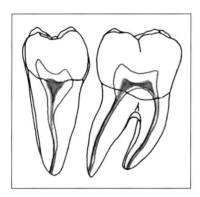

**Fig. 2.80** Schematic representation of the pulp morphology of the mandibular second permanent molar.

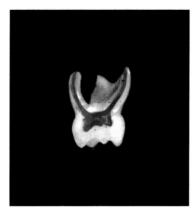

**Fig. 2.81** Sectioned maxillary second deciduous molar demonstrating pulp morphology.

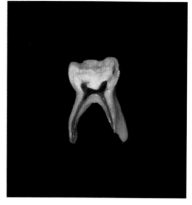

**Fig. 2.82** Sectioned mandibular second deciduous molar demonstrating pulp morphology.

mesiolingual canal is straighter; both are circular in cross-section. In 30% of teeth, the distal root has two canals. The distal canal, especially when single, is considerably larger and more oval in cross-section than the mesial root canals and follows a straighter course.

## Mandibular second permanent molar

The pulp morphology of the mandibular second permanent molar (Fig. 2.80) closely resembles that of the adjacent first molar, although there are only four pulp horns and only rarely (8% of cases) two canals in the distal root.

## SHAPE OF THE PULP CHAMBER IN DECIDUOUS TEETH

As in permanent teeth, the shape of the deciduous pulp chamber reflects the shape of the crown but, in the deciduous teeth, the chamber is relatively larger and the pulp horns longer and closer to the surface of the tooth. All incisors and canines have single canals that are either round or oval (being compressed mesiodistally). In 10% of deciduous mandibular incisors there are two root canals. The pulp chambers of deciduous mandibular molars are proportionately larger than those of the deciduous maxillary molars. The mesiobuccal pulp horn in deciduous molars is particularly near to the occlusal surface and thus highly vulnerable to exposure by dental caries, trauma or cavity preparation. Small canals running from the pulp chamber to the furcation region are common in deciduous molars. In the slender roots of deciduous molars, the root canals are narrower mesiodistally and more ribbon-shaped than those in permanent teeth. This, and the severe curvature of deciduous roots, makes complete debridement and obturation of the root canal system difficult. Although pulpotomy is the more common treatment for the diseased deciduous pulp, pulpectomy and canal obturation is feasible. When resorption of the deciduous root begins, it commences on the lingual surfaces of the anterior teeth and furcal surfaces of molars; this complicates root canal therapy as the exit to the canal system becomes very wide and may be some distance from the root end as visualized radiographically. Other features to bear in mind are:

- The maxillary first deciduous molar has two to four root canals, with two canals in the mesiobuccal root in 75% of cases. The palatal and distobuccal roots are often fused (one-third of cases) but contain distinct canals.
- The maxillary second deciduous molar has two to five root canals (Fig. 2.81). The mesiobuccal root usually bifurcates or contains two canals (90% of cases). Palatal and distobuccal roots sometimes fuse and contain a single, common canal.

- The mandibular first deciduous molar may have two to four canals (Fig. 2.82). Most mesial roots (75%) have two canals, 25% of distal.
- The mandibular second deciduous molar usually has three canals but can vary from two to five. Two canals are seen in 85% of mesial roots but only 25% of distal roots have two canals.

## ALIGNMENT AND OCCLUSION OF THE PERMANENT TEETH

The relationships of the teeth, both within and between the dental arches, are of fundamental importance to an understanding of mastication and for such clinical disciplines as orthodontics and restorative dentistry. Tooth alignment is the term that refers to the arrangement of the teeth within the dental arches; occlusion refers to the relationship of the dental arches when tooth contact is made.

Traditionally, textbooks describe a standard set of tooth relationships that is called 'normal' (i.e. normal alignment and normal occlusion). Normal is a term that is generally used to describe situations that are the ordinary or most frequent; alternatively, normal may define an authoritative standard or ideal that, in medical terms, is the healthy state. In these terms, malocclusions could be regarded as normal, for they are more commonly found in the population than 'normal' occlusion (approximately 75% of the population of the USA have some degree of occlusal 'disharmony').

Malocclusions do not always predispose to dental disease and, in most cases, are not associated with masticatory dysfunction, speech defects, bruxism or pain in and around the temporomandibular joint. Furthermore, our knowledge of the association between the structure and function of the dental arches during mastication is not yet sufficient to provide an authoritative standard for tooth relationships; in structural terms, the ideal occlusion is a rather subjective concept. If there is an ideal occlusion, it can presently be defined only in broad functional terms. We believe therefore that the occlusion is 'ideal' when:

- the teeth are aligned such that the masticatory loads are within physiological range and act through the long axes of as many teeth in the arch as possible
- mastication involves alternating bilateral jaw movements (and not habitual, unilateral biting preferences as a result of adaptation to occlusal interference)
- lateral jaw movements occur without undue mechanical interference
- in the rest position of the jaw, the gap between teeth (the freeway space; see page 41) is correct for the individual concerned
- the tooth alignment is aesthetically pleasing to its possessor.

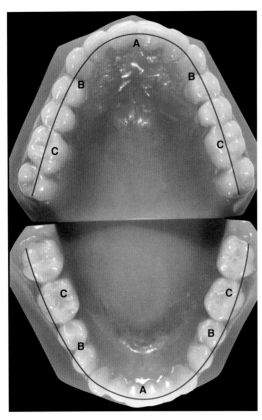

**Fig. 2.83** The form of the maxillary and mandibular dental arches showing the anatomical alignment of the teeth and Angle's lines of occlusion.

Despite our reservations, the traditional descriptions of 'normal' tooth relationships provide a convenient model for the classification of malocclusions in clinical situations. However, we have chosen to use the terms 'anatomical alignment' and 'anatomical occlusion' instead of 'normal alignment' and 'normal occlusion' in order to avoid the difficulties of defining normality with respect to tooth relationships. The occlusion of the deciduous dentition and the development of occlusion is considered in Chapter 26.

## ANATOMICAL ALIGNMENT OF TEETH

Each dental arch (maxillary/upper and mandibular/lower) generally takes the form of a catenary curve (Fig. 2.83). Such a curve is described when a rope or chain is hung at both ends. There are no spacings or rotations of teeth within the arch and therefore all teeth are in contact with neighbouring teeth along the arch.

Superimposed on the occlusal surfaces of the teeth shown in Figure 2.83 are Angle's 'lines of occlusion'. Because the maxillary arch is broader than the mandibular arch, the line of occlusion for the maxillary arch passes through the cingula of the anterior teeth and through the central fossae of the posterior teeth. However, the line of occlusion for the mandibular arch runs along the incisal edges of the anterior teeth and along the buccal cusps of the posterior teeth.

The well aligned dental arch may be divided into different segments. A curved line in the coronal plane describes the anterior segment. This segment extends across the midline from canine to canine. The middle segments are described by straight lines extending from the distal edges of the canines to the mesiobuccal cusps of the first molars. The posterior segments extend from the mesiobuccal cusps of the first molars backwards. Both the middle and posterior segments lie in the sagittal plane, the posterior segments being more nearly parallel to this plane than the middle segments.

The positions of the teeth within the dental arch are determined by numerous factors and forces. Indeed, the spatial configuration of the arches

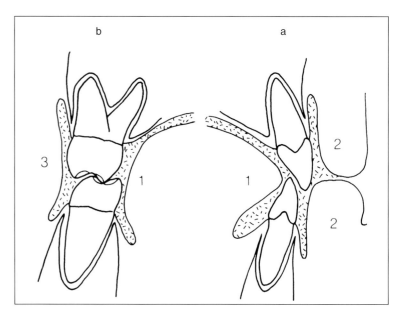

**Fig. 2.84** The configuration of the neutral zone (the stippled area) in the incisor region (a) and the molar region (b). 1 = tongue; 2 = lips; 3 = cheek. Redrawn after Professors B.J. Kraus, R.E. Jordan and L. Abrams.

**Table 2.4** *Average widths of the dental arches (males)*

| Age (years) | Between maxillary canines (mm) | Between mandibular canines (mm) | Between maxillary first molars (mm) | Between mandibular first molars (mm) |
|---|---|---|---|---|
| 6 | 28 | 23 | 42 | 40 |
| 18 | 32 | 25 | 47 | 43 |

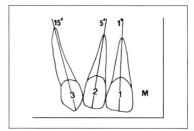

**Fig. 2.85** The alignment of the maxillary incisors and canine viewed labially. The teeth are not drawn to scale and the numerical dental shorthand is used to identify the tooth. All angles quoted are average figures. M = mesial.

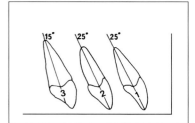

**Fig. 2.86** The alignment of the maxillary incisors and canine viewed distally. The teeth are not drawn to scale and the numerical dental shorthand is used to identify the tooth. All angles quoted are average figures.

is dependent upon an interaction between the eruptive movements carrying the teeth into their functional positions and, once erupted, the forces brought to bear upon each tooth. The term 'neutral zone' (Fig. 2.84) is used to describe that space in which there is an equilibrium of forces so that the teeth attain a position of relative stability. A change in balance in this system, such as that produced by abnormal tongue-thrusting behaviour and abnormal lip posture, can result in malalignment of the teeth.

The size of the dental arches varies considerably between individuals. Table 2.4 provides the average widths of the dental arches for the completed deciduous dentition (6 years) and the completed permanent dentition (18 years) for males. Averages for females are usually 1 mm less.

Figures 2.85–2.92 describe the angulation or axial positioning of individual teeth within the alveolus relative to perpendiculars dropped from a hypothetically flat occlusal plane. In these diagrams, the angles quoted are average figures, although variation is considerable.

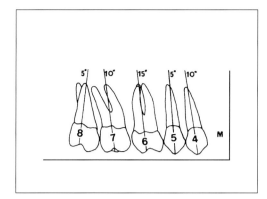

**Fig. 2.87** The alignment of the maxillary premolars and molars viewed buccally. The teeth are not drawn to scale and the numerical dental shorthand is used to identify the tooth. All angles quoted are average figures. M = mesial.

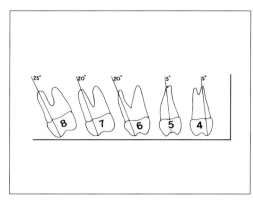

**Fig. 2.88** The alignment of the maxillary premolars and molars viewed distally. The teeth are not drawn to scale and the numerical dental shorthand is used to identify the tooth. All angles quoted are average figures.

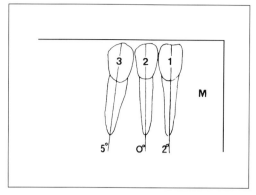

**Fig. 2.89** The alignment of the mandibular incisors and canine viewed labially. The teeth are not drawn to scale and the numerical dental shorthand is used to identify the tooth. All angles quoted are average figures. M = mesial.

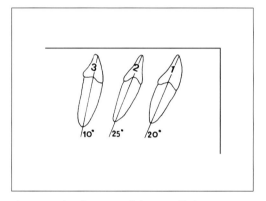

**Fig. 2.90** The alignment of the mandibular incisors and canine viewed distally. The teeth are not drawn to scale and the numerical dental shorthand is used to identify the tooth. All angles quoted are average figures.

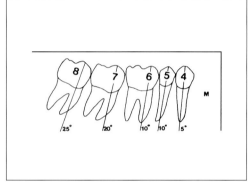

**Fig. 2.91** The alignment of the mandibular premolars and molars viewed buccally. The teeth are not drawn to scale and the numerical dental shorthand is used to identify the tooth. All angles quoted are average figures. M = mesial.

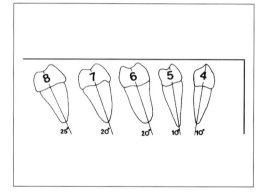

**Fig. 2.92** The alignment of the mandibular premolars and molars viewed distally. The teeth are not drawn to scale and the numerical dental shorthand is used to identify the tooth. All angles quoted are average figures.

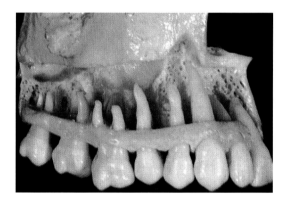

**Fig. 2.93** The curvatures of the maxillary teeth within the alveolar bone of the maxilla.

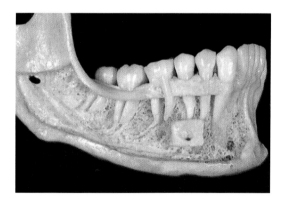

**Fig. 2.94** The curvatures of the mandibular teeth within the alveolar bone of the mandible.

Viewed labially, the maxillary incisors have slight distal inclinations whereas the canine has a distinct mesial angulation. When these teeth are viewed distally, all show pronounced proclinations into the lip (although the canine is slightly more vertical). For the mandibular incisors and canine, when viewed labially, the incisors are more or less vertical and the canine has a slight mesial inclination. When viewed distally, these anterior mandibular teeth, like the anterior maxillary teeth, are proclined.

When viewed buccally, the maxillary premolars and molars change from a slight mesial angulation (premolars) to a distal inclination (the third molar). This contrasts with the mandibular posterior teeth, which show increasing mesial inclination moving back through the arch. When the maxillary premolars and molars are viewed distally, the teeth change from being essentially vertical in the premolar region to being distinctly buc-

cally inclined in the molars. This again contrasts with the mandibular premolars and molars, where the teeth become more lingually inclined moving through the arch.

## Curvatures of the teeth and arches

The impression could readily be gained from Figures 2.85–2.92 that the axes of the teeth are straight and run perpendicular to a horizontal, flat, occlusal plane. However, neither the axes of the teeth nor the occlusal planes are straight but are curved in all directions (Figs 2.93, 2.94). The curved axes of the teeth have a tendency to parallelism and are inclined mesially. It is often thought, mistakenly so, that the forces of mastication are at right angles to the occlusal surfaces of the teeth. If this were so, and

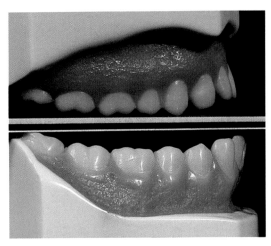

**Fig. 2.95** Curvatures of the occlusal plane – the curves of Spee.

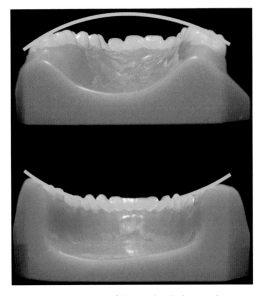

**Fig. 2.96** Curvatures of the occlusal plane – the curves of Wilson.

if the occlusal planes and axes of the teeth were not curved, the arches might not be stable and the masticatory loads might be at an unfavourable angle to the teeth. Indeed, it is thought that, during mastication, the loads strike the teeth such that there is a mesial component of force (see pages 373, 374). The occlusal plane shows two types of curvature – the curve of Spee and the curve of Wilson.

The teeth align themselves such that the occlusal plane is not flat but describes a relatively linear curve in the anteroposterior direction, the curve of Spee (Fig. 2.95). The mandibular curve of Spee is concave whereas the maxillary curve is convex. An appreciation of the contribution of each tooth to the curve of Spee may be gained from analysis of the alignment of the long axes of the posterior teeth viewed buccally (Figs 2.87, 2.91) and from the axes of the anterior teeth viewed distally (Figs 2.86, 2.90). Although the maxillary and mandibular curves of Spee are different, they are nevertheless complementary and thereby may help achieve occlusal balance during mastication by encouraging simultaneous contact in more than one area of the dental arches. If the curves are exaggerated, however, there will be crowding in the mandibular arch and increased spacing in the maxillary arch.

The occlusal curves of Wilson (Fig. 2.96) are aligned in the transverse plane. Analysis of the alignment of the long axes of the posterior teeth (Figs 2.88, 2.92) shows that the curves of Wilson are such that the occlusal surfaces of the mandibular molars are directed lingually, while those of the maxillary molars are directed buccally. As for the curves of Spee, the curves of Wilson for the maxillary and mandibular posterior teeth are opposite but complementary. The curves of Spee and Wilson were once

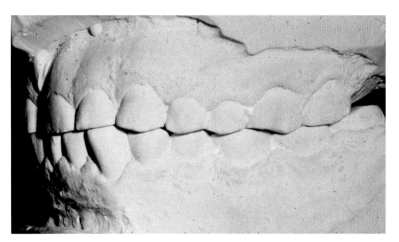

**Fig. 2.97** Effects of wear on the curvatures of the occlusal plane, which becomes flat.

thought to be related three-dimensionally, the occlusal surfaces of the teeth being aligned on the curved surface of a segment of a sphere having a radius of about 10 cm. However, attempts to demonstrate, and then measure, the spherical curves (of Monson) have been unsuccessful.

With age, and as a result of wear (attrition), the cusps of the teeth are worn away so that the curvatures of the occlusal plane are lost and the plane becomes flat (Fig. 2.97). In addition, wear will affect the overjet and overbite for the anterior teeth (see page 37) and the nature of the tooth contacts (see centric stops, page 38).

## ANATOMICAL OCCLUSION OF TEETH

The relationships of the jaws in function are so variable that our understanding of the functional articulation of teeth remains poor. To simplify analysis, several occlusal positions have been strictly defined. These positions may be classified into those that are symmetrical and those that are asymmetrical. This corresponds with the classification of mandibular movements into symmetrical and asymmetrical movements. The symmetrical occlusal positions include centric occlusion and bilaterally protrusive position. The asymmetrical occlusal positions are those associated with lateral (side-to-side) movements. Within the clinic, centric occlusal position is regarded as the 'standard' or 'model' for orthodontic and prosthetic diagnoses and treatments. While it is important in the dental clinic to be confident that oral examinations are based upon an accurate recording of tooth relationships in centric occlusion, the consistent attainment of centric occlusal position for some patients is notoriously difficult. Clinicians have consequently developed a variety of strategies to attain this position, including palpating the mandibular condyles within the mandibular fossae, pronouncing certain sounds, words or phrases, fatiguing the mandible by making the patient make rapid movements of the lower jaw, and even hypnosis!

### Centric occlusal position

The centric occlusal position (Fig. 2.98) is defined as the terminal position of physiological jaw movements. It is the relationship between the two arches when the teeth are brought into contact with the mandibular condyles centrally positioned, at rest, in the mandibular fossae.

According to the pioneer orthodontist Edward Angle, the key to the intercuspal relationships between the teeth in the centric occlusal position is to be found in the relative positions of the maxillary and mandibular first permanent molars. In the 'normal' or anatomical condition, each arch is bilaterally symmetrical. Because the anterior maxillary segment is slightly larger than the corresponding mandibular segment (because of the unequal sizes of the maxillary and mandibular first incisors), each maxillary tooth will contact its corresponding mandibular antagonist and its

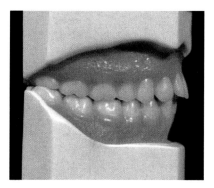

**Fig. 2.98** Lateral view of the arrangement of teeth in anatomical centric occlusion.

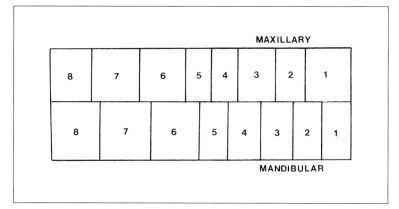

**Fig. 2.99** Diagram illustrating the relationships between maxillary and mandibular permanent teeth in anatomical centric occlusal position. The teeth are identified according to the Palmer-Zsigmondy system.

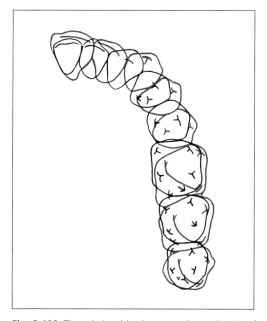

**Fig. 2.100** The relationships between the occlusal surfaces of the maxillary (red) and mandibular (black) permanent teeth in anatomical centric occlusion.

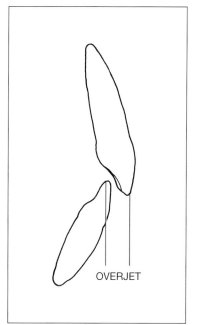

**Fig. 2.101** The buccolingual incisor relationships in anatomical centric occlusion – overjet.

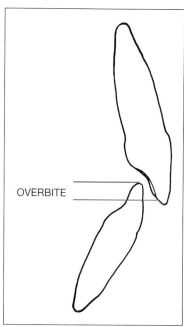

**Fig. 2.102** The buccolingual incisor relationships in anatomical centric occlusion – overbite.

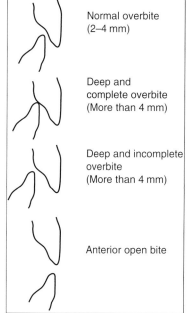

**Fig. 2.103** Classification of overbite.

distal neighbour. Thus, the maxillary first permanent molar will contact the distal part of the mandibular first permanent molar and the mesial part of the mandibular second permanent molar. The only exceptions are the mandibular first incisor and the maxillary third molar. The relationships between maxillary and mandibular permanent teeth in anatomical centric occlusal position are shown in Figure 2.99.

Figure 2.100 illustrates the relationships between the maxillary and mandibular permanent teeth in anatomical centric occlusion by superimposing the occlusal surfaces of the teeth in the maxillary arch on those of the mandibular arch. This diagram shows not only the general anteroposterior relationships of the maxillary teeth and their antagonists but also the buccolingual relationships of the arches. As the maxillary arch is a little larger and broader than the mandibular arch, there is a slight overlap of the mandibular arch by the maxillary arch such that the buccal cusps of the maxillary teeth extend a few millimetres beyond the buccal occlusal edge of the mandibular teeth. This overlap is termed overjet.

When the buccolingual incisor relationships in anatomical centric occlusion are considered (Figs 2.101, 2.102), two types of 'overlap' of the mandibular incisors by the maxillary incisors can be discerned. The overlap in the horizontal plane (overjet) is approximately 2–3 mm. The vertical overlap, specific to the incisors and canines, is termed overbite (and is also approximately 2–3 mm). The overbite in anatomical centric occlusion is such that the palatal surfaces of the maxillary incisors on average overlap the incisal third of the labial surfaces of the mandibular incisors. Furthermore, the incisal edges of the mandibular incisors are related to the cingulum areas of the maxillary incisors. Figure 2.103 provides a classification of overbite used in the orthodontic clinic.

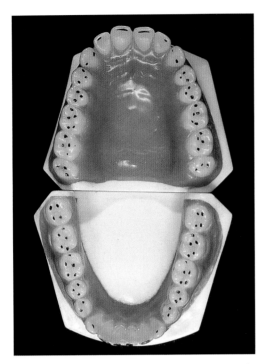

**Fig. 2.104** The occlusal surfaces of the permanent dentition marked to show the position of centric stops in anatomical centric occlusion.

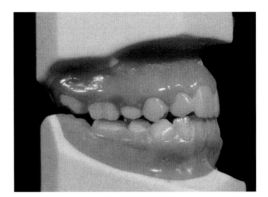

**Fig. 2.105** Angle's class I malocclusion.

With age, and as a result of attrition, the dimensions of the overjet and overbite decrease.

Figure 2.104 shows the occlusal surfaces of the permanent dentition marked with the positions of hard contact in anatomical centric occlusion. These contacts are termed 'centric stops' (also sometimes referred to as 'holding contacts') and represent the intercuspal contact positions. When the 32 teeth within the permanent dentition occlude, there are 138 centric stops, although this is seldom achieved during the normal bite. The major markings register on the occlusal surfaces of the posterior teeth (Fig. 2.104). The slopes of the maxillary palatal cusps make stops coincident with the stops within the central fossae of the mandibular posterior teeth. The stops in the central fossae of the maxillary teeth coincide with the stops on the slopes of the buccal cusps of the mandibular posterior teeth. The cusps seated in the central fossae are sometimes referred to as 'supporting cusps'. As befits the anatomical overjet relationships, the tips of the maxillary buccal cusps and the mandibular lingual cusps remain relatively unmarked. For the anterior teeth, the mandibular incisors have the centric stops on the incisal edges whereas the stops on the maxillary incisors are positioned down their palatal surfaces.

Similar marks to centric stops can be made in the clinic by interposing articulating paper between the teeth and then instructing the patient to go into centric occlusal position. With age, and with attrition, the occlusal surfaces become flattened as the cusps are worn and consequently the centric stops are significantly altered.

## Variations in the relationships of the dental arches in centric position

Malocclusions should be regarded as anatomical variations rather than abnormalities for, although they may be aesthetically displeasing, they are rarely involved in masticatory dysfunction. Our lack of understanding of the relationships between masticatory efficiency and tooth and arch form is responsible for the classification of malocclusion in terms of variations in the anatomical centric position and not in more functional terms.

Malocclusions result from malposition of individual teeth, malrelationship of the dental arches and/or variation in skeletal morphology of the jaws. Techniques for determining the skeletal relationships of the jaws are described on pages 46, 47. Two classifications describing malposition of teeth and malrelationship of the arches are in general use – Angle's classification and a classification based upon the relationships of the incisors. A classification of malocclusion based upon canine relationships is also available for clinical use. However, this is much less employed than Angle's classification and the incisor relationship classification.

### Angle's classification

Angle's classification of malocclusion was derived at the end of the 19th century. It relies upon the relationship of the arches in the anteroposterior plane using the maxillary and mandibular first permanent molars as key teeth (with some additional information regarding incisor positions). Nowadays, clinicians will consider the relationship of the molars, canines and incisors as three separate elements but, perhaps confusingly, still use Angle's original terminology.

***Angle's class I malocclusion.*** Although one or more of the teeth are malpositioned, this does not affect the 'standard' anatomical relationship of the first permanent molars. Thus, the mesiobuccal cusp of the permanent maxillary first molar tooth occludes with the mid-buccal groove of the permanent mandibular first molar tooth. Recently, Andrews has added two further elements to this:

1. The distal surface of the distal marginal ridge of the maxillary molar contacts, and occludes with, the mesial surface of the mesial marginal ridge of the mandibular second molar.
2. The mesiopalatal cusp of the maxillary molar sits in the central fossa of the mandibular molar.

In the models shown in Figure 2.105, the maxillary canine is missing and the premolars are malaligned but the maxillary first molar tooth occludes correctly with the mandibular first and second molar teeth.

***Angle's class II malocclusion.*** Angle's class II malocclusion is characterized by a 'prenormal' maxillary arch relationship, the maxillary first permanent molars occluding at least half a cusp more mesial to the mandibular first permanent molars than the standard anatomical position. Thus, the mesiobuccal cusp of the permanent maxillary first molar tooth occludes mesial to the mid-buccal groove of the permanent mandibular first molar tooth.

Angle's class II malocclusion also takes into consideration incisor position.

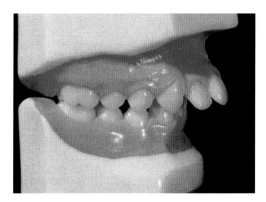

**Fig. 2.106** Angle's class II malocclusion (division 1).

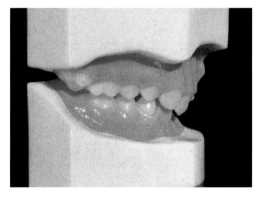

**Fig. 2.107** Angle's class II malocclusion (division 2).

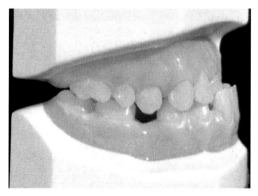

**Fig. 2.108** Angle's class III malocclusion.

Angle's class II malocclusion (division 1) indicates that the maxillary incisors are proclined (Fig. 2.106).

Angle's class II malocclusion (division 2) indicates that the maxillary incisors are retroclined (Fig. 2.107). Frequently only the first incisors are retroclined, the second being proclined. For this malocclusion it is not uncommon to see increased overbite in the incisor region.

**Angle's class III malocclusion.** This malocclusion is characterized by a 'postnormal' maxillary arch relationship, the maxillary first permanent molars occluding at least half a cusp more distal to the mandibular first permanent molars than the 'standard' anatomical position. Thus, the mesio-buccal cusp of the permanent maxillary first molar tooth occludes distal to the mid-buccal groove of the permanent mandibular first molar tooth. The incisor relationship varies from 'normal' overjet to an 'edge-to-edge' bite to reverse overjet (where the mandibular incisors lie labially to the maxillary incisors – as shown in Figure 2.108).

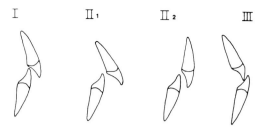

**Fig. 2.109** Classification of malocclusion using incisor relationships.

### Classification based on canine relationships

**Class I.** The cusp of the permanent maxillary canine tooth occludes in the embrasure between the permanent mandibular canine and first premolar teeth.

**Class II.** The permanent maxillary canine tooth occludes mesial to that in Class I.

**Class III.** The permanent maxillary canine tooth occludes distal to that in Class I.

### Classification based on incisor relationships

As for Angle's classification, the classification of malocclusions based upon incisor relationships uses the categories class I, class II (division 1), class II (division 2) and class III. However, care must be taken not to confuse these classifications – for example, an Angle's class I molar relationship might exist alongside an incisor class III relationship in the same person!

As the permanent molars do not have a fixed relationship in the arch, and may migrate following early loss of deciduous teeth, the classification of malocclusion based upon incisor relationships (Fig. 2.109) is often preferred to Angle's classification. Furthermore, a classification of malocclusion related to the incisors is seen by many clinicians as being more appropriate because a major objective of orthodontic treatment is to establish an anatomical incisor relationship (patients being more concerned about, and aware of, the aesthetics of the incisor relationship than they are of the molar relationship). Thus, a classification based on incisor relationships is a much more informative method of describing the malocclusion. Furthermore, it avoids the confusion that can sometimes occur when trying to use Angle's original classification to describe a patient who presents with class I molars with class II canines and class III incisors (such as may occur in a patient with normal buccal segment relationships, missing maxillary second incisors and first incisors that are retroclined).

The incisor relationship classification was devised by Ballard and Wayman in the 1960s and relies upon the relationship of incisors relative to a specific landmark – the cingulum plateau on the maxillary central incisor.

**Class I incisor relationship.** This represents the relationship where the incisors do not show any malposition. The incisal margins of the permanent mandibular incisors occlude with, or lie directly below, the middle third of the palatal surfaces of the permanent maxillary incisors (i.e. on or below the cingulum plateau area).

**Class II incisor relationship.** The incisal margins of the mandibular incisors lie behind the cingulum plateau area on the palatal surfaces of the maxillary incisors. Thus, the incisal margins of the mandibular incisors are related to the gingival third of the palatal surfaces of the maxillary incisors. Division 1 indicates that the maxillary central incisors are proclined with an increased overjet; division 2 indicates that the maxillary central incisors are retroclined and there is increased overbite.

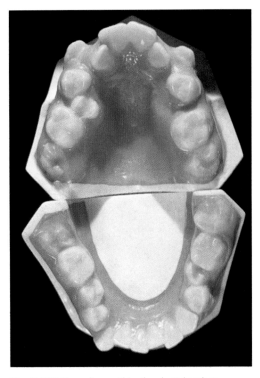

**Fig. 2.110** Crowding within the dental arches.

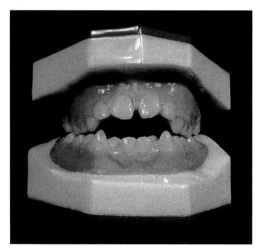

**Fig. 2.111** Anterior open bite.

***Class III incisor relationship.*** The incisal margins of the permanent mandibular incisors lie in front of the cingulum plateau area on the palatal surfaces of the permanent maxillary incisors. Thus, the incisal margins of the mandibular incisors are related to the incisal third of the palatal surface of the maxillary incisors and there is a reduced, or even a reverse, overjet (the lower incisors lying anterior to the maxillary incisors).

## Forms of malocclusion

Three common forms of malocclusion are: crowding, anterior open bite and crossbite.

**Crowding** is the term used to describe the condition where teeth are markedly out of the line of the dental arch because there is disproportion between the size of the arch and the size of the teeth. The severe crowding illustrated in Figure 2.110 reflects the developmental positions of the teeth before eruption (note that the second incisors develop inside the dental arch and the canines develop outside the arch). Spacing within an arch occurs where the teeth are small in relation to the size of the arch (or where there are missing teeth). The site of crowding also reflects the timing of eruption. The last teeth to erupt usually manifest the crowding – hence buccally displaced maxillary canines and impacted mandibular second premolars.

**Anterior open bite** (Fig. 2.111) occurs where there is no incisor contact and no incisor overbite. It may be caused by thumb-sucking habits, by abnormal swallowing patterns or by skeletal anomalies. Skeletal anterior open bites sometimes result from lack of development of the anterior alveolar region but are more often associated with an increase in anterior intermaxillary height (i.e. the distance between the maxillary and mandibular dental bases; see Fig. 2.124). Anterior open bite may also be 'physiological' and related to the stage of eruption (incomplete eruption) of the incisors.

Crossbite (Fig. 2.112) is a transverse abnormality of the dental arches where there is an asymmetrical bite. It may be unilateral or, as illustrated in Figure 2.112, bilateral. Crossbites are frequently related to discrepancies in the widths of the dental bases and may involve the displacement of the mandible to one side to obtain maximal intercuspation.

Table 2.5 provides data indicating the severity and type of malocclusion in the population of the USA. Approximately 80% of children and

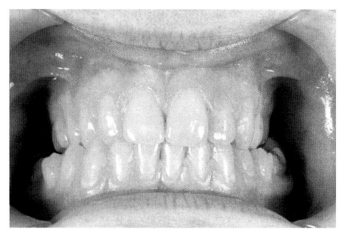

**Fig. 2.112** Bilateral crossbite.

**Table 2.5** *Severity and types of malocclusions in the general population of the USA*

| | Distribution (%) | |
| --- | --- | --- |
| | Age 6–11 years | Age 12–17 years |
| **Severity** | | |
| Near-ideal occlusion | 23 | 10 |
| Mild malocclusion | 40 | 35 |
| Moderate malocclusion | 23 | 26 |
| Severe or very severe malocclusion | 14 | 29 |
| **Type** | | |
| **Crowding/malalignment problems** | | |
| Ideal | 57 | 13 |
| Moderate | 39 | 44 |
| Severe | 4 | 43 |
| **Anteroposterior problems** | | |
| Overjet (6 mm or more) | 17 | 15 |
| Reverse overjet (1 mm or more) | 1 | |
| **Vertical problems** | | |
| Open bite (2 mm or more) | 1 | 1 |
| Overbite (6 mm or more) | 8 | 12 |
| **Transverse problems** | | |
| Lingual crossbite (two or more teeth) | 5 | 6 |
| Buccal crossbite (two or more teeth) | 1 | 2 |

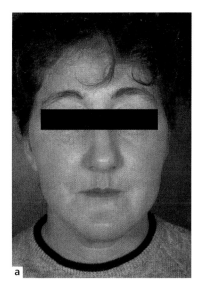 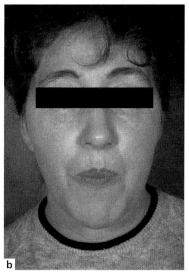 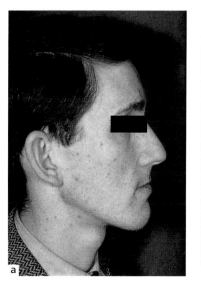 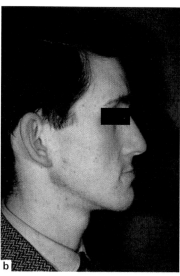

**Fig. 2.113** The appearance produced as a result of over-opening. (a) Normal resting position and facial profile for a patient without dentures. (b) Over-opened appearance produced typically by wearing dentures without provision of adequate freeway space. Courtesy of Professor D.C. Berry.

**Fig. 2.114** The appearance produced by over-closure. (a) Normal resting position and facial profile of a patient who displays over-closure with an ill-fitting denture (b). Courtesy of Professor D.C. Berry.

adolescents in the USA thus show some degree of malocclusion. Most commonly there are problems of crowding (for about 40% of children and 80% of adolescents). The second most common type of malocclusion is excessive overjet of the maxillary incisors (about 15% of both children and adolescents).

## MANDIBULAR POSTURE

When the mandible is at rest, a gap of a few millimetres remains between the occlusal surfaces of the teeth – the so-called 'freeway space'. The opinion has long been held that the position of rest is innate and unalterable throughout life. However, the concept of a fixed mandibular resting posture is an oversimplification. Indeed, psychological state, body posture and fatigue are well known short-term influences that can change the resting interocclusal distance. Furthermore, research shows that, following speech, mastication or swallowing, the mandible appears to return to whatever position of rest it can find. In the long term, ageing and the removal of occlusal contacts affect the resting position. Although the physiological mechanisms responsible for maintaining a rest position are not fully understood, evidence suggests that the physical properties of the soft tissues are responsible for the rest position, and not the tonic activity of the elevator muscles of the jaw.

Several instruments and techniques have been devised to measure freeway space – some elaborate, some relatively simple. All suffer from inaccuracies produced by examiner bias and misconceptions about the nature of the mandibular resting posture. The use of measuring techniques relies upon the concept that the mandibular resting position is innate and unalterable. Consequently, the removal of teeth is deemed not to affect the rest position. Thus, when a patient has lost all natural occlusal contacts, it is considered necessary only to put a prosthesis into the mouth at a level which reproduces the freeway space to restore the original occlusal vertical dimension.

Although most clinicians would prefer objective criteria for determining vertical jaw relationships, many realize that, because of the relative instability of such relationships, at best one has to rely upon such subjective assessments as overall facial appearance, mandibular position during deglutition, jaw posture giving greatest comfort, position allowing the development of maximum biting force, and lip and tongue posture. Nevertheless, however one gauges the mandibular resting position, if prosthetic appliances are to be placed in the mouth, it is necessary to ensure that the vertical dimensions of the jaws are not adversely affected. Figure 2.113 shows the appearance produced as a result of over-opening and Figure 2.114 the appearance produced by over-closure. The result of over-opening is an elongation of the face, a parting of the lips at rest, and a 'strained' facial appearance. The general effect of over-closure on facial appearance is to produce features of increased age. There is a closer approximation of the nose and chin than normal. The greater the degree of over-closure, the more the soft tissues of the face appear to sag and fall in, and the more pronounced are the lines on the face.

## RADIOGRAPHIC APPEARANCE OF JAWS AND TEETH

Dental radiography and radiology are concerned with the techniques of producing and interpreting photographic images of orodental tissues taken with X-rays. X-rays, being part of the spectrum of electromagnetic radiation, have a wavelength of approximately $10^{-8}$ cm (compared with wavelengths of around $10^{-4}$ cm for visible light). It is the short wavelength that allows X-rays to penetrate materials that would otherwise absorb or reflect light. However, X-rays do not pass through all matter with similar ease: materials composed of elements with low atomic numbers are readily penetrated and are described as being radiolucent, whereas elements with high atomic numbers absorb X-rays and are termed radio-opaque. Thus, gases and soft tissues are radiolucent while calcified materials such as bone and teeth are radio-opaque. X-rays produce a photosensitization reaction when they strike a silver-salt emulsion. When a radio-opaque structure is placed between a beam of X-rays and a photographic plate that is subsequently developed, the radio-opaque structure is 'mapped out' as a white area on the negative. It is because of the properties of tissue penetration and photosensitization that X-rays can be used in dentistry to provide

**Table 2.6** *Extraoral radiographic projections describing jaws and teeth*

| Projection/technique | Purpose |
|---|---|
| Posteroanterior skull (PA) (Fig. 2.115) | Survey of facial bones and mandible |
| Anteroposterior skull (AP) (Fig. 2.116) | Survey of posterior part of cranium, mandible and temporomandibular articulation |
| Reverse Towne's (Fig. 2.117) | Anatomy of mandibular condyles and temporomandibular articulation |
| Occipitomental skull (Fig. 2.118) | Survey of facial bones and air sinuses |
| Lateral skull (Fig. 2.119) | Survey of lateral regions of face, cranium and mandible. View of facial profile and covering soft tissues |
| Lateral skull with cephalostat (Fig. 2.123) | Recording of relationships between teeth, jaws and cranial base |
| Lateral oblique view of mandible (Fig. 2.120) | Survey of posterior regions of body and ramus of mandible |
| Orthopantomogram (Fig. 2.121) | A tomogram to display both maxillae, the mandible and the dentition on a single film |
| Transcranial temporomandibular joint (Fig. 2.122) | Movement of mandibular condyles in mandibular fossae |
| Sialography (Figs 2.133, 2.134) | Infusion of radio-opaque material into the main salivary ducts to study their structure and distribution |
| Tomography (Fig. 2.135) | Technique for the radiography of selected areas that, under standard radiographic technique, are obscured by superimposition of other structures (e.g. temporomandibular joint and air sinuses) |

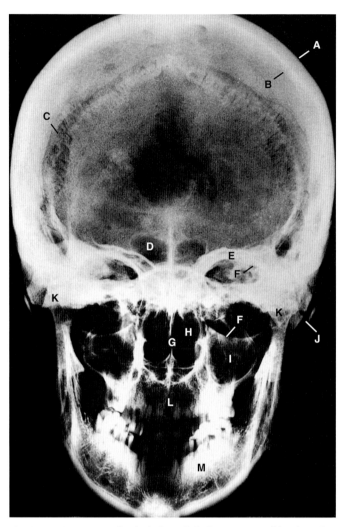

**Fig. 2.116** Anteroposterior (AP) view of skull. A = outer table of cranium; B = inner table of cranium; C = lambdoid suture; D = frontal air sinus; E = superimposed sphenoid, petrous and supraorbital ridges; F = rim of orbit; G = nasal septum; H = nasal fossa; I = maxillary air sinus; J = zygoma; K = condyle of mandible; L = maxilla and teeth; M = body of mandible and teeth.

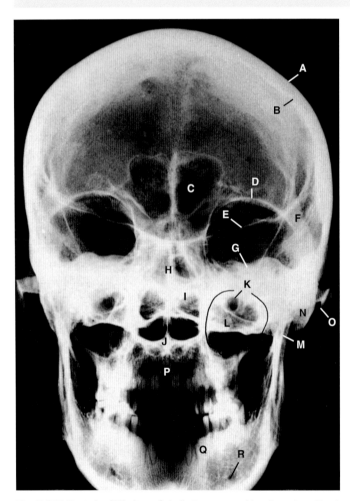

**Fig. 2.115** Posterior (PA) view of skull. A = outer table of cranium; B = inner table of cranium; C = frontal air sinus; D = superior rim of orbit; E = sphenoid ridge in middle cranial fossa; F = zygomatic process of frontal bone; G = petrous ridge; H = nasal septum; I = nasal fossa; J = anterior nasal spine; K = infra-orbital foramen; L = maxillary air sinus; M = neck of mandibular condyle; N = mastoid process of temporal bone; O = zygomatic arch; P = maxilla and teeth; Q = body of mandible and teeth; R = mental foramen.

valuable information concerning underlying hard tissue structures not otherwise visible.

X-rays produce a shadow picture without a focus; therefore the features of a large object such as a skull are not shown equally distinctly on a radiograph. As a general rule, structures nearest the photographic plate appear clearer than those some distance from it. Superimposition may also make interpretation of radiographs difficult, because most radiographs are two-dimensional representations of three-dimensional objects. Care must be taken not to overinterpret radiographs by diagnosing pathological conditions without recourse to other diagnostic aids or clinical findings. The prime use of a radiograph is therefore to describe gross topographic features.

## EXTRA-ORAL RADIOGRAPHIC PROJECTIONS OF JAWS AND TEETH

Table 2.6 outlines the major extra-oral radiographic projections used to view the human jaws and dentition. In this context, 'extra-oral' indicates that the radiographic plate is positioned outside the mouth.

Among the specialized techniques worthy of fuller description here, Figures 2.123–2.135 are concerned with cephalometric radiography, sialography and tomography.

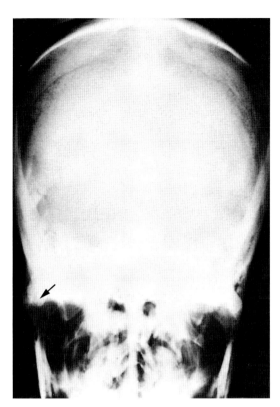

**Fig. 2.117** Reverse Towne's view showing position of mandibular condyle (arrowed).

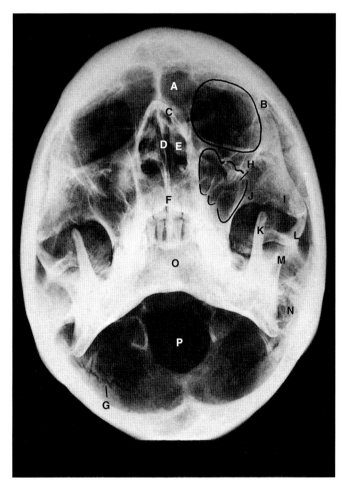

**Fig. 2.118** Occipitomental view of skull (OM 30°). A = frontal air sinus; B = outline of orbit; C = nasal bones; D = nasal septum; E = nasal fossa with superimposed shadows of ethmoidal air cells; F = maxilla and teeth; G = lambdoid suture; H = malar (zygomatic) extension of maxillary sinus; I = zygoma; J = outline of maxillary air sinus; K = coronoid process of mandible; L = zygomatic process of temporal bone; M = condyle of mandible; N = mastoid air cells; O = body of mandible and teeth; P = foramen magnum.

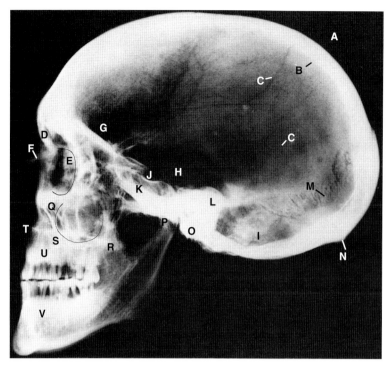

**Fig. 2.119** Lateral skull radiograph. A = outer table of cranium; B = inner table of cranium; C = depressions in cranium related to middle meningeal vessels; D = frontal air sinus; E = margins of orbit; F = nasal bone; G = anterior cranial fossa; H = middle cranial fossa; I = posterior cranial fossa; J = hypophyseal (pituitary) fossa; K = sphenoid air sinus; L = petrous ridge; M = lambdoid suture; N = external occipital protuberance; O = mastoid process; P = condyle of mandible; Q = margin of maxillary air sinus; R = coronoid process of mandible; S = hard palate; T = anterior nasal spine; U = maxilla and teeth; V = body of mandible and teeth.

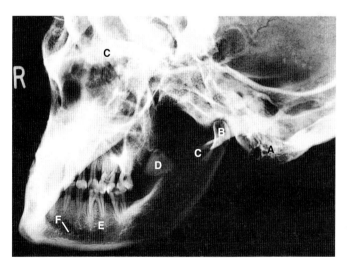

**Fig. 2.120** Lateral oblique view of mandible. A = mastoid process of temporal bone; B = condyle of mandible lying in mandibular fossa of temporomandibular joint; C = zygomatic arch; D = shadow of mandibular coronoid process on maxillary tuberosity; E = body of mandible showing teeth posterior to premolars; F = mental foramen.

**Fig. 2.121** Orthopantomogram (OPG). A panoramic radiographic survey of the jaws and teeth. Dentition is radiographed at 6 years of age. A = external acoustic meatus; B = mandibular condyle; C = coronoid process of mandible; D = maxillary air sinus; E = nasal cavity; F = vertebral column.

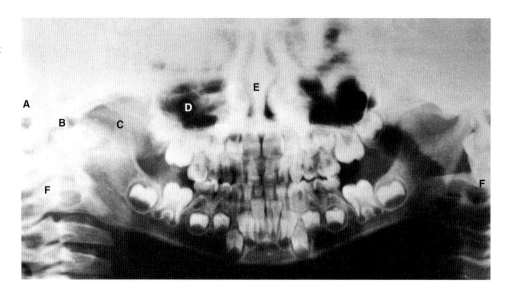

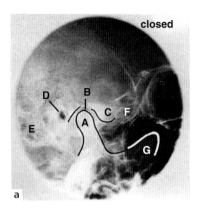
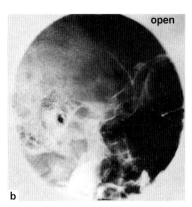

**Fig. 2.122** Transcranial temporomandibular articulation (a, mouth closed; b, mouth open). A = mandibular condyle; B = temporomandibular joint cavity space; C = articular tubercle; D = external acoustic meatus; E = mastoid air cells; F = zygomatic arch; G = coronoid process.

**Table 2.7** *Normal values for cephalometric measurements*

| | |
|---|---|
| Maxillary-mandibular plane angle | 27 (±5)° |
| SNA angle | 82 (±3)° |
| ANB angle | 3 (±1)° |
| Maxillary incisor/maxillary plane angle | 109 (±5)° |
| Mandibular incisor/mandibular plane angle | 90 (±5)° |
| Maxillary incisor/mandibular incisor angle | 135 (±9)° |
| N–S–Ba angle | 130° (150° at birth) |

For abbreviations see Table 2.8.

## Cephalometric analysis of lateral skull radiographs

Lateral skull radiographs (Fig. 2.123) are often used in dentistry to assess by measurement general skeletal morphology, particularly for recording relationships between the jaws and the cranial base. They are also of value for the evaluation of the direction and the amount of growth, for determining dentoskeletal relationships, and even for soft tissue analysis. In order to provide the most meaningful measurements, cephalometric radiographs are taken under standard conditions to enable comparisons between patients and for the same patient at different times. Thus, the position of the head must be standardized using a cephalostat (head holder) such that the beam of X-rays is shot in a predetermined plane to the head from a standard distance. This necessitates that the Frankfort plane (between the ear and orbit; see Fig. 2.125) is horizontal, that the dentition is in centric occlusion (see pages 36–38) and that the lips are in their habitual position. Lateral skull radiographs are preferred for dental cephalometry primarily because the facial variations of greatest importance are located in the sagittal plane. Normal values for cephalometric measurements are given in Table 2.7.

Figure 2.124 shows a lateral view of a skull and tracing taken from a lateral skull radiograph and illustrates the most common cephalometric landmarks used in dentistry (see also Table. 2.8).

**Table 2.8** *The most common cephalometric landmarks used in dentistry*

| | |
|---|---|
| Basion (Ba) | The most inferior and posterior point on the basi-occiput, lying on the anterior margin of the foramen magnum |
| Sella point (S) | Centre of shadow of sella turcica (pituitary fossa) |
| Nasion (N) | Junction between frontal and nasal bones in the midline on the frontonasal suture |
| Porion (Po) | Highest bony point of the margin of the external acoustic meatus |
| Orbitale (Or) | Lowest point of the infra-orbital margin |
| Anterior nasal spine (ANS) | |
| Posterior nasal spine (PNS) | |
| Subspinale (A point) | Position of greatest concavity of the maxillary alveolus in the midline |
| Supramentale (B point) | Position of greatest concavity of the mandibular alveolus in the midline |
| Pogonion (Pog) | Most anterior point on the chin |
| Menton (Me) | Lowest point of the chin |
| Gnathion (Gn) | Point between the most anterior and inferior points of chin established by bisecting the angle formed between the N–Pog and mandibular planes |
| Gonion (Go) | Most inferior and posterior point at the angle of the mandible established by bisecting the angle formed between the planes through the lower border of the mandible and posterior border of ramus |

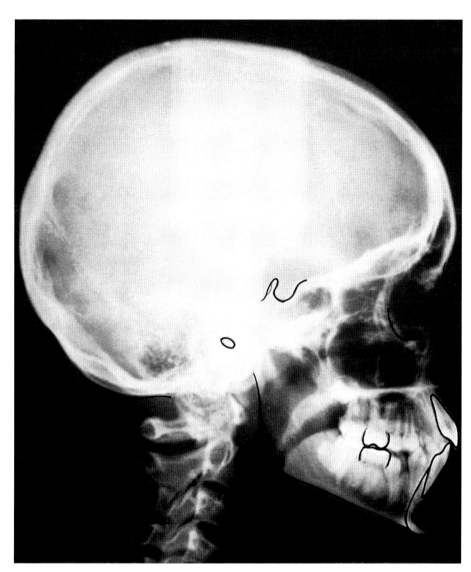

Fig. 2.123

Fig. 2.123

**Fig. 2.123** Lateral skull radiograph taken using a cephalostat.

**Fig. 2.124** Lateral view of skull (a) and tracing taken from a lateral skull radiograph (b), illustrating the most common cephalometric landmarks used in dentistry.
Ba = basion (the most inferior and posterior point on the basi-occiput, lying on the anterior margin of the foramen magnum);
S = sella point (centre of shadow of sella turcica (pituitary fossa));
N = nasion (junction between frontal and nasal bones in midline on the frontonasal suture);
Po = porion (highest bony point of margin of external acoustic meatus);
Or = orbitale (lowest point of the infra-orbital margin);
ANS = anterior nasal spine;
PNS = posterior nasal spine;
A = subspinale (A point: position of greatest concavity of maxillary alveolus in the midline);
B = supramentale (B point: position of greatest concavity of mandibular alveolus in the midline);
Pog = pogonion (most anterior point on the chin);
Me = menton (lowest point of the chin);
Gn = gnathion (point between the most anterior and inferior points of chin, established by bisecting the angle formed between the N-Pog and mandibular planes);
Go = gonion (most inferior and posterior point at the angle of the mandible, established by bisecting the angle formed between the planes through the lower border of the mandible and posterior border of ramus).

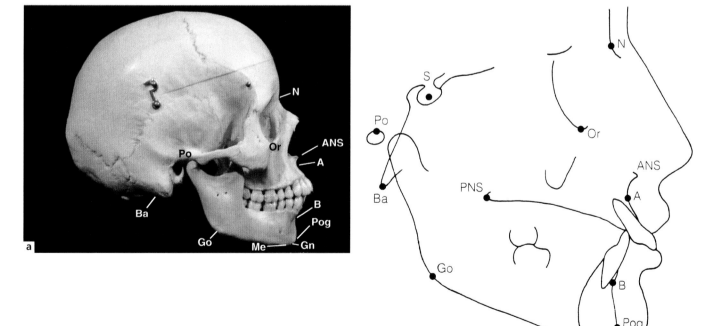

Fig. 2.124

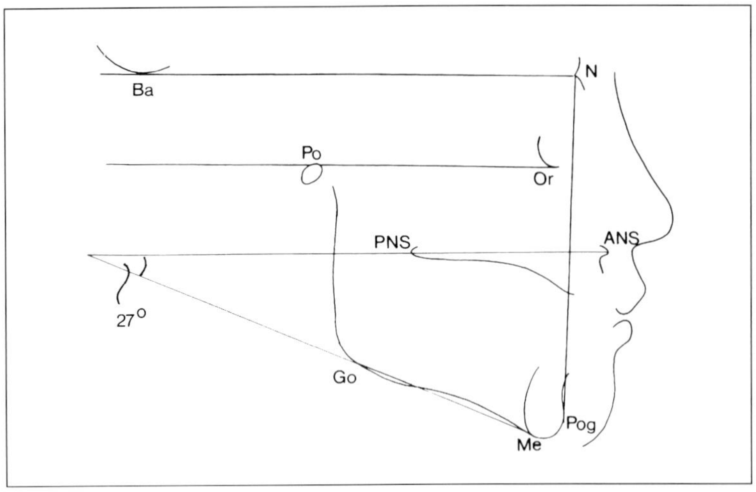

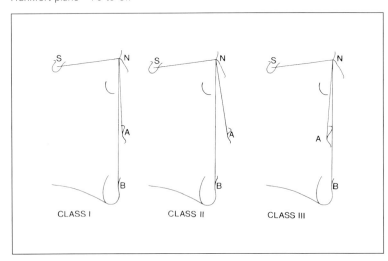

**Fig. 2.125** Cephalometric analysis of jaw relationships and facial form. Ba = basion; N = nasion; Po = porion; Or = orbitale; PNS = posterior nasal spine; ANS = anterior nasal spine; Go = gonion; Me = menton; Pog = pogonion. Frankfort plane = Po to Or.

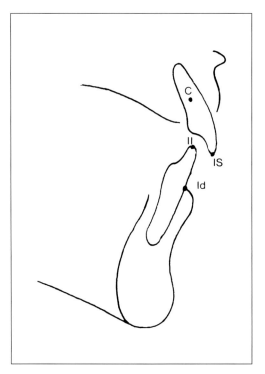

**Fig. 2.127** Cephalometric landmarks used for assessing dentoskeletal relationships. C = centroid of the maxillary incisor root (the midpoint along the root axis of the most prominent maxillary incisor); IS = incision superius (the incisal tip of the most prominent maxillary incisor); II = incision inferius (the incisal tip of the most prominent mandibular incisor); Id = infradentale (the junction of alveolar crest with the outline of the most prominent mandibular incisor).

**Fig. 2.126** The use of SNA and SNB angles to record maxillary–mandibular skeletal relationships. S = sella point; N = nasion; A = subspinale (A point); B = supramentale (B point).

**Table 2.9** *Cephalometric landmarks for assessing dentoskeletal relationships*

| | |
|---|---|
| Centroid of the maxillary incisor root (C) | The midpoint along the root axis of the most prominent maxillary incisor |
| Incision superius (IS) | The incisal tip of the most prominent maxillary incisor |
| Incision inferius (II) | The incisal tip of the most prominent mandibular incisor |
| Infradentale (Id) | The junction of the alveolar crest with the outline of the most prominent mandibular incisor |

## Cephalometric analysis of jaw relationships and facial form

The mandibular plane passes through the menton and gonion (Fig. 2.125). It is used in conjunction with the Frankfort, maxillary and Ba–N (Table 2.8) planes to assess the vertical development of the anterior part of the face. The Frankfort plane extends from the orbitale to the porion. The Frankfort-mandibular angle in 'normal' subjects is said to be approximately 27°. The maxillary plane extends through the anterior and posterior nasal spines (ANS, PNS) and is easier to identify on a lateral skull radiograph than the Frankfort plane. Both the maxillary–mandibular plane angle and the mandibular–cranial base (Ba–N) angle are of the same order as the Frankfort–mandibular plane angle. A plane termed the facial line can be drawn between the nasion and the pogonion. This plane aids the assessment of facial profile and the angle it makes with the Frankfort plane indicates whether the profile is orthognathic, prognathic or retrognathic.

Figure 2.126 describes the use of SNA and SNB angles to record maxillary–mandibular skeletal relationships. SNA measures the degree of prognathism of the maxillary alveolar base: its average value is 82°; SNB assesses the degree of prognathism of the mandibular alveolar base. The angle SNA–SNB (i.e. ANB) is frequently used to determine the skeletal pattern for the jaws because the cranial base (SN plane) is thought to undergo very little change from the later years of childhood. Where ANB is 2–5°, the skeletal pattern is designated to be class I. Where ANB is greater than 5°, the jaws show a class II relationship with maxillary prog-

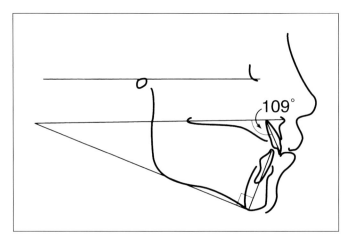

**Fig. 2.128** The inclinations of the incisors to the planes of the jaws.

nathism. Where ANB is less than 2°, the jaws show a class III relationship with mandibular prognathism. Should SNA be significantly different from its normal value, a correction must be made before assigning an ANB value to a specific skeletal class.

Figure 2.127 and Table 2.9 provide the cephalometric landmarks used for assessing dentoskeletal relationships.

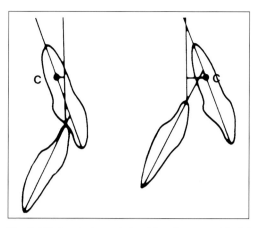

**Fig. 2.129** Interincisor relationships. C = centroid of the maxillary incisor root. Redrawn after Professors N.J.B. Houston and W.S. Tulley.

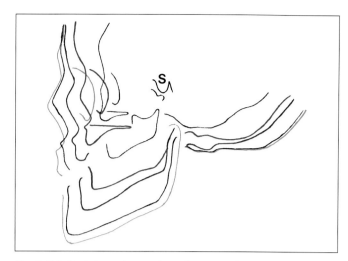

**Fig. 2.131** Cephalometric growth studies – superimposition of tracings at different ages. S = sella point.

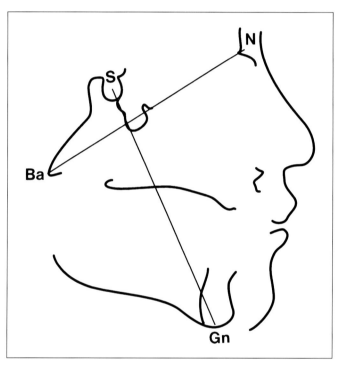

**Fig. 2.130** Cephalometric growth studies – the Y-axis. Ba = basion; S = sella point; N = nasion; Gn = gnathion.

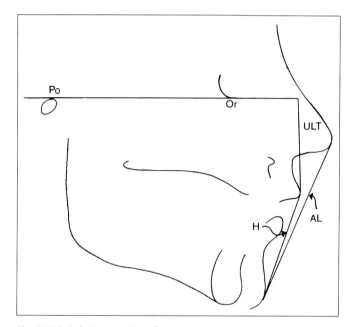

**Fig. 2.132** Soft tissue analysis from cephalometric radiographs. Po = porion; Or = orbitale; H = the harmony line of Holdaway (H line); ULT = the upper lip tangent; AL = the aesthetic line.

The inclinations of the incisors to the planes of the jaws are illustrated in Figure 2.128. The inclination of the maxillary incisor can be determined by measuring the angle between a line drawn through its root axis and the Frankfort (or maxillary) plane. On average, this angle is 109°. The inclination of the mandibular incisor is assessed by the angle formed between its root axis and the mandibular plane: it is approximately a right angle. Interincisor relationships are described in Figure 2.129. The angle formed by the junction of the longitudinal axes of the maxillary and mandibular central incisors is of the order of 135°; however, its clinical usefulness is limited because the anteroposterior relationship of the incisal edges is of greater importance. This is assessed by analysing the distance between the mandibular incisal edge and the centroid of the maxillary incisor root. Two examples are shown in Figure 2.129. In both, the maxillary and mandibular incisors meet at the same angle of approximately 135°. However, they differ markedly in terms of the distances between the mandibular incisal edges and the centroids.

## Cephalometric growth studies

Every bone of the skull in the growing child shows some degree of growth and consequently no point can be considered 'fixed'. For analytical convenience, however, several landmarks and strategies are defined and

adopted to study the degree and direction of cranial growth. The Y-axis is a line from the sella point to the gnathion and is used to describe the general direction of facial growth relative to the cranial base (Fig. 2.130). The angle between the Y-axis and the Ba–N plane is used to assess changes in growth direction.

A frequently employed strategy to assess growth relies upon the superimposition of successive cephalometric tracings of the same individual at different ages (Fig. 2.131). A reasonably reliable picture of growth of the facial skeleton can be obtained by superimposition at the S–N planes with registration of the sella point. Growth at the maxillary region is notoriously difficult to assess but can be analysed by superimposition at the maxillary plane with registration of the anterior surface of the zygomatic process of the maxilla. For the mandibular region, it is necessary to superimpose at the mandibular canal and at the inner surface of the mandible behind the chin.

### Soft-tissue analysis

Soft-tissue analysis (Fig. 2.132) is possible from cephalometric radiographs provided that the soft-tissue outlines are sufficiently clear and that the lips are in their habitual posture. To undertake such analysis, reference is often made to the following three planes:

**Fig. 2.133** Sialogram showing a normal parotid gland (arrow). Courtesy of Dr N. Drage.

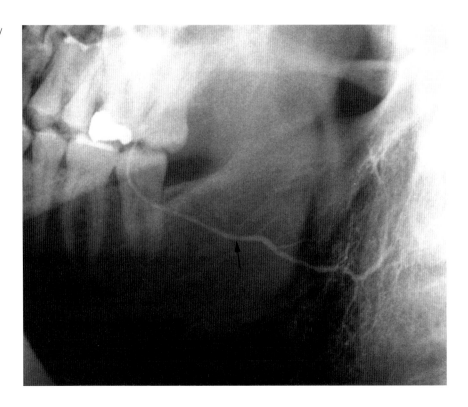

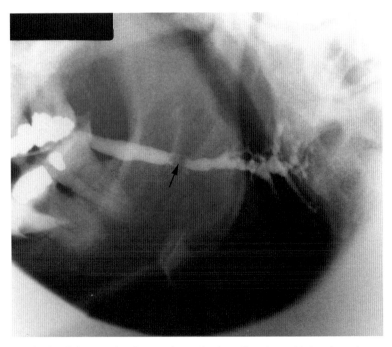

**Fig. 2.134** Sialogram showing an obstruction in a dilated parotid duct (arrow). Courtesy of Dr N. Drage.

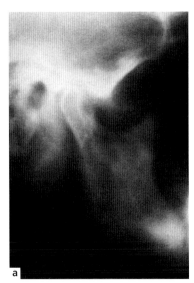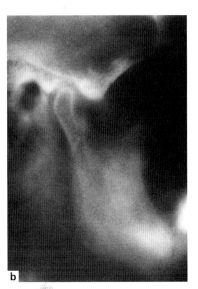

**Fig. 2.135** Tomographic examination of the temporomandibular joint. The two images (a and b) are about 0.5 cm apart.

- The H line (the Harmony line of Holdaway) is drawn between the chin and the vermilion border of the upper lip. It can be used to assess the degree of lower lip pout. The vermilion border of the lower lip should be within 1 mm of the H line.
- The upper lip tangent (ULT) describes the plane perpendicular to the Frankfort plane and tangential to the vermilion border of the upper lip. It is used to assess the amount of upper lip curl, the concavity of the upper lip profile normally being 1–4 mm behind the upper lip tangent.
- The aesthetic line (AL) extends from the tip of the nose to the chin. The vermilion borders of both upper and lower lips usually lie close to the aesthetic line.

## Sialography

Sialography is the technique whereby the duct systems of the major salivary glands are visualized by injecting an iodine-based contrast medium into the duct orifice (Fig. 2.133). This technique is used to identify obstructions (Fig. 2.134).

## Tomographic examination of the temporomandibular joint

Tomography is a radiographic technique used to study layers within a volume of tissue, in a way analogous to the examination of a single portion of bread within a whole loaf without physically slicing it. The two pictures of the temporomandibular joint illustrated here (Fig. 2.135) represent two layers in this region approximately 0.5 cm apart.

## INTRA-ORAL RADIOGRAPHIC PROJECTIONS OF JAWS AND TEETH

Table 2.10 outlines the major intra-oral radiographic projections used to view the human jaws and dentition. In this context, 'intra-oral' indicates that the radiographic plate is positioned inside the mouth.

There are two maxillary occlusal views – the vertex approach (Fig. 2.136) and the nasal approach (Fig. 2.137). As the names suggest, these views of the maxilla essentially differ in the positioning of the X-ray tube, which is either to the vertex of the skull or to the nasion. Differences in the radiographic pictures obtained relate to the degree of superimposition (greater in the vertex occlusal) and the direction and proportions of the longitudinal axes of the teeth (more vertical and less distorted roots with the vertex occlusal). In addition to surveying the maxillary dentition, the maxillary occlusal views may also be used to define the nasal fossae and maxillary air sinuses. Figure 2.138 illustrates a mandibular occlusal view.

**Table 2.10** *Intra-oral radiographic projections describing jaws and teeth*

| Projection/technique | Purpose |
| --- | --- |
| Maxillary and mandibular occlusal views of teeth in buccolingual plane (Figs 2.136–2.138) | Relationships of structures |
| Periapical view of teeth (Fig. 2.139) | Examination of apices of teeth. Relationships of structures in the mesiodistal plane |
| Bitewing examination of teeth (Fig. 2.140) | Survey of crowns of teeth and the alveolar crests |

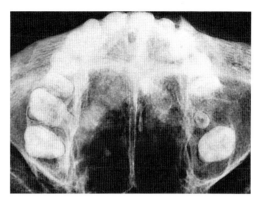

**Fig. 2.136** Maxillary occlusal view – vertex approach.

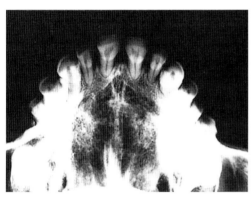

**Fig. 2.137** Maxillary occlusal view – nasal approach.

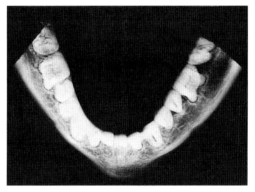

**Fig. 2.138** Mandibular occlusal view.

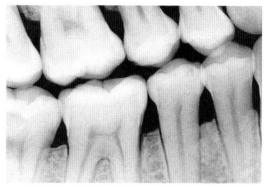

**Fig. 2.140** Examination of the crowns of the permanent molars and associated alveolar crests using bitewing radiographs.

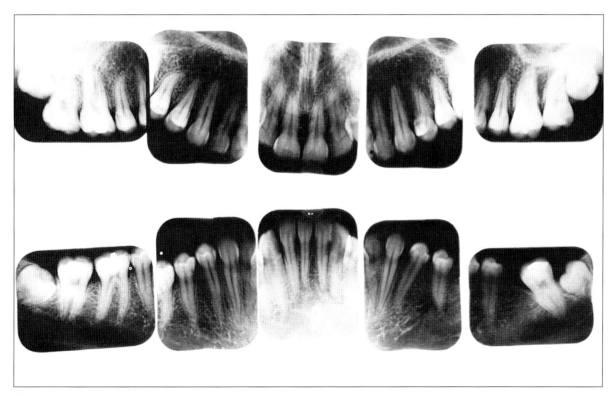

**Fig. 2.139** Intra-oral survey of the permanent dentition with periapical views of the teeth.

## Anatomical features seen on intra-oral radiographs

The importance of appreciating the radiographic appearance of the teeth and their supporting tissues need hardly be emphasized. However, equally essential for the interpretation of an apparent divergence from the normal is an awareness of non-dental anatomical structures, which, to the unwary, may simulate pathological lesions on intra-oral radiographs. The radio-opacities of normal anatomical structures seen on intra-oral radiographs are given in Table 2.11.

The radiographic image of a tooth is illustrated in Figure 2.141. Tooth substance absorbs more X-rays than any other tissue of comparable size and thickness. Enamel is the most radio-opaque and is easily distinguished covering the anatomical crown of the tooth. In normal teeth, the enamel is of uniform density, although in some areas where the enamel is thin (e.g. the cervical regions) it may appear relatively radiolucent. Such an appearance may easily be misinterpreted as dental caries. Dentine and cementum cannot be readily distinguished from each other radiographically because of their similar capacity to absorb X-rays. Owing to the lower radio-opacity of dentine, it appears comparatively 'greyer' than

the enamel and thus the enamel–dentine junction is clearly demarcated. The pulp of a tooth, being soft tissue, is readily penetrated by X-rays and consequently on a radiograph the pulp cavity is clearly defined as the central radiolucent region of the tooth. However, because of distortion, foreshortening and superimposition, care should be taken in assessing the pulpal anatomy from radiographs. The tooth is supported in the bony alveolus. In this text, the alveolus refers to the whole of the bony supporting tissue of the tooth, and the lamina dura refers to the compact bone lining the tooth socket. The morphology of the margins of the alveolus (alveolar crest) is important in the diagnosis of periodontal disease. As a general rule, the width of the crest depends upon the distance the teeth are separated. Consequently, between the molars the crests are flat and horizontal, while between the incisors the crests rise only as points or spines. In the healthy situation, the crest rises to just below the level of the cementum–enamel junction. The lamina dura is considered to be a very important structure in the radiographic interpretation of periodontal and periapical pathologies. It appears as a continuous radio-opaque lining of the socket and usually is continuous over the alveolar crests. However, the radio-opacity of the lamina dura does not indicate any hypermineralization, being a consequence of superimposition. Discontinuity of the lamina dura in the root region is usually indicative of abnormality or disease. Between the root of the tooth and the lamina dura of the socket is the connective tissue of the periodontal ligament, which appears as a thin radiolucent region. Figure 2.142 shows the appearance of developing and erupting teeth (molars and premolars) where there are radiolucent regions around the emerging crowns and around the developing root apices.

With respect to anatomical structures that appear in association with the maxillary dentition, Figure 2.143 describes some radiolucent, anatomical

**Table 2.11** *Radio-opacity of normal anatomical structures seen on intra-oral radiographs*

| Radiolucent | Radio-opaque |
|---|---|
| Dental pulp | Enamel |
| Gingiva and periodontal ligament | Dentine |
| Bone marrow | Cementum |
| | Cortical bony plates |
| | Lamina dura |
| Maxillary sinus | Bony walls of maxillary sinus |
| Nasal cavity | Bony walls of nasal cavity |
| Incisive foramen | Nasal septum |
| Median palatine suture | Anterior nasal spine |
| Intermaxillary suture | Maxillary tuberosity |
| Nasolacrimal canal | Zygomatic arch |
| | Coronoid process |
| Mandibular canal | Pterygoid hamulus |
| | Internal and external oblique lines of mandible |
| Mental foramen | Borders of mandibular canal |
| Mandibular symphysis | Mental and canine prominences |
| | Genial spines |
| Bony depressions (e.g. mental and submandibular fossa) | |
| Nutrient canals | |

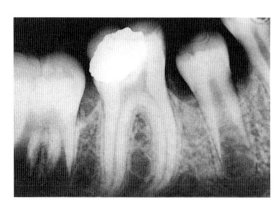

**Fig. 2.142** Radiograph of developing and erupting molars and premolars.

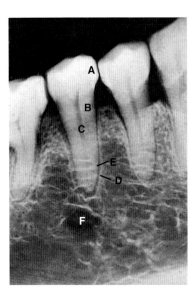

**Fig. 2.141** Radiographic image of a tooth. A = enamel; B = dentine; C = dental pulp; D = lamina dura; E = periodontal space; F = mental foramen.

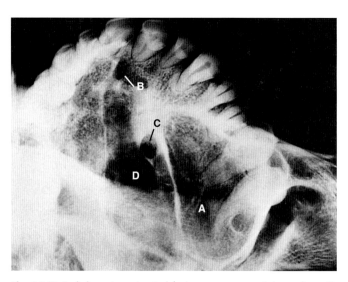

**Fig. 2.143** Radiolucent, anatomical features seen on an intra-oral maxillary occlusal oblique view. A = maxillary antrum; B = incisive foramen; C = nasolacrimal canal; D = nasal fossa.

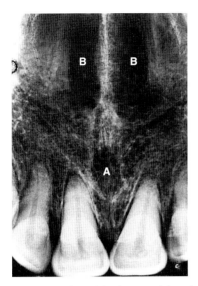

**Fig. 2.144** The incisive foramen (A) and nasal fossae (B) seen on an intra-oral periapical view of the maxillary first incisors.

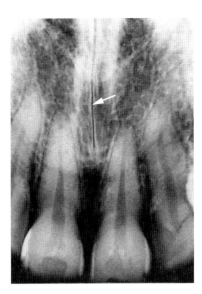

**Fig. 2.145** The median palatine suture (arrowed) seen on an intra-oral periapical view of the maxillary first incisors.

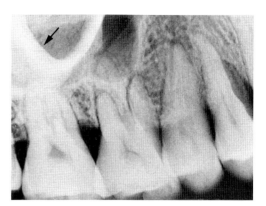

**Fig. 2.146** Malar (zygomatic) shadow (arrowed).

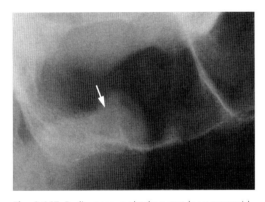

**Fig. 2.147** Radio-opaque shadow cast by a coronoid process (arrowed).

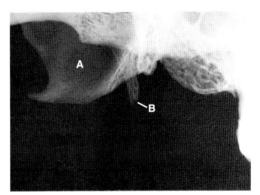

**Fig. 2.148** Shadows of the pterygoid plates (A) and pterygoid hamulus (B) near the maxillary tuberosity.

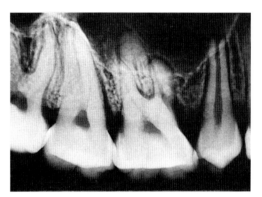

**Fig. 2.149** The floor of the maxillary air sinus seen on an intra-oral periapical view of the maxillary premolars and molars.

features seen on an intra-oral maxillary occlusal oblique view – i.e. the maxillary air sinus, the incisive foramen, the nasolacrimal canal and the nasal fossae. Figure 2.144 shows how the incisive foramen and the nasal fossae can be seen on an intra-oral periapical view of the maxillary first incisors. The medial palatine suture seen on an intra-oral periapical view of the maxillary first incisors is illustrated in Figure 2.145. The malar (zygomatic) shadow viewed on an intra-oral periapical view of the maxillary molars is seen in Figure 2.146 and Figure 2.147 shows the radio-opaque shadow cast by a coronoid process of the mandible superimposed on a maxillary tuberosity. In Figure 2.148, the shadows of the pterygoid plates and pterygoid hamulus of the sphenoid bone near the maxillary tuberosity are shown.

Of particular importance in the upper jaw is the appearance of the maxillary air sinus or antrum. The floor of the sinus viewed on an intra-oral periapical view of the maxillary premolars and molars is shown in Figure 2.149. The maxillary air sinus is an air-filled cavity of varying dimensions; it appears radiographically as a dark, radiolucent shadow bounded by radio-opaque lines representing the lining layers of cortical bone. The radiolucency is not usually uniform because of superimposition of the zygomatic process and the soft tissues of the cheek. The air sinus often presents not as a single sinus but as several compartments because of bony septation. It is said that the cortical lining of the air sinus is not continuous but exhibits numerous, small, linear interruptions associated with nutrient canals (Fig. 2.150). This radiographic characteristic may be important in

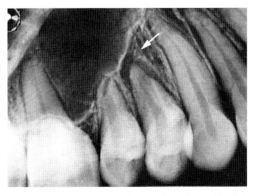

**Fig. 2.150** Nutrient canals (arrowed) in the walls of the maxillary air sinus.

avoiding misinterpretation of the sinus as a pathological lesion. The floor of the maxillary air sinus is closely related to the root apices of the maxillary teeth. Generally, the sinus extends from the premolars to the tuberosity, although variations are frequent. Because of the close relationship of the teeth to the maxillary air sinus, communication between the sinus and the oral cavity (oro-antral fistula) following tooth extractions is unfortunately all too frequent. Because of the problems of interpreting three-dimensional situations on a two-dimensional radiograph, care must be taken to avoid misreading the relationship of the teeth to the sinus.

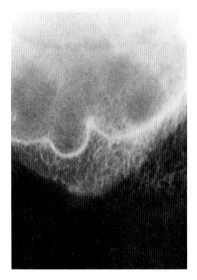

**Fig. 2.151** The maxillary antrum seen on an intra-oral view of an edentulous maxillary tuberosity.

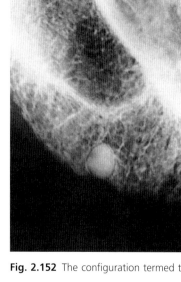

**Fig. 2.152** The configuration termed the Y of Ennis.

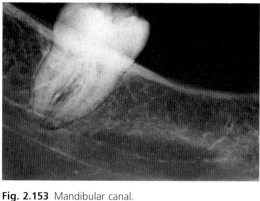

**Fig. 2.153** Mandibular canal.

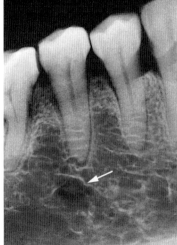

**Fig. 2.154** Mental foramen (arrowed).

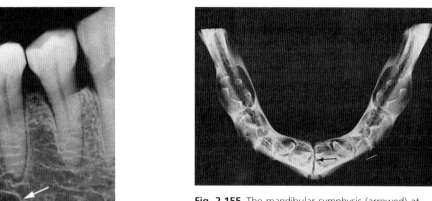

**Fig. 2.155** The mandibular symphysis (arrowed) at birth.

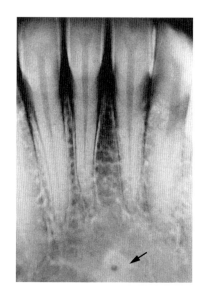

**Fig. 2.156** The genial spines (arrowed).

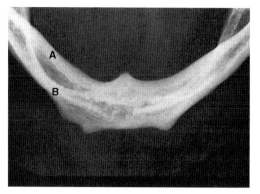

**Fig. 2.157** Internal (A) and external (B) oblique lines of the mandible.

Figure 2.151 shows the maxillary sinus seen on an intra-oral view of an edentulous maxillary tuberosity and Figure 2.152 illustrates the configuration termed the 'Y of Ennis' that is formed by the abutment of the anterior wall of the maxillary air sinus and the floor of the nasal fossa.

With respect to anatomical structures that appear in association with the mandibular dentition, of particular importance is the radiographic appearance of the mandibular canal. The mandibular canal in the region of the mandibular third molar tooth is shown in Figure 2.153. The mandibular canal commences at the mandibular foramen and passes downwards and forwards from the ramus into the body of the mandible where, near the root apices of the premolars, it terminates by dividing into the mental and incisive canals. The radiographic appearance of the mandibular canal is generally that of a radiolucent shadow bounded superiorly and inferiorly by radio-opaque lines. The width and position of the canal varies considerably. Most commonly, it is closely related to the roots of the molars, although it lies some distance from the roots of the premolars. Generally, the canal lies buccal to the root apices, a feature that should be remembered when interpreting the relationship of the root apices to the canal. The precise relationship of the teeth to the canal is difficult to determine from radiographs, although some hint of a very close relationship can be obtained by reference to the densities of shadows cast by the roots and canal, the position and densities of the lamina dura and the radio-opaque margins of the canal, and the dimensions of the lumen of the canal. The appearance of the mental foramen near the apices of the mandibular premolars is shown in Figure 2.154.

The mandibular symphysis at birth is shown on an intra-oral mandibular occlusal radiograph in Figure 2.155. This symphysis closes by the age of 3 years. Figure 2.156 illustrates the genial spines seen on an intra-oral periapical view of the mandibular central incisors. Note the characteristic radiographic appearance of the genial spines (i.e. a radiolucent dot surrounded by a distinct radio-opaque region). The internal and external oblique lines of the mandible are seen in Figure 2.157, where an occlusal view of an edentulous mandible demonstrates the prominent radio-opacities associated with these lines.

## CLINICAL CONSIDERATIONS

### FACIAL FRACTURES

Fractures of the facial skeleton (including the jaws) are very common, often as a result of road traffic accidents (RTAs), physical violence (i.e. interpersonal violence), work accidents and sports injuries. Fractures affecting the face are often complex, particularly for the middle third of the face. In order to appreciate fractures of the central middle third of the face, it is necessary to understand the extent to which this region is supported by the maxillary bones. These bones not only form the alveolar processes (i.e. the upper jaws housing the maxillary dentition) but also contribute to the palate, the nasal aperture, the zygomatic complex (i.e. cheek bone region), the floor of the orbit and part of the bridge of the nose extending up to the forehead. Fractures of the central middle third of the face are categorized according to a Le Fort system of classification (Fig. 2.158). Le Fort I fractures have a fracture line running horizontally above the level of the floor of the nose and produce a mobile segment comprising the alveolar process, the palate and the lower region of the pterygoid plates. Le Fort II fractures have a more extensive involvement of the maxillary bones. Le Fort III fractures separate the entire facial skeleton from the cranial base, the fracture lines running parallel with the base of the skull.

It should be borne in mind that fractures of the central middle third of the face are not always bilaterally symmetrical and separation of the fracture segments does not usually result from muscle pull. The fracture segments are generally displaced downwards and backwards, resulting in a 'dished-in' appearance of the face. Furthermore, the airway may become obstructed.

Fractures of the mandible, a bone that constitutes the lower third of the face, are also very common. In most instances, the mandible fractures at two (or more) sites and consequently isolated fractures are unusual. In order of frequency, most fractures of the mandible occur at the neck of the condyle (Figs 2.159, 2.160), the angle (and ramus) of the mandible, and

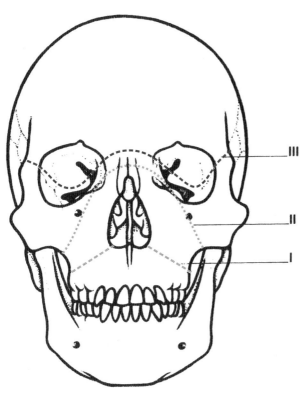

**Fig. 2.158** Le Fort classification of fractures of the face I, II and III.

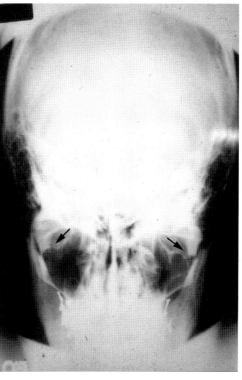

**Fig. 2.160** Posteroanterior radiograph showing bilateral fracture of the condyles (arrows).

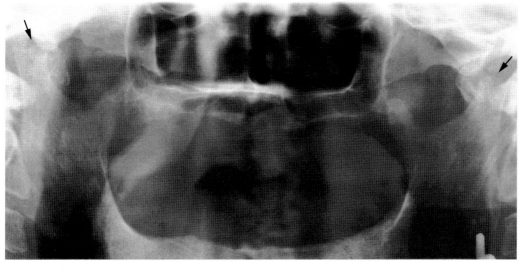

**Fig. 2.159** Orthopantomogram of edentulous patient showing bilateral fracture of condyles (arrows). Courtesy of Dr J. Jones.

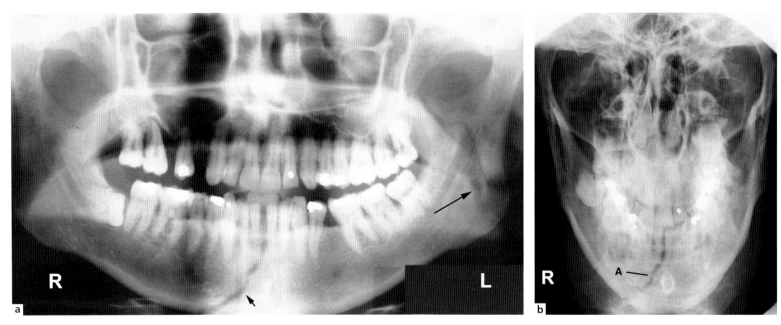

**Fig. 2.161** (a) OPG of patient with a bilateral fracture of the body near the midline (small arrow) and angle and ramus (large arrow) of the left side of the mandible. (b) Posteroanterior radiograph showing favourable fracture line at angle of mandible with no displacement of left ramus. A = Line of fracture of body of mandible. Courtesy of Dr J. Jones.

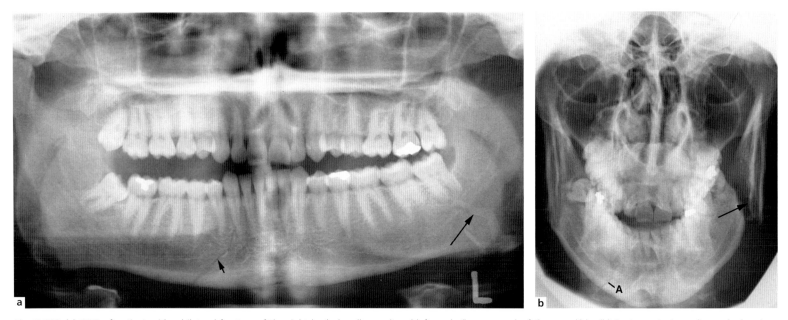

**Fig. 2.162** (a) OPG of patient with a bilateral fracture of the right body (small arrow) and left angle (large arrow) of the mandible. (b) Posteroanterior radiograph showing unfavourable fracture line at angle of mandible with displacement of ramus (arrow). A = line of fracture of the body on the right side. Courtesy of Dr J. Jones.

the body of the mandible (Figs 2.161, 2.162). Fractures at the neck of the condyle can occur when a patient receives a blow to the chin or to the body of the mandible on the contralateral side. When this occurs, the condyle is usually displaced anteromedially, as a result of the pull of the lateral pterygoid muscle. With a fracture of the angle of the mandible, the fracture line usually extends downwards and backwards from the alveolar bone and could involve the third molar tooth (and its socket). The posterior fragment would then be displaced upwards, inwards and forwards because of the pull of the masseter, temporalis and medial pterygoid muscles. Fractures of the body of the mandible are usually found in the canine or first molar regions as a result of a direct blow to these parts. Should the fracture line pass downwards and forwards, the fragments will not be greatly displaced because the upward pull of the masseter, temporalis and medial pterygoid muscles is counteracted by the downward and backward pull of the anterior belly of the digastric and geniohyoid muscles. However, if the fracture line runs downwards and backwards, the fragments may be considerably displaced, particularly if the patient is edentulous.

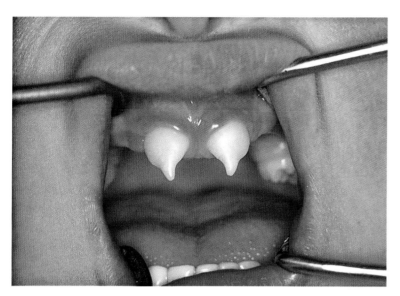

**Fig. 2.163** Hereditary ectodermal dysplasia showing absent teeth and conically shaped teeth. Courtesy of Dr P. Smith.

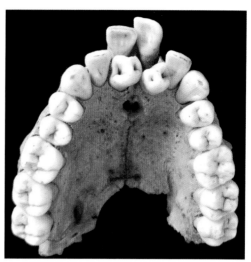

**Fig. 2.165** Upper jaw showing the presence of two mesiodens. Courtesy of the Royal College of Surgeons of England.

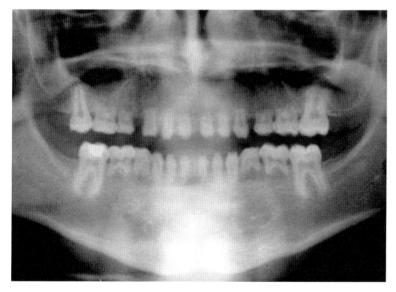

**Fig. 2.164** Radiograph of patient with a complete deciduous dentition but with absence of the permanent dentition. Courtesy of Dr P. Smith.

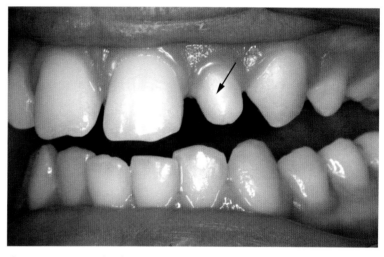

**Fig. 2.166** An example of microdontia in the form of a 'peg' maxillary lateral incisor (arrow). Courtesy of Dr M. Cobourne.

## VARIATION IN TOOTH MORPHOLOGY

### Number of teeth

Although a full dentition numbers 32 teeth, a tooth may fail to develop, giving a reduced number. This condition is commonly known as hypodontia (partial anodontia). The tooth most commonly absent (in about 25% of cases) is the third molar tooth, followed by the second premolar, and the maxillary lateral incisor in about 2.5% of cases. From this distribution, it can be seen that the tooth most affected is the last tooth of molar, premolar and incisor series. The maxillary second incisor is also susceptible to a reduction in size in about another 2.5% of individuals, giving rise to the 'peg-shaped' incisor (see Fig. 2.47).

In rarer cases more than one tooth type is missing. In rare congenital disorders, such as ectodermal dysplasia, all the teeth may be missing (anodontia). In ectodermal dysplasia, some teeth are generally present and may have a simplified morphology (Fig. 2.163). Figure 2.164 is a radiograph illustrating a patient in which the permanent dentition is entirely absent.

As well as teeth being reduced in number, there may be additional teeth present. Where they resemble the normal tooth morphology they are referred to as supplemental teeth. Most commonly, however, they have a simpler morphology and are termed supernumerary teeth. They are most often found in the midline between the maxillary central incisors and are called **mesiodens** (Fig. 2.165). Their presence may obstruct the eruption of the permanent central incisors, in which case they will need to be surgically removed (see Fig. 26.50).

### Size of teeth

There is considerable variation in the size of the dentition in different individuals. Where a tooth (or teeth) is unusually small, the condition is referred to as **microdontia** (Fig. 2.166). Microdontia generally affects individual teeth, usually the maxillary second incisor and the third molar. Occasionally, however, many teeth in the same dentition may be affected, in which case the teeth may be spaced apart. Where a tooth is unusually large, the condition is referred to as **macrodontia (megadontia)**

(Fig. 2.167). During early tooth development, the enamel organ may partially divide, resulting in the appearance of a large 'double tooth'. This is known as a **geminated tooth** and can be found in most tooth positions (Figs 2.168–2.169). The number of teeth present in these situations is normal.

## Fusion and transposition of teeth

Rarely two adjacent teeth may be joined, giving rise to a **fused tooth**. In this situation, the total number of teeth would be one less than normal, distinguishing it from a geminated tooth. **Tooth transposition** refers to the positional interchange of two adjacent teeth. The tooth most commonly involved is the permanent canine, the maxillary being more frequently encountered than the mandibular. The maxillary canine is most frequently transposed with the first premolar (Fig. 2.170) rather than with the lateral incisor. When the mandibular canine is involved, it is invariably transposed with the lateral incisor. Patients exhibiting transpositions also show a higher incidence of congenitally absent teeth, peg-shaped lateral incisors and/or supernumerary teeth.

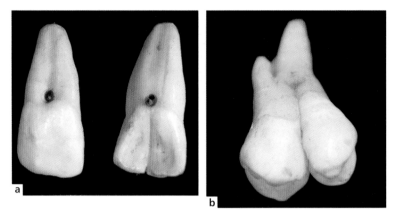

**Fig. 2.168** (a) Geminated maxillary permanent incisor tooth. Courtesy of the Royal College of Surgeons of England. (b) Geminated maxillary premolar tooth. Courtesy of the Royal College of Surgeons of England.

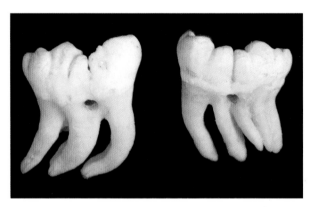

**Fig. 2.169** Geminated mandibular permanent molar tooth. Courtesy of the Royal College of Surgeons of England.

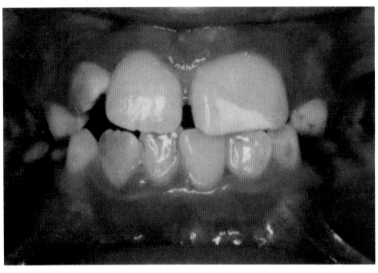

**Fig. 2.167** An example of macrodontia affecting the maxillary left first incisor.

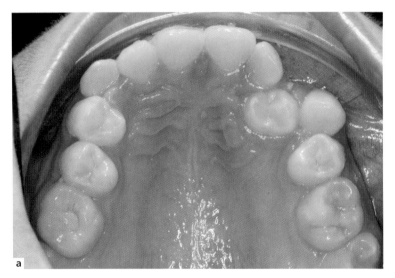

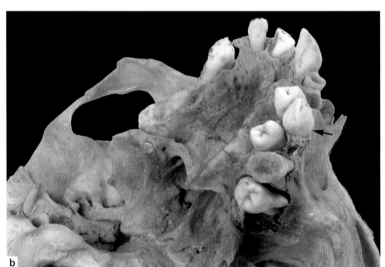

**Fig. 2.170** (a) Transposition of a left maxillary canine with a first premolar. Courtesy of Professor F. McDonald. (b) Skull showing transposition of left permanent canine (arrow) with first premolar. On the right side there is an accompanying severe abnormality in the alignment of the permanent canine and the first permanent molar tooth. Courtesy of the Royal College of Surgeons of England.

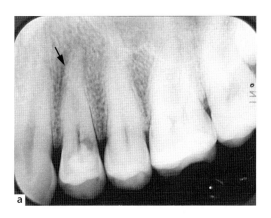

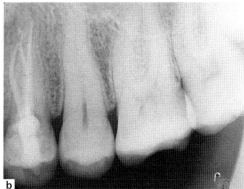

**Fig. 2.171** (a) Radiograph showing evidence of three root canals (arrow) associated with a maxillary first premolar before endodontic treatment. (b) Same tooth after endodontic treatment. Courtesy of Dr S. Patel.

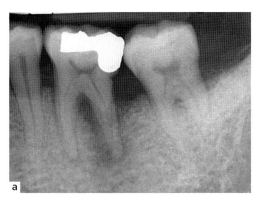

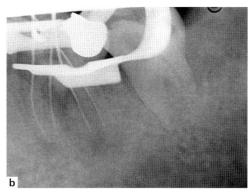

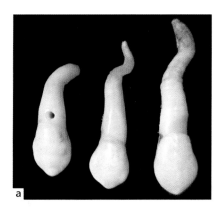

**Fig. 2.172** (a) Radiograph showing evidence of an extra root on mandibular first permanent molar before endodontic treatment. (b) Same tooth during endodontic treatment.

**Fig. 2.173** Radiograph showing the presence of a three-rooted mandibular first permanent molar.

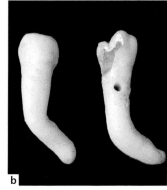

**Fig. 2.174** Dilacerated roots in (a) permanent maxillary canine teeth; (b) mandibular premolars. Courtesy of the Royal College of Surgeons of England.

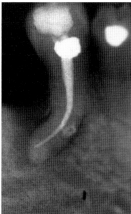

**Fig. 2.175** A radiograph showing dilacerated mandibular premolar roots. Courtesy of Dr N. McDonald.

## Root and pulp morphology

There is extensive detailed information available on root canal morphology obtained by examining and dissecting extracted teeth, by making casts of the canal system and by filling the system with fluids that can be visualized after clearing the teeth or that are radiopaque. In the clinical setting the information available from an individual tooth is much more restricted. Radiographs are the main source but are only two dimensional shadows suffering seriously from superimposition. This can be lessened somewhat by taking multiple radiographs at different angles. In the future, three-dimensional techniques such as computed tomography will reduce this limitation.

There is considerable variation in root morphology, but it is important to know the more common patterns, including the number of roots and root canals (see pages 28–33). Indeed, initial radiographs may alert the dental surgeon to the presence of extra roots and/or extra root canals (Figs 2.171–2.173).

Variation in root morphology will have clinical implications. The root may be unduly curved or show sudden bending (dilacerations), generally due to trauma encountered during development (Figs 2.174, 2.175), or

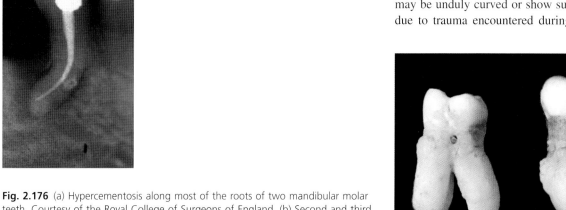

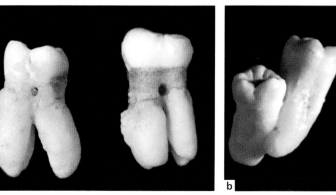

**Fig. 2.176** (a) Hypercementosis along most of the roots of two mandibular molar teeth. Courtesy of the Royal College of Surgeons of England. (b) Second and third molar teeth fused at their roots via cementum (concrescence). Courtesy of Professor J. Freher.

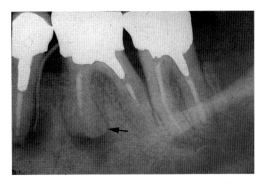

**Fig. 2.177** Radiograph showing hypercementosis associated with the mesial root of a mandibular first permanent molar (arrow). Courtesy of Dr T. Botero.

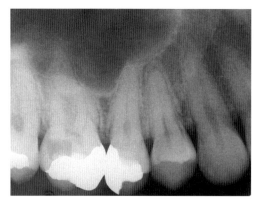

**Fig. 2.178** Radiograph showing roots of cheek teeth invaginating the maxillary sinus. Courtesy of Dr N. McDonald.

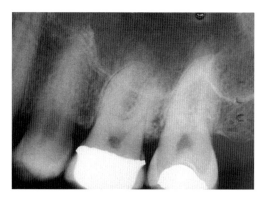

**Fig. 2.179** Radiograph showing roots of cheek teeth invaginating the maxillary sinus.

**Fig. 2.180** (a) Radiograph indicating that the mandibular canal and its contents are closely related to the roots of the mandibular permanent third molar (arrow). Courtesy of Professor D. Smith. (b) Grooves in apical part of the roots of the mandibular third molar (arrows) due to close association with inferior alveolar nerve and vessels. Courtesy of Professor J. Freher.

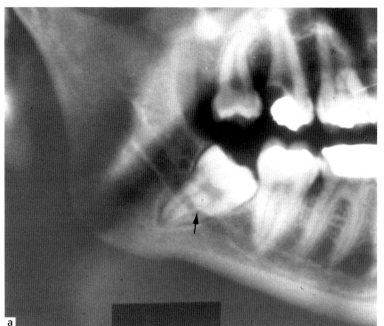

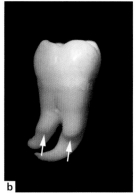

present thickenings at the apex due to hypercementosis (Figs 2.176a, 2.177 and Fig. 11.31). Rarely the roots of adjacent teeth may be joined by cementum (Fig. 2.176b). This is known as concrescence and usually affects second and third permanent molars. Such teeth will require special surgical treatment should tooth extraction be required.

The root apices of the upper cheek teeth are close to and may even invaginate the maxillary sinus (Figs 2.178, 2.179; see also Fig. 2.5). During removal of fractured root apices in this region, care must be taken to ensure that the root fragment is not pushed into the sinus. A clear periapical radiograph is required before any tooth extraction is undertaken as it may alert the dental surgeon to any problems that may be encountered. Thus, although normally lying beneath the roots of third permanent molar teeth, the inferior alveolar nerve and vessels lying in the mandibular canal may occupy a higher position and even run between the roots. Evidence of this close relationship may be evident in radiographs as a constriction of the mandibular canal or the radiolucent canal overlying the roots of the third molar (Fig. 2.180). In this situation, the neurovascular structures are at risk during extraction of third molars. The root of a mandibular premolar may occasionally be unusually long and can be in close relationship to the mental nerve and its parent branch, the inferior alveolar nerve, and these nerves are at risk during extraction of this tooth.

An understanding of the morphology of the pulp chamber and the root canal system is clearly essential in endodontic treatment (root canal therapy), in which a diseased pulp is removed and replaced with an inert

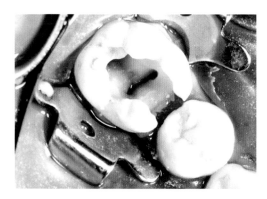

**Fig. 2.181** Access cavity prepared on lower molar to provide good access to see the distal root canal.

filling material. As well as the number and shape of the root canals, it is important to know where the orifices of the root canals may be found on the floor of the pulp chamber so that the correct cavity (access cavity) is cut on the crown to gain the best access (Fig. 2.181). With advancing age, the continued deposition of secondary and perhaps tertiary dentine leads to a reduction in size of the pulp chamber and root canals (Fig. 2.182).

The cementum–dentine junction at the root apex is a biologically significant point as it marks the junction of the dental pulp and the periodontal tissues. As such, it is the level to which a filling replacing the dental pulp should extend. The cementum at the junction forms a constriction, the apical constriction (see Fig. 26.9) against which, in ideal circumstances, a filling material may be packed. This constriction is found a short but variable distance within the canal back from its exit on the root surface. The root canal exits on to the root surface a short distance below the anatomical apex of the root. Care must be taken to ensure that root filling material is not introduced into the tissues beyond the root apex as in the case of the maxillary canine and the cheek teeth, for example, it may pass into maxillary sinus (Fig. 2.183) and in the case of a mandibular molar into the mandibular canal (Fig. 2.184).

Occasionally a taurodont tooth may be evident on radiographs. In this type of tooth, the broad root only bifurcates near its apex and therefore the pulp chamber extends a significant distance into the root. The taurodont tooth will require a different mode of treatment from that for a tooth with normal root canals (Fig. 2.185).

## AESTHETICS, THE SMILE, AND THE ALIGNMENT AND OCCLUSION OF ANTERIOR TEETH

The abnormalities described under malocclusion (see pages 38–40) will probably require orthodontic treatment, with or without the necessity of tooth extraction to provide any necessary space. However, many patients are not particularly concerned about occlusal dysfunction (unless it is particularly severe) and are generally more concerned about the aesthetics of their anterior teeth. Consequently, they may be specifically dissatisfied with their appearances when they smile. Many factors need to be considered when applying cosmetic dentistry to such situations as the smile is

formed from the interaction of three components: the teeth (primarily the maxillary anterior teeth), the lips and the gingivae.

Some of dimensions of the teeth seen in a 'desirable' smile would be as follows:

- The height of the maxillary first (central) incisors would be approximately 11 cm, with the width being between 0.7 and 0.8 of the

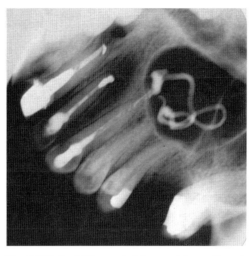

**Fig. 2.183** Root filling material present in maxillary sinus because of over-zealous force applied to upper permanent canine tooth. Courtesy of Professor J.D. Langdon.

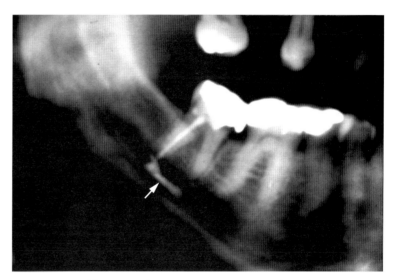

**Fig. 2.184** Root filling material present in mandibular canal (arrow) due to over-zealous force applied to mandibular second permanent molar. Courtesy of Professor J.D. Langdon.

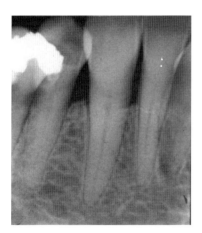

**Fig. 2.182** Radiograph showing absence of radiolucency of pulp chamber in the mandibular incisor teeth due to continued deposition of secondary dentine formation. Courtesy of Dr T. Botero.

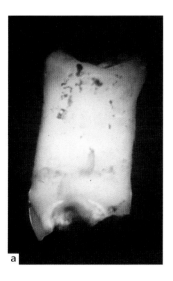
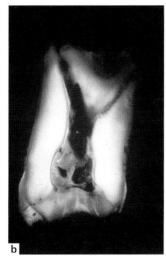
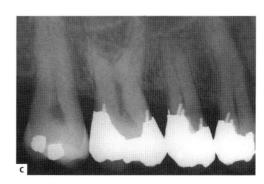

**Fig. 2.185** (a) Taurodont molar tooth. Note lack of root bifurcation until near root apex. (b) Bisected taurodont tooth showing lack of division of pulp chamber until near root apex. (c) Radiograph of taurodont upper first permanent molar. (a, b) Courtesy of Professor C. Franklin.

height. These first incisors need to be more than 2 cm shorter than normal before a difference is noticeable.

- The ratios of the width of the maxillary first (central) incisor, second (lateral) incisor and canine teeth as seen from the front would be 1.6:1.0:0.6, each tooth's width being about two-thirds that of the tooth in front. (This rule also applies to the premolar teeth behind, which are also visible in the smile; Fig. 2.186). The maxillary second incisors need to be about 3 mm narrower than the maxillary first incisors before a difference is noticeable.
- The long axis of the maxillary first (central) incisors should be parallel to the facial midline and to each other. The long axis of the second (lateral) incisor should slope about 5° distal and the canine and premolars about 10–12° distal to that of the first incisor (Fig. 2.187). Note that if the midline between the first incisors does not coincide with the facial midline, it needs to be more than about 4 mm off centre before this difference is noticeable.
- The visible areas of contact between the teeth (connectors) should be 50% of the height between the two maxillary first (central) incisors, 40% of the height of the first incisor between the first and second incisors and 30% of the height of the first incisor between the second incisor and canine (Fig. 2.188).

With regard to the lips, about 3–4 mm of the maxillary incisors should ideally be visible at rest, although this decreases with age. During smiling,

a normal lip line (seen in about 45% of patients) is present when the upper lip is at the level of the gingival margins and the interdental gingivae are exposed. A low lip line (in about 45% of patients) is where the lip covers the interdental gingivae. A high lip line (in about 10% of patients) occurs when the lip exposes the gingivae above the gingival margin (Fig. 2.189).

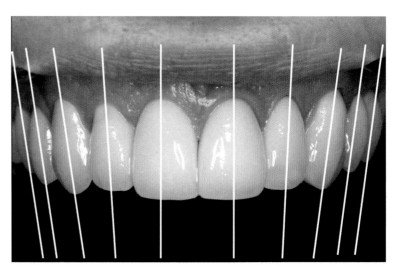

**Fig. 2.187** Ideal arrangement of the long axis of the crowns of the maxillary teeth. Courtesy of Dr C. Orr.

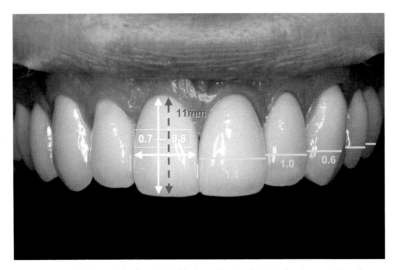

**Fig. 2.186** Ideal length (red) and width:length ratio (white) for the maxillary first incisor, and width proportions for the teeth as seen from the front (yellow). Courtesy of Dr C. Orr.

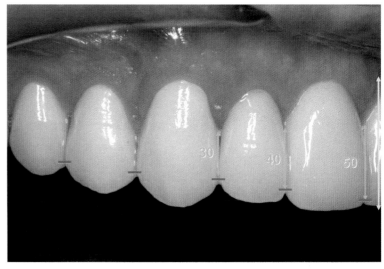

**Fig. 2.188** Percentage comparisons of the contact lengths (connectors) of the anterior maxillary teeth (blue) compared with that between the two maxillary first incisors (yellow). Courtesy of Dr C. Orr.

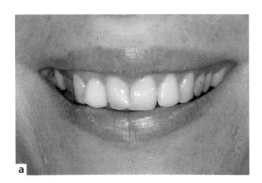
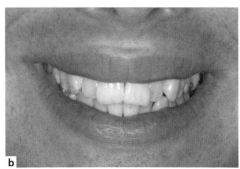
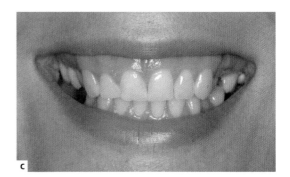

**Fig. 2.189** (a) Normal lip line. (b) Low lip line. (c) High lip line. Courtesy of Dr C. Orr.

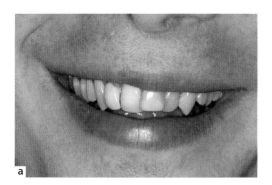

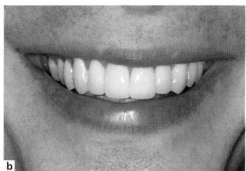

**Fig. 2.190** (a) Patient before treatment, showing many irregularities of the anterior teeth when smiling. (b) Patient after treatment, showing a greatly improved appearance. Courtesy of Dr C. Orr.

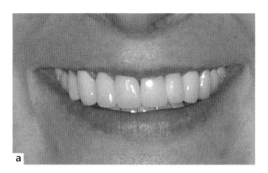

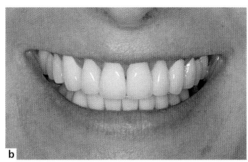

**Fig. 2.191** (a) Patient before treatment, with a sloping (canted) midline between the maxillary first incisors. (b) Patient after treatment; crowns have been made for the two maxillary first incisors to correct the canted midline. Courtesy of Dr C. Orr.

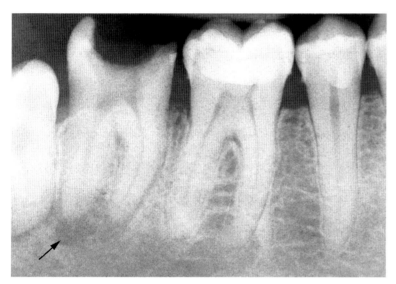

**Fig. 2.192** Bitewing radiograph of cheek teeth. In the healthy second premolar and first permanent molar teeth, the lamina dura is continuous. However, in the case of the second permanent molar tooth, the bulk of the crown has been lost because of dental caries and an abscess has formed at the root apex (arrow) with loss of continuity of the lamina dura. From Standring S (ed) 2004 *Gray's anatomy*, 39th edn, Churchill Livingstone, Edinburgh. Courtesy of Ms N. White.

Figures 2.190 and 2.191 show examples of patients with unaesthetic smiles (before and after treatment).

## RADIOGRAPHIC ANATOMY

Cephalometric radiography measures and assesses growth patterns of the skull and jaws and also jaw relationships (see pages 44–48). To provide an example, the orthodontist would use cephalometry to determine whether a reverse overjet of the incisors (see Fig. 2.108 and pages 39, 40) is the consequence of tooth malalignment and/or jaw malformation; the results of such investigations greatly influencing the treatment plan.

Examination of the teeth by radiography is often accomplished to discern the presence of dental caries or inflammatory periodontal disease. To this end, intra-oral bitewing radiographs (see page 50) may be used or, more frequently nowadays, orthopantomography (see Fig. 2.121). Intra-oral periapical views may be used for assessing the progress of root canal therapy or determining the presence of a dental abscess at the root apex (Fig. 2.192). It is often stated that to determine whether a radiolucency in the region of the root apex is a dental abscess, it is necessary to assess whether the lamina dura at the alveolar socket is continuous or discontinuous (as is more likely in the presence of the abscess) (see also page 206).

# 3 Regional topography of the mouth and related areas

This chapter considers aspects of the gross anatomy of orodental regions, principally the temporomandibular joint, the muscles of mastication, palate and tongue, the salivary glands of the oral cavity, and the tissue spaces around the jaws.

## TEMPOROMANDIBULAR JOINT

The temporomandibular joint (TMJ) is the synovial articulation between the mandible and the cranium. For this reason, the joint is sometimes referred to as the craniomandibular joint. It is formed by the condylar process of the mandible articulating in the mandibular (glenoid) fossa of the temporal bone (Fig. 3.1). The TMJ, although basically a hinge joint, also allows for some gliding movements. Movement of the condylar head occurs within the mandibular fossa and down a bony prominence immediately anterior to the mandibular fossa, the articular eminence of the temporal bone.

Although having a number of features typical of synovial joints in other regions (e.g. a joint capsule, a synovial membrane secreting synovial fluid, ligaments to limit movement), the TMJ also has some unusual features:

- The joint space is divided into two joint cavities (upper and lower) by an intra-articular disc (see Fig. 15.1): the upper joint space allows for gliding movements, the lower joint space for hinge movements.
- The articular surfaces are not composed of hyaline cartilage but of fibrous tissue. This reflects the joint's intramembranous (rather than endochondral) development – see pages 293–294.
- A secondary condylar cartilage is present in the head of the condyle until adolescence.
- Movement of the joint is influenced by the teeth.
- There are two TMJs associated with a single mandible: this has

considerable functional significance as movement at one joint is accompanied by movement at the other.

The histology of the TMJ is considered in Chapter 15.

## MANDIBULAR FOSSA

The mandibular fossa (Fig. 3.2) is an oval depression in the temporal bone lying immediately anterior to the external acoustic meatus. Its mediolateral dimension is greater than its anteroposterior one in order to accommodate the mandibular condyle, and it is wider laterally than medially. The curvature of the mandibular fossa varies and may show some relationship to the nature of the occlusion. The mandibular fossa is bounded anteriorly by the articular eminence, laterally by the zygomatic process and posteriorly by the tympanic plate. The posterior margin is elevated to form the posterior auricular ridge, which may be enlarged laterally as the postglenoid tubercle just anterior to the external auditory meatus. Medially, the mandibular fossa may be defined by a ridge, the medial glenoid plane. The squamous and tympanic parts of the temporal bone are delineated laterally by the squamotympanic fissure. This fissure bifurcates medially due to the presence of a small component of the petrous portion, the tegmen tympani, giving rise to the petrosquamous fissure anteriorly and the petrotympanic fissure immediately behind. The petrotympanic fissure is the site at which the chorda tympani nerve exits from the cranium into the infratemporal fossa.

The shape of the mandibular fossa does not exactly conform to the shape of the mandibular condyle, the intra-articular disc moulding together the joint surfaces. The bone of the central part of the fossa is thin. This indicates that masticatory loads are not dissipated through the mandibular fossa but through the teeth and thence the facial bones and base of the cranium.

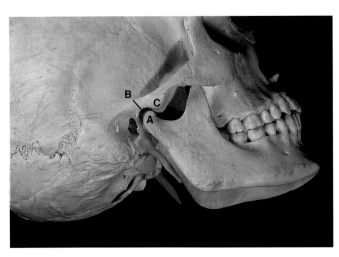

**Fig. 3.1** The osteology of the temporomandibular joint. A = mandibular condyle; B = mandibular fossa of temporal bone; C = articular eminence of temporal bone.

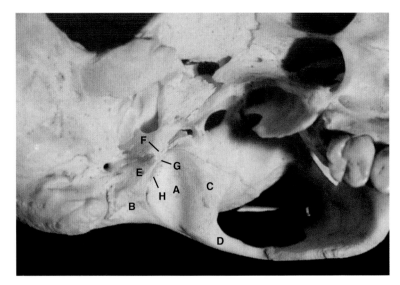

**Fig. 3.2** The osteology of the mandibular fossa. A = mandibular fossa; B = external acoustic meatus; C = articular eminence; D = zygomatic process of temporal bone; E = tympanic plate; F = petrotympanic fissure; G = petrosquamous fissure; H = squamotympanic fissure.

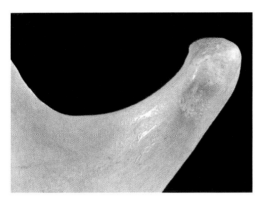

**Fig. 3.3** The mandibular condyle viewed laterally.

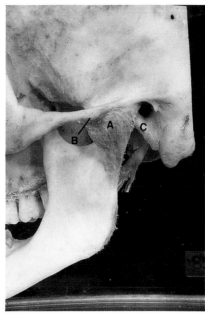

**Fig. 3.5** The capsule of the temporomandibular joint (A). B = articular eminence; C = tympanic plate. Courtesy of Professor C. Dean.

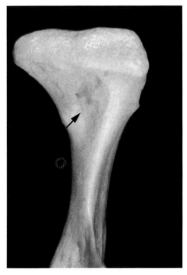

**Fig. 3.4** The mandibular condyle viewed from above. The pterygoid fovea is arrowed.

## MANDIBULAR CONDYLE

The mandibular condyle varies considerably (Figs 3.3, 3.4). When viewed from above, the condyle is roughly ovoid in outline, the anteroposterior dimension (approximately 1 cm) being about half the mediolateral dimension. The medial aspect is wider than the lateral. The long axis of the condyle is not, however, at right angles to the ramus, but diverges posteriorly from a strictly coronal plane. Thus the lateral pole of the condyle lies slightly anterior to the medial pole – if the long axes of the two condyles were extended, they would meet at an obtuse angle of approximately 145° at the anterior border of the foramen magnum. The convex anterior and superior surfaces of the head of the condyle are the articular surfaces. The articular surface area of the condyle is of the order of 200 mm², which is about half that of the mandibular fossa. The non-articular posterior surface of the condyle is broad and flat. The articular surface may be separated from the non-articular surface by a slight ridge, indicating the site of attachment of the joint capsule. The broad articular head of the condyle joins the ramus through a thin bony projection termed the neck of the condyle. A small depression, the pterygoid fovea, marks part of the attachment of the inferior head of the lateral pterygoid muscle and is situated on the anterior part of the neck below the articular surface of the condyle.

## JOINT CAPSULE

The capsule of the TMJ is a thin, slack cuff that does not limit mandibular movements and is too weak to provide much support for the joint (Fig. 3.5). Above, it is attached to the mandibular fossa, extending anteriorly to just in front of the crest of the articular eminence, posteriorly to the squamotympanic and petrotympanic fissures, medially to the medial glenoid plane and laterally between the lateral margin of the articular eminence and the postglenoid process. Below, it is attached to the neck of the condyle of the mandible. The upper fibres of the capsule are more loosely arranged than the lower. Posteriorly, the capsule is associated with the thick, vascular, but loosely arranged connective tissue of the bilaminar zone of the intra-articular disc (the retrodiscal pad). Internally, it is attached to the intra-articular disc and is lined by synovial membrane. The collagen fibres of the capsule run predominantly in a vertical direction. The capsule is richly innervated. There is debate as to whether muscle fibres of the superior head of lateral pterygoid insert into the capsule or whether they also pass through to attach to the medial aspect of the anterior border of the intra-articular disc itself.

## SYNOVIAL MEMBRANE

The synovial membrane lines the inner surface of the fibrous capsule and the margins of the intra-articular disc but does not cover the articular surfaces of the joint. The synovial membrane secretes the synovial fluid that occupies the joint cavities, lubricates the joint and presumably also has nutritive functions. Important components of the synovial fluid are the proteoglycans, which aid lubrication. At rest, the hydrostatic pressure of the synovial fluid has been reported as being subatmospheric, but this is greatly elevated during mastication.

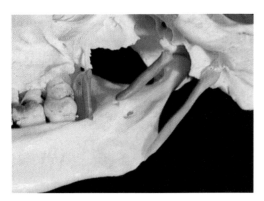

**Fig. 3.6** Model showing accessory ligaments associated with the temporomandibular joint. Yellow = stylomandibular ligament; red = pterygomandibular raphe; green = sphenomandibular ligament.

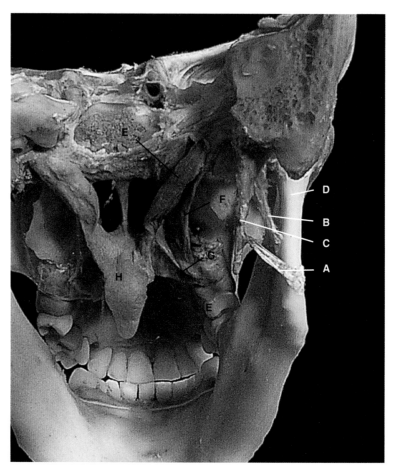

**Fig. 3.7** Posterior view of the jaw apparatus showing the stylomandibular (A) and sphenomandibular (B) ligaments. C = styloid process; D = posterior border of ramus of mandible; E = levator veli palati muscle; F = tensor veli palati muscle; G = pterygoid hamulus; H = soft palate. Courtesy of the Museums of the Royal College of Surgeons of England.

## TEMPOROMANDIBULAR LIGAMENT

The joint capsule is strengthened by the temporomandibular (lateral) ligament. This ligament cannot be readily separated from the capsule. It takes origin from the lateral surface of the articular eminence of the temporal bone at the site of a small bony protrusion, the articular tubercle. The temporomandibular ligament inserts onto the posterior surface of the condyle. This ligament provides the main means of support for the joint, restricting backward and inferior movements of the mandible and resisting dislocation during functional movements. The temporomandibular ligament is reinforced by a horizontal band of fibres running from the articular tubercle to the lateral surface of the condyle. These horizontal fibres restrict posterior movement of the condyle. The temporomandibular ligament is believed also to convert the potentially separating forces generated by the muscles opening the jaws into a force that compresses the condyle of the mandible on to the articular eminence. There is little evidence of any comparable ligament on the medial aspect of the joint capsule, so medial displacement is likely to be prevented by the temporomandibular ligament of the opposite side.

## ACCESSORY LIGAMENTS

The accessory ligaments of the TMJ traditionally described are the stylomandibular ligament, the sphenomandibular ligament and the pterygomandibular raphe (Figs 3.6, 3.7). However, only the sphenomandibular ligament is likely to have any significant influence on mandibular movements.

The *sphenomandibular ligament* is a remnant of the perichondrium of Meckel's cartilage (the cartilage of the embryonic first branchial arch; see page 293) and extends from the spine of the sphenoid bone to the lingula near the mandibular foramen. The sphenomandibular ligament is slack when the jaws are closed but becomes tense at about the time when the condyle has passed in front of the temporomandibular ligament.

The *stylomandibular ligament* is a reinforced lamina of the deep cervical fascia as it passes medially to the parotid salivary gland. It extends from the top of the styloid process of the temporal bone and from the stylohyoid ligament to the angle of the mandible.

The *pterygomandibular raphe* (from which the buccinator and superior constrictor muscles arise) extends from the pterygoid hamulus to the posterior end of the mylohyoid line in the retromolar region of the mandible.

An additional ligament, the retinacular ligament, has been described in association with the temporomandibular ligament. This arises from the articular eminence, descends along the ramus of the mandible and inserts into the fascia overlying the masseter muscle at the angle of the mandible. As this ligament is connected with the posterolateral aspect of the retrodiscal tissues and contains an accompanying vein, it may function in maintaining blood circulation during masticatory movements.

## INTRA-ARTICULAR DISC

The intra-articular disc (meniscus) is of a dense, fibrous consistency and is moulded to the bony joint surfaces above and below (Figs 3.8–3.10). Blood vessels are evident only at the periphery of the intra-articular disc, the bulk of it being avascular. Above, the disc covers the slope of the articular eminence in front while below it covers the condyle. When viewed in sagittal section the upper surface of the disc is concavo-convex from front to back and the lower surface is concave. Viewed superiorly, the disc is somewhat rectangular or oval in outline. The disc is of variable thickness, being thinnest in its central part, with a thickness of about 1 mm, and thickest posteriorly in the region above and behind the mandibular condyle, where its thickness is about 3 mm. The lateral half of the disc

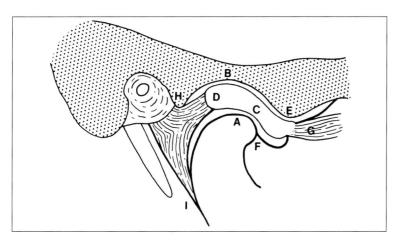

**Fig. 3.8** Diagrammatic representation of the intra-articular disc.
A = mandibular condyle
B = mandibular fossa
C = central part of intra-articular disc
D = posterior part of intra-articular disc
E = articular eminence
F = attachment of anterior part of intra-articular disc to anterior margin of mandibular condyle
G = lateral pterygoid muscle
H = attachment of upper part of bilaminar zone
I = attachment of the lower part of bilaminar zone.

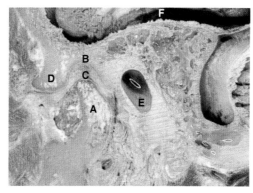

**Fig. 3.10** Sagittal section of head showing the intra-articular disc (C).
A = mandibular condyle
B = mandibular fossa
D = articular eminence
E = external acoustic meatus
F = floor of middle cranial fossa.

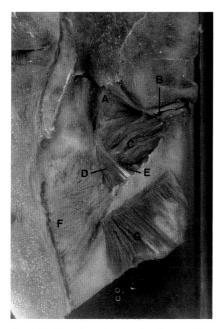

**Fig. 3.9** Dissection showing the fibres of the upper head of the lateral pterygoid muscle (A) attaching to the intra-articular disc (B) of the temporomandibular joint. C = fibres of the inferior head of the lateral pterygoid muscle inserting into the pterygoid fovea of the mandibular condyle; D = superficial head of medial pterygoid muscle; E = deep head of medial pterygoid muscle; F = buccinator muscle; G = cut edge of masseter muscle. Courtesy of Professor L. Garey.

The intra-articular disc has been subdivided into three portions: anterior, intermediate and posterior (Fig. 3.8). The intermediate zone is the thinnest. In the intermediate part the collagen bundles have been described as running preferentially in an anteroposterior direction, while in the anterior and posterior bands they run both anteroposterior and mediolaterally. The overall shape of the intra-articular disc is thought to provide a self-centering mechanism, which automatically acts to maintain its correct relationship to the articular surface of the mandibular condyle during mandibular movements.

The margin of the intra-articular disc merges peripherally with the joint capsule. Anteriorly, fibrous bands connect the disc to the anterior margin of the articular eminence above and to the anterior margin of the condyle below. Medially and laterally the disc is attached to the joint capsule just below the medial and lateral poles of the condyle by triangular zones of connective tissue. Posteriorly, it is attached to the capsule by a bilaminar zone (retrodiscal tissue/pad – see also page 257). The superior lamina is loose and possesses numerous vascular elements and elastin fibres. It attaches to the anterior margin of the squamotympanic fissure. The inferior lamina is relatively avascular and less extensible (as it has few elastin fibres), and is attached to the posterior margin of the condyle. The volume of the retrodiscal tissue appears to increase about five times during jaw opening as a result of venous engorgement, because of its continuity with the pterygoid venous plexus lying medial to the condyle. This activity fills the vacated space in the mandibular fossa and rapidly equilibrates any changes in intracapsular pressures that may hinder jaw movement. Changes in tissue fluid pressure during mandibular movements could also help regulate the flow of blood in the retrodiscal pad. As the mandibular condyle moves backwards during jaw closure, blood leaves the retrodiscal tissues. The close relationship of elastin fibres to the walls of blood vessels in the retrodiscal tissues has led to the view that the fibres function as a pump, facilitating blood flow during venous dilatation and compression.

The return of the intra-articular disc to its original position may be aided by the elastic recoil of the superior lamella. The return could be passive, because of the shape of the disc and its firm insertion to the lateral and medial poles of the condyle of the mandible. There is evidence that the superior head of the lateral pterygoid is active only on final closure.

The intra-articular disc divides the TMJ cavity into superior and inferior joint cavities. About 1 ml of synovial fluid occupies the inferior joint cavity, while a little more occupies the superior joint cavity.

is thinner than the medial half. The medial and lateral margins of the disc are slightly thickened. In centric occlusal position, the articular surface of the condyle lies against the thinner intermediate part of the intra-articular disc and faces the posterior slope of the articular eminence (Fig. 3.8).

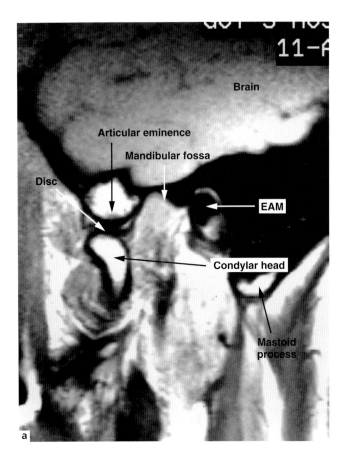
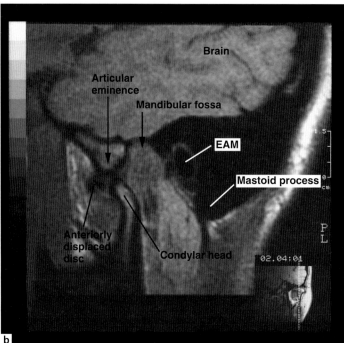

**Fig. 3.11** (a) MRI showing normal position of intra-articular disc with the jaw in the open position; (b) MRI showing anterior displacement of disc (internal derangement) with the jaw in the open position. EAM = external acoustic meatus. Courtesy of Dr N. Drage.

During jaw opening, two types of movement occur at the joint. The first is a hinge movement in the lower joint cavity of the head of the mandibular condyle around a horizontal axis. The second movement involves the upper joint cavity and is a forward or translatory movement of the condyle and the intra-articular disc. During opening and closing of the jaws, a combination of rotation and translation occurs: during wide opening about 75% of the movement can be explained by rotation in the lower compartment. The condyle and disc move together anteriorly beneath the articular eminence. With the mouth closed, the condyle is in contact with the posterior band immediately above. As the condyle translates forward, it contacts the thinner intermediate zone of the intra-articular disc that separates it from the articular eminence. With the mouth fully opened, the condyle may lie beneath the anterior band of the disc.

Among the functions attributed to the intra-articular disc are to improve the fit between the bony articulating surfaces, to provide stability during mandibular movements, to act as a shock absorber and distribute loads over a large area, to protect the articular surfaces, especially from shear forces generated during condylar movements, and to spread the synovial fluid. Although some regard the functions of the intra-articular disc as helping to stabilize the condyle, others see it as primarily destabilizing the condyle and permitting it to move more freely.

Apart from being prone to disorders affecting other synovial joints, such as arthritis, the TMJ is affected in the condition referred to as internal derangement. In internal derangement, the posterior band of the intra-articular disc comes to lie in front of the condyle (Fig. 3.11). This is associated with stretching of the bilaminar zone. The intra-articular disc may return to its correct relationship to the condyle. This is referred to as anterior displacement with reduction and may be associated with a clicking joint. However, the intra-articular disc may remain anteriorly displaced. This is referred to as anterior displacement without reduction.

Degenerative changes in the disc may lead to its perforation and there may be a limitation of jaw movements.

## NERVES AND VESSELS OF THE TEMPOROMANDIBULAR JOINT

The TMJ is richly innervated. Innervation for the joint is provided by the auriculotemporal, masseteric and deep temporal nerves of the mandibular division of the trigeminal nerve. The largest is the auriculotemporal nerve, supplying the medial, lateral and posterior parts of the joint. The remaining two nerves supply the anterior parts of the joint. Although free nerve endings associated with nociception are found everywhere in the joint capsule, of particular functional importance are more complex endings (e.g. Ruffini-like, Golgi tendon organs) associated with proprioception and important in the reflex control of mastication. The blood supply to the joint is mainly from the superficial temporal and maxillary arteries.

## MUSCLES OF MASTICATION

Although many muscles, both in the head and the neck, are involved in the process of mastication, 'the muscles of mastication' is a collective term reserved for the masseter, temporalis and medial and lateral pterygoid muscles. All the muscles of mastication develop from the mesenchyme of the first branchial (pharyngeal) arch. They therefore receive their innervation from the mandibular branch of the trigeminal nerve. Closely associated functionally and developmentally with the muscles of mastication is the digastric muscle. The masseter and temporalis muscles lie on the superficial face, while the lateral and medial pterygoid muscles lie deeper within the infratemporal fossa.

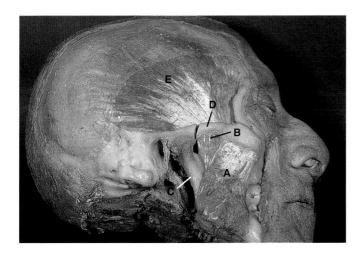

**Fig. 3.12** The masseter muscle showing superficial (A) and deep (B) heads. C = posterior border of ramus of mandible; D = zygomatic arch; E = temporalis muscle.

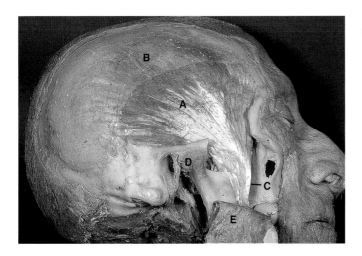

**Fig. 3.13** The temporalis muscle (A) arising in part from the overlying temporal fascia (B) and inserting into the coronoid process (C) of the mandible. D = mandibular condyle; E = deep surface of masseter muscle revealed following reflection of the zygomatic arch.

## MASSETER

The masseter muscle consists of two overlapping heads (Fig. 3.12). The superficial head arises from the zygomatic process of the maxilla and from the anterior two-thirds of the lower border of the zygomatic arch. The deep head arises from the deep surface of the zygomatic arch. Internally, the muscle has many tendinous septa that greatly increase the area for muscle attachment and provide a multipennate arrangement, thereby increasing its power. The superficial head passes downwards and backwards to insert into the lower half of the lateral surface of the mandibular ramus. The deep head, whose posterior fibres are more vertically oriented, inserts into the upper half of the lateral surface of the ramus, particularly over the coronoid process. The muscle elevates the mandible and is primarily active when grinding tough food. Indeed, the muscle exerts considerable power when the mandible is close to the centric occlusal position. On the basis of its fibre orientation, the posterior fibres of the deep head may have some retrusive capability for the mandible.

## TEMPORALIS

The temporalis muscle is the largest muscle of mastication. It takes origin from the floor of the temporal fossa on the lateral surface of the skull and from the overlying temporal fascia. The muscle is considered as a bi-pennate muscle. The attachment is limited above by the inferior temporal line. From this wide origin, the fibres of the temporalis muscle converge towards their insertion on the apex, the anterior and posterior borders, and the medial surface of the coronoid process of the mandible (Fig. 3.13).

Indeed, the insertion extends down the anterior border of the mandibular ramus almost as far as the third molar tooth. The posterior fibres of the muscle pass horizontally forwards while the anterior fibres pass vertically downwards on to the coronoid process. To reach the coronoid process, the muscle runs beneath the zygomatic arch. The anterior (vertical) part elevates the mandible, while the posterior (horizontal) part retracts the protruded mandible. In certain sites, the masseter and temporalis muscles are joined. This is particularly so for the deep fibres of the deep head of the masseter and the overlying temporalis muscle. The functional significance of this 'zygomatico-mandibular mass' is unclear.

Both the masseter and the temporalis muscles are innervated by branches of the anterior division of the mandibular nerve (see page 88). Both receive their blood supply from the maxillary artery (masseteric and deep temporal branches), the superficial temporal artery (transverse facial and middle temporal branches) and, for the masseter muscle, the facial artery.

## PTERYGOIDS

In order to fully appreciate the anatomy of the pterygoid muscles, an understanding of the osteology of the infratemporal fossa is required as both muscles arise from bony landmarks within this fossa. The reader is therefore referred to page 75 and Fig. 3.30.

### Lateral pterygoid

The lateral pterygoid muscle lies in the roof of the infratemporal fossa and has essentially a horizontal alignment. It has two heads, superior and

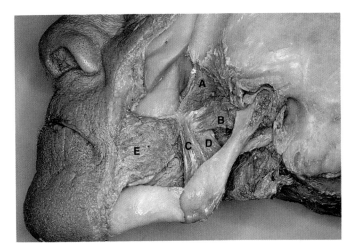

**Fig. 3.14** Lateral view of the pterygoid muscles. A = superior head of lateral pterygoid; B = inferior head of lateral pterygoid; C = superficial head of medial pterygoid; D = deep head of lateral pterygoid; E = buccinator muscle.

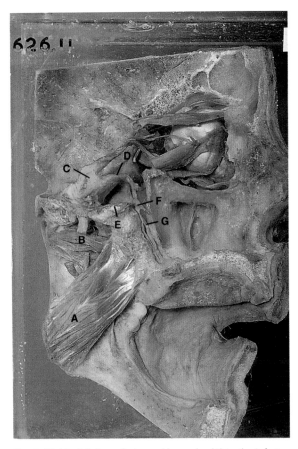

**Fig. 3.15** Medial view of pterygoid muscles (A) in the infratemporal fossa. B = lateral pterygoid muscle; C = trigeminal ganglion; D = maxillary nerve; E = nerve of pterygoid canal; F = pterygopalatine ganglion; G = greater and lesser palatine nerves. Courtesy of Professor L. Garey.

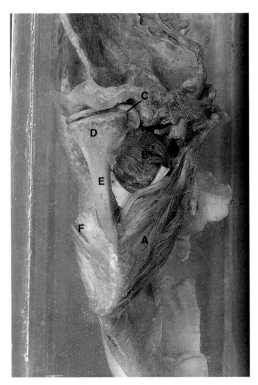

**Fig. 3.16** Posterior view of the medial (A) and lateral (B) pterygoid muscles. C = Intra-articular disc of temporomandibular joint; D = mandibular condyle; E = posterior border of ramus of mandible; F = cut edge of masseter muscle. Courtesy of Professor L. Garey.

inferior (Figs 3.14–3.16). The superior (upper) head is the smaller and arises from the infratemporal surface of the greater wing of the sphenoid bone (see Fig. 3.30). The inferior (lower) head forms the bulk of the muscle and takes origin from the lateral surface of the lateral pterygoid plate of the sphenoid bone (Fig. 3.30). Both heads pass backwards and outwards and appear to merge before their areas of insertion. The fibres of the superior head insert into the capsule and possibly the medial aspect of the anterior border of the intra-articular disc of the TMJ. The fibres of the inferior head of the lateral hterygoid muscle insert into the pterygoid fovea of the mandibular condyle. However, the precise insertions of the muscle are still controversial and may have clinical relevance with regard to TMJ disorders, particularly internal derangement where the disc is dis-

placed, usually in an anteromedial position, and the jaw may become locked (Fig. 3.11). Such conditions may be associated with clicking joints, limited jaw movements and pain and some anatomists have attributed variations in the attachment, and therefore the function, of the superior head as an aetiological factor in the condition. Some anatomists consider the superior and inferior heads as two separate muscles, the inferior head being concerned with mandibular protrusion, depression and lateral excursions while the superior head is activated during mandibular retrusion (providing controlled movements) and during clenching of the mandible. However, others consider the two heads as forming a single functional muscle, with its activities shaded according to the biomechanical demands of the task.

## Medial pterygoid

The medial pterygoid muscle consists of two heads (Figs 3.14–3.16). The bulk of the muscle arises as a deep head from the medial surface of the lateral pterygoid plate of the sphenoid bone (see Fig. 3.30). The smaller superficial head arises from the maxillary tuberosity and the neighbouring part of the palatine bone (pyramidal process). From these sites of origin, the fibres of the medial pterygoid pass downwards, backwards and laterally to insert into the roughened surface of the medial aspect of the angle of the mandible. Tendinous septa within the muscle increase the surface area for muscle attachment, providing a multipennate arrangement and therefore increasing the power the muscle can exert. The main action of the muscle is to elevate the mandible but it also assists in lateral and protrusive movements. An accessory medial pterygoid muscle has been described as a separate slip of muscle close to the deep surface of the medial pterygoid. This takes origin from the base of the skull close to the foramen ovale and merges with the deep head of the medial pterygoid. Its function is unknown. The masseter and medial pterygoid muscles together form a muscular sling that supports the mandible on the cranium.

The medial pterygoid muscle is innervated by a branch of the mandibular nerve that arises proximal to the division of the mandibular nerve into anterior and posterior trunks (see Fig. 4.17). The lateral pterygoid receives its nerve supply from the anterior trunk. Both muscles receive their blood supply as muscular branches from the maxillary artery.

## SPHENOMANDIBULAR

A fifth muscle of mastication has recently been described. It appears to take origin from the greater wing of the sphenoid bone (at the base of the temporal fossa) and extends downwards and backwards to be inserted on to the inner and anterior aspect of the mandibular coronoid process and the anterior edge of the mandibular ramus. From its orientation, the muscle would aid elevation (and perhaps protrusion) of the mandible. An alternative explanation for the muscle is that it is a previously 'unidentified' component of a known muscle. Indeed, it may therefore be linked to the medial pterygoid muscle or be considered part of the temporalis muscle.

## DIGASTRIC

Because of its functional associations, the digastric muscle is described here although it is not usually strictly classified as a 'muscle of mastication'. This muscle is located below the inferior border of the mandible and consists of anterior and posterior bellies connected by an intermediate tendon (Fig. 3.17). The posterior belly arises from the mastoid notch immediately behind the mastoid process of the temporal bone; it passes downwards and forwards towards the hyoid bone, where it becomes the digastric tendon. The digastric muscle passes through the insertion of the stylohyoid muscle and is attached to the greater horn of the hyoid bone by a fibrous loop. The anterior belly of the digastric muscle is attached to the digastric fossa on the inferior border of the mandible and runs downwards and backwards to the digastric tendon. The digastric muscle depresses and retrudes the mandible and is involved in stabilizing the position of the hyoid bone and in elevation of the hyoid during swallowing.

The anterior belly of the digastric muscle is innervated by the mylohyoid branch of the mandibular division of the trigeminal nerve, the posterior belly by the digastric branch of the facial nerve. This reflects different embryological origins, from first and second branchial arch mesenchyme respectively. The anterior belly receives its blood supply from the facial artery, the posterior belly from the posterior auricular and occipital arteries.

## MUSCLES OF THE SOFT PALATE

The soft palate is supported by the fibrous palatine aponeurosis, the shape and position of which is altered by the activity of four pairs of muscles: the tensor veli palatini, the levator veli palatini, the palatoglossus and the palatopharyngeus muscles. In addition, there is the musculus uvulae.

## TENSOR VELI PALATINI

The tensor veli palatini muscle (Figs 3.18–3.20) arises from the scaphoid fossa of the sphenoid bone at the root of the pterygoid plates and from the

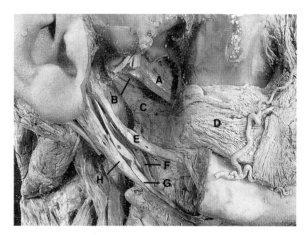

**Fig. 3.18** Deep dissection of the infratemporal fossa to reveal tensor veli palatini muscle (A). B = partially obscured levator veli palatini muscle; C = superior constrictor muscle; D = buccinator muscle; E = styloglossus muscle; F = stylopharyngeus muscle; G = stylohyoid muscle; H = posterior belly of digastric muscle. Courtesy of Professor C. Dean.

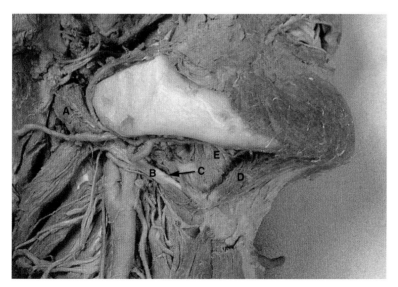

**Fig. 3.17** The digastric muscle. A = posterior belly; B = tendon of digastric; C = stylohyoid muscle splitting around digastric tendon; D = anterior belly of digastric; E = mylohyoid muscle.

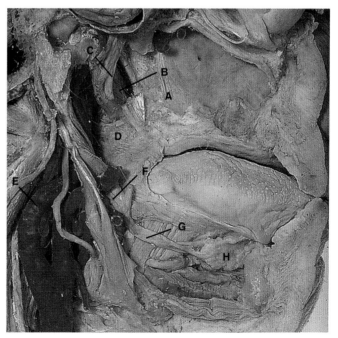

**Fig. 3.19** Deep dissection of the infratemporal fossa with the tensor palati muscle (A) cut to reveal the levator palati muscle (B). C = mandibular nerve; D = superior constrictor; E = internal carotid artery; F = styloglossus muscle; G = lingual nerve on hyoglossus muscle; H = sublingual gland. Courtesy of Professor L. Garey.

**Fig. 3.20** Diagrammatic representation of palatal and pharyngeal muscles. (a) Posterior view, (b) Medial view.
A = tensor veli palatini
B = levator veli palatini
C = palatoglossus
D = palatopharyngeus
E = auditory (pharyngotympanic or Eustachian) tube
F = pterygoid hamulus
G = musculus uvulae
H = salpingopharyngeus muscle
I = superior constrictor muscle.

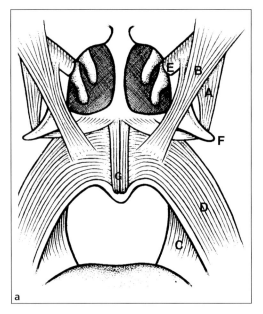

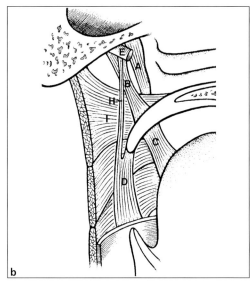

lateral side of the cartilaginous part of the auditory (pharyngotympanic) tube. From its origin, the fibres converge towards the pterygoid hamulus, whence the muscle becomes tendinous (the tendon bending at right angles around the hamulus to become the palatine aponeurosis). The anterior border of the aponeurosis is attached to the posterior border of the hard palate. Medially, it merges with the aponeurosis of the other side. Posteriorly, it becomes indistinct, merging with submucosa at the posterior edge of the soft palate. When the tensor veli palatini muscle contracts, the aponeurosis becomes a taut, horizontal plate of tissue upon which other palatine muscles may act to change the position of the soft palate.

The motor innervation of the tensor veli palatini is derived from the mandibular branch of the trigeminal nerve (via the nerve to the medial pterygoid muscle and the otic ganglion).

## LEVATOR VELI PALATINI

The levator veli palatini muscle (Figs 3.18–3.20) originates from the base of the skull at the apex of the petrous part of the temporal bone, anterior to the opening of the carotid canal, and from the medial side of the cartilaginous part of the auditory tube. The muscle curves downwards, medially and forwards to enter the palate immediately below the opening of the auditory tube.

The levator muscles of the palate form a U-shaped muscular sling (Fig. 3.20). When the palatine aponeurosis is stiffened by the tensor muscles, contraction of the levator muscles produces an upwards and backwards movement of the soft palate. In this way, the nasopharynx is shut off from the oropharynx by the apposition of the soft palate on to the posterior wall of the pharynx.

## PALATOPHARYNGEUS

The palatopharyngeus muscle (Fig. 3.20) arises from two heads: one from the posterior border of the hard palate, the other from the upper surface of the palatine aponeurosis (Fig. 3.20). The two heads unite after arching over the lateral edge of the palatine aponeurosis, where the muscle passes downwards beneath the mucous membrane of the lateral wall of the oropharynx as the palatopharyngeal fold (see Fig. 1.11). The muscle is inserted into the posterior border of the thyroid cartilage of the larynx. The main action of the palatopharyngeus muscle is to elevate the larynx and pharynx but it may also arch the relaxed palate and depress the tensed palate.

## PALATOGLOSSUS

The palatoglossus muscle (Fig. 3.20) arises from the aponeurosis of the soft palate and descends to the tongue in the palatoglossal fold (see Fig. 1.11), whence its fibres intercalate with the transverse fibres of the tongue. The action of the palatoglossus is to raise the tongue in order to narrow the transverse diameter of the oropharyngeal isthmus.

## MUSCULUS UVULAE

The musculus uvulae (Fig. 3.20) arises from the posterior nasal spine at the back of the hard palate and from the palatine aponeurosis. It passes backwards and downwards to insert into the mucosa of the uvula. It moves the uvula upwards and laterally and helps to complete the seal between the soft palate and pharynx in the midline region when the palate is elevated.

## NERVE AND BLOOD SUPPLY

With the exception of the tensor veli palatini muscle, the nerve supply to the muscles of the palate is derived from the cranial part of the accessory nerve via the pharyngeal plexus. The arterial supply to the muscles of the soft palate is derived from the facial artery (ascending palatine branch), the ascending pharyngeal artery and the maxillary artery (palatine branches).

## PASSAVANT'S MUSCLE

Passavant's muscle is a sphincter-like muscle that encircles the pharynx at the level of the palate, inside the fibres of the superior constrictor muscles. It is formed by fibres arising from the anterior and lateral part of the upper surface of the palatine aponeurosis. Contraction of this muscle forms a ridge (Passavant's ridge), against which the soft palate is elevated.

## MUSCLES OF THE TONGUE

The tongue is composed of intrinsic and extrinsic muscles. The intrinsic muscles are restricted to the substance of the tongue and change its shape, while the extrinsic muscles arise outside the tongue and are responsible for bodily movement of the tongue.

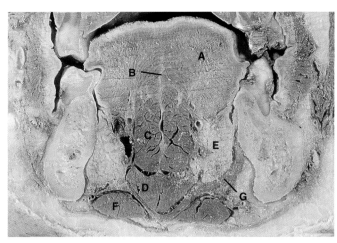

**Fig. 3.21** Coronal section through the tongue and floor of the mouth. Note the interlacing of the intrinsic muscles in the body of the tongue (A). B = lingual septum; C = genioglossus muscle; D = geniohyoid muscle; E = sublingual gland above mylohyoid; F = anterior belly of digastric muscle; G = mylohyoid muscle.

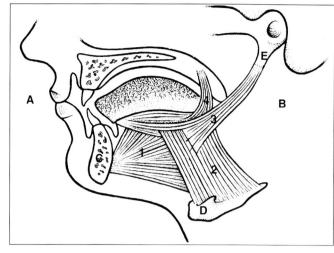

**Fig. 3.22** Diagrammatic representation of the extrinsic muscles of the tongue. A = anterior; B = posterior; C = mandible; D = hyoid bone; E = styloid process; 1 = genioglossus; 2 = hyoglossus; 3 = styloglossus; 4 = palatoglossus.

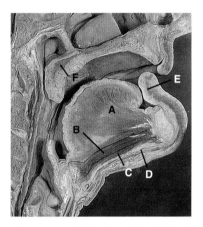

**Fig. 3.23** Sagittal section of head showing genioglossus muscle (A). B = geniohyoid muscle; C = mylohyoid muscle; D = platysma muscle; E = orbicularis oris muscle; F = levator veli palatini muscle.

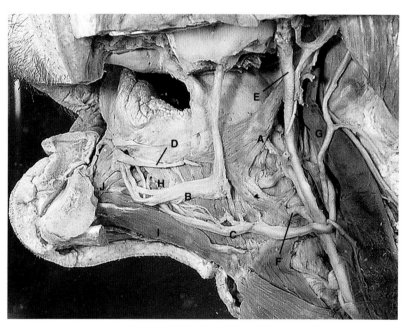

**Fig. 3.24** Lateral view of tongue showing styloglossus muscle (A). B = lingual nerve; C = hypoglossal nerve; D = submandibular duct (cut); E = external carotid artery; F = lingual artery; G = glossopharyngeal nerve; H = hyoglossus muscle; I = geniohyoid muscle; J = genioglossus muscle. Courtesy of Professor C. Dean.

## INTRINSIC MUSCLES

The intrinsic muscles of the tongue can be divided into three fibre groups: transverse, longitudinal and vertical. Rarely can these three groups be distinguished in dissections, but their interlacing gives the tongue its characteristic appearance in cross-section (Fig. 3.21). The *transverse fibres* arise from a sheet of connective tissue called the lingual septum, running longitudinally through the midline of the tongue. These transverse fibres pass laterally from the septum to intercalate with fibres of the other groups of intrinsic muscles. The *longitudinal fibres* may be subdivided into upper and lower groups, the superior and inferior longitudinal muscles of the tongue. The *vertical fibres* pass directly between the upper and lower surfaces, particularly at the lateral borders of the tongue. Contraction of the vertical fibres would make the tongue thinner (and wider). Contraction of the longitudinal fibres would shorten (and thicken) the tongue. Contraction of the transverse fibres would narrow (and widen) the tongue. The

intrinsic muscles receive their motor innervation from the hypoglossal cranial nerve.

## EXTRINSIC MUSCLES

The extrinsic muscles of the tongue arise from the skull and hyoid bone and thence spread into the body of the tongue. The extrinsic musculature is composed of four groups of muscles: genioglossus, hyoglossus, styloglossus and palatoglossus.

### Genioglossus

The genioglossus muscle (Figs 3.21–3.24) arises from the superior genial spine on the medial surface of the body of the mandible. At this level, the two genioglossus muscles cannot readily be separated. As the muscles enter the tongue, a thin strip of connective tissue intervenes between the right and left genioglossus muscles. The bulk of the fibres fan out into the body of the tongue but the superior fibres pass upwards and anteriorly to the tip of the tongue and some of its inferior fibres insert on to the body of the hyoid bone. The genioglossus muscle is mainly a protractor and depressor of the tongue.

## Hyoglossus

The hyoglossus muscle (Figs 3.22, 3.24) originates from the superior border of the greater horn of the hyoid bone and passes vertically upwards into the tongue. Its function is to depress the tongue. At its origin, the hyoglossus muscle is separated from the attachment of the middle constrictor muscle of the pharynx beneath by the lingual artery.

## Styloglossus

The styloglossus muscle (Figs 3.18, 3.19, 3.22, 3.24) arises from the anterior surface of the styloid process of the temporal bone, from which the muscle runs downwards and forwards to enter the tongue below the insertion of the palatoglossus muscle. At this point, its fibres intercalate with the fibres of the hyoglossus before continuing forwards towards the tip of the tongue. The styloglossus muscle is a retractor of the tongue.

## Palatoglossus

The palatoglossus muscle (Figs 3.20, 3.22) arises from the aponeurosis of the soft palate and descends to the tongue in the anterior pillar of the fauces, whence its fibres intercalate with the transverse fibres of the tongue. The action of the palatoglossus muscles is to raise the tongue in order to narrow the transverse diameter of the oropharyngeal isthmus.

The extrinsic muscles of the tongue are innervated by the hypoglossal nerve (except for the palatoglossus, which is innervated by the cranial part of the accessory nerve via the pharyngeal plexus). The main source of the blood supply to the tongue is the lingual artery.

## MUSCLES IN THE FLOOR OF THE MOUTH

The floor of the mouth is the region located between the medial surface of the mandible, the inferior surface of the tongue and the mylohyoid muscles. The mylohyoid muscles are attached to the mylohyoid lines of the mandible and consequently structures above these lines are related to the floor of the mouth, whereas structures below the lines are related to the upper part of the neck (supralyoid region). This concept is of considerable clinical importance with respect to the spread of inflammation from infected teeth within the mandible (see pages 79, 80). The two mylohyoid muscles form a muscular diaphragm for the floor of the mouth (Figs 3.17, 3.21, 3.23). Above this diaphragm are found the genioglossus and geniohyoid muscles medially and the hyoglossus muscles laterally. Below the diaphragm lie the digastric and stylohyoid muscles.

## MYLOHYOID

The mylohyoid muscle (Figs 3.21, 3.23) arises from the mylohyoid line on the inner surface of the body of the mandible. Its fibres slope downwards, forwards and inwards. The anterior fibres of the mylohyoid muscle interdigitate with the corresponding fibres on the opposite side to form a median raphe. This raphe is attached above to the chin and below to the hyoid bone. The posterior fibres are inserted on to the anterior surface of the body of the hyoid bone. The muscle raises the floor of the mouth during the early stages of swallowing. It also helps to depress the mandible when the hyoid bone is fixed. The mylohyoid muscle is supplied by the mylohyoid branch of the inferior alveolar branch of the mandibular division of the trigeminal nerve. Its blood supply is derived from the lingual artery (sublingual branch), the maxillary artery (mylohyoid branch of the inferior alveolar artery) and the facial artery (submental branch).

## GENIOHYOID

The geniohyoid muscle (Figs 3.21, 3.23, 3.24) originates from the inferior genial spine. It passes backwards and slightly downwards to insert on to the anterior surface of the body of the hyoid bone. The geniohyoid muscle elevates the hyoid bone and is a weak depressor of the mandible. Its innervation is from the first cervical spinal nerve travelling with the hypoglossal nerve. Its blood supply is derived from the lingual artery (sublingual branch).

## SUPERFICIAL MUSCLES OF THE FACE

The muscles of facial expression (Figs 3.25, 3.26) are characterized by their superficial arrangement in the face, by their activities on the skin (brought about directly by their attachment to the facial integument) and

**Fig. 3.25** Schematic diagram of the muscles of facial expression.
a = levator labii superioris alaeque nasi
b = levator labii superioris
c = orbicularis oculi
d = zygomaticus minor
e = zygomaticus major
f = risorius
g = platysma
h = depressor anguli oris
i = depressor labii inferioris
j = mentalis
k = orbicularis oris
m = masseter
n = buccinator
o = levator anguli oris
p = mental foramen
q = position of the parotid duct piercing the buccinator.

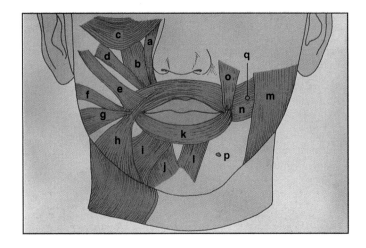

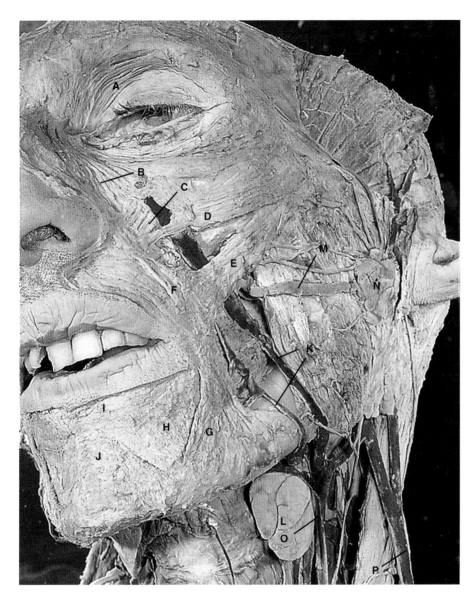

**Fig. 3.26** The muscles of facial expression.
A = orbicularis oculi
B = levator labii superioris alaeque nasi
C = levator labii superioris
D = zygomaticus minor
E = zygomaticus major
F = levator anguli oris
G = depressor anguli oris
H = depressor labii inferioris
I = orbicularis oris
J = mentalis
K = facial vessels
L = submandibular gland
M = parotid duct
N = parotid gland with facial nerve branches
O = facial vein receiving the anterior retromandibular vein
P = external jugular vein formed by the anterior branch of the retromandibular and the posterior auricular vein.
Courtesy of Professor C. Dean.

by their common motor innervation, the facial nerve. They are all derived embryologically from mesenchyme of the second branchial arch. Functionally, the muscles of facial expression are grouped around the orifices of the face (the orbit, nose, ear and mouth) and should be considered primarily as muscles controlling the degree of opening and closing of these apertures: the expressive functions of the muscles have developed secondarily. The muscles of facial expression vary considerably between individuals in terms of size, shape and strength.

The superficial muscles around the lips and cheeks may be subdivided into two groups: the various parts of the orbicularis oris muscle and muscles that are radially arranged from the orbicularis oris muscle. The fibres of orbicularis oris pass around the lips. The muscle is divided into four parts, each part corresponding to a quadrant of the lips. Its muscle fibres do not gain attachment directly to bone but occupy a central part of the lip. Muscle fibres in the philtrum insert on to the nasal septum. The range of movement produced by orbicularis oris includes lip closure, protrusion and pursing. The radial muscles can be divided into superficial and deep muscles of the upper and lower lips. The levator labii superioris,

levator labii superioris alaeque nasi and zygomaticus major and minor are superficial muscles of the upper lip. The levator anguli oris is a deep muscle of the upper lip. The depressor anguli oris is a superficial muscle of the lower lip and the depressor labii inferioris and mentalis muscle are deep muscles of the lower lip. As their names suggest, the levator labii superioris elevates the upper lip, the depressor labii inferioris depresses the lower lip and the corners of the mouth are raised and lowered by the levator and depressor anguli oris muscles respectively.

Two muscles extend to the corner of the mouth: the risorius and buccinator muscles, risorius lying superficial to buccinator. The risorius muscle stretches the angles of the mouth laterally. The buccinator muscle (see Fig. 3.9) arises from the pterygomandibular raphe and from the buccal side of the maxillary and mandibular alveoli above the molar teeth. Most of its fibres insert into mucous membrane covering the cheek; other fibres intercalate with orbicularis oris in the lips. As the fibres of buccinator converge towards the angle of the mouth, the central fibres decussate. The main function of the buccinator muscle is to maintain the tension of the cheek against the teeth during mastication.

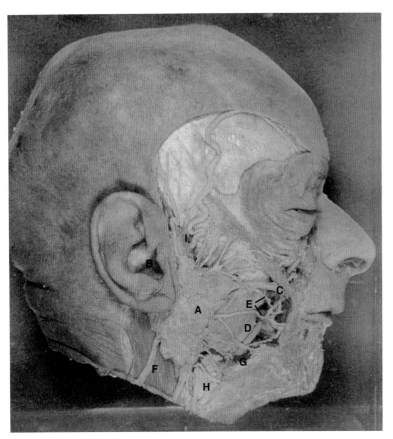

**Fig. 3.27** The shape and relations of the parotid gland (A). B = external acoustic meatus; C = parotid duct; D = masseter muscle; E = branches of facial nerve; F = great auricular nerve; G = facial vessels coursing through muscles of facial expression; H = superficial part of submandibular gland; I = superficial temporal vessels and auriculotemporal nerve.

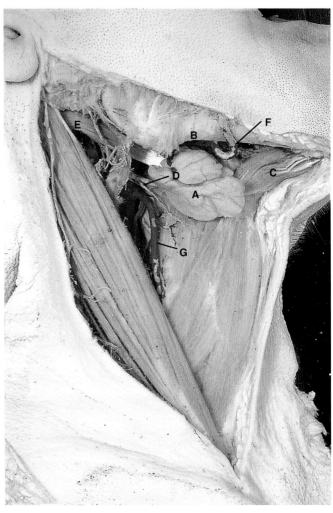

**Fig. 3.28** The superficial part of the submandibular gland (A) seen in the upper part of the neck; B = inferior border of mandible; C = anterior belly of the digastric muscle; D = hypoglossal nerve; E = posterior belly of the digastric muscle; F = facial artery on the mylohyoid muscle; G = superior thyroid artery. Courtesy of Professor C. Dean.

## SALIVARY GLANDS

### PAROTID GLAND

The parotid gland (Fig. 3.27) is the largest of the major salivary glands and secretes a serous saliva. It occupies the region between the ramus of the mandible and the mastoid process. The parotid is pyramidal in shape; its apex extends beyond the angle of the mandible and the base is closely related to the external acoustic meatus. A deep surface of the gland rests anteriorly on the ramus and masseter muscle and extends around the posterior border of the mandible, where it can reach the pharynx. The gland is surrounded by an unyielding tough fibrous capsule (the parotid capsule). The parotid duct (Stensen's duct) appears at the anterior border of the gland and passes horizontally across the masseter muscle before piercing the buccinator to terminate in the oral cavity opposite the maxillary second molar. Lying with the duct on the masseter may be an accessory parotid gland.

Within the parotid gland are found the external carotid artery, retromandibular veins and the facial nerve. Branches of the facial nerve are seen emerging from the anterior and inferior margins of the gland. Appearing at the superior border of the gland are the superficial temporal vessels and the auriculotemporal nerve. From the inferior border of the gland may be seen the anterior and posterior retromandibular veins. The former joins the facial vein, the latter joining the posterior auricular to form the external jugular vein (Fig. 3.26). Lymph nodes are also associated with the parotid gland.

The parasympathetic innervation of the parotid gland is from the lesser petrosal branch of the glossopharyngeal nerve (see Fig. 4.13). The pre-ganglionic fibres synapse in the otic ganglion and postganglionic fibres reach the gland by travelling with the auriculotemporal branch of the mandibular nerve. The sensory innervation of the parotid capsule is by the great auricular nerve, a branch of the cervical plexus (Fig. 3.27). The roots of this nerve are formed from the anterior primary rami of the second and third cervical nerves. The sensation of pain in mumps caused by enlargement of the gland (with subsequent tension on the unyielding parotid capsule) is mediated by the great auricular nerve.

### SUBMANDIBULAR GLAND

The submandibular gland produces both serous and mucous saliva (in a 3:2 ratio). It is found in the floor of the mouth and in the suprahyoid region of the neck. A large part of the gland (the superficial part) is visible just beneath the inferior border of the mandible (Figs 3.26–3.28). The gland has an important relationship with the mylohyoid muscle, wrapping around the free posterior border (not unlike the letter C). This gives rise to the smaller deep portion of the gland (Fig. 3.29). Posteriorly, the submandibular gland comes close to the apex of the parotid gland, with only the stylomandibular ligament intervening. The submandibular duct (Wharton's duct) appears from the deep part of the gland and wraps around the lingual nerve, as it crosses the hyoglossus muscle, to terminate on the sublingual papilla in the floor of the mouth (Figs 1.13, 3.29).

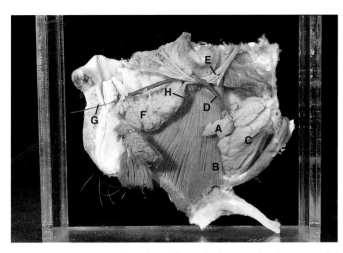

**Fig. 3.29** Medial view of the floor of mouth showing the deep part of the sub-mandibular gland (A) passing around the free posterior border of the mylohyoid muscle (B). C = superficial part of submandibular gland; D = submandibular duct wrapping around lingual nerve (E); F = sublingual gland; G = bristle in opening of the submandibular duct at the sublingual papilla; H = branches of the lingual nerve to the sublingual gland carrying parasympathetic fibres. Courtesy of Professor C. Dean.

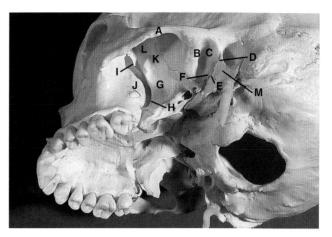

**Fig. 3.30** The osteology of the infratemporal fossa. A = zygomatic arch; B = articular eminence; C = mandibular fossa; D = squamotympanic fissure; E = petrotympanic fissure; F = petrosquamous fissure; G = lateral pterygoid plate; H = pterygomaxillary fissure leading into the pterygopalatine fossa; I = inferior orbital fissure; J = posterior border of maxilla; K = infratemporal crest of sphenoid bone; L = infratemporal surface of greater wing of sphenoid bone; M = tympanic plate.

## SUBLINGUAL GLAND

The sublingual gland, the smallest of the three major pairs of salivary glands, produces serous and mucous saliva in the approximate ratio of 1:3. It is located on the hyoglossus muscle in the floor of the mouth (Fig. 3.19), adjacent to the sublingual fossa of the mandible. The gland is associated with the sublingual folds beneath the tongue. In coronal section, the gland rests on the mylohyoid muscle (Fig. 3.21). The sublingual gland may be joined to the deep part of the submandibular gland to form a single sublingual–submandibular complex. The sublingual gland is subdivided into anterior and posterior parts. The ducts of the anterior part may unite to form a large main duct (Bartholin's duct), which either joins the sub-mandibular duct or drains directly on to the sublingual papilla. The ducts from the posterior part of the sublingual gland drain through the sub-lingual fold (see Fig. 1.13).

The parasympathetic innervation of both the submandibular and sublin-gual glands is the chorda tympani branch of the facial nerve. Preganglionic fibres are carried with this nerve (via the lingual nerve) to the submandib-ular ganglion. Postganglionic fibres pass from this ganglion to the sub-mandibular and sublingual glands (Fig. 3.14).

### INFRATEMPORAL FOSSA

The infratemporal fossa is the space located deep to the ramus of the mandible. Together with the temporal fossa, pterygoid processes and maxillary tuberosity, the infratemporal fossa has been thought of by some anatomists as part of a 'masticatory muscle compartment' or 'masticatory space'.

The infratemporal fossa (Fig. 3.30) is bounded anteriorly by the poste-rior surface of the maxilla, posteriorly by the styloid apparatus, carotid sheath and deep part of the parotid gland. Medially lie the lateral pterygoid plate and the superior constrictor of the pharynx. The roof is formed by the infratemporal surface of the greater wing of the sphenoid. The infra-temporal fossa has no floor, being continuous with the neck. It communi-cates with the temporal fossa deep to the zygomatic arch; also with the pterygopalatine fossa through the pterygomaxillary fissure. At the base of

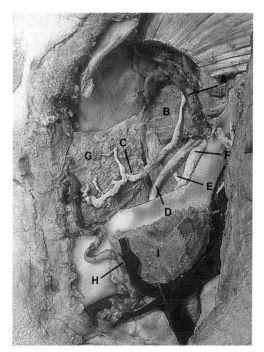

**Fig. 3.31** Contents of the infratemporal fossa. A = maxillary artery; B = lateral pterygoid (lower head); C = buccal branch of mandibular division of trigeminal nerve; D = lingual nerve; E = medial pterygoid muscle; F = inferior alveolar nerve; G = buccinator muscle; H = facial blood vessels; I = masseter muscle. Courtesy of Professor L. Garey.

the cranium, the foramen ovale and foramen spinosum enter the fossa through the sphenoid bone. The foramen lacerum and the petrotympanic, squamotympanic and petrosquamous fissures are also found close to the infratemporal fossa. On the medial surface of the ramus of the mandible is the mandibular foramen.

The major structures within the infratemporal fossa (Fig. 3.31) are the lateral pterygoid and medial pterygoid muscles (see pages 67–69 for details), branches of the mandibular nerve (including the inferior alveolar, buccal and lingual nerves; see page 88), the chorda tympani branch of the facial nerve, the otic ganglion, the maxillary artery and the pterygoid venous plexus.

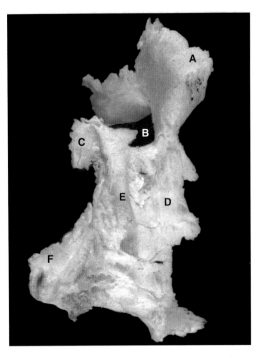

**Fig. 3.32** Lateral view of palatine bone forming the medial wall of the pterygopalatine fossa. A = orbital process; B = sphenopalatine notch; C = sphenoidal process; D = perpendicular plate; E = greater palatine groove; F = pyramidal process.

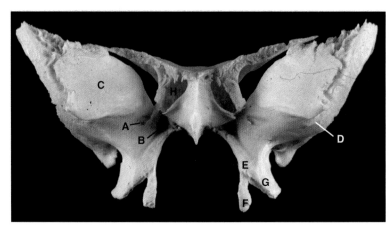

**Fig. 3.33** Anterior surface of the sphenoid bone showing the foramen rotundum (A) and pterygoid canal (B). C = orbital surface of greater wing; D = infratemporal crest of greater wing; E = pterygoid process; F = pterygoid hamulus surmounting the medial pterygoid plate; G = lateral pterygoid plate; H = sphenoidal air sinus.

## PTERYGOPALATINE FOSSA

The pterygopalatine fossa lies between the infratemporal (posterior) surface of the maxilla and the pterygoid process of the sphenoid bone. The pterygopalatine fossa contains three major structures: the maxillary nerve, the maxillary artery (third part) and the pterygopalatine parasympathetic ganglion.

The elongated cleft between the posterior surface of the maxilla and the pterygoid process of the sphenoid bone is the pterygomaxillary fissure (Fig. 3.30), which forms the lateral aspect of the pterygopalatine fossa. The anterior wall of the fossa is the infratemporal surface of the maxilla. The posterior wall of the fossa is the pterygoid process below and the greater wing of the sphenoid above. The medial wall is formed by the perpendicular plate of the palatine bone (Fig. 3.32). The pyramidal process of the palatine bone is situated inferiorly and articulates with the tuberosity of the maxilla. It fills the triangular gap between the lower ends of the medial and lateral pterygoid plates.

Laterally, the pterygopalatine fossa communicates with the infratemporal fossa through the pterygomaxillary fissure. The fissure continues above with the posterior end of the inferior orbital fissure in the floor of the orbit (Fig. 3.30).

The pterygomaxillary fissure transmits the maxillary artery from the infratemporal fossa, the posterior superior alveolar branches of the maxillary division of the trigeminal nerve and the sphenopalatine veins. Passing through the inferior orbital fissure from the pterygopalatine fossa are the infra-orbital and zygomatic branches of the maxillary nerve, the orbital branches of the pterygopalatine ganglion and the infra-orbital vessels.

Entering the pterygopalatine fossa posteriorly are the foramen rotundum from the middle cranial fossa, and the pterygoid canal from the region of the foramen lacerum at the base of the skull (Fig. 3.33). The foramen rotundum occupying the greater wing of the sphenoid bone lies above and lateral to the pterygoid canal. The maxillary division of the trigeminal nerve passes through the foramen rotundum. The pterygoid canal transmits the greater petrosal and deep petrosal nerves (which combine to form the nerve of the pterygoid canal) and an accompanying artery derived from the maxillary artery.

High up on the medial wall of the pterygopalatine fossa lies the sphenopalatine foramen. It is formed by the notch between the orbital and sphenoid processes of the perpendicular plate of the palatine bone (Fig. 3.32) articulating with the body of the sphenoid bone. This foramen communicates with the lateral wall of the nasal cavity. It transmits the nasopalatine and posterior superior nasal nerves (from the pterygopalatine ganglion) and the sphenopalatine vessels.

At the base of the pterygopalatine fossa is found the opening of the anterior (greater) palatine canal. This canal is formed when the greater palatine groove running down the posterior margin of the lateral surface of the perpendicular plate of the palatine bone articulates with the posterior surface of the maxillary bone (see Fig. 2.3) and the medial pterygoid plate. In the lower part of the anterior palatine canal a smaller canal, the posterior palatine canal, is given off to run backwards in the pyramidal process of the palatine bone. The anterior palatine canal enters the hard palate at the anterior (greater) palatine foramen in the region of the transverse palatine suture (see Fig. 2.6). The posterior palatine canal enters the hard palate at the posterior (lesser) palatine foramen (foramina) (see Fig. 2.6). The anterior palatine canal transmits the greater and lesser palatine nerves (and the posterior inferior nasal branches from the pterygopalatine ganglion), together with accompanying vessels, and these pass to the hard palate to emerge at the anterior and posterior palatine foramina.

## TISSUE SPACES AROUND THE JAWS

Knowledge of the tissue spaces around the jaws is necessary to understand the possible spread of infections (including oedema and pus) from a dental site into the rest of the head and neck.

Most structures in the body are ensheathed by a connective tissue covering of varying thickness. If thin and delicate, this connective tissue presents little resistance to the spread of infection; if the connective tissue layer is thick, tendinous or membranous, it resists the spread of infection (particularly over certain muscles). Such thick connective tissues, capable of holding surgical sutures, are sometimes referred to as 'true fascia'. From clinical experience, it is evident that certain predictable pathways exist along which infection may spread. The loose connective tissue uniting fascial planes may be destroyed and the potential space delineated by adjacent structures considerably enlarged as inflammatory exudate accumulates. Such potential spaces are referred to as 'tissue spaces'.

The dissemination of infection in soft tissues is influenced by the natural barriers presented by bone, muscle and fascia. Around the jaws are body compartments, the so-called tissue spaces, the boundaries of which are primarily defined by the mylohyoid, buccinator, masseter, medial ptery-

**Table 3.1** *The most important tissue spaces around the jaws*

| Lower jaw | Upper jaw |
|---|---|
| 1. Submental | 10. Palatal |
| 2. Submandibular | 11. Canine fossa |
| 3. Sublingual | 12. Infratemporal |
| 4. Buccal | |
| 5. Submasseteric | |
| 6. Parotid | |
| 7. Pterygomandibular | |
| 8. Parapharyngeal | |
| 9. Peritonsillar | |

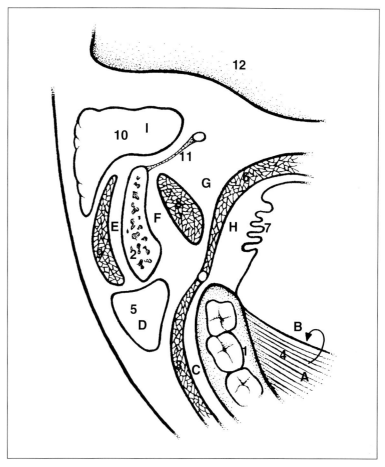

**Fig. 3.34** The relationships of tissue spaces around the mandibular ramus. 1 = body of mandible bearing the molar teeth; 2 = ramus of mandible; 3 = buccinator muscle; 4 = mylohyoid muscle; 5 = buccal pad of fat; 6 = superior constrictor muscle; 7 = mucosa overlying palatal tonsil; 8 = medial pterygoid muscle; 9 = masseter muscle; 10 = parotid gland; 11 = stylomandibular ligament; 12 = base of skull; A = sublingual space in the floor of the mouth above the mylohyoid muscle, which, over its posterior margin, leads to B = submandibular space; C = buccal vestibule, delineated by the buccinator from D = buccal space; E = submasseteric spaces formed by the multiple insertion of the masseter muscle on the lateral surface of the ramus; F = pterygomandibular space bounded by the lateral surface of the medial pterygoid muscle and the medial surface of the ramus; G = parapharyngeal space bounded by the superior constrictor of the pharynx and the medial surface of the medial pterygoid muscle; H = peritonsillar space bounded by the medial surface of the superior constrictor of the pharynx and its mucosa; I = parotid space (in and around the parotid gland).

goid, superior constrictor and orbicularis oris muscles. The fascial layers of the neck are less important in influencing the spread of infection around the jaws. None of the 'spaces' are actually empty; they are potential spaces normally occupied by loose connective tissue. It is only when inflammatory products (or bleeding or tumours) destroy the loose connective tissue that an anatomically defined space is produced.

Infection may spread from one tissue space to another where the spaces are in direct communication or along the side of structures that pass from one tissue space to another (such as blood vessels or nerves). Infection can also invade tissue spaces by directly eroding the intervening fascia. In addition to such direct pathways, infection may also spread through the lymphatics and the blood vessels.

The most important potential tissue spaces around the jaws are shown in Table 3.1. With the exception of the submental, submandibular and palatal spaces, all the tissue spaces listed in the table are paired.

Figure 3.34 shows the relationships of tissue spaces around the mandibular ramus. Because of the occurrence of inflammation in the soft tissues associated with partially impacted mandibular third molars (pericoronitis) and, less commonly, of dental abscesses of these teeth, the infratemporal fossa region is significant in terms of tissue spaces. This is due to the fact that the infratemporal fossa lies in a pivotal position, being intermediate between the tissue spaces of the face above and the tissue spaces of the neck below. The term **masticator tissue space** is sometimes used to describe the space enclosed by the investing layer of fascia ensheathing the muscles of mastication and the ramus of the mandible. The submasseteric, pterygomandibular, infratemporal and temporal tissue spaces are all part of this masticator tissue space.

## SUBMASSETERIC SPACE

The submasseteric space(s) may take the form of a series of spaces between the lateral surface of the ramus of the mandible and the masseter muscle. These spaces may form because the fibres of the masseter muscle have multiple insertions on to most of the lateral surface of the ramus and spaces may be found between the attachment of the superficial and deep parts of the muscle. Alternatively, they may relate to the passage of the neurovascular bundles. Whatever the true explanation, abscesses may develop between the masseter and the ramus of the mandible.

## PTERYGOMANDIBULAR SPACE

The pterygomandibular space lies between the ramus of the mandible laterally and the medial pterygoid muscle medially. Above lies the inferior head of the lateral pterygoid muscle. Anteriorly, beneath the overlying oral mucosa, lie fibres of the buccinator muscle, which arise from the pterygomandibular raphe. Immediately beneath the buccinator lies the tendon of the temporalis muscle. Posteriorly, the investing layer of deep cervical fascia covering the masseter and medial pterygoid muscles merges with the posterior border of the ramus, behind which lies the parotid gland. The

pterygomandibular space is a prominent component of the infratemporal fossa. Between the ramus of the mandible and the medial pterygoid muscle lie the inferior alveolar and lingual nerves: the pterygomandibular space is therefore the site of injection for an inferior alveolar nerve block. It also contains the maxillary artery and pterygoid venous plexus.

## INFRATEMPORAL SPACE

The infratemporal space is the upper extremity of the pterygomandibular space. It lies behind the maxilla and is bounded medially by the lateral pterygoid plate and above by the base of the skull. It is in continuity with the deep temporal space laterally.

## TEMPORAL SPACE

The temporal space consists of superficial and deep components that are found in relation to the temporalis muscle. The superficial temporal space lies on the lateral surface of the muscle, beneath the skin and the superficial (temporal) fascia. The deep temporal space lies between the medial (deep) surface of the muscle and the adjacent temporal bone.

Unlike infections involving odontogenic tissues that drain directly into the oral cavity (via the buccal or lingual sulci), those involving the tissue spaces around the infratemporal fossa do not drain directly into the oral cavity and have the potential to spread some distance through the head and neck. Of particular relevance in this regard are the tissue spaces around the pharynx, as involvement of these spaces may affect the larynx and thus compromise the airway. Symptoms associated with such conditions may include trismus, fever, dysphagia (difficulty in swallowing) and dyspnoea (difficulty in breathing), and patients must be treated quickly because of the potential development of life-threatening situations. In the most extreme situation, inflammation will eventually spread to involve the thorax.

## PHARYNGEAL SPACE

The pharyngeal tissue spaces can be subdivided into the peripharyngeal spaces around, and external to, the pharynx and the intrapharyngeal space within it. With regard to the peripharyngeal spaces there is the parapharyngeal space laterally and the retropharyngeal space posteriorly. Some anatomists also include the submental and submandibular spaces as pharyngeal tissue spaces because they lie immediately anteriorly.

Each *parapharyngeal space* (or lateral pharyngeal space) passes laterally around the pharynx and is continuous posteriorly with the retropharyngeal space. Unlike the retropharyngeal space, however, it is a space that is restricted to the suprahyoid region. It contains loose connective tissue and is bounded medially by the pharynx (superior constrictor muscle) and laterally by the pterygoid muscles and the parotid gland. Superiorly, it is bounded by the base of the skull. Inferiorly, it does not extend right down the neck but is limited by the suprahyoid structures, such as the fascia associated with the styloid group of muscles and the submandibular gland. Behind is situated the carotid sheath. The lateral pharyngeal space is partly divided by the styloid process and associated group of muscles into an anterior compartment containing muscle and a posterior compartment containing the carotid sheath and cranial nerves IX–XII.

The *retropharyngeal space* is the area of loose connective tissue lying behind the pharynx and in front of the prevertebral fascia. It extends upwards to the base of the skull and downwards to the retrovisceral space in the infrahyoid part of the neck.

An *intrapharyngeal* space potentially exists between the inner surface of the constrictor muscles of the pharynx and the pharyngeal mucosa. Infections at this site are either restricted locally or spread through the pharynx into the retropharyngeal or parapharyngeal spaces. An important part of the intrapharyngeal space is the peritonsillar space. This lies around the palatine tonsil, between the pillars of the fauces. Infections here (quinsy) usually spread up or down the intrapharyngeal space, or through the pharynx into the parapharyngeal space.

The parapharyngeal space is particularly prone to infections from the jaws and teeth. This space is restricted to the suprahyoid region of the neck and the infratemporal region. For infection to spread inferiorly from the parapharyngeal space, it must first pass into the retropharyngeal region because suprahyoid structures (particularly the sheath around the submandibular gland formed by the investing layer of deep cervical fascia) provide a restrictive inferior boundary.

The tissue spaces below the inferior border of the mandible and in the suprahyoid region of the neck (i.e. the submental and submandibular tissue spaces) are illustrated in Figure 3.35.

## SUBMENTAL SPACE

The submental space lies beneath the chin in the midline, between the mylohyoid muscles below and the investing layer of deep cervical fascia and platysma muscle superficially. It is bounded laterally by the two anterior bellies of the digastric muscles. The submental space communi-

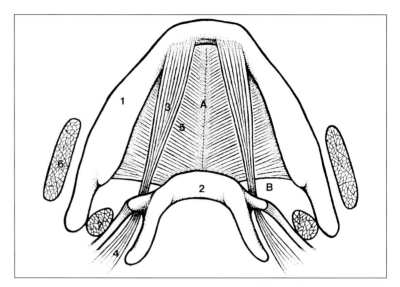

**Fig. 3.35** Inferior view of the submental and submandibular tissue spaces. 1 = body of mandible; 2 = hyoid bone; 3 = anterior belly of digastric muscle; 4 = posterior belly of digastric muscle; 5 = mylohyoid muscle; 6 = masseter muscle; 7 = medial pterygoid muscle; A = submental space lying between the mylohyoid muscle and the investing layer of deep cervical fascia. Laterally, it is bounded by the two anterior bellies of the digastric muscles. The submental space communicates posteriorly with the submandibular space (B) around the posterior border of the mylohyoid muscle.

cates posteriorly over the anterior bellies of the digastric muscles with the two submandibular spaces.

## SUBMANDIBULAR SPACE

The submandibular space is situated between the anterior and posterior bellies of the digastric muscle and is bounded above and laterally by the body of the mandible. It lies superficial to (below) the mylohyoid muscle (and more posteriorly the hyoglossus and styloglossus muscles) and is covered by the platysma muscle and by the investing layer of deep cervical fascia, which explains why abscesses in this region do not readily drain through the skin. The submandibular space communicates with the sublingual space around the posterior free border of the mylohyoid muscle and via small deficiencies within the muscular tissue of the mylohyoid muscle. The submandibular space contains the submandibular gland, facial vessels and submandibular lymph nodes. A submandibular abscess is commonly caused by spread of infection from the second or third mandibular molar tooth (see Fig. 3.39).

The suprahyoid spaces (*submental* and *submandibular spaces*) are bounded inferiorly by the attachment of the investing layer of deep cervical fascia to the hyoid bone. Consequently, if oedema or pus accumulates in the suprahyoid region there will be a restriction in the spread into the rest of the neck. This is potentially very dangerous because the suprahyoid region will swell markedly and restrict the airway (Ludwig's angina).

## SUBLINGUAL SPACE

Figure 3.36 illustrates the relationships of tissue spaces to the tongue. The *sublingual space* lies in the floor of the mouth, above the mylohyoid muscles and below the oral mucosa. It is delineated in front, and at the sides, by the body of the mandible and behind (and below) by the attachment of the mylohyoid muscle to the hyoid bone. The sublingual space contains the sublingual gland and the submandibular duct.

In the anterior region of both the upper and lower jaws, the orbicularis oris muscle presents a barrier to pus between the vestibule on the oral side and the skin of the lip on the facial side. In the upper jaw, pus may accumulate between the muscles of facial expression, particularly in the canine fossa between the levator labii superioris and zygomaticus muscles.

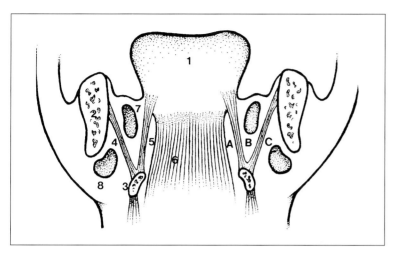

**Fig. 3.36** The relationships of a number of tissue spaces to the tongue. 1 = tongue; 2 = body of mandible; 3 = hyoid bone; 4 = mylohyoid muscle; 5 = hyoglossus; 6 = genioglossus; 7 = sublingual salivary gland; 8 = submandibular salivary gland; A = cleft between genioglossus and hyoglossus muscles that communicates directly with the parapharyngeal space; B = sublingual space between the mylohyoid and hyoglossus muscles; C = submandibular space below the mylohyoid muscle.

## OTHER TISSUE SPACES AROUND THE MOUTH

Other spaces around the mouth that need to be described are the buccal, parotid and palatal tissue spaces.

## BUCCAL SPACE

The buccal space is located in the cheek. It has the buccinator muscle (covered by a delicate connective tissue layer called the buccopharyngeal fascia) medially, the skin of the cheek laterally, the pterygomandibular raphe (giving origin to the buccinator muscle) posteriorly and some muscles of orbicularis oris anteriorly. The buccal space contains the parotid duct accompanied by blood vessels and branches of the facial nerve as well as the buccal pad of fat.

## PAROTID SPACE

The parotid space surrounds the parotid gland and its contents. It is defined by the parotid capsule. The superficial layer of the parotid capsule is of variable thickness and is not a typical fascia as it contains muscle fibres that parallel those of the platysma muscle. It appears to be continuous with the fascia associated with the platysma muscle. The deep surface of the parotid capsule is derived from the investing layer of deep cervical fascia. Above the level of the stylomandibular ligament, the deep surface of the parotid capsule may be thin and may serve as a communicating pathway into the lateral pharyngeal space.

## PALATAL SPACE

The palatal space in the hard palate exists only when pus strips the muco-periosteum from the underlying bone of the hard palate.

The way in which infections of dental origin spread through the bone of the jaws into the tissue spaces naturally depends upon the site at which the pus escapes the bone. Thus, pus from a periapical abscess in a mandibular incisor that escapes inferior to the mylohyoid muscle will enter the submental space, while pus escaping superior to this muscle will enter the sublingual space. It should also be borne in mind that the tissue spaces are not discrete regions; they intercommunicate. Thus, a sublingual abscess may spread from the sublingual space over the posterior margin of the mylohyoid muscle into the submandibular space (Figs 3.34, 3.35).

Furthermore, none of the muscle or fascial barriers defining the spaces is impenetrable.

## CLINICAL ASPECTS OF TISSUE SPACES

Infection of the infratemporal fossa is commonly met in dental practice and, because of the associated tissue spaces, is potentially dangerous. It is most commonly associated with a pericoronitis affecting a partially impacted mandibular third molar tooth. It may also be associated with a dental abscess of this tooth or occur as a result of infection following tooth extraction (dry socket). Rarely, it may result from an infected needle used during an inferior alveolar nerve block. Infection of the infratemporal region may be secondary, due to spread from an adjacent infected tissue space. An important determinant of the subsequent spread of infection from teeth depends on the relationship of the root apices to muscle. For example, if the discharge of a dental abscess from a cheek tooth is below the attachment of the buccinator muscle it will enter into the vestibule and drain harmlessly (Fig. 3.37). If, however, it drains above the attachment and into the buccal space, it will produce a fluctuant swelling over the cheek that will need surgical drainage (Fig. 3.38). Similarly, if an infected

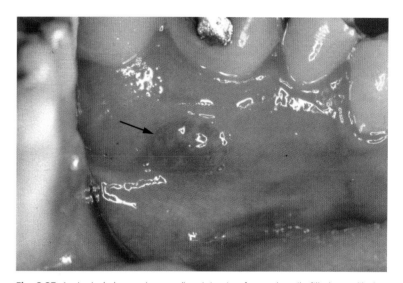

**Fig. 3.37** A gingival abscess (arrowed), originating from a heavily filled mandibular first permanent molar, which will discharge into the vestibular sulcus. Courtesy of Dr J. Potts.

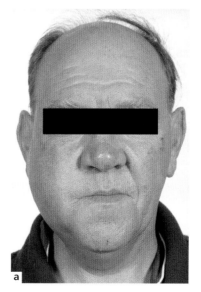 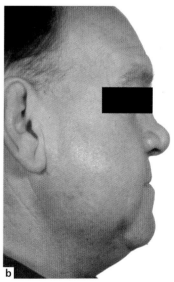

**Fig. 3.38** Buccal space infection on the right side. (a) Front view. (b) View from right side. Courtesy of Professor J. Langdon.

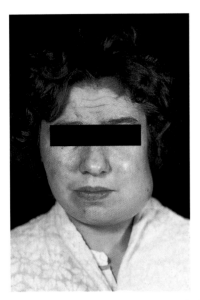

**Fig. 3.39** Abscess within the submandibular tissue space. Courtesy of Professor J. Langdon.

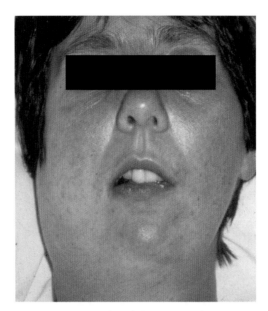

**Fig. 3.40** Patient with Ludwig's angina. There is sublingual and submandibular cellulites, with a painful swelling of the upper part of the neck and the floor of the mouth on both sides. Courtesy of Professor J. Langdon.

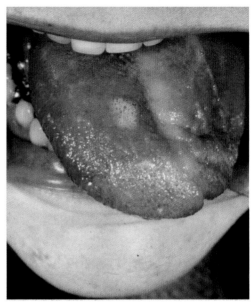

**Fig. 3.41** Patient with damage to the left hypoglossal nerve following removal of a malignant tumour associated with the submandibular gland. There has been wasting of muscles on the left side of the tongue. On protrusion of the tongue, there is deviation to the affected side due to unopposed activity of the unaffected musculature on the right side. Courtesy of Professor J. Langdon.

mandibular tooth drains above the attachment of the mylohyoid muscle, the infection would drain favourably into the oral cavity. If it drains below the attachment of mylohyoid, especially in the case of second and third mandibular molars, it may enter the submandibular tissue space and produce a swelling centred upon the upper part of the neck, mainly along the lower border of the mandible (Fig. 3.39).

As the tissue spaces are interconnected, infection may spread from the submandibular space into the sublingual or parapharyngeal spaces. Ludwig's angina is characterized by rapid development of sublingual and submandibular cellulitis with a painful, brawny swelling of the upper part of the neck and the floor of the mouth on both sides (Fig. 3.40). When the parapharyngeal tissue space becomes involved, the swelling tracks down the neck and oedema readily spreads into the loose connective tissue around the glottis. There is difficulty in swallowing, opening the mouth may be limited and the tongue may be pushed up against the soft palate. Oedema of the glottis can cause increasing respiratory obstruction. The patient soon becomes seriously ill, with fever, headache and malaise.

Cavernous sinus thrombosis is a serious complication that can also arise from spread of infection from a maxillary anterior tooth. Infected thrombi in the anterior facial vein communicate with the cavernous sinus via the ophthalmic veins (a less common spread is through infection in the ptery-goid plexus of veins reaching the cavernous sinus via emissary veins). Infection may also spread via the facial vein from infected spots or boils on the upper lip or in the anterior nares. In a cavernous sinus thrombosis, there is gross oedema of the eyelids together with pulsatile exophthalmos due to venous obstruction. The venous stasis also leads to cyanosis. The patient is seriously ill with rigors and a high, swinging pyrexia. Initially one side of the face is affected but, without treatment, both sides quickly become affected.

Lymphatic drainage of the infratemporal fossa region is into the sub-mandibular and upper deep cervical group of nodes, so that enlargement of the nodes in this region should alert the clinician to the possibility of infection arising in the infratemporal fossa.

Paralysis of the hypoglossal nerve, the XIIth cranial nerve, affects both the extrinsic and intrinsic muscles of the tongue on the affected side. When this occurs, and on asking a patient to protrude his/her tongue, the tongue deviates to the affected side (because the muscles on the unaffected side are still active; analogous to a ship turning in water as a result of the pro-

peller functioning on one side only) (Fig. 3.41). With time, there may be wasting of the tongue musculature on the paralysed side. The most common complaint is difficulty with speech, particularly for lingual sounds. With an upper motor neurone lesion, the tongue becomes spastic but does not waste. Thus, wasting is associated with a lower motor neurone lesion. The causes of hypoglossal nerve paralysis are many and may be associated with the course of the nerve either intracranially or extracranially. Tumours near the anterior condylar canal may be responsible, as may Paget's disease where the foramen is severely reduced in size. Hypoglossal nerve paralysis can also arise with trauma, with excessive stretching of the neck, with intradural synovial cysts, following tonsillectomy, with trauma and even as an unusual result of giving influenza vaccine!

The muscles of mastication may be damaged or become non-functional under some situations as a result of otherwise normal clinical procedures. For example, following 'blocking' of the inferior alveolar nerve with local anaesthetic solution injected into the infratemporal fossa, there may be painful reflex muscle spasm associated with the lateral and medial pterygoid muscles. This is termed 'trismus' and can result from bleeding into the muscles (haematoma) or from infection in the pterygomandibular space between the ramus of the mandible and the medial pterygoid muscle as a result of pericoronitis around an erupting third molar tooth. Externally, there may be little evidence of tissue swelling. Trismus may also result from TMJ dysfunction, from tetanus, from fracture of the mandibular condyle, or following a course of radiotherapy. Trismus nowadays is often used to describe any restriction to opening of the mouth. The inabil-ity to open the mouth can affect a patient's oral hygiene and ability to eat and chew. Furthermore, there may be problems with swallowing (particularly where there has been radiotherapy in the head and neck region). Additionally, and not surprisingly, a patient may have difficulty in speaking.

A pain reflex is elicited when a muscle is damaged; this is termed 'muscle guarding'. This pain results in muscle contraction and a restriction of the range of movements for the damaged muscle. This, being a reflex cannot readily be controlled by the patient. Should the trismus persist, there may be signs of atrophy of the muscles involved. Treatment should involve gentle passive movements of the jaw.

# Vasculature and innervation of the mouth

# 4

## BLOOD SUPPLY TO ORODENTAL TISSUES

The face is supplied mainly through the facial artery (Figs 4.1, 4.2; see also Fig. 3.27), a branch of the external carotid artery in the neck. The facial artery first appears on the face as it hooks round the lower border of the mandible, at the anterior edge of the masseter. It then runs a tortuous course between the facial muscles towards the medial angle of the eye. There is a rich anastomosis with the artery of the opposite side and with additional vessels supplying the face (transverse facial branch of the superficial temporal artery; infra-orbital and mental branches of the maxillary artery; dorsal nasal branch of the ophthalmic artery).

The main arteries to the teeth and jaws are derived from the maxillary artery, a terminal branch of the external carotid, which runs in the infra-temporal fossa (see Figs 3.31, 4.2). The alveolar arteries follow essentially the same course as the alveolar nerves.

## MANDIBULAR TEETH AND PERIODONTIUM

The inferior alveolar artery, which supplies the mandibular teeth, is derived from the maxillary artery before it crosses the lateral pterygoid muscle in the infratemporal fossa (Fig. 4.2). A mylohyoid branch is given off before the inferior alveolar artery enters the mandibular foramen in the ramus of the mandible. The inferior alveolar artery passes through the mandibular foramen to enter the mandibular canal and terminates as the mental and incisive arteries.

Posteriorly, the buccal gingiva is supplied by the buccal artery (a branch of the maxillary artery as it crosses the lateral pterygoid muscle) and by perforating branches from the inferior alveolar artery. Anteriorly, the labial gingiva is supplied by the mental artery and by perforating branches of the incisive artery. The lingual gingiva is supplied by perforating branches from the inferior alveolar artery and by the lingual artery, a branch of the external carotid artery.

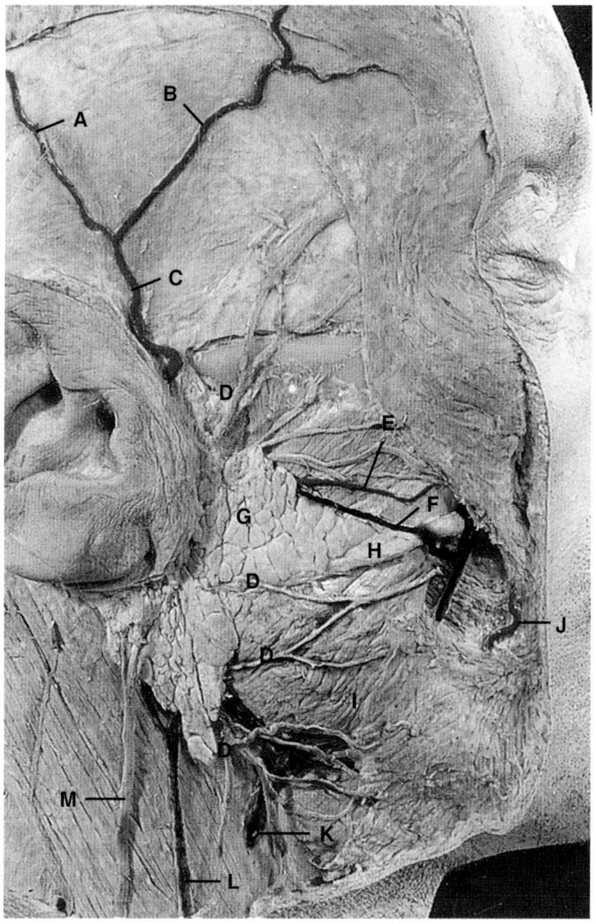

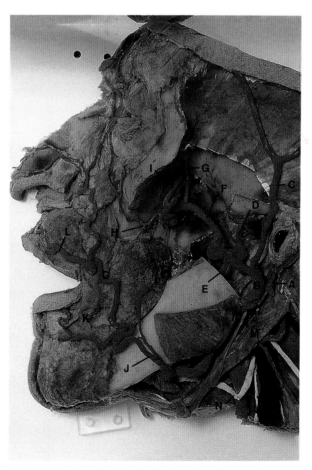

**Fig. 4.1** Blood supply to the face. A = parietal branch of superficial temporal artery; B = frontal branch of superficial temporal artery; C = superficial temporal artery; D = branches of facial nerve; E = transverse facial branch of superficial temporal artery; F = transverse facial vein; G = parotid gland; H = parotid duct; I = masseter muscle; J = facial artery; K = facial vein formed by anterior branch of the retromandibular vein and facial veins; L = external jugular vein formed by posterior branch of the retromandibular and posterior auricular veins; M = great auricular nerve on sternocleidomastoid muscle. Courtesy of Professor C. Dean.

**Fig. 4.2** Dissection showing the facial and maxillary arteries. A = posterior auricular artery; B = external carotid artery; C = superficial temporal artery; D = middle meningeal artery; E = inferior alveolar artery; F = maxillary artery; G = deep temporal artery; H = posterior superior alveolar artery; I = third part of maxillary artery entering the pterygopalatine fossa; J = facial artery; K = inferior labial artery; L = superior labial artery; M = posterior belly of the digastric muscle; N = hypoglossal nerve. Courtesy of Professor L. Garey.

## MAXILLARY TEETH AND PERIODONTIUM

The posterior superior alveolar artery arises from the maxillary artery in the pterygopalatine fossa. Occasionally, the posterior superior alveolar artery is derived from the buccal artery. It courses tortuously over the maxillary tuberosity before entering bony canals to supply molar and premolar teeth. The artery also gives off branches to the adjacent buccal gingiva, maxillary sinus and cheek.

The middle superior alveolar artery, when present, arises from the infra-orbital artery (which is itself a branch of the third part of the maxillary artery in the pterygopalatine fossa). The middle superior alveolar artery runs in the lateral wall of the maxillary sinus, terminating near the canine tooth where it anastomoses with the anterior and posterior superior alveolar arteries. The anterior superior alveolar artery also arises from the infra-orbital artery and runs downwards in the anterior wall of the maxillary sinus to supply the anterior teeth. As for the superior alveolar nerves, the superior alveolar arteries form plexuses above the root apices.

The buccal gingiva around the posterior maxillary teeth is supplied by gingival and perforating branches from the posterior superior alveolar artery and by the buccal artery. The labial gingiva of anterior teeth is supplied by labial branches of the infra-orbital artery and by perforating branches of the anterior superior alveolar artery.

The palatal gingiva around the maxillary teeth is supplied primarily by branches of the greater palatine artery, a branch of the third part of the maxillary artery in the pterygopalatine fossa.

## PALATE, CHEEK, TONGUE AND LIPS

The palate derives its blood supply from the greater and lesser palatine branches of the maxillary artery. The greater palatine artery passes through the incisive fossa, where it anastomoses with the nasopalatine artery. The cheek is supplied by the buccal branch of the maxillary artery and the floor of the mouth and the tongue by the lingual arteries. The lips are mainly supplied by the superior and inferior labial branches of the facial arteries.

### VENOUS DRAINAGE OF ORODENTAL TISSUES

The venous drainage of this region is extremely variable. The facial vein is the main vein draining the face (see Figs 3.27, 4.1). It begins at the medial corner of the eye by confluence of the supra-orbital and supra-trochlear veins and passes across the face behind the facial artery. Below the mandible, it receives the anterior branch of the retromandibular vein before draining into the internal jugular vein.

## TEETH AND PERIODONTIUM

Small veins from the teeth and alveolar bone pass into larger veins surrounding the apex of each tooth, or into veins running in the interdental septa. In the mandible, the veins are then collected into one or more inferior alveolar veins, which themselves may drain anteriorly through the mental foramen to join the facial vein or posteriorly through the mandibular foramen to join the pterygoid plexus of veins in the infratemporal fossa. In the maxilla, the veins may drain anteriorly into the facial vein or posteriorly into the pterygoid plexus. No accurate description is available concerning the venous drainage of the gingiva, although it may be assumed that the buccal, lingual, greater palatine and nasopalatine veins are involved; apart from the lingual veins (which pass directly into the internal jugular veins), these veins run into the pterygoid plexuses.

## PALATE, CHEEK, TONGUE AND LIPS

The veins of the palate are rather diffuse and variable. However, those of the hard palate generally pass into the pterygoid venous plexus, those of the soft palate into the pharyngeal venous plexus. The buccal vein of the cheek drains into the pterygoid plexus. Venous blood from the lips drains into the facial veins via the superior and inferior labial veins. The veins of the tongue follow two different routes: those of the dorsum and sides of the tongue form the lingual veins, which, accompanying the lingual arteries, empty into the internal jugular veins; those of the ventral surface form the deep lingual veins (see Fig. 1.14), which ultimately join the facial, internal jugular or lingual veins.

### LYMPHATIC DRAINAGE OF ORODENTAL TISSUES

As with the venous system, the lymphatic drainage is extremely variable: Figure 4.3 provides a 'consensus' view of the lymphatic drainage of the oral structures.

Lymphatics from the lower part of the face generally pass through, or around, the buccal lymph nodes to reach the submandibular lymph nodes. However, lymphatics from the medial portion of the lower lip drain into the submental nodes.

The lymph vessels from the teeth usually run directly into the submandibular nodes on the same side. However, lymph from the mandibular incisors drains into the submental nodes. Occasionally, lymph from the molars passes directly into the jugulodigastric group of nodes.

The lymph vessels of the labial and buccal gingivae of the maxillary and mandibular teeth unite to drain into the submandibular nodes, although in the labial region of the mandibular incisors they may drain into the submental nodes. The lingual and palatal gingivae drain into the jugulodigastric group of nodes, either directly or indirectly through the submandibular nodes.

Lymphatics from most areas of the palate terminate in the jugulodigastric group of nodes. Vessels from the posterior part of the soft palate terminate in pharyngeal lymph nodes. Lymph from the floor of the mouth region can drain directly to the jugulodigastric nodes.

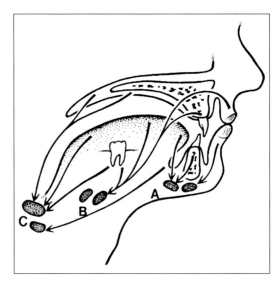

**Fig. 4.3** Lymphatic drainage of oral structures. A = submental nodes; B = submandibular nodes; C = jugulodigastric nodes.

Lymphatics from the anterior two-thirds of the tongue may be sub-divided into two groups: marginal and central vessels. The marginal lymphatic vessels drain the lateral third of the dorsum of the tongue and the lateral margin of its ventral surface. The remaining regions drain into the central vessels. The marginal vessels pass to the submandibular lymph nodes of the same side. The central vessels at the tip of the tongue pass to the submental lymph nodes. Central vessels behind the tip drain into ipsilateral and contralateral submandibular lymph nodes. Some marginal and central lymph vessels pass directly to the jugulodigastric group of nodes (or even the jugulo-omohyoid nodes). Lymphatics from the posterior third of the tongue drain into the deep cervical group of nodes, vessels centrally draining both ipsilaterally and contralaterally. Knowledge of the ipsilateral and contralateral drainage from the tongue is important clinically where, for example, a tumour near the central part of the tongue may be associated with spread into lymph nodes on both sides.

At the oropharyngeal isthmus lie the palatine tonsils between the pillars of the fauces (see Fig. 1.11) and the lingual tonsils on the pharyngeal surface of the tongue (see Fig. 1.15). These tonsils form part of a ring of lymphoid tissue known as Waldeyer's tonsillar ring. The other components are the tubal tonsils and adenoid tissue (pharyngeal tonsils) located in the nasopharynx.

## INNERVATION OF ORODENTAL TISSUES

Excepting regions around the oropharyngeal isthmus, the oral mucosa receives sensory innervation from the maxillary and mandibular divisions of the trigeminal nerve. The trigeminal nerve also supplies the teeth and their supporting tissues (Table 4.1). Both the major and minor salivary glands are supplied by secretomotor parasympathetic fibres from the facial and glossopharyngeal nerves. The motor innervation of the muscles of the jaws and oral cavity is from the trigeminal, facial, accessory and hypoglossal nerves.

Figure 4.4 illustrates the cutaneous innervation of the face. All three divisions of the trigeminal nerve are involved, the ophthalmic division supplying the upper part of the face, forehead and scalp, and the maxillary and mandibular divisions essentially supplying the upper and lower jaw regions, respectively. Knowledge of these areas, and of the specific branches involved, is important clinically for assessing the effects of nerve damage and for an understanding of the successful anaesthetizing of the buccal, infra-orbital and inferior alveolar (mental) nerves during dental treatment. The areas supplied by the three divisions of the trigeminal nerve also relate to aspects of the development of the face (see pages 278–279).

**Table 4.1** *Nerve supply to the teeth and gingivae*

| | | | | | | | | | |
|---|---|---|---|---|---|---|---|---|---|
| | Nasopalatine nerve | Greater palatine nerve | | | | | | | Palatal gingiva |
| Maxilla | Anterior superior alveolar nerve | Middle superior alveolar nerve | | | Posterior superior alveolar nerve | | | | Teeth |
| | Infra-orbital nerve | Posterior superior alveolar nerve and buccal nerve | | | | | | | Buccal gingiva |
| | 1 | 2 | 3 | 4 | 5 | 6 | 7 | 8 | Tooth position (Palmer-Zsigmondy system) |
| | Mental nerve | Buccal nerve and perforating branches of inferior alveolar nerve | | | | | | | Buccal gingiva |
| Mandible | Incisive nerve | Inferior alveolar nerve | | | | | | | Teeth |
| | Lingual nerve and perforating branches of inferior alveolar nerve | | | | | | | | Lingual gingiva |

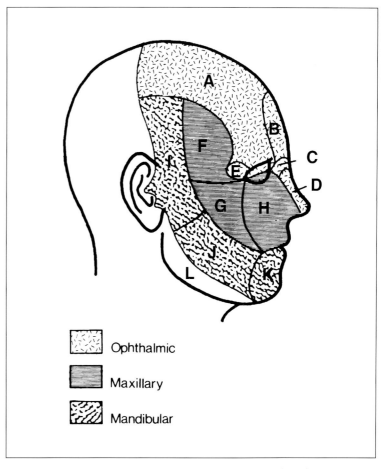

**Fig. 4.4** Schematic diagram showing cutaneous innervation of the face. A = supra-orbital nerve; B = supratrochlear nerve; C = infratrochlear nerve; D = external nasal nerve; E = lacrimal nerve; F = zygomaticotemporal nerve; G = zygomaticofacial nerve; H = infra-orbital nerve; I = auriculotemporal nerve; J = buccal nerve; K = mental nerve; L = great auricular nerve.

Ophthalmic

Maxillary

Mandibular

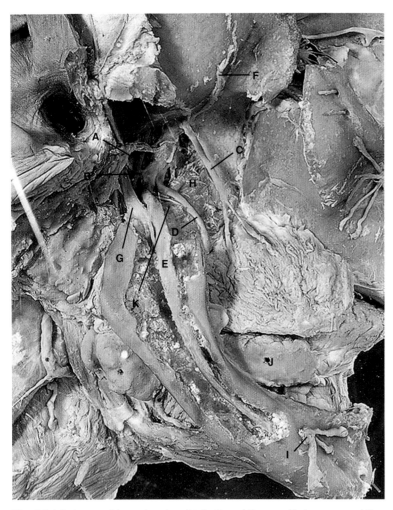

**Fig. 4.5** Infratemporal fossa showing distribution of the mandibular nerve and the course of its inferior alveolar branch.
A = auriculotemporal nerve
B = middle meningeal artery
C = buccal branch
D = lingual nerve
E = inferior alveolar nerve with mylohyoid branch
F = deep temporal nerve
G = sphenomandibular ligament
H = medial pterygoid muscle
I = mental nerve
J = sublingual gland
K = chorda tympani.
Courtesy of Professor C. Dean.

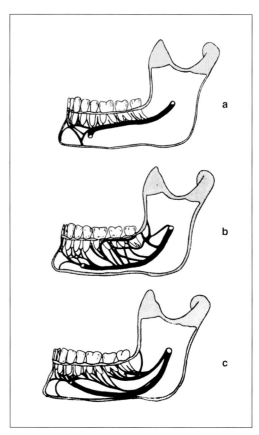

**Fig. 4.6** Schematic diagram showing variation in the course of the inferior alveolar nerve through the mandible. Redrawn after Drs R.B. Carter and E.N. Keen.

## INFERIOR ALVEOLAR NERVE

The course of the inferior alveolar nerve through the mandible is illustrated in Figures 4.5 and 4.6. The distribution of nerves to the mandibular premolars and molars is variable, dental branches coming either directly from the inferior alveolar nerve by short (Fig. 4.6a) or long (Fig. 4.6b) branches or indirectly through several alveolar branches (Fig. 4.6c). In rare instances, the nerve to the mandibular third molar may arise from the inferior alveolar nerve before it enters the mandibular canal. Communications between the inferior alveolar nerve and nerves from the temporalis and lateral pterygoid muscles have been described, the nerves penetrating the mandible through foramina in the region of muscle attachments. It has been suggested that such nerve connections might explain why, in approxi-

mately 5% of patients, the teeth may not be anaesthetized after the main trunk of the inferior alveolar nerve has been blocked at the mandibular foramen by the injection of local anaesthetic solution.

It is said that, in any one individual, the mandibular canal remains in a relatively fixed position with respect to the lower border of the mandible. The canal is often closely related to the roots of the mandibular molars. Indeed, the roots of lower third molars may even be perforated by the mandibular canal.

In the premolar region the main trunk of the inferior alveolar nerve divides into mental and incisive nerves. The mental nerve runs for a short distance in a mental canal before leaving the body of the mandible at the mental foramen to emerge on to the face. In about 50% of cases, the mental foramen lies on a vertical line passing through the mandibular second premolar. However, in negroid ethnic groups, the mental foramen may be situated slightly more posteriorly, midway between the roots of the second premolar and first permanent molar. In an adult with a full dentition, the mental foramen usually lies midway between the upper and lower borders of the mandible. During the first and second years of life, as the prominence of the chin develops, the opening of the mental foramen alters in direction, from facing forwards to facing upwards and backwards. As well as supplying the skin of the lower lip, the mental nerve provides fibres to an incisor plexus that innervates the labial periodontium of the mandibular incisors. The incisive nerve runs forwards in an intraosseous incisive canal. This nerve primarily supplies the incisors and canines but may also supply the first premolar. In some instances, the canine may be supplied directly from the inferior alveolar nerve.

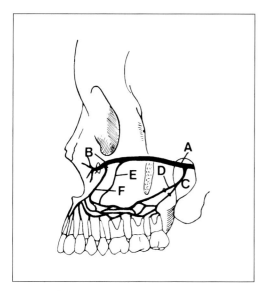

**Fig. 4.7** The superior alveolar nerves and associated dental plexuses.
A = trunk of maxillary division of the trigeminal nerve
B = infra-orbital nerve
C = pterygopalatine fossa
D = posterior superior alveolar nerves
E = middle superior alveolar nerve
F = anterior superior alveolar nerve.

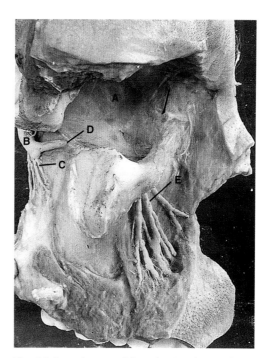

**Fig. 4.8** Frontal aspect of face showing the maxillary nerve;
A = orbit
B = maxillary nerve
C = posterior superior alveolar nerve
D = infra-orbital nerve in floor of orbit
E = infra-orbital nerve entering the face at the infra-orbital foramen.

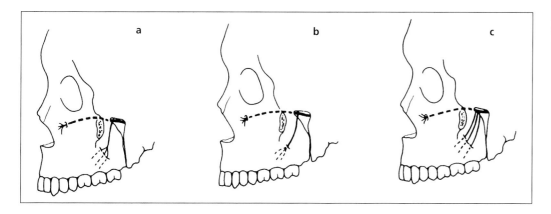

**Fig. 4.9** Three different patterns for the posterior superior alveolar nerves on the tuberosity of the maxilla.

## SUPERIOR ALVEOLAR NERVES

The superior alveolar nerves and associated dental plexuses are shown in Figure 4.7. The posterior superior alveolar nerve arises from the maxillary nerve in the pterygopalatine fossa, whence it passes through the pterygomaxillary fissure to descend on the posterior wall (tuberosity) of the maxilla (Fig. 4.8). The dental branches of the nerve enter the maxilla and run in narrow posterior superior alveolar canals above the roots of the molar teeth. A gingival branch does not enter the bone, however, but runs downwards and forwards along the outer surface of the maxillary tuberosity. The dental branches of the posterior superior alveolar nerve may arise from a common nerve trunk within the bone (Fig. 4.9b) or on the tuberosity before entering bone (Fig. 4.9a), or alternatively may appear as separate nerve trunks from the main trunk of the maxillary nerve in the pterygopalatine fossa (Fig. 4.9c). The middle superior alveolar nerve is found in about 70% of subjects. The nerve generally arises from the infraorbital nerve in the floor of the orbit/roof of the maxillary air sinus, although it may arise from the maxillary nerve in the pterygopalatine fossa.

The nerve may run in the posterior, lateral or anterior walls of the maxillary sinus. It terminates above the roots of the premolar teeth. The anterior superior alveolar nerve arises from the infra-orbital nerve within the infraorbital canal, generally as a single nerve but occasionally as two or three small branches. The nerve leaves the infra-orbital canal near its termination and then, diverging laterally from the infra-orbital nerve, runs in the anterior wall of the maxillary sinus. It terminates near the anterior nasal spine after giving off a small nasal branch. Note that the posterior superior alveolar nerve has an extra-bony course that permits anaesthesia of the nerve trunk(s) as it passes across the maxillary tuberosity, whereas the middle and anterior superior alveolar nerves are entirely intra-bony in their course and cannot be 'blocked' with an anaesthetic injection.

The superior alveolar nerve forms a plexus above the root apices of the maxillary teeth (Fig. 4.7). From this plexus, nerves pass to the teeth, although it is difficult to trace the precise innervation of the teeth from specific superior alveolar nerves. As a general rule, however, the incisors and canines are supplied by the anterior nerve, the molars by the posterior nerve and intermediate areas by the middle nerve.

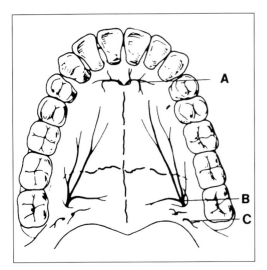

**Fig. 4.10** The sensory nerve supply to the palate. A = nasopalatine nerves; B = greater palatine nerve; C = lesser palatine nerve.

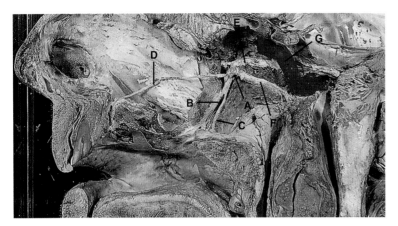

**Fig. 4.11** The pterygopalatine ganglion (A) giving rise to the greater (B) and lesser (C) palatine nerves and the nasopalatine nerve (D). E = maxillary nerve; F = nerve of pterygoid canal; G = internal carotid artery.

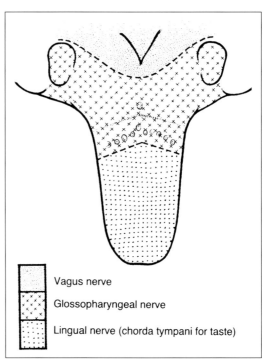

**Fig. 4.12** Schematic representation of the sensory innervation of the tongue.

Vagus nerve

Glossopharyngeal nerve

Lingual nerve (chorda tympani for taste)

## SENSORY NERVES TO ORAL CAVITY

The sensory nerve supply to the palate is described in Figures 4.10 and 4.11. The nerve supply is derived from the maxillary division of the trigeminal nerve via branches of the pterygopalatine ganglion. A small area behind the maxillary incisor teeth is supplied by terminal branches of the nasopalatine nerves. These nerves emerge on to the palate at the incisive fossa. The remainder of the hard palate is supplied by the greater palatine nerves emerging on to the palate at the greater palatine foramina. The soft palate is supplied by the lesser palatine nerves emerging on to the palate via the lesser palatine foramina. Although the maxillary division of the trigeminal nerve supplies most of the palate, there is evidence to suggest that some areas supplied by the lesser palatine nerves may also be innervated by fibres from the facial nerve. The posterior part of the soft palate and the uvula may be supplied by the glossopharyngeal nerve.

The sensory innervation of the tongue is illustrated in Figure 4.12. Three distinct nerve fields can be recognized on the dorsum of the tongue. The anterior part of the tongue, in front of the circumvallate papillae, is supplied by the lingual branch of the mandibular division of the trigeminal nerve (Fig. 4.5). However, its accompanying chorda tympani fibres from the nervus intermedius part of the facial nerve are those associated with the perception of taste. Figure 4.5 shows the chorda tympani joining the lingual nerve in the infratemporal fossa. Behind, and including the circum-

vallate papillae, the tongue is supplied primarily by the glossopharyngeal nerve (providing both general sensation and taste). A small area on the posterior part of the tongue around the epiglottis is supplied by the vagus nerve (via its superior laryngeal branch). The mucosa on the ventral surface of the tongue is supplied by the lingual nerve.

The mucosa of the upper lip is supplied by the infra-orbital branch of the maxillary division of the trigeminal nerve. That of the lower lip is supplied by the mental branch of the mandibular division of the trigeminal nerve (Fig. 4.5). The mucosa of the cheeks is supplied by the buccal branch of the mandibular division of the trigeminal. The mucosa on the floor of the mouth is innervated by the lingual branch of the mandibular division of the trigeminal nerve. The mucosa over the pillars of the fauces (the oropharyngeal isthmus) is supplied by the glossopharyngeal nerve.

## SECRETOMOTOR INNERVATION OF THE SALIVARY GLANDS

### PAROTID GLAND

The secretomotor supply of the parotid gland (Fig. 4.13) is derived through the otic parasympathetic ganglion. This ganglion is situated in the roof of the infratemporal fossa, close to the foramen ovale and the mandibular division of the trigeminal nerve. Like other parasympathetic ganglia in the head, three types of nerve fibre are associated with it: parasympathetic, sympathetic and sensory. However, only the parasympathetic fibres synapse in the ganglion. The preganglionic parasympathetic fibres to the otic ganglion originate from the inferior salivatory nucleus in the brainstem and pass with the glossopharyngeal nerve via its lesser petrosal branch. The sympathetic root of the otic ganglion is derived from postganglionic fibres from the superior cervical ganglion and reaches the otic ganglion via the plexus around the middle meningeal artery in the infratemporal fossa. The sensory root is derived from the auriculotemporal branch of the mandibular division of the trigeminal nerve. The postganglionic parasympathetic fibres (with sensory and sympathetic fibres) reach the parotid gland through the auriculotemporal branch of the mandibular nerve.

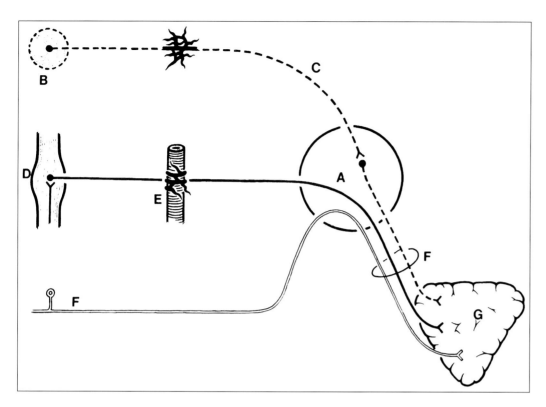

**Fig. 4.13** The secretomotor supply to the parotid salivary gland.
A = otic parasympathetic ganglion; B = inferior salivary nucleus; C = lesser petrosal branch of the glossopharyngeal nerve; D = postganglionic fibres from the superior cervical ganglion; E = sympathetic plexus around the middle meningeal artery; F = auriculotemporal branch of mandibular division of trigeminal nerve; G = parotid gland.

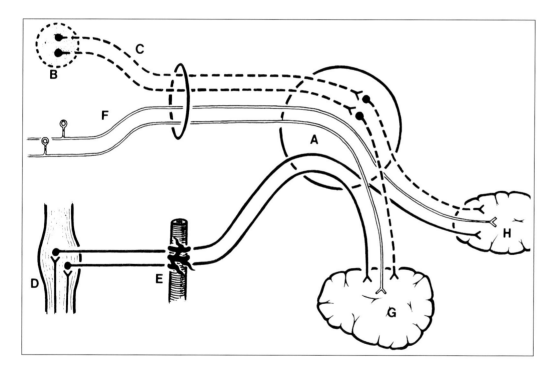

**Fig. 4.14** The secretomotor supply to the submandibular and sublingual salivary glands.
A = submandibular parasympathetic ganglion; B = superior salivatory nucleus; C = chorda tympani branch of facial nerve; D = postganglionic fibres from the superior cervical ganglion; E = sympathetic plexus around the facial artery; F = lingual nerve; G = submandibular gland; H = sublingual gland.

## SUBMANDIBULAR AND SUBLINGUAL GLANDS

The secretomotor supply of the submandibular and sublingual glands (Fig. 4.14) is derived through the submandibular parasympathetic ganglion. This ganglion is situated, with the lingual nerve, on the hyoglossus muscle in the floor of the mouth above the deep part of the submandibular gland. The preganglionic parasympathetic fibres to the ganglion originate from the superior salivatory nucleus in the brainstem and pass with the nervus intermedius of the facial nerve, and subsequently its chorda tympani branch, to reach the lingual nerve in the infratemporal fossa (Fig. 4.5). It is via the lingual nerve that the preganglionic fibres are conveyed to the submandibular ganglion. The sympathetic root of the ganglion is derived from postganglionic fibres from the superior cervical ganglion and reaches the submandibular ganglion via the plexus around the facial artery. The sensory root is derived from the lingual nerve. The postganglionic parasympathetic fibres (with sensory and sympathetic fibres) pass directly to the adjacent submandibular gland but reach the sublingual gland after re-entering the lingual nerve.

**Table 4.2** *Innervation of the oral musculature*

| Region | Muscle | Nerve |
|---|---|---|
| Lips | Orbicularis oris | Facial |
| Cheeks | Buccinator | Facial |
| Tongue (intrinsic musculature) | Transverse Longitudinal Vertical | Hypoglossal |
| Tongue (extrinsic musculature) | Genioglossus Hyoglossus Styloglossus Palatoglossus | Hypoglossal Accessory (cranial part) |
| Floor of mouth | Mylohyoid Geniohyoid | Mandibular division of trigeminal Hypoglossal (CI fibres) |
| Palate | Tensor veli palatini Levator veli palatini Palatoglossus Palatopharyngeus Musculus uvulae | Mandibular division of trigeminal Accessory (cranial part) |

## INNERVATION OF THE ORAL MUSCULATURE

The functions of mastication, swallowing and speech are among the most complex in the body. This is reflected in the number and variety of muscles found around the mouth and by the range of cranial nerves that innervate them. Table 4.2 summarizes the innervation of the oral musculature.

## TRIGEMINAL NERVE (MAXILLARY AND MANDIBULAR DIVISIONS)

### MAXILLARY DIVISION

The maxillary division of the trigeminal nerve (Figs 4.15, 4.16; see also Figs 4.8 and 4.11) contains only sensory fibres. It supplies the maxillary teeth and their supporting structures, the palate, the maxillary air sinus, much of the nasal cavity and the skin overlying the middle part of the face. The nerve emerges into the pterygopalatine fossa through the foramen rotundum of the sphenoid bone. Its subsequent branches can be subdivided into branches from the main nerve trunk (Fig. 4.15) and branches from the pterygopalatine ganglion (Fig. 4.16). From the main trunk are the meningeal, ganglionic, zygomatic, posterior superior alveolar and infra-

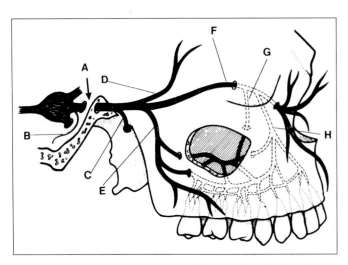

**Fig. 4.15** Diagrammatic representation of the maxillary division of the trigeminal nerve and the branches that are derived directly from the nerve trunk.
A = maxillary nerve trunk passing through the foramen rotundum into the pterygopalatine fossa; B = meningeal branch; C = ganglionic branch; D = main zygomatic nerve; E = posterior superior alveolar nerve; F = infra-orbital nerve; G = middle superior alveolar nerve; H = anterior superior alveolar nerve.

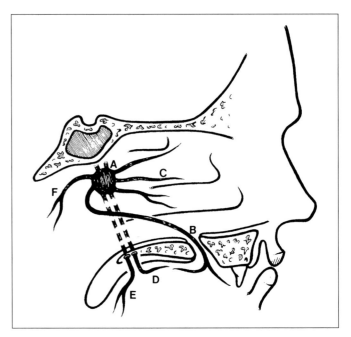

**Fig. 4.16** Diagrammatic representation of the maxillary division of the trigeminal nerve and the branches that are derived via the pterygopalatine ganglion. A = pterygopalatine ganglion; B = nasopalatine nerve; C = posterior superior nasal nerve; D = greater palatine nerve; E = lesser palatine nerve; F = pharyngeal nerve.

orbital nerves. The infra-orbital nerve gives rise to the middle and anterior superior alveolar nerves. The branches of the maxillary nerve that arise via the pterygopalatine ganglion contain a mixture of sensory, parasympathetic (secretomotor) and sympathetic (vasomotor) fibres. The branches arising from the ganglion are the orbital, nasopalatine, posterior superior nasal, greater and lesser palatine, and pharyngeal nerves. Thus, the branches supplying the teeth and their supporting structures and the palate and the upper lip are the posterior, middle and anterior superior alveolar nerves, the nasopalatine and the greater and lesser palatine nerves, and the infra-orbital nerve.

### MANDIBULAR DIVISION

The mandibular division of the trigeminal nerve (Fig. 4.17; see also Figs 3.31 and 4.5) is the largest division of the trigeminal nerve. It is the only division that contains motor fibres as well as sensory fibres. Its sensory fibres supply the mandibular teeth (and their supporting structures), the mucosa of the anterior two-thirds of the tongue and the floor of the mouth, the skin of the lower part of the face, and parts of the temple and auricle. Its motor fibres supply the muscles of mastication, the mylohyoid, the anterior belly of the digastric, and the tensor veli palatini and tensor tympani muscles. The mandibular nerve emerges into the infratemporal fossa through the foramen ovale of the sphenoid bone. It lies deep to the lateral pterygoid muscle, where it gives off all its branches, dividing into anterior (mainly motor) and posterior (mainly sensory) trunks. Proximal to this division, it gives off the meningeal branch and the nerve to the medial pterygoid.

The meningeal branch passes back into the middle cranial fossa through the foramen spinosum of the sphenoid bone (accompanied by the middle meningeal artery). The nerve to the medial pterygoid muscle passes through the otic ganglion (without synapsing) and, after supplying the muscle, continues on to supply the tensor veli palatini and tensor tympani muscles. The anterior trunk gives motor branches to the masseter, temporalis and lateral pterygoid, and the sensory buccal nerve. The posterior trunk gives off the sensory auriculotemporal, lingual and inferior alveolar nerves, and the motor mylohyoid nerve. Note that the chorda tympani branch of the facial nerve joins the lingual nerve and that postganglionic

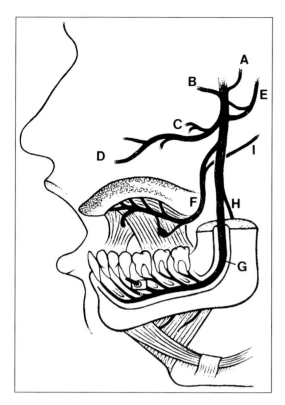

**Fig. 4.17** Schematic diagram of the mandibular division of the trigeminal nerve. A = meningeal branch; B = nerve to medial pterygoid; C = anterior trunk giving motor branches to masseter, temporalis and lateral pterygoid muscles; D = buccal nerve; E = auriculotemporal nerve; F = lingual nerve; G = inferior alveolar nerve; H = mylohyoid nerve; I = chorda tympani branch of facial nerve joining the lingual nerve.

fibres from the otic parasympathetic ganglion run with the auriculotemporal nerve to provide secretomotor fibres to the parotid gland.

## CENTRAL CONNECTIONS

Central connections of the trigeminal nerve are summarized in Figure 4.18. The trigeminal nerve conveys discriminative tactile information from the ipsilateral half of the face and the top of the head; the axons of the trigeminal ganglion cells pass to the principal sensory nucleus and to the pars oralis of the spinal tract of the trigeminal nerve. Proprioceptive information from the ipsilateral muscles of mastication and the temporomandibular joint reaches the mesencephalic nucleus of the trigeminal. However, recent evidence suggests that proprioceptive information from the teeth also passes to the principal sensory nucleus. Direct and indirect connections of these nuclei form the basis of cranial nerve reflexes. Signals from the principal sensory and mesencephalic nuclei are transmitted mainly via the contralateral ventral trigeminothalamic tract (trigeminal lemniscus) and the ipsilateral dorsal trigeminothalamic tract to the nucleus ventralis posterior medialis of the thalamus. Axons from this nucleus

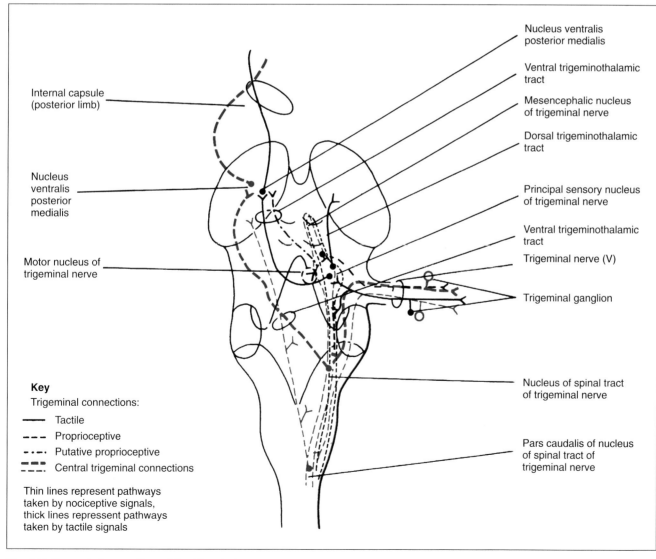

**Fig. 4.18** The central connections of the trigeminal nerve.

pass through the posterior limb of the internal capsule to the inferior part of the postcentral gyrus and frontoparietal operculum. The nucleus of the spinal tract of the trigeminal nerve is subdivided into the pars oralis, pars interpolaris and pars caudalis. The pars oralis deals mainly with tactile signals. The pars interpolaris receives cutaneous and proprioceptive information and sends fibres to the cerebellum. The pars caudalis deals particularly with nociceptive signals (but also with tactile and thermal information). Fibres from the nucleus of the spinal tract pass to the reticular formation (for cranial nerve reflexes). Some fibres run near the medial lemniscus in the contralateral ventral trigeminothalamic tract to reach the various thalamic nuclei. The motor nucleus of the trigeminal nerve lies close to the principal central nucleus in the central part of the pons. It receives fibres from the other sensory trigeminal nuclei, the reticular formation, the cerebellum and the cerebral cortex via bilateral corticonuclear fibres.

## CLINICAL CONSIDERATIONS OF THE INNERVATION OF THE MOUTH

In anaesthetizing the teeth during various dental procedures, local infiltration techniques are usually adequate where the surrounding alveolar bone is thin (such as in the maxilla and anterior region of the mandible). However, when treating the mandibular cheek teeth, which are surrounded by thicker bone, it is necessary to anaesthetize the inferior alveolar nerve in the infratemporal fossa, before it enters the mandibular canal. This involves placing the needle in the pterygomandibular space in a procedure known as an inferior alveolar nerve block (Fig. 4.19). In the routine open-mouth direct method, the patient is asked to open their mouth widely and, with the syringe held over the opposite mandibular first premolar tooth, the needle is inserted into the triangular fossa situated between the ridges overlying the base of the pterygomandibular raphe medially and the internal oblique ridge of the ramus of the mandible laterally. The needle is advanced about 1 cm where it comes close to the ramus and the inferior

alveolar (and lingual) nerve. The needle should lie about 1 cm above the occlusal surface of the mandibular teeth. An alternative method intended to anaesthetize the whole of the mandibular nerve seeks to inject the anaesthetic solution at a higher level within the pterygomandibular space and is known as the intra-oral 'high condyle' (Gow–Gates) technique.

From a knowledge of the anatomy of the infratemporal fossa (Fig. 4.19), the following common complications may arise following an inferior alveolar nerve block:

- If the needle (and anaesthetic solution) is injected too far medially it may penetrate the medial pterygoid muscle; if placed too far laterally, it may penetrate the temporalis muscle. In either case, there will be an absence of anaesthesia that may be followed by trismus (painful spasm of the muscle).
- If the needle is advanced too deeply, the facial nerve may be affected and a temporary unilateral facial palsy may result.
- The needle may rupture a vein(s) associated with the pterygoid venous plexus, resulting in a haematoma.
- If the needle directly encounters the inferior alveolar nerve, the patient may experience the sensation of an 'electric shock'. The needle must be withdrawn before injecting the anaesthetic solution.
- Local anaesthetic solution may pass into the pterygomandibular space and thence into the inferior orbital fissure. The closest nerve is the abducent nerve, which may be temporarily anaesthetized, resulting in diplopia (double vision) due to paralysis of the lateral rectus muscle.
- The needle may penetrate the inferior alveolar artery, but to prevent the dire consequences of injecting anaesthetic solution directly into the artery, the needle should always be aspirated first.

If a careful aseptic technique is not attained during anaesthesia, the possibility arises of introducing infective agents into the pterygomandibular space. From here, infection may spread to adjacent tissue spaces (see pages 76–80). Infection may spread via emissary veins from the pterygoid venous plexus to the cavernous sinus.

Even if a correct inferior alveolar nerve block is administered to anaesthetize a molar tooth, pain may still be felt by a patient undergoing a clinical procedure. This 'escape from anaesthesia' may be related to anatomical variation. For example, a nerve branch supplying the tooth may arise high up from the parent inferior alveolar nerve in the infratemporal fossa and be unaffected by the normal nerve block injection given lower down. Occasionally, additional branches supplying the tooth pass with the buccal or temporal branches of the mandibular nerve. Additional local infiltration of anaesthetic solution around the tooth may solve the problem.

Knowledge of the anatomy of the inferior alveolar nerve is important when extracting teeth. The mental nerve exits the mental foramen, which lies close to the root apices of the mandibular premolar teeth (see Fig. 2.154) and may be at risk when surgically removing the roots of such teeth. A clear radiograph of the region must be available to alert the operator of any problems, such as the presence of an abnormally long root. Damage to the mental nerve will manifest itself as paraesthesia in the lower lip of the affected side.

During the surgical removal of impacted mandibular third molars the inferior alveolar and lingual nerves are at risk of damage. The inferior alveolar nerve may sometimes lie close to or even between the roots. This close relationship may be evident in radiographs, with the radiolucent nerve canal being superimposed on roots or being constricted (see Fig. 2.180) as one of the warning signs. Symptoms of damage affecting its terminal mental branch include paraesthesia to the lower lip on the affected side.

The close relationship of the lingual nerve to the alveolar process of the third molar tooth makes the nerve susceptible to damage during removal

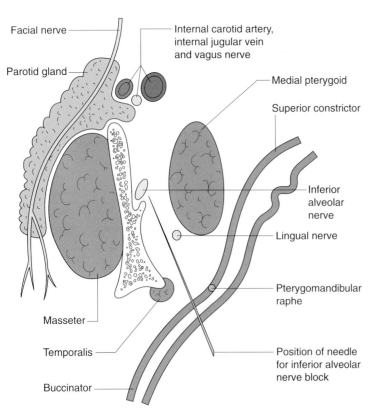

Facial nerve

Parotid gland

Internal carotid artery, internal jugular vein and vagus nerve

Medial pterygoid

Superior constrictor

Inferior alveolar nerve

Lingual nerve

Pterygomandibular raphe

Masseter

Temporalis

Position of needle for inferior alveolar nerve block

Buccinator

**Fig. 4.19** Diagram showing position of needle in an inferior alveolar nerve block.

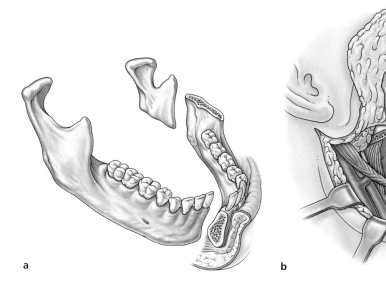

a b

**Fig. 4.20** The transmandibular surgical approach to the infratemporal fossa. (a) The site for mandibular osteotomies. (b) The medial and lateral pterygoid muscles and the sphenomandibular ligament are detached, allowing the mandibular segment to be reflected superiorly to expose the infratemporal fossa while preserving the inferior alveolar nerve and vessels. Redrawn from Tiwari RM 2002 Tumours and tumour-like disorders of the infratemporal fossa. In: Langdon JD, Berkovitz BKB, Moxham BJ (eds) *Surgical anatomy of the infratemporal fossa*. Dunitz, London, pp 125–140.

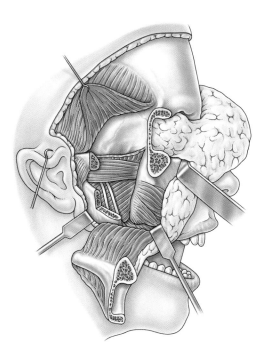

**Fig. 4.21** The lateral transzygomatic surgical approach to the infratemporal fossa. This follows the reflection of the zygomatic arch inferiorly, coronoidectomy and the superior reflection of the temporalis muscle. Redrawn from Evans BT, Wiesenfeld D, Clauser L, Curioni C 2002 Surgical approaches to the infratemporal fossa. In: Langdon JD, Berkovitz BKB, Moxham BJ (eds) *Surgical anatomy of the infratemporal fossa*. Dunitz, London, pp 141–180.

of the tooth. This may be more likely if the procedure is carried out with a lingual rather than a buccal approach. In addition, in about one in seven cases, the lingual nerve is actually located above the lingual bony plate in the third molar region and may be more at risk of damage during surgery. The symptoms of lingual nerve damage are paraesthesia in the distribution of the nerve (i.e. tongue, floor of mouth and gingiva).

A detailed knowledge of the infratemporal and pterygopalatine fossae is important in understanding and then treating the damage that may occur from bony disruptions following maxillofacial trauma and orthognathic surgery. Of particular importance is consideration of the sphenoid bone that contributes to the roof and medial wall. Knowledge of the region is essential in gaining sufficient and clear surgical access in order to remove tumours and other pathologies from the region (the majority of tumours being contiguous or metastatic rather than primary). Neurosurgery may also require an approach to the cranial base via the infratemporal fossa.

A number of different surgical approaches are now available to expose the infratemporal fossa. These new approaches are possible because of advances in imaging and surgical techniques, including the development of rigid fixation systems that enable accurate replacement and retention of mobilized skull bones. Each surgical technique will involve the detachment and reflection of various skeletal elements (osteotomies). Two are illustrated here.

- In the transmandibular approach (Fig. 4.20), the mandible is divided in the midline and along the ramus and is then reflected to expose the infratemporal fossa.
- In the (subcranial) lateral transzygomatic approach, the zygomatic arch is reflected inferiorly, following which a coronoidectomy is undertaken and the temporalis muscle is reflected superiorly (Fig. 4.21).

# 5

# Sectional anatomy of the oral cavity and related areas

The study of anatomical sections has become increasingly important in medicine with the advent of imaging techniques such as computed tomography (CT) and magnetic resonance imaging (MRI). Although these specialized techniques are available for some disciplines in dentistry, knowledge of sectional anatomy is important for all dentists because many of the procedures (surgical and anaesthetic) require a good knowledge of the relationships of structures around the mouth. Thus, the illustrations in this chapter provide transverse sections through the head at various levels relative to the oral cavity and alongside corresponding MRI images.

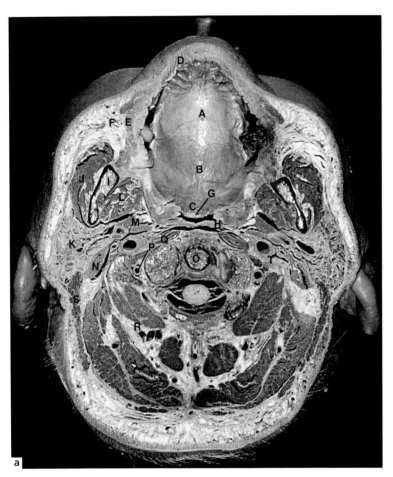

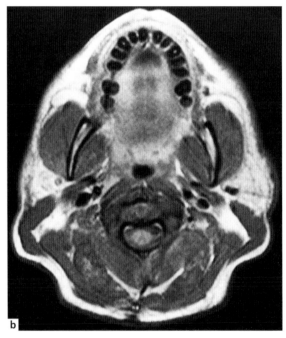

**Fig. 5.1** (a) Transverse section through the head to show the palate and its topographic relationships.
A = hard palate
B = soft palate
C = uvula
D = upper lip
E = buccinator muscle
F = buccal pad of fat
G = nasopharynx
H = superior constrictor muscle of pharynx
I = ramus of mandible
J = masseter muscle
K = parotid gland
L = medial pterygoid muscle
M = styloid group of muscles: stylopharyngeus, stylohyoid, styloglossus
N = posterior belly of digastric muscle
O = axis (second cervical vertebra)
P = vertebral artery
Q = prevertebral muscles
R = postvertebral muscles
S = sternocleidomastoid muscle
T = internal carotid artery and internal jugular vein.
(b) MRI scan of the head at the level of the palate. Courtesy of Squadron Leader S.C.P. Blease.

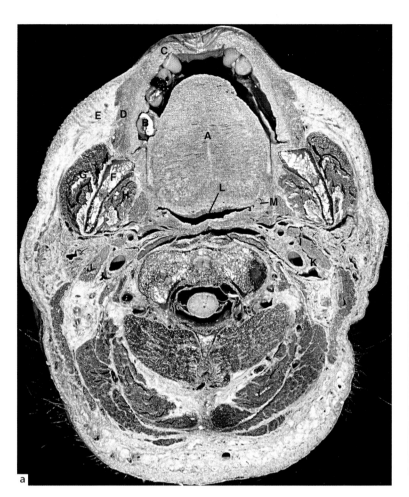

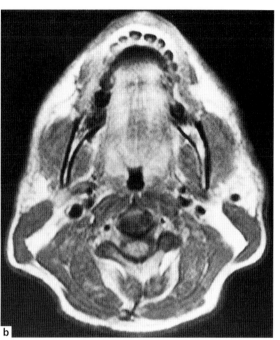

**Fig. 5.2** (a) Transverse section through the head at the level of the palatine tonsil to show the tongue and its topographic relationships. A = tongue; B = mandibular molar; C = lower lip; D = buccinator muscle; E = buccal pad of fat; F = ramus of mandible; G = masseter muscle; H = medial pterygoid muscle; I = styloid group of muscles; J = posterior belly of digastric muscle; K = carotid sheath containing internal carotid artery, internal jugular vein and vagus nerve; L = oropharynx; M = palatopharyngeus muscle. (b) MRI scan of the head at the level of the tongue and palatine tonsil. Courtesy of Squadron Leader S.C.P. Blease.

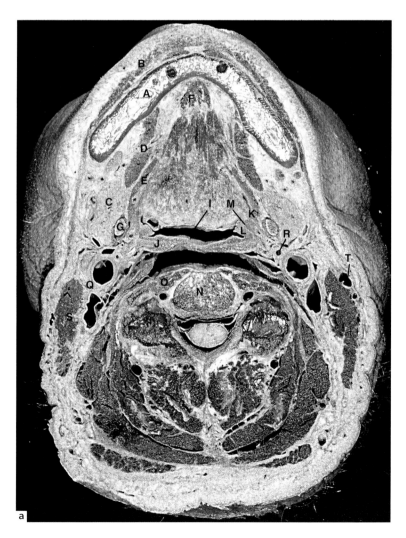

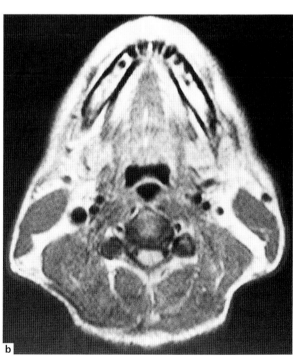

**Fig. 5.3** (a) Transverse section through the head to show the floor of the mouth and its topographic relationships. A = body of mandible; B = depressor labii superioris and depressor anguli oris muscles; C = submandibular gland; D = mylohyoid muscle; E = hyoglossus muscle; F = genioglossus muscle; G = tendon of digastric muscle; I = oropharynx; J = middle constrictor muscle of pharynx; K = palatoglossal fold – anterior pillar of the fauces; L = palatopharyngeal fold – posterior pillars of the fauces; M = tonsillar crypt; N = cervical vertebra; O = prevertebral group of muscles; Q = carotid sheath containing internal carotid artery, internal jugular vein and vagus nerve; R = external carotid artery; S = sternocleidomastoid muscle; T = external jugular vein. (b) MRI scan of the head at the level of the floor of the mouth. Courtesy of Squadron Leader S.C.P. Blease.

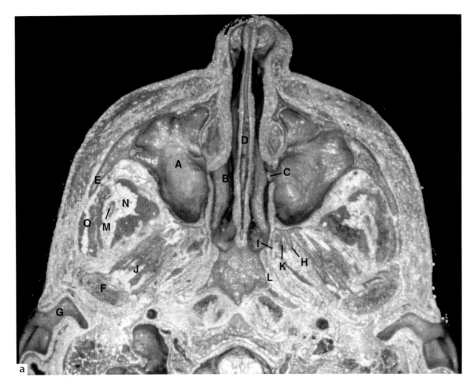
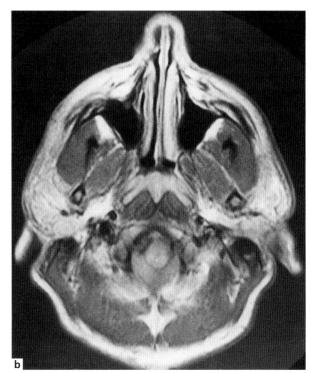

**Fig. 5.4** (a) Transverse section through head to show the maxillary air sinuses and their topographic relationships.

A = floor of maxillary air sinus

B = nasal fossa

C = ostium – opening of maxillary sinus into middle meatus on the lateral wall of the nose

D = nasal septum

E = zygomatic arch

F = condyle of mandible

G = external acoustic meatus

H = lateral pterygoid plate of sphenoid bone

I = medial pterygoid plate of sphenoid bone

J = lateral pterygoid muscle

K = medial pterygoid muscle

L = superior constrictor of pharynx

M = coronoid process of mandible

N = temporalis muscle

O = masseter muscle.

(b) MRI scan of the head to show maxillary air sinuses. Courtesy of Squadron Leader S.C.P. Blease.

# Functional anatomy  6

## MASTICATION

Mastication is the process whereby ingested food is cut or crushed into small pieces, mixed with saliva and formed into a bolus in preparation for swallowing. It is characteristic of mammals, which possess teeth of different forms (heterodonty) adapted to the comminution of food. In non-mammalians, the teeth are used mainly for prehension, the prey generally being seized head first and swallowed whole.

Various functions have been ascribed to mastication in humans. It:

- enables the food bolus to be easily swallowed
- mixes the food with saliva, initiating digestion by the activity of salivary amylase
- enhances the digestibility of food by:
    - decreasing the size of particles to increase the surface area for enzyme activity
    - reflexly stimulating the secretion of digestive juices (e.g. saliva and gastric juice)
- prevents irritation of the gastrointestinal system by large food masses
- ensures healthy growth and development of the oral tissues.

Of all these, the increase in digestive efficiency is usually considered to be the primary purpose of mastication. Indeed, it has been suggested that there is an enormous gain in digestive efficiency without which the high rate of metabolism associated with homeothermy in mammals could not be sustained. However, some experimental evidence indicates that mastication produces little gain in digestive efficiency in humans. Table 6.1 classifies different foods according to the value of mastication in their digestion. The information in the table was obtained by research in which 1 g of either premasticated or unmasticated food was placed in cotton net bags, swallowed and subsequently collected from the faeces. Category 1 foods were those that left some large residues if swallowed with or without pre-mastication. Category 2 foods left some residues when unchewed but were usually completely digested when chewed. Category 3 foods were likely to be fully digested with or without pre-mastication. Thus, it is only for the few types of food in Category 2 that mastication improves

digestion. That these results suggest that mastication produces little gain in digestive efficiency may simply be a reflection of the Western ability to select, grow and prepare foods so that all socially acceptable items of diet are inherently easily digestible.

Mastication occurs by the convergent movements of maxillary and mandibular teeth. In humans, most foods are first crushed by vertical movements of the mandible before being sheared by lateral to medial movements of the mandible. The initial crushing of the food does not require full occlusion of the teeth. Indeed, it is often only after the food has been well softened that the maxillary and mandibular teeth eventually contact. Once the cusps can interdigitate, the ridges on the slopes of the cusps shear the food as the mandibular teeth move across the maxillary teeth. As the cusps cross the depressions within the opposing occlusal surfaces, there is grinding of food, which has been likened to the action of a pestle and mortar. The food particles are progressively formed into a bolus by the tongue.

Figure 6.1 relates the morphology of the cheek teeth to the displacement of food during mastication. Several features common to all the cheek teeth provide protection for the adjacent gingiva during chewing. The marginal ridges bounding the interproximal edges of the occlusal surfaces of the teeth are important protective features. These ridges deflect most of the food, potentially driven between adjacent teeth by their opponents, on to the occlusal surfaces. The contact points beneath the marginal ridges should abut firmly to prevent food being wedged between the teeth and above the interdental papillae. These contacts are maintained by the process

### Table 6.1 *(Modified after J.H. Farrell)*

| Category 1 | Category 2 | Category 3 |
|---|---|---|
| Roast and fried pork | Roast chicken | Fried and stewed beef fat |
| Fried bacon | Stewed lamb | Fried and boiled cod |
| Roast, fried and stewed beef | | Fried kipper |
| Roast and stewed mutton | | Hard-boiled egg |
| Roast and fried lamb | | Boiled rice |
| Fried and boiled potatoes | | White and wholemeal bread |
| Boiled garden peas | | Cheddar cheese |
| Boiled carrots | | |

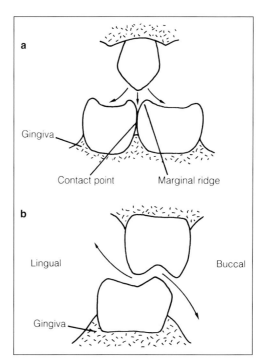

**Fig. 6.1** Morphology of the cheek teeth in relation to the displacement of food (arrows). (a) Buccal view. (b) Interproximal view.

of mesial drift (pages 373–374), despite the constant attrition of inter-proximal dental tissue. The buccal cusps of the mandibular cheek teeth bite between the buccal and palatal cusps of the maxillary cheek teeth, with the result that food trapped between them is forced up over the palatal sides of the maxillary teeth and down over the buccal sides of the man-dibular teeth. The palatal gingiva for the maxillary teeth is thus protected by the marked curvature of these teeth. In addition, it is the buccal surfaces of the mandibular cheek teeth that are the most curved.

Mastication is not simply a result of rhythmically closing teeth of a particular form on a piece of food. This would simply produce random breakage of food. Two other functions are essential. Firstly, the placement of food between the occluding surfaces of the teeth by the tongue. Secondly, the selection by the tongue of those pieces of food in the mouth that require further physical reduction. Other structural features associated with mastication that are peculiar to mammals include:

- temporomandibular jaw articulation
- serous salivary glands
- prismatic enamel
- secondary palate
- significant muscle development associated with lips, cheeks, tongue and muscles of mastication
- diphyodonty
- gomphosis type of tooth attachment.

The development of an increased mass of the muscles of mastication allows the force of the bite to be increased, while the development of the temporomandibular articulation is associated with increased precision of more complex movements. Saliva adds to the moistening and lubrication of food during mastication and its enzymes allow some carbohydrate digestion to commence at an early stage in the mouth. The prismatic arrangement of dental enamel (pages 108–111) and its greater thickness in mammals are said to be more efficient in resisting both masticatory loads and attrition than non-prismatic enamel. The development of a sec-ondary palate is thought to be related to the necessity of maintaining ventilation during prolonged masticatory periods. The development of muscles within the lips, cheeks and tongue is associated with manipulation of the bolus within the mouth. The change from polyphyodonty (i.e. multiple tooth succession) to diphyodonty (two dentitions: deciduous and permanent) may be related to two factors: 1) a 'grinding-in' period necessary to produce an efficient cutting or grinding tooth surface, or possibly 2) the formation of a particular pattern of jaw movement by conditioned reflexes originating from stimulation of the periodontal receptors; it seems inefficient to replace such teeth too frequently. The gomphosis type of attachment (with a periodontal ligament; see Ch. 12) may be associated with the increased stresses and strains brought to bear on the tooth during mastication; it also allows for tooth movement. Such movement stimulates sensory receptors in the periodontal ligament, so providing information on the loading and movement of individual teeth.

Mastication is dependent upon a complex chain of events that produce rhythmic opening and closing movements of the jaws and correlated tongue movements. The forces that are exerted on the teeth and jaws are very large and physiologically significant. Experiments involving the implantation of force transducers into the occlusal surfaces of teeth have shown that the bite force exerted on the food during human mastication is of the order of 5–15 kg. This force varies according to the texture of the food. When conscious bite force is measured with a gnathodynamometer, maximum pressures of the order of 50 kg can be readily recorded.

Rhythmic jaw movements (Fig. 6.2) are now generally accepted as being generated by a centre within the brainstem. This is referred to as an oral rhythm/pattern generator and is activated both by drive from the higher centres and by peripheral sensory input. The pattern of activity is

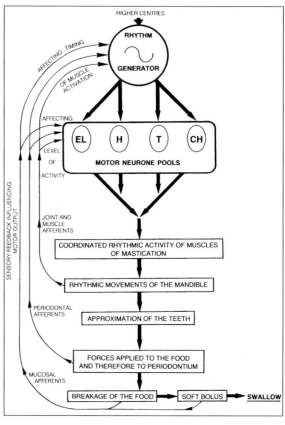

**Fig. 6.2** A diagrammatic representation of the way jaw movements are thought to operate. EL = jaw elevator musculature; H = hyoid and associated musculature; T = tongue and associated musculature; CH = cheek and associated musculature. Courtesy of Dr A. Thexton.

distributed to the motor neurone pools, which also receive excitatory or inhibitory sensory inputs from a variety of peripheral structures. The hypothesis is that the sensory input generated by closing on hard food supports the generation of rhythmic jaw activity, whereas closure on a softened bolus promotes tongue movement and food transport, eliciting a swallow: the effect is to terminate the rhythmic jaw activity.

## CHEWING CYCLE

Mammals generally chew on one side at a time. Two methods of chewing have been distinguished, depending upon the initial texture of the food and the stage in its breakdown.

- **Puncture/crushing**. Hard food is first crushed and pierced between the teeth without direct tooth-to-tooth contact. This results in wear (attrition) of the teeth, especially at the tips of the cusps.
- **Shearing stroke**. This method involves tooth contacts that take place only after the food has been sufficiently reduced. This type of move-ment produces attrition facets with characteristic directional scratch lines on the faces of the cusps.

The action of the teeth during mastication depends on their morphology, the movements of the mandible and the nature of the forces generated by the muscles of mastication. The chewing cycle involves three basic phases (or strokes) of the mandible in relation to the maxilla. From a posi-tion in which the jaw is open, the closing stroke results in the teeth being brought into initial contact with the food; the work done in this phase is really against gravity. This is followed by the power stroke, when the food undergoes reduction. Movement of the mandible in this phase is slower than in the closing stroke because of the resistance caused by the food, even though there may be vastly greater masseter and temporalis muscle activity during this time. Finally, there is the opening stroke, when the mandible is lowered, with an initial slower stage followed by a faster stage.

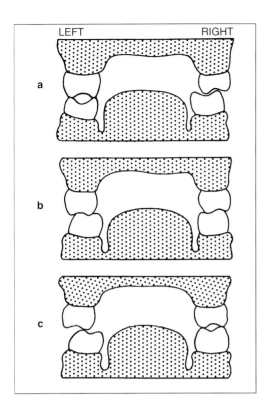

**Fig. 6.3** Occlusal relationships of the cheek teeth during chewing on the left side. (a) Buccal phase on working (left) side. (b) Intercuspal position. (c) Lingual phase. Note the positions of the teeth on the balancing side (right).

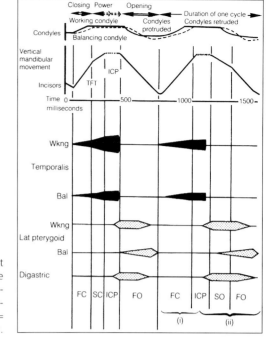

**Fig. 6.4** Patterns of chewing cycle during two different cycles of jaw movement (cycle 1 for solid food; cycle 2 for soft food). FC = fast-closing phase; SC = slow-closing phase; ICP – intercuspal phase; SO = slow-opening phase; FO = fast-opening phase; TFT = tooth–food–tooth contact. Courtesy of Dr A. Thexton.

Figure 6.3 shows the occlusal relationships of the cheek teeth during chewing (shearing) on the left side. From an open position the mandible is moved upwards and outwards, bringing the buccal cusps of the maxillary and mandibular teeth on the working (left) side in contact (Fig. 6.3a). As mentioned previously, the teeth may not contact each other during the initial masticatory cycles. In the power stroke the mandibular teeth then slide upwards and medially against the maxillary teeth to momentarily attain intercuspal position (Fig. 6.3b). Following attainment of the intercuspal position, the mandibular teeth continue downwards and inwards against the maxillary teeth (the lingual phase, Fig. 6.3c). The opening stroke then follows and the cycle is repeated. The relationships of the teeth on the balancing side are also illustrated in Fig. 6.3. Note that, while the teeth on the working side are moving through the buccal phase (Fig. 6.3a), those on the balancing (right) side are in the lingual phase but in the reverse direction. Although the diagrams in Figure 6.3 show tooth contact, it is probable that any contact on the balancing side is only transient.

In primates (including humans), the chewing cycle differs depending upon whether the food is solid or soft (Fig. 6.4). Note that the vertical component of condylar movement is due to its movement up and down the slope of the articular eminence (page 62). The first cycle has a profile that is commonly found when solid food is chewed. After a previous opening, the jaw accelerates into relatively fast closing (phase labelled 'FC'). At this stage, the food is being accelerated only against gravity, and the electromyographic activity in the jaw-closing muscles is of low amplitude. As tooth–food–tooth ('TFT') contact is made, activity in the jaw-closing muscles increases and force is exerted on the food. The food resistance slows the jaw closing ('SC'). As the cusps continue to interdigitate, closing velocity slows to zero. The duration of this stationary phase is a matter of dispute. Because of uncertainty, the intercuspal phase ('ICP') is shown as a dashed line. The jaw subsequently opens with a relatively constant velocity. There is relatively little movement of the tongue producing food transport towards the pharynx. The second cycle shown in the figure is characteristic of the ingestion of soft food. The closing phase consists largely of fast closing because the food offers little resistance to jaw closure. Opening now consists of two phases – slow opening followed by fast opening. The duration of the first phase of

opening (slow opening) correlates with the amplitude of tongue movement and with food transport towards the pharynx.

A main feature of the chewing cycle described above is that its form is variable, depending upon the sensory feedback (see pages 98, 99).

## Envelope of motion

The pathway followed by the mandible during chewing is termed 'the envelope of motion' (Fig. 6.5). This demonstrates the symmetrical mandibular movements produced during opening and closing of the jaw.

The envelope of motion is the volume of space within which all movements of a specified point on the mandible occur. The envelope is limited by anatomical considerations such as ligaments and tooth contacts. Most natural movements do not utilize this maximum volume but occur well

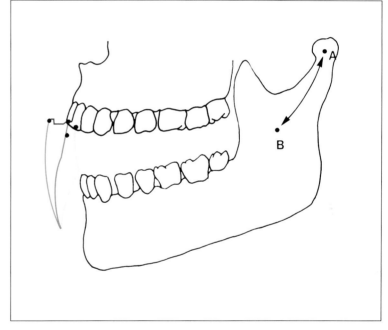

**Fig. 6.5** The envelope of motion of the contact point between the mandibular incisors when viewed from the side (laterally and in the sagittal plane). See text for explanation of coloured trajectories and for the change in the fulcrum of movements from point A to point B.

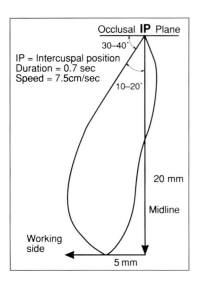

**Fig. 6.6** Profile/envelope of motion showing the average incisal movements in the frontal plane during a masticatory cycle. Redrawn after Professor J. Ahlgren.

**Fig. 6.7** Transverse movements of the lower jaw (lateral excursions or side-to-side movements). The thick lines represent the horizontal band of the temporomandibular ligament. A = articular eminence. Redrawn after Professors H. Sicher and E.L. Dubrul.

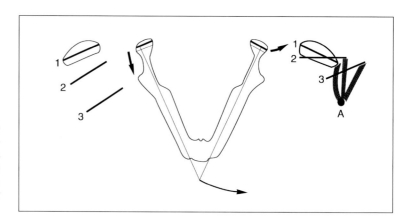

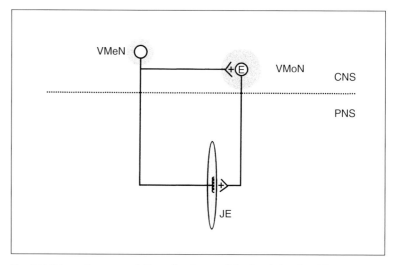

**Fig. 6.8** Schematic representation of pathway of the jaw jerk reflex. There are monosynaptic connections between afferent nerves and from spindles in the jaw elevator muscles (JE) and the motor neurones to these same muscles. Shaded areas represent brainstem nuclei. VMeN = trigeminal mesencephalic nucleus; VMoN = trigeminal motor nucleus; CNS = central nervous system; PNS = peripheral nervous system; + = excitatory synapse; E = jaw elevator motor neurone. Orchardson R, Cadden SW 1998 Mastication. In: Linden RWA (ed) *The scientific basis of eating: taste and smell, salivation, mastication and swallowing and their dysfunctions.* Frontiers of Oral Biology Series Vol 9. Karger, Basel, pp 76–121.

within the 'envelope'. The yellow trajectory shown in Figure 6.5 depicts a two-phased, conscious movement from the rest position to the fully opened position. The first phase is a hinge-like movement during which the condyles remain retruded within the mandibular fossae. When the teeth become separated by approximately 25 mm, the second phase of opening occurs and involves anterior movement or protrusion of the condyles down the articular eminences. The blue and red trajectories shown in the figure describe a biphasic path of closure from the fully opened mandibular position, which can be performed only with conscious effort. The first phase (the blue trajectory) takes the mandible up to a protruded closed position, while the second phase (the red trajectory) takes the mandible from this protruded contact position to a retruded contact position. The green trajectory describes the free, habitual, unconscious movement during both mandibular opening and closing. The points on the ramus of the mandible in the figure represent the centres of rotation during opening and closure. Point A is the fulcrum associated with simple hinge movements. The path described between points A and B represents the shift of the centre of rotation of the mandible; this shift occurs because of the transition from a pure hinge movement at the condyle to protrusion and rotation during opening (with the reverse during closing). Point B has been described as representing the point of rotation around the attachment of the sphenomandibular ligament at the lingula.

A 'profile' or 'envelope of motion' showing the average incisal movements in the frontal plane during a masticatory cycle is shown in Figure 6.6. In this coronal plane (i.e. viewed from in front) the opening movement rarely goes straight down but deviates to one side. There is a wide variation in profiles between individuals and also continuous variation between consecutive chewing cycles in the same individual: for example, the initial deviation may be towards the chewing side or away from it (as shown in Fig. 6.6). Furthermore, the profiles differ according to the type of occlusion and the texture of the food.

The transverse movements of the lower jaw (i.e. lateral excursions or side-to-side movements as viewed from above) are illustrated in Figure 6.7. These movements involve bilaterally asymmetric movements of the mandible. They are produced by protrusion of the mandibular condyle down the articular eminence of the temporal bone on one side with reactive movements of the other condyle (rotation around a laterally shifting axis). The illustration describes the changing positions of the long axes of the mandibular condyles during lateral movements of the mandible to the left. The figure also shows the change in the horizontal band of the temporomandibular ligament passing from the articular tubercle to the lateral surface of the condyle during lateral movements. A slight lateral shift in the condyle (Bennett shift) produces tension in the horizontal band.

## CONTROL OF MASTICATION

There has in the past been much controversy concerning the origin and control of the rhythmic activity of the jaws during mastication. One older view, the cerebral hemispheres theory, held that mastication was a conscious act, a patterned set of instructions originating in the higher centres of the central nervous system (in particular the motor cortex) and descending to directly drive the motor neurones within the brainstem (trigeminal, facial and hypoglossal motor neurones). Another older idea, the reflex chain theory, held that mastication involved a series of interacting chains of reflexes. Accordingly, sensory input from the region of the mouth (e.g. pressure on the teeth) triggered the motor neurones in the brainstem to elicit a jaw opening movement. In turn, this movement produced another sensory input (e.g. from stretch receptors in the jaw muscles), which resulted in a jaw closing reflex. Although there are several well recognized types of jaw reflex (Figs 6.8–6.10), objections to the reflex chain theory have been raised on the basis that mastication involves prolonged bursts of muscle activity and not the brief and abrupt behaviour usually associated with reflex activation of muscle. A third theory, the rhythm (pattern) generator theory, has recently been updated to explain rhythmic jaw functioning. This theory is based upon the proposition that there are central pattern generators (CPGs) within the brainstem that can be stimulated from either higher centres or sensory inputs in the region from the mouth, so

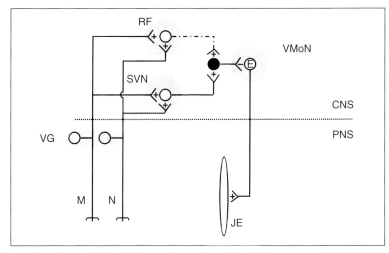

**Fig. 6.9** Inhibitory exteroceptive jaw reflexes: schematic representation of probable pathways. These reflexes can be produced most effectively by stimulation of mechanoreceptors (M) or nociceptors (N) from the mouth and face. Two responses can be identified: a short-latency one mediated by a di- or trisynaptic pathway through the supratrigeminal nucleus and a long-latency one mediated by a polysynaptic pathway through the reticular formation. Shaded areas represent ganglia or nuclei. VG = trigeminal ganglion; SVN = supratrigeminal nucleus; RF = reticular formation; VMoN = trigeminal motor nucleus; CNS = central nervous system; PNS = peripheral nervous system; + = excitatory synapse; − = inhibitory synapse; E = jaw elevator motor neurone; JE = jaw elevator muscle. Broken line represents uncertainty about the number of synapses involved in that pathway. Orchardson R, Cadden SW 1998 Mastication. In: Linden RWA (ed) *The scientific basis of eating: taste and smell, salivation, mastication and swallowing and their dysfunctions.* Frontiers of Oral Biology Series Vol 9. Karger, Basel, pp 76–121.

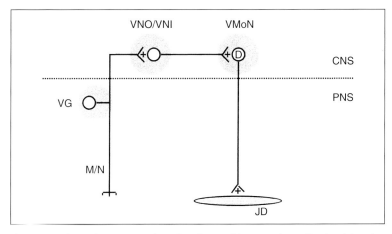

**Fig. 6.10** Schematic representation of pathway of jaw opening reflex involving the digastric muscle. There are disynaptic connections between afferent nerves from orofacial mechanoreceptors and nociceptors (M/N) through the trigeminal sensory nuclei oralis (VNO) and/or interpolaris (VNI) to jaw depressor motor neurones (D). Shaded areas represent ganglia or brainstem nuclei. VG = trigeminal ganglion; VMoN = trigeminal motor nucleus; CNS = central nervous system; PNS = peripheral nervous system; + = excitatory synapse; JD = jaw depressor muscle. Orchardson R, Cadden SW 1998 Mastication. In: Linden RWA (ed) *The scientific basis of eating: taste and smell, salivation, mastication and swallowing and their dysfunctions.* Frontiers of Oral Biology Series Vol 9. Karger, Basel, pp 76–121.

that they are driven into rhythmic activity. This idea could account for rhythmic activity obtained by stimulating either the motor cortex or, in decerebrate animals and anencephalics (where the cerebral hemispheres are congenitally absent), the oral cavity. This theory, supported by comparisons with other physiological systems that require pattern generators (e.g. respiration), is now generally accepted.

A CPG is a set of closely interconnected neurones that generates a series of rhythmic outputs passing to the different groups of motor neurones involved in a particular movement (e.g. suckling, chewing). Consequently, each motor neurone group, and therefore each muscle, is activated at the

correct time for that rhythmic movement. The activity of this generator depends upon excitation descending in pathways from cerebral cortical areas and upon excitation deriving from peripheral stimulation (i.e. the rhythmic activity can be generated by conscious drive and/or by the presence of food in the mouth). However, the relative importance of the two sources of excitation seems to vary with age. The human adult may be unable to feed at all after damage to the cerebral cortex while, in the anencephalic infant (one born without any cerebral hemispheres), suckling movements can be elicited simply by stimulating the lips.

During mastication, the cycles of jaw movement differ, depending upon the consistency of the food initially ingested and upon the stage of breakdown of that food. This indicates that the cyclic activity generated by the CPG is subject to modification by sensory input from the mouth. However, if equivalent types of sensory input are generated experimentally by controlled stimuli applied to oral sites, then reflex responses can be generated quite independently of any pre-existing rhythmic activity. Whether a particular sensory input elicits a reflex, fails to elicit a reflex or whether it modifies ongoing activity simply depends upon what else is going on in the central nervous system.

In the last 100 years, at least a dozen oral reflexes have been described, forgotten and redescribed. Only the two least contentious and most commonly known are described here: the jaw jerk and the jaw opening reflex.

## Jaw jerk

The jaw jerk is produced when the jaw closing muscles are stretched by tapping the chin downwards so that the jaw opens suddenly. The monosynaptic reflex is due to stimulation of stretch-sensitive receptors (muscle spindles) in the masseter and temporalis muscles. The stretch produces a burst of impulses in the sensory nerves that is conveyed back to the motor neurones of those muscles. The muscles are consequently activated briefly to produce a short-lived contraction (Fig. 6.8).

## Jaw opening reflex

The jaw opening reflexes are more complex (polysynaptic) and can be produced by applying mechanical or electrical stimuli to oral mucosa, periodontal ligament or teeth; the stimuli do not have to be painful to elicit the reflex but stronger stimuli do produce correspondingly more vigorous responses. In humans, the reflex is characterized by a brief period of inhibition of activity in the motor neurones of the jaw closing muscles (Fig. 6.9). However, in other mammals (and in some neurological disorders in humans) there is in addition a simultaneous activation of the jaw opening muscles (e.g. digastric and infrahyoid muscles) (Fig. 6.10).

## SWALLOWING

Swallowing (deglutition) involves an ordered sequence of events that carry food (or saliva) from the mouth into the stomach. Although a continuous activity, swallowing is subdivided into stages for descriptive convenience. Humans swallow approximately 600 times every 24 hours, but only about 150 of these are concerned with food and drink; the rest simply clear saliva from the mouth. It is important to appreciate that, alongside muscle activity required to move the bolus, there must be mechanisms to protect the airway (e.g. closure of the nasopharynx by the soft palate, elevation of the larynx, closure of the laryngeal inlet by the epiglottis).

In preparation for swallowing, a softened food bolus or liquid is moved through the mouth by the action of the tongue. The bolus is first moved to lie in a longitudinal midline furrow formed in the dorsum of the tongue; the floor of this furrow is then progressively raised from before backwards,

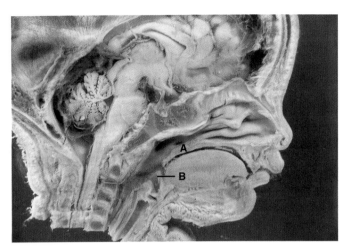

**Fig. 6.11** Sagittal section of the head of a neonate. Note the relatively high position of the larynx, the opening being at the level of the soft palate (A). B = epiglottis.

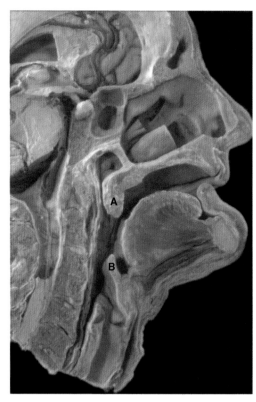

**Fig. 6.12** Sagittal section of an adult head. Compared with Fig. 6.11, the opening of the larynx lies well below the level of the soft palate (A). B = epiglottis.

squeezing the bolus back against the hard palate. The kinetic energy imparted to the bolus moves it into and through the pharynx, where contractions of the circularly arranged pharyngeal constrictor muscles complete the movement of the bolus down to the oesophagus. Peristalsis (a moving wave of contraction) then conveys the bolus onwards to the stomach. The process requires that the upper (cricopharyngeal) and lower (cardiac) sphincters of the oesophagus relax at the correct time to allow the bolus to pass. The classical division of the above components of the swallow in the human adult is into three phases: the oral phase, the pharyngeal phase and the oesophageal phase.

In the adult human, the process of swallowing is complicated by the fact that the pharynx also forms part of the airway leading from the nose to the larynx. Consequently, swallowing and breathing cannot safely occur at the same time. In contrast, in the human newborn and generally in other mammals (both infant and adult), the larynx occupies a relatively higher position (Fig. 6.11). In these cases, the laryngeal opening is usually above the level of the soft palate, the lateral part of which extends around the larynx. In this situation, there is a degree of anatomical separation of the respiratory tract and the alimentary tract (in some animals the high larynx completely divides the pharynx into two passages, which pass laterally on either side of the larynx, rejoining behind and below it). The timed separation of swallowing and breathing is consequently less critical in this situation than it is in adult humans.

The anatomical differences between adults and neonates also produce differences in the way that the swallow is executed. In the case of the high larynx in the infant, the epiglottis contacts the posterior edge of the U-shaped soft palate, so that a potential space is formed, bounded above by the soft palate, behind by the anterior surface of the epiglottis/larynx and in front and below by the dorsum of the tongue. During feeding, this space accumulates food before its onward passage via the pharynx and oesophagus to the stomach. The potential space (filled by the posterior part of the tongue, Fig. 6.11) includes the valleculae (the pockets formed between the epiglottal base and the surface of the back of the tongue). For convenience, this storage area will be referred to as the 'vallecular space'.

Growth in length of the human pharynx (starting a few months after birth) causes the larynx to take up a relatively lower position in the pharynx so that its contact with the soft palate is lost (Fig. 6.12). There is consequently no longer an enclosed space in which food can be stored or accumulated and the airway is no longer anatomically separated from the food passage. A variety of measures operate to protect the airway during swallowing in this situation, including interruption of breathing, closure of the glottis, tipping the larynx forward so that the back of the tongue bulges over it during swallowing, plus bending of the epiglottis back and down

over the laryngeal opening. At the same time the nasal airway is closed by elevation of the soft palate against an upper pharynx narrowed by the pharyngeal constrictor muscles. Because of the low position of the larynx, the pattern of swallowing in the adult human is the exception to the general pattern in mammals (at least in non-primate mammals).

In most mammalian (and human infant) feeding, the 'vallecular space' is gradually filled during the course of a number of food transport cycles (which may include mastication where appropriate). Adequate filling of the 'vallecular space' appears to be the trigger for its periodic emptying. The contents then pass down the pharynx and oesophagus. Unless one includes all of the tongue and jaw movements involved in suckling, lapping or chewing that are associated with filling the vallecular space, the true swallow consists only of emptying that space and the subsequent movement of the bolus down the pharynx and oesophagus. In animals, the ratio of the number of cycles filling the vallecular space to the number of cycles in which swallowing (vallecular emptying) occurs varies from about 2:1 to 14:1. The situation is different in the human adult, where the descent of the larynx means that the vallecular space no longer exists as a potentially closed cavity and storage area. In this situation, a swallow is initiated immediately the first trace of food material or saliva enters the true valleculae. The question then becomes one of how vallecular emptying is triggered so readily in the adult human when (unlike other mammals where a significant amount of food is transported into the vallecular space over a number of cycles) only a trace of food or liquid may have reached the region. Furthermore, in humans the movement of the bolus backwards from the mouth to the valleculae is followed by vallecular emptying generally on a 1:1 basis. Consequently, the transport of the bolus into the valleculae is regarded as part of the swallow and is classically described as the first (oral) phase of the swallow in adult humans.

In mammals generally, the neural mechanisms involved in swallowing depend upon sensory input from branches of the glossopharyngeal and vagus nerves that supply the mucous membrane of the vallecular space. Through its internal laryngeal branch, the superior laryngeal nerve (a branch of the vagus) carries important sensory inputs from the larynx, epiglottis and valleculae; this is one of the most powerful sensory pathways involved in eliciting a swallow. In the case of the high larynx, swallowing can be elicited reflexly by fluid in the vallecular space even when the brainstem has no connections with those parts of the brain above the brainstem (as in decerebrate animals and in infants with anencephaly). It can therefore be assumed, firstly, that all the necessary neural components for swallowing are located in the brainstem. Secondly, it can be assumed that sensory input from the surface of the palate, epiglottis and tongue (the walls of the vallecular space of animals and human infants) is alone sufficient to elicit a swallow. The generally accepted view is that the peripheral sensory input activates a set of neural circuits within the brainstem that collectively produce the pattern of motor activity constituting a swallow. These circuits constitute a CPG for the activity involving the 30 or so muscles that take part in a swallow. The relevant network of brainstem neurones receives not only peripheral sensory input but also excitatory fibres descending from the cerebral cortex, in this way being similar to the CPG for mastication.

In the adult human, where there is no longer an enclosed vallecular space and no possibility of significant storage of food, the level of sensory input from the periphery must be less than that arising in other mammals. The initiation of swallowing in adult humans can, however, be explained on the basis of high levels of activity in the excitatory pathway descending from the cerebral cortex exciting the swallowing CPG, so that it requires only a trace more sensory input from the peripheral nerves to trigger the swallow. In other words, the descending drive lowers the threshold for reflex emptying of the valleculae. Because only a weak sensory input is necessary, only a trace of material has to reach the vallecula to elicit its emptying and all the subsequent components of the swallow. The lower threshold does, however, mean that other sensory inputs (e.g. glossopharyngeal) play a larger role in eliciting the swallow.

## STAGES OF SWALLOWING

Although the act of swallowing is not discontinuous, classically it has been divided into three stages for descriptive convenience: the oral stage, the pharyngeal stage and the oesophageal stage (Fig. 6.13). At each stage it is necessary to consider not only the movement of the bolus but also how the airway is isolated from the food.

### Stage 1 – Oral stage

The jaw is elevated by the action of the masseter and temporalis muscles, and the lips are approximated by the circumoral muscles, forming the anterior oral seal. A longitudinal furrow is produced in the dorsum of the tongue by the bilateral action of the styloglossus muscles inserted into the lateral edges of the tongue, by the vertical fibres of the intrinsic musculature and by the action of the genioglossus muscles inserted close to the midline. The tongue is then elevated against the palate by the action of the mylohyoid muscles and the groove in the tongue is progressively emptied from before backwards, moving the bolus rapidly towards the pharynx. The airway remains open at this stage, with the soft palate lying away from the posterior wall of the pharynx and contacting the back of the tongue, so forming a posterior oral seal.

### Stage 2 – Pharyngeal stage

The bolus passes through the oropharyngeal isthmus into the pharynx because of the kinetic energy imparted by the tongue; as the bolus leaves the oral cavity the palatoglossal folds contract behind the bolus. The tensor veli palatini and levator veli palatini muscles are activated so that the soft palate elevates to contact the posterior wall of the pharynx, closing the nasopharynx. The larynx is elevated and its opening is protected by the bulge of the back of the tongue and by being covered by the epiglottis, which is flexed partly by the drag of the bolus and partly by the action of the aryepiglottic muscles. The laryngeal inlet is also protected by closure of the glottis. A wave of contraction within the pharyngeal constrictor muscles then clears the bolus from the pharynx.

### Stage 3 – Oesophageal stage

Relaxation of the cricopharyngeal part of the inferior constrictor muscle allows the food into the oesophagus, where a peristaltic wave moves the bolus on towards the stomach. Once the bolus is in the oesophagus, the cricopharyngeal sphincter closes to prevent reflux. The passage of the bolus into the stomach requires relaxation of the lower oesophageal (or cardiac) sphincter. The airway is re-established during the oesophageal phase, i.e. the soft palate, tongue and epiglottis return to their normal positions and the glottis opens.

## SPEECH

The acquisition of language is probably the most complex sensorimotor developmental process in a person's life. Indeed, individuals can be readily recognized and distinguished by the distinctive features of their voice, which, in turn, relate to the special anatomical and functional characteristics of that person's 'vocal tract' (the region from the larynx to the mouth).

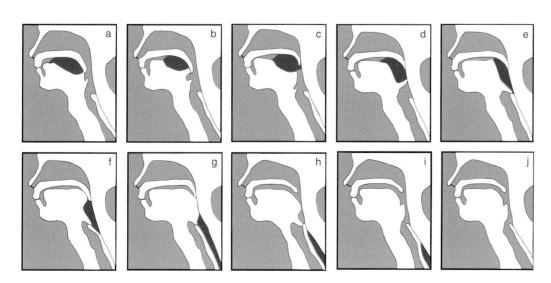

**Fig. 6.13** The stages of swallowing. (a–c) = oral stage; (d–f) = pharyngeal stage; (g–j) = oesophageal stage.

Sounds are produced during exhalation and initially within the larynx ('voice box'), a structure that has evolved from its original purpose of protecting the trachea from inhaling food substances to enable the production of very complex sound patterns. This process is called phonation and involves the coordinated movements of abdominal, thoracic and laryngeal muscles. Subsequent modification of this laryngeal sound to generate meaningful speech occurs principally within the resonating chambers of the pharyngeal, oral and nasal cavities (a process termed articulation). This section primarily describes the role of oral structures in speech and the reader is referred elsewhere for detailed accounts of the role of the larynx.

The fundamental laryngeal note has a thin and reedy quality. This sound therefore contains a limited amount of speech information and so is modified within resonating chambers (Table 6.2) acting as acoustic filters (amplifying selected frequencies and attenuating others by a process of sympathetic vibration) and by the activity of organs such as the lips, cheeks, teeth, tongue and palate. In addition, the relative positions of the maxillary and mandibular teeth (and therefore the position of the mandible) have important effects.

## CLASSIFICATION OF SOUNDS

Phonetics is the linguistic science dealing with pronunciation and features the way in which phonemes are produced by the vocal apparatus. Phonemes are defined as the essential sequential contrastive units within a language and they therefore vary considerably between languages.

Sounds may be voiced (i.e. the vocal folds in the larynx vibrate for sound production) or breathed (i.e. the vocal folds do not vibrate). The two main groups of speech sounds are vowels and consonants.

Vowel sounds are modified by resonance and all vowel sounds are voiced. They are produced without interruption of the air flow, the air being channelled or restricted by the position of the tongue and lips (Fig. 6.14). The range of higher harmonics define or characterize the vowel sound. Close vowels are those produced when the tongue is positioned high in the mouth and open vowels result when the tongue is low in the mouth. Furthermore, front and back vowels are generated when the tongue is located forwards or backwards in the mouth.

A consonant is produced when the air flow is impeded before it is released. Consonants may be voiced (e.g. b, d, z) or breathed (e.g. p, t, s). Consonant sounds are of low amplitude (vowels are created by high-amplitude waves) and are classified in two ways: according to the place of articulation or according to the manner of articulation.

For the classification based upon the place of articulation (Table 6.3), consonants are categorized into bilabial, labiodental, linguodental, linguopalatal and glottal sounds. In bilabial sounds (e.g. b, p, m) the two lips are used. In labiodental sounds, the lower lip meets the maxillary incisors (e.g. f, v). Linguodental sounds (e.g. d, t) involve the tip of the tongue contacting the maxillary incisors and the adjacent hard palate; for linguopalatal sounds the tongue meets the palate away from the region of the maxillary incisors (e.g. g, k).

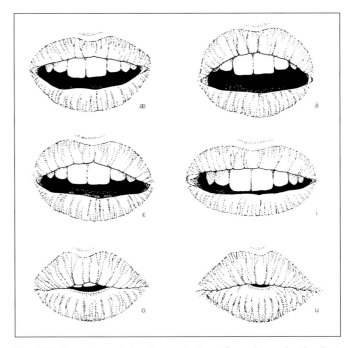

**Fig. 6.14** Lip postures during the production of vowel sounds. The short vowel sounds are shown on the left and the long vowel sounds on the right.

---

**Table 6.2** *The vocal resonators*

The following spaces are present in the vocal apparatus, any or all of which might be available as variable resonating chambers.
1. Between the true and false vocal cords
2. Between the larynx and the root of the tongue, possibly involving the epiglottis
3. Between the pharyngeal wall and the soft palate and uvula
4. Between the dorsum of the tongue and the posterior surface of the hard palate
5. Between the dorsum of the tongue and the anterior surface of the hard palate
6. Between the tip of the tongue and the teeth
7. Between the teeth and the lips
8. The nasal passages

---

**Table 6.3** *Classification of consonant sounds based upon place and manner of articulation*

| Manner of articulation | Place of articulation | | | | | | | | | | | |
|---|---|---|---|---|---|---|---|---|---|---|---|---|
| | Bilabial | | Labiodental | | Linguodentals | | | | Linguopalatals | | | | |
| | | | | | Dental | | Alveolar | | Alveolar | | Palatal | | Glottal |
| Voicing | − | + | − | + | − | + | − | + | − | + | − | + | − | + |
| Plosives | p | b | | | | | t | d | | | k | g | | |
| Fricatives | | | f | v | θ | ð | s | z | ʃ | ʒ | | | h | |
| Affricatives | | | | | | | tʃ | | | | j | | | |
| | | | | | | | tr | dr | | | | | | |
| Nasals | m | | | | | | | n | ng | | | | | |
| Laterals | | | | | | | | l | | | | | | |
| Semi-vowels | w | | | | | | | | | | | | | |

For the classification of consonant sounds based upon the manner of articulation (Table 6.4), the degree of stoppage of the air flow is an important criterion. For example, a plosive consonant (e.g. b, p) requires sudden release of air. Note that, although one may describe the position of articulators for a particular vowel or consonant, there are no fixed positions during speech, only continuous movement. Both systems for classifying consonant sounds can be linked, as in Table 6.3. The configuration of the oral structures during consonant articulations is illustrated in Figure 6.15. From this it can be seen that the tongue has a significant role during speech, although all oral structures (including the soft palate) are important.

**Table 6.4** *Classification of consonant sounds based upon manner of articulation*

| | | |
|---|---|---|
| Plosives | (p, b, t, d, g, k) | Require a complete stoppage of air |
| Fricatives | (f, v, th) | Require only a partial stoppage of air |
| Affricatives | (c, h, j) | Although involving only a partial stoppage of air, they require a rapid release of this air |
| Nasals | (m, n) | Require obstruction of the mouth with the nasal passages open |
| Laterals | (l) | Air forced to leave sides of mouth |
| Rolled | (r) | |

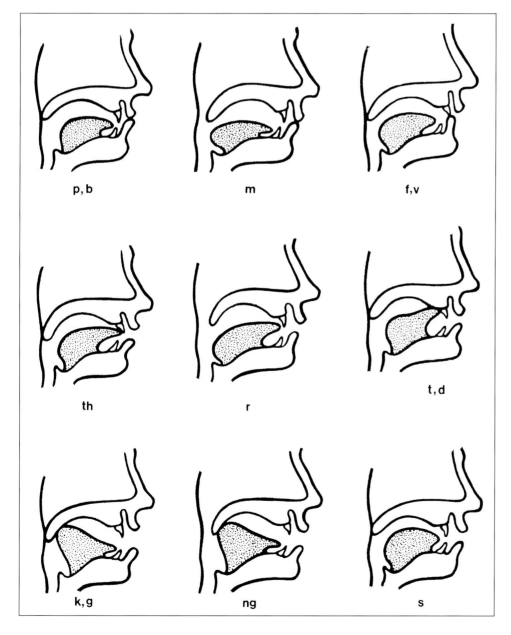

**Fig. 6.15** Configuration of the oral structures during consonant articulations.

**Fig. 6.16** The principal sensory and motor mechanisms in speech.

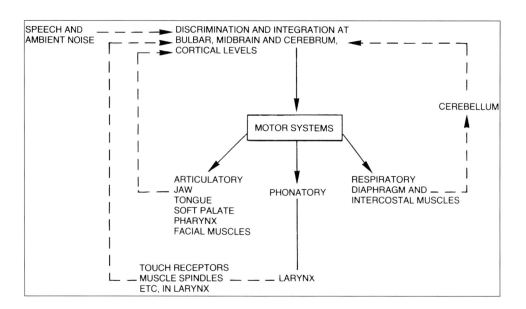

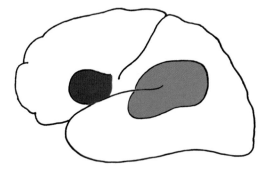

**Fig. 6.17** Speech areas of the brain are located in the dominant cerebral hemisphere (i.e. left hemisphere for right-handed persons). The main areas are Broca's area (red), which is concerned with speech production, and Wernicke's area (blue), which is concerned with ensuring that spoken language is comprehensible. A third area (not illustrated), around the angular gyrus and posterior to Wernicke's area, is concerned with 'meaning'. In addition, the insula of the brain coordinates the activities of the speech areas. Note the large amount of the cerebral hemisphere given to speech.

Figure 6.16 summarizes the principal sensory and motor mechanisms in speech. The main speech area of the brain is located within the temporoparietal region of the dominant cerebral hemisphere (i.e. the left cerebral hemisphere for a right-handed person) (Fig. 6.17). Figure 6.16 indicates the many monitoring systems involved in the control of speech (such as hearing, proprioceptive information from the various muscles involved). Note that there has to be coordinated activity of respiration, laryngeal behaviour and oral structures to produce effective speech.

That speech is probably the most complex movement in the body is indicated by the range of muscles involved, by the great number of nerves implicated and by the large areas of the cerebral hemispheres of the brain associated with speech (Fig. 6.17). The muscles involved include those in the chest that control breathing, the intrinsic muscles of the larynx that are concerned with phonation (i.e. those required to close the rima glottidis between the cords, to put tension in the cords, and to change the shape of the cords), the muscles in the pharynx and soft palate that help in resonance, and the muscles of the tongue, palate, jaws and facial musculature that produce meaningful speech. The nerves involved may include the intercostals and phrenic nerves, the recurrent laryngeal and superior (external) laryngeal branches of the vagus, nerves associated with the pharyngeal plexus, and the trigeminal, facial and hypoglossal cranial nerves.

The complexity of speech is further indicated by the fact that, although meaningful speech results from the bringing together of very simple sounds so that phonemes become syllables become words become whole sentences and concepts, the brain has to work in the opposite manner, so that whole concepts and ideas, if not entirely coherent sentences, have to be established before the physiological process of phonation and articulation. In addition, speech occurs alongside other means of communication – facial expression, hand movements, body posture – and requires feedback from the person(s) to whom one is speaking so that visual and auditory signals must be coordinated with speech.

Before describing enamel, a few introductory remarks are required concerning the dental and supporting tissues. The teeth are composed of three mineralized tissues (enamel, dentine and cementum) surrounding an inner core of loose connective tissue, the dental pulp. Enamel is of ectodermal origin; dentine, cementum and the dental pulp are of ectomesenchymal origin.

The appearance of the tissues depends upon the method of specimen preparation: in ground sections the hard, mineralized tissues remain intact but the soft connective tissues and epithelia are lost; in demineralized sections the soft connective tissues and the organic matrices of the mineralized tissues remain. Because enamel is almost entirely mineral it is lost completely after most demineralization procedures and its structural features are mainly described in ground sections (Fig. 7.1).

Dentine forms the bulk of the tooth and is covered in the crown with enamel and in the root with cementum (Figs 7.1, 7.2). The dental pulp derives from the dental papilla and is responsible for the production of dentine, which continues throughout life. It also acts as a sensory organ, detecting significant stimuli and toxins that may affect it. It has a positive, but limited, ability to respond to noxious stimuli by laying down additional dentine.

The tissues that support the teeth, known collectively as the periodontium (Figs 7.1, 7.2), include the alveolar bone forming the tooth sockets, the periodontal ligament (a connective tissue that attaches the tooth to the alveolar bone) and the gingivae (the component of the oral mucosa that forms a collar around the tooth).

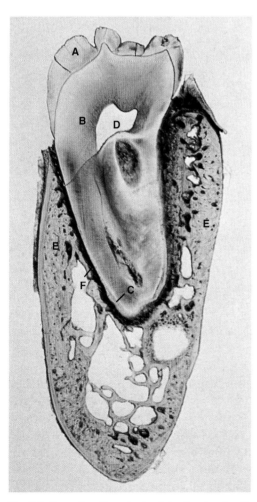

**Fig. 7.1** Ground section of a tooth in situ showing the distribution of the dental tissues. A = enamel; B = dentine; C = cementum; D = dental pulp; E = alveolar bone. As the section was embedded in plastic, part of the periodontal ligament (F) has been fortuitously retained (×4).

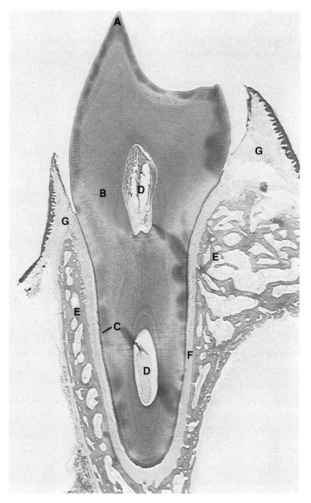

**Fig. 7.2** Demineralized section of a tooth in situ. A = enamel; B = dentine; C = cementum; D = dental pulp; E = alveolar bone; F = periodontal ligament; G = gingiva. Compared with Fig. 7.1, the enamel has been lost (×6). Courtesy of Dr D.A. Lunt.

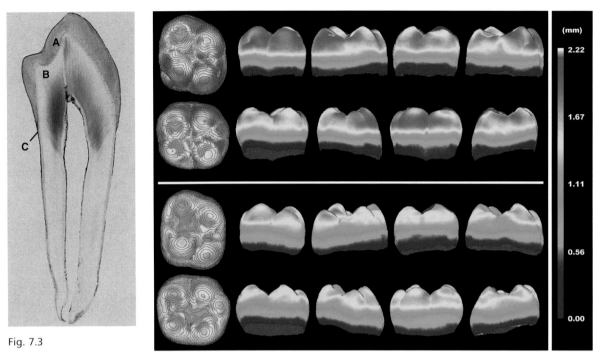

Fig. 7.3

Fig. 7.4

**Fig. 7.3** The distribution of enamel. A = enamel; B = dentine; C = cementum (×3).

**Fig. 7.4** Enamel thickness patterns of lateral and occlusal molar crown surfaces shown by colour grading. The colour scale to the right is common to all images. These images are obtained by taking an impression of each crown both before and after the enamel is removed by acid. Casts are made from these impressions and laser-scanned. The inner and outer surface of the enamel of each crown is reassembled using three-dimensional reconstruction software and the thickness of the enamel is measured and colour-coded. The images show the lateral crown surfaces of two individuals. Each individual is shown in either the top or bottom rows, with the maxillary and mandibular molars in the left and the right quadrants respectively (L = lingual, D = distal, B = buccal, M = mesial). The variation in thickness within each tooth is clearly seen and follows a similar pattern in each tooth. The numerical values for thickness vary substantially between individuals and to a lesser extent between teeth from the same individual. From Kono et al 2002 *Archives of Oral Biology* 47: 867–875, with permission.

## PHYSICAL PROPERTIES

Enamel covers the crown of the tooth (Fig. 7.3). It is thickest over cusps and incisal edges and thinnest at the cervical margin. Over the cusps of unworn permanent teeth it is about 2.5 mm thick (over the cusps of decid-uous teeth 1.3 mm), and on lateral surfaces up to 1.3 mm (Fig. 7.4). The thickness declines gradually to become a very thin layer at the cervical margin. Enamel thickness varies between individuals and between teeth (Fig. 7.4), increasing from first to third molar. While thickest in parts of the tooth that will suffer most attrition it is also relatively thick in some protected areas where it will add to the overall strength of the cusp and reduce the likelihood of fracture. Enamel is the hardest biological tissue and, while highly mineralized, withstands both shearing and impact forces well. Its abrasion resistance is high, allowing it to wear down only slowly, an important property as enamel can undergo neither repair nor replacement. Although enamel has a low tensile strength and is brittle, it has a high modulus of elasticity and this, together with the flexible support of the underlying dentine, minimizes the possibility of fracture. Enamel has a high specific gravity ($\approx$3).

The properties of enamel vary at different regions within the tissue. Surface enamel is harder, denser and less porous than subsurface enamel. Hardness and density also decrease from the surface towards the interior and from the cuspal/incisal tip towards the cervical margin.

Enamel is a birefringent crystalline material, the crystals refracting light differently in different directions. Young enamel is white because, although light enters it readily, it is almost entirely internally reflected with no wavelengths differentially absorbed. This results in low translucency and the white colour. The translucency of enamel increases with age and some of the colour of the underlying dentine is then transmitted, resulting in a more yellow appearance. The tissue has an average refractive index of 1.62. These optical properties considerably influence the histological appearance of enamel (e.g. explaining why there are differences with various mounting media). Some of the physical properties of enamel (and, for comparison, dentine) are listed in Table 7.1. Though softer than the geological materials enamel resists fracture three times as well (Table 7.2) because of the arrangement of the crystals into prisms and the incorpora-tion of an organic matrix.

**Table 7.1** *A comparison of the physical properties of enamel and dentine (typical values)*

|  | Enamel | Dentine |
|---|---|---|
| Specific gravity | 2.9 | 2.14 |
| Hardness (Knoop no.) | 296 | 64 |
| Stiffness (Young's modulus) | 131 GN/m² | 12 GN/m² |
| Compressive strength | 76 MN/m² | 262 MN/m² |
| Tensile strength | 46 MN/m² | 33 MN/m² |

GN = giganewtons (N × 10⁹), MN = meganewtons (N × 10⁶)

## CHEMICAL PROPERTIES

### HYDROXYAPATITE CRYSTALS

The principal mineral component of enamel is calcium hydroxyapatite, $Ca_{10}(PO_4)_6(OH)_2$, but in a form that contains impurities such as carbonate substituting for phosphate in the crystal lattice. This mineral comprises about 88–90% of the tissue by volume, corresponding to about 95–96% by weight. The remainder of the tissue is organic material and water. The mineral content increases from the dentine–enamel junction to the surface. Hydroxyapatite is present in the form of crystallites (Figs 7.5, 7.6) about 70 nm in width, 25 nm thick and of great length and generally extend across the full width of the tissue. Most crystallites are regularly hexagonal in cross-section (Figs 7.7, 7.8), although some are distorted by crowding during development. The cores of the crystallites differ slightly in composition from the periphery, being richer in magnesium and carbonate. The core of the crystallite is more soluble than the periphery. A comparison of some of the characteristics of enamel in comparison to geological hydroxyapatite and fluorapatite is shown in Table 7.2.

The molecular arrangement within each unit cell of the crystallite consists of a hydroxyl group surrounded by three uniformly spaced calcium ions, which in turn are surrounded by three similarly spaced phosphate ions. Six calcium ions in a uniform hexagon enclose the phosphate ions. The crystal consists of this arrangement of planes of ions repeated side by side and in

**Table 7.2** *Mechanical properties of enamel, hydroxyapatite and fluorapatite*

| | Fracture toughness (MPa m$^{1/2}$) | Vickers microhardness (GPa) |
|---|---|---|
| Enamel along prisms | 0.90 | – |
| Enamel across prisms | 1.30 | – |
| Enamel | – | 3.0 |
| Geological hydroxyapatite | 0.37 | 5.4 |
| Geological fluorapatite | 0.39 | 5.1 |

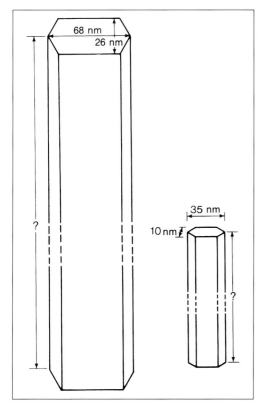

Fig. 7.5

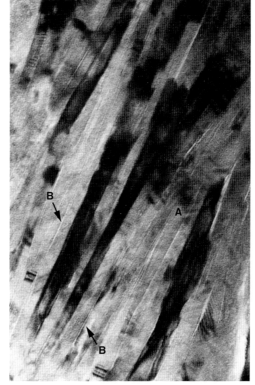

Fig. 7.6

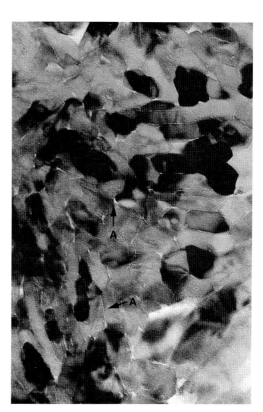

Fig. 7.7

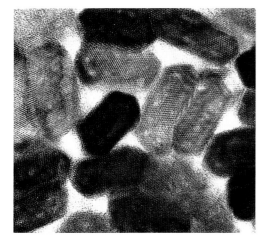

Fig. 7.8

**Fig. 7.5** The dimensions of an enamel crystallite (left) and a dentine crystallite (right). Both are impure hydroxyapatite.

**Fig. 7.6** Enamel crystallites in longitudinal section prepared by ion-beam thinning. For this technique a beam of ionized argon is directed obliquely onto the section so that is etched. In such specimens, crystallites (A) up to 100 μm long are seen and it is possible that some crystallites cross the full thickness of the enamel. B = Pores between crystallites (TEM; ×100 000). Courtesy of Drs H.J. Orams, P.P. Phakey and W. Rachinger, and the editor of *Advances in Dental Research*.

**Fig. 7.7** TEM showing enamel crystallites in cross-section prepared by ion-beam thinning, showing the hexagonal pattern of the enamel crystallites (×120 000). Small gaps or pores (A), which may contain water and organic material, occur between crystallites. Courtesy of Drs H.J. Orams, P.P. Phakey and W. Rachinger, and the editor of *Advances in Dental Research*.

**Fig. 7.8** TEM of isolated hexagonal enamel crystallites containing many hydroxyapatite molecules organized in a repeating pattern or lattice (×800 000). Courtesy of Professor H. Warshawsky.

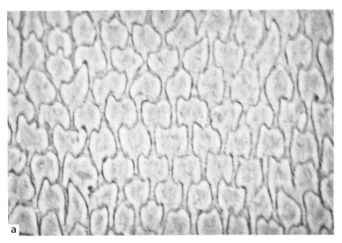
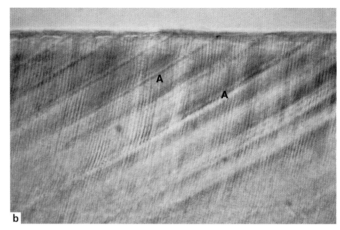

**Fig. 7.9** (a) Enamel prisms in transverse section demonstrating the keyhole pattern seen in most regions of human enamel (phase contrast ×14 500). (b) Enamel prisms cut longitudinally and running towards the surface in the direction of the arrow (×250). The lines running obliquely (A) are enamel striae. Courtesy of Dr D.F.G. Poole.

stacked layers. Although the basic molecular arrangement of the crystal is highly organized, it is subject to variation. 'Normal' ions may be replaced by different ionic species. Carbonate may occur at a phosphate or hydroxyl site (about 90% being found at the phosphate position). Magnesium may occur in the place of a calcium ion or elsewhere in the lattice. Fluoride may substitute for hydroxyl ions, conferring greater stability and resistance to acidic dissolution. Fluoride levels (unlike magnesium and carbonate) decline from the outer surface towards the dentine, perhaps because the fluoride is acquired during enamel maturation. Chloride, lead, zinc, sodium, strontium and aluminium ions may also substitute into the apatite lattice. Another change in the molecular arrangement occurs if one plane of ions 'slips' from the usual uniform arrangement with its neighbour.

It has been suggested, although not established with certainty, that small quantities of non-apatitic minerals may also be present in mature enamel. These possibly include octacalcium phosphate, which may be a hydroxy-apatite precursor.

## WATER

Water constitutes about 2% by weight of enamel, corresponding to 5–10% by volume. The presence of water is related to the porosity of the tissue. Some of the water may lie between crystals and surround the organic material, some may be trapped within defects of the crystalline structure and the remainder forms a hydration layer coating the crystals. As ions such as fluoride would travel through the water component its distribution is of clinical importance (see page 120).

## ORGANIC MATRIX

Mature enamel contains only 1–2% by weight of organic matrix. The organic component of regions where the crystallite arrangement is straight and regular may be as low as 0.05% w/w; where the prisms and crystallites are more irregular it may be as high as 3%. The most important components comprising the organic matrix are the enamel proteins.

Classically, the protein constituents of the enamel matrix have been divided into two groups: the amelogenins and the non-amelogenins. Those present in adult enamel are the remnants of a component that is very much larger during development, particularly during mineralization, and is best discussed during a description of this process (Ch. 22).

Although little studied, the lipid content of enamel appears to be a little less than that of protein. It too may represent the remnants of cell membranes remaining from development. Lipid material has been identified in the cross-striations, the lines of Retzius, the Hunter–Schreger bands, in the prism sheath and prism core in mature human enamel.

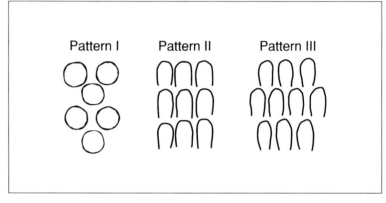

**Fig. 7.10** The three prism patterns seen in human enamel. In pattern I enamel the prisms are circular. In pattern II enamel the prisms are aligned in parallel rows. In pattern III enamel the prisms are arranged in staggered rows such that the tail of a prism lies between two heads in the next row, giving a keyhole appearance.

## ENAMEL PRISMS

Enamel is best described as a composite ceramic with the crystallites oriented in a complex three-dimensional continuum. The basic structural unit of enamel is the enamel prism or rod (Fig. 7.9), consisting of several million crystallites packed into a long thin rod 5–6 μm in diameter and up to 2.5 mm in length. Although the units are not strictly prismatic in outline, this term for the enamel unit has become accepted by widespread usage. Prisms run from the enamel–dentine junction to the surface. The boundaries of the prisms reflect sudden changes in crystallite orientation that give an optical effect different from that of the prism core or body: at the boundaries, the crystallites deviate by 40–60° from those inside the prism. Because of the resultant increased microporosity at the prism boundary, slightly more organic material can be accommodated.

Atomic force microscopy and nanoindentation techniques have been used to measure hardness and elastic modulus within single enamel prisms and the surrounding prism boundaries. The nanohardness and elastic modulus of the prism boundaries were approximately 75% and 50% lower than those within the prism cores.

In cross-section, the shape of an enamel prism approximates to one of three main patterns (Fig. 7.10). The distribution of the three pattern types varies between mammalian species. All three patterns are present in humans, but pattern III (Figs 7.9a and 7.11), the keyhole pattern, predominates. In pattern I enamel the prisms appear circular. The enamel between the prisms has been termed 'interprismatic'. Its composition is similar to that inside the prisms but it has a different optical effect because

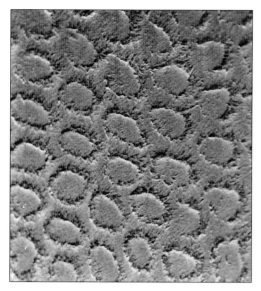

**Fig. 7.11** Circular pattern I prisms (SEM ×4300). Courtesy of Professor A. Boyde.

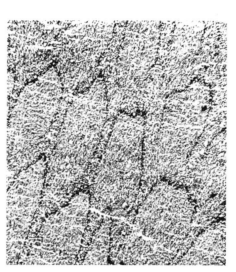

**Fig. 7.12** Transverse section of prisms showing type III keyhole pattern (TEM with silver staining ×2000). Courtesy of Dr D.F.G. Poole.

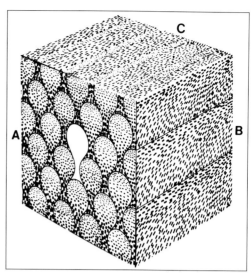

**Fig. 7.13** Crystallite orientation and prism structure in a diagrammatic representation of a block of enamel. A = cross-sectional view; B – lateral surface; C = top surface. The cross-sectional view reveals the characteristic keyhole arrangement of enamel prisms with the tails pointing cervically and the heads occlusally. In the head of the prism the crystallites run parallel to the long axis of the prism. In the tail, the crystallites gradually diverge from this to become angled 65–70° to the long axis. The change within a single prism is gradual such that no clear division between head and tail of the same prism is seen. However, the crystallites in the tail of one prism show a sudden divergence from the crystallites in the head of an adjacent prism. The sudden change in crystallite orientation at the prism boundary can be seen most clearly in the lateral surface of the block (B). On this surface, where the prisms have been cut exactly centrally through the head–tail axis, there are rows of equal but wide prisms. On the top surface (C), where the plane of section has passed through adjacent heads and tails, there is the appearance of broad prisms separated by narrower bands of 'interprismatic' enamel. It must be noted that in preparing histological material the enamel will be sectioned with varying degrees of obliquity, producing a wide variety of prism appearances and crystallite orientations. Courtesy of Drs A.H. Meckel, W.J. Griebstein and R.N. Neal, and John Wright, Publishers.

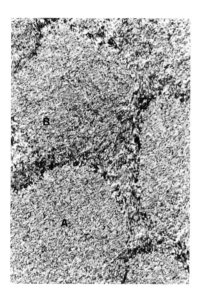

**Fig. 7.14** TEM showing enamel prisms cut transversely showing variations in crystal orientation between head (A) and tail (B) regions (×7000). Courtesy of Dr D.F.G. Poole.

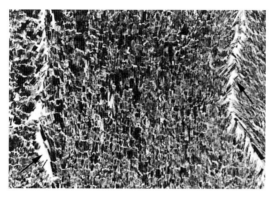

**Fig. 7.15** TEM showing enamel prisms cut longitudinally showing sudden change in orientation (arrow) at the prism boundary. The apparent space at the prism boundary represents a preparation artefact (×13500). Courtesy of Dr D.F.G. Poole.

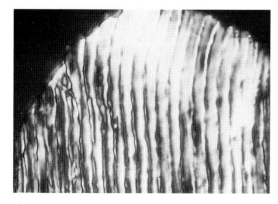

**Fig. 7.16** In polarized light, enamel cut longitudinal to the prisms shows a series of light and dark lines that distinguish the prism cores from the prism boundaries. This appearance is due to the abrupt change in orientation of the crystals at the prism boundary (and not to differential degrees of mineralization). Indeed, the presence of the enamel prism as a subunit of enamel is entirely due to these changes in crystal orientation (×600). Courtesy of Dr D.F.G. Poole.

the crystals deviate by 40–60° from those in the prism. Pattern 1 (Fig. 7.12) is found near the enamel–dentine junction and near the surface, possibly because the enamel in these regions is formed slowly.

The keyhole pattern III of enamel shows clear 'head' and 'tail' regions, the tail of one prism lying between the heads of the adjacent prisms and pointing cervically. There is an abrupt change in crystal orientation (Figs 7.13–7.15), which is responsible for the refraction of light and the appearance of the prism boundary. As polarized light identifies changes in crystallite orientation, it is useful in highlighting features in enamel such as prisms (Fig. 7.16).

In the head of the prism the crystals run parallel to the long axis of the prism. In the tail the crystals gradually diverge from this to become angled 65–70° to the long axis (Fig. 7.13, face A). The change within a single prism is gradual such that there is no clear division between head and tail of the same prism; however, the crystals in the tail of one prism show a sudden divergence from the crystals in the head of an adjacent prism (Figs 7.13, 7.14). In preparing histological material the enamel will be sectioned with varying degrees of obliquity, producing a wide variety of prism appearances. Although some areas may be termed interprismatic, what appears 'interprismatic' is often the tail of a prism from an adjacent row and prismatic and interprismatic enamel are really continuous. In fractured enamel observed by scanning electron microscopy peripheral crystallites

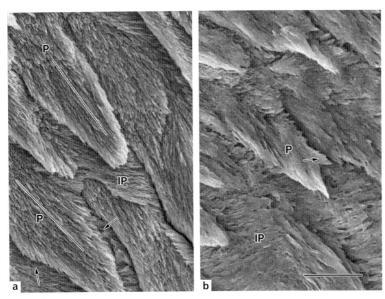

**Fig. 7.17** SEMs of prismatic (P) and interprismatic (IP) enamel in sagittal section (bar = 5 µm). Peripheral crystallites (arrow in (a)) deviate from the long axes of the prisms to form a continuum with interprismatic enamel (arrow in (b)). Interprismatic crystallites cross prisms at an angle of approximately 60°. Courtesy of Dr. S. White and the *Journal of Dental Research*.

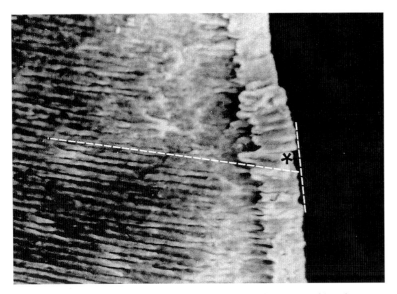

**Fig. 7.18** SEM of lightly etched enamel showing enamel prisms reaching the surface at 60° (*) (×320). Courtesy of Dr R.C. Shore and the CRC Press.

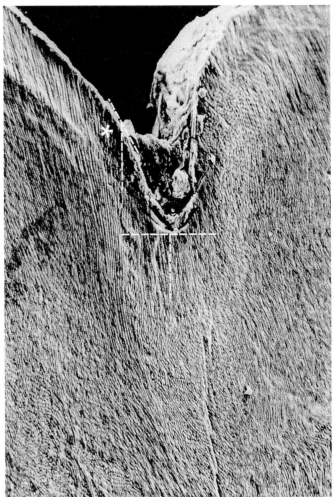

**Fig. 7.19** SEM showing the orientation of enamel prisms within an occlusal fissure. Note the acute angle (*) at which the prisms reach the surface in this region (×100). Courtesy of Dr R.C. Shore and the CRC Press.

(arrow in Fig. 7.17a) deviate from the long axes of the rods to form a continuum with interprismatic enamel (arrow in Fig. 17.7b). Interprismatic crystallites cross prisms at an angle of approximately 60°.

When viewed in enamel fractured or sectioned parallel to the long axis of the tooth (Fig. 7.9b), most prisms appear to travel in a sinusoidal line from the enamel–dentine junction to the surface (however, see Hunter–Schreger bands, below). The prisms meet the surface at varying angles, depending on the relative shape of the enamel–dentine junction and the outer surface. Just above the cervical margin prisms meet the surface at right angles whereas more occlusally they meet the surface at an angle of about 60° (Fig. 7.18). Within fissures, prisms make surface angles as acute as 20° (Fig. 7.19).

## HUNTER–SCHREGER BANDS

Between 10 and 13 layers of prisms follow the same direction but blocks above and below follow paths in different directions (Figs 7.20–7.22). These periodic changes in prism direction give rise to a banding pattern

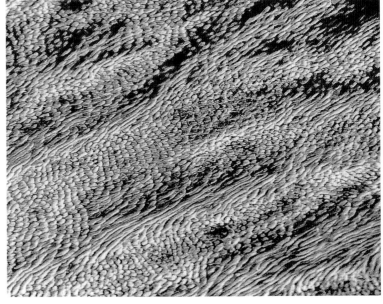

**Fig. 7.20** SEM of longitudinally sectioned enamel lightly etched to show alternating bands of transversely sectioned (diazones) and longitudinally sectioned (parazones) prisms (×160). Courtesy of Dr R.C. Shore and the CRC Press.

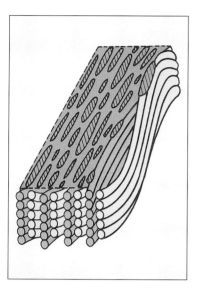

Fig. 7.21

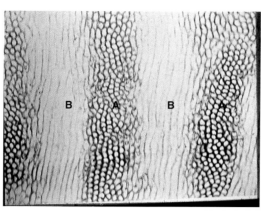

Fig. 7.22

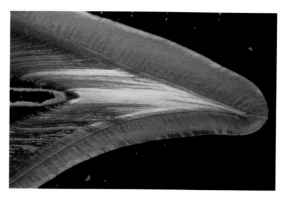

Fig. 7.23

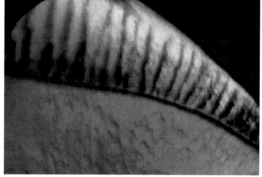

Fig. 7.24

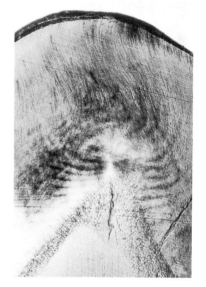

Fig. 7.25

**Fig. 7.21** The sinusoidal direction of the enamel prisms in alternating sheets results in alternately reflecting bands on the cut surface. Different sheets exhibit different crystal orientations and thus different degrees of polarization.

**Fig. 7.22** Longitudinal section of enamel showing alternating regions with groups of prism sectioned more transversely (A) or more longitudinally (B) that give rise to the appearance of Hunter–Schreger bands (×300). Courtesy of Dr B.A.W. Brown.

**Fig. 7.23** Longitudinal section of enamel showing Hunter–Schreger bands in reflected light (×12).

**Fig. 7.24** Longitudinal section of enamel showing Hunter–Schreger bands in polarized light. Note that the bands do not completely reach the outermost surface of the enamel (×25).

**Fig. 7.25** Longitudinal section of a cusp showing gnarled enamel (×25).

**Fig. 7.26** (a) SEM showing a layer of aprismatic enamel (A) of even thickness overlying a layer of prismatic enamel (B) (×63). (b) SEM showing a layer of aprismatic enamel (arrow) of uneven thickness overlying prismatic enamel. Courtesy of Dr D.K. Whittaker.

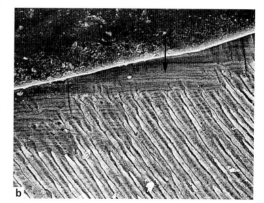

Fig. 7.26

termed the Hunter–Schreger bands (Fig. 7.23). These bands are approximately 50 μm wide and are visible because the different bands of prisms reflect or transmit light in different directions. In sections of enamel cut parallel to the long axis of the tooth, the individual crystallites will be oriented differently in the groups of prism cut more transversely or more longitudinally. The bands of prisms that are cut longitudinally are known as parazones and those cut transversely as diazones. The angle between parazones and diazones is about 40°. This complex pattern of prisms makes enamel resistant to fracture and, when exposed on the surface, leads to a micro-ridged grinding surface. In approximately the outer quarter of enamel, the prisms all run in the same direction and no Hunter–Schreger bands are present (Fig. 7.24).

As prisms are arranged in a spiral pattern, in some areas beneath the cusps and incisal edges the changes in direction of the prisms appear more marked and irregular. Groups of prisms seem to spiral around others, giving the appearance of 'gnarled' enamel (Fig. 7.25).

## NON-PRISMATIC (APRISMATIC/PRISMLESS) ENAMEL

The outer 20–100 μm of enamel of newly erupted deciduous teeth and the outer 20–70 μm of newly erupted permanent teeth is non-prismatic. Here, the enamel crystallites are all aligned at right angles to the surface and parallel to each other. This surface layer is more highly mineralized than the rest of the enamel because of the absence of prism boundaries, where more organic material is located. Its thickness is variable (Fig. 7.26). A very thin layer of non-prismatic enamel, just a few microns wide, has also been reported to be present in the first enamel formed at the enamel–dentine junction. Non-prismatic enamel occurs as a result of the absence of Tomes processes from the ameloblasts in the first and final stages of enamel deposition (see Ch. 22).

## INCREMENTAL LINES

During development changes in the enamel secretory rhythm, chemical composition and/or the position of the developing enamel front are recorded as incremental features. There are two main types of incremental line: short period (cross-striations) and long period (enamel striae).

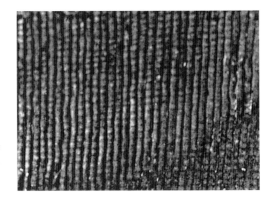

**Fig. 7.27** Phase-contrast microscopy of longitudinal section of enamel showing cross-striations (horizontal lines) along the enamel prisms (×400). Courtesy of Dr D.F.G. Poole.

## CROSS-STRIATIONS

Cross-striations are lines that cross enamel prisms at right angles to their long axes (Fig. 7.27) with a common interval of about 3–6 μm being closer together near the enamel–dentine junction.

These are diurnal being formed every 24 hours parallel to the secretory face of the ameloblast. Their appearance may relate to regular variations in prism width (Figs 7.28, 7.29). It has also been suggested that the appearance of cross-striations is the result of subtle changes in the nature of the organic matrix and/or crystallite orientation.

**Fig. 7.28** SEM of fractured enamel surface showing cross-striations along the length of prisms seemingly corresponding to sites of narrowing of the prism width (×600). Courtesy of Professor M.C. Dean.

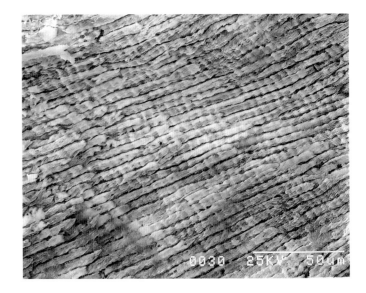

**Fig. 7.29** SEM of lightly etched enamel showing individual enamel crystallites (arrows) terminating at constrictions of prisms (*) (×1600). Courtesy of Dr R.C. Shore and the CRC Press.

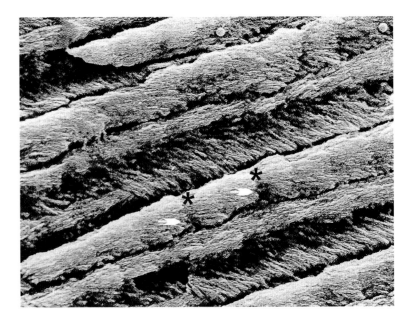

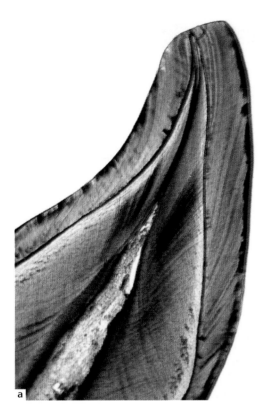

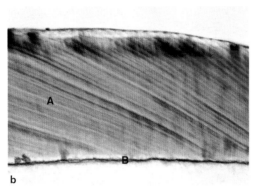

**Fig. 7.30** (a) Longitudinal section of enamel showing enamel striae running obliquely across the tissue. Wear at the tip of the cusp has exposed some of the striae on the surface at this site. Along the slopes of the tooth the striae naturally reach the surface (×15). (b) Higher-power view (×40) of enamel striae in enamel (A) along the side of the tooth running from the enamel–dentine junction (B) to the surface.

## ENAMEL STRIAE

In sections of enamel cut along the longitudinal axis of the crown the enamel striae (or striae of Retzius) are seen as prominent lines that run obliquely across the enamel prisms to the surface (Fig. 7.30). In horizontal sections they form concentric rings (Fig. 7.31). They represent the successive positions of the enamel-forming front. The periodic nature of this feature, which may be assessed by the number of cross-striations between successive enamel lines has been one of the more contentious topics in the study of enamel microstructure.

Although following routine demineralization all enamel structure is lost because of the low content of the organic matrix, leaving an enamel space (Fig. 7.2), controlled (and probably incomplete) demineralization will allow retention of some organic material for subsequent staining. Many of the structural features seen in ground sections will be retained. The keyhole pattern of the prisms can be clearly seen (Fig. 7.32a). Although it is known that the prism lacks an organic sheath, the level of organic material and water is likely to be higher at the prism boundary because of the larger

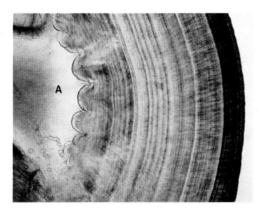

**Fig. 7.31** Transverse section of enamel showing enamel striae running circumferentially. A = dentine (×120). Courtesy of Dr M.E. Atkinson.

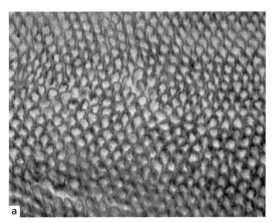

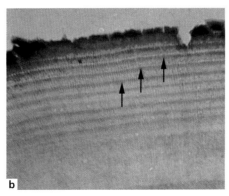

**Fig. 7.32** (a) Demineralized section of enamel prisms cut transversely showing retained enamel matrix presenting a prismatic appearance (Light blue stain; ×600). (b) Demineralized transverse section of enamel showing enamel striae patterns (arrows) in the retained enamel matrix (Light blue stain; ×150).

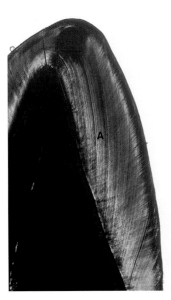

**Fig. 7.33** Longitudinal section of unworn enamel (A) showing that striae passing over the cusp do not reach the outer tooth surface, but those more laterally do (×20). Courtesy of Drs R.J. Hillier and G.T. Craig.

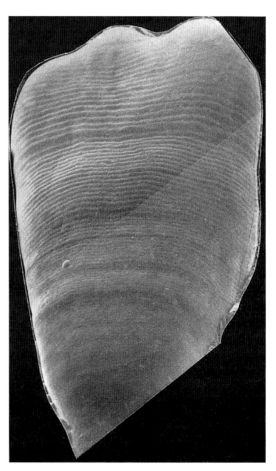

**Fig. 7.35** SEM of enamel surface of a human lower incisor showing numerous transversely running perikymata grooves and ridges (×10). Courtesy of Professor M.C. Dean and the *Journal of Human Evolution*.

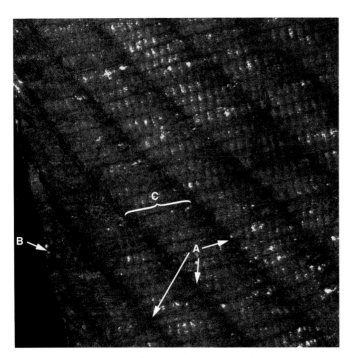

**Fig. 7.34** Confocal image of a longitudinal section of enamel showing enamel striae (A) reaching the surface at perikymata grooves (B). Between adjacent striae, about seven cross-striations (C) are evident as vertical lines (×850). Courtesy of Professor M.C. Dean.

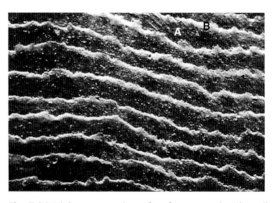

**Fig. 7.36** Higher power view of surface enamel with perikymata grooves (A) separated by perikymata ridges (B) (SEM, ×400). Courtesy of Dr D.F.G. Poole.

pores produced by the abutment of hydroxyapatite crystallites at this junction. This, and the apparently lower solubility of the organic matrix at the prism boundary, can explain the deeper staining at these sites. Enamel striae are also observed in demineralized sections (Fig. 7.32b).

Due to the manner in which enamel is deposited (see page 320), the striae overlying the cusps and incisal edges do not reach the surface (Fig. 7.33) unless there has been enamel loss (Fig. 7.30a). In the case of unworn incisors, the first 25–30 striae do not reach the surface.

In human teeth there are seven to 10 cross-striations between adjacent striae in any one individual (Fig. 7.34). The striae are therefore formed at about weekly intervals. As the average distance between two cross-striations is about 4 μm, enamel striae in the middle portion of enamel are about 25–35 μm apart. In cervical enamel, where enamel is formed more slowly and cross-striations may be only about 2 μm apart, the striae are

closer together and may be separated by only 15–20 μm. Accentuated striae may be due to metabolic disturbances occurring during the time of mineralization.

Over the whole of the lateral enamel, enamel striae reach the surface in a series of fine grooves running circumferentially around the crown. These features are known as the perikymata grooves and are separated by ridges, the perikymata ridges (Figs 7.35–7.37, 7.40). The distance between perikymata reflects the data already given for that of enamel striae: they are close together near the cervical margin (about 15–20 μm) but as they reach the surface obliquely may be up to 100 μm apart towards the cusp of the tooth. The process that results in the production of the enamel striae is unknown.

In deciduous teeth, enamel striae and perikymata are only ever clearly seen in the cervical enamel of deciduous second molars.

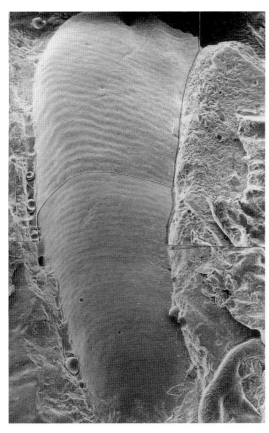

**Fig. 7.37** SEM showing perikymata on the surface of a mandibular incisor from *Paranthropus robustus* (×10). Courtesy of Professor M.C. Dean.

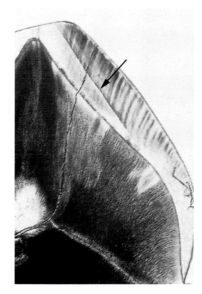

**Fig. 7.38** Longitudinal section of a deciduous tooth showing a neonatal line (arrow) (×6). Courtesy of Drs R.J. Hillier and G.T. Craig.

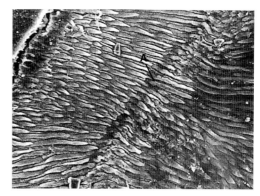

**Fig. 7.39** SEM of an etched longitudinal section of deciduous enamel showing enamel prisms changing in both thickness and direction at the neonatal line (A) (×400). Courtesy of Dr D.K. Whittaker.

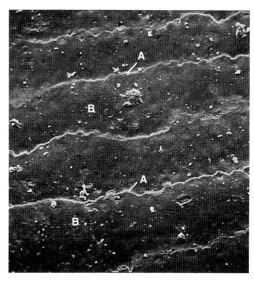

**Fig. 7.40** SEM of enamel surface showing perikymata grooves (A) separated from each other by perikymata ridges (B) (×500). Courtesy of Professor H.N. Newman.

The exaggeration of striae in different teeth forming at the same time suggests a common systemic influence. One hypothesis is that there may be a rhythm with a 27-hour cycle in addition to a diurnal daily rhythm. The two rhythms would coincide approximately every 7 or 8 days, producing a fault in the developing enamel. The underlying reason for the structural feature apparent as a stria in ground section is differential light-scattering effects at this fault line, possibly due to a slight change in prism direction/thickness, or slight differences in crystallite composition/orientation, and/or differences in organic content. That the striae are seen in partially demineralized sections has been interpreted by some as being due to the site of striae having a higher carbonate content, which causes greater solubility of the crystals and greater porosity.

It is possible to use the incremental markings in enamel (cross-striations, enamel striae and perikymata) to assess the time taken to form the crown of the tooth and to help age material. As impressions of the surface enamel can record the perikymata, rare teeth of fossil hominids have also been studied without the need to prepare destructive ground sections (Fig. 7.37). Assuming adjacent perikymata are separated by approximately 7-day intervals, the total number of perikymata on a crown indicates the time taken for the crown to form, if about 6–9 months are added to this total to account for the 25–30 striae over the top of the crown that do not reach the surface (Fig. 7.33). From such studies it has been found, for example, that the teeth of apes and many extinct hominids develop more quickly than those of modern humans. There is some evidence in primates that the number of cross-striations between two adjacent striae reflects body size: in monkeys, there are only four to five cross-striations between striae.

Enamel striae are less pronounced or absent from enamel formed before birth. A particularly marked stria is formed at birth – this is the neonatal line (Fig. 7.38) and reflects the metabolic changes at birth. Prisms appear to change both direction and thickness at the time of this event (Fig. 7.39).

## SURFACE ENAMEL

The surface of the enamel is, perhaps, its most clinically significant region. It is here that the tooth comes into contact with food, dental caries is initiated, restorations are attached or abutted, orthodontic brackets are cemented and toothpaste, bleaches and fluoride/remineralization preparations applied.

Both physically and chemically, surface enamel differs markedly from subsurface enamel. Surface enamel is harder, less porous, less soluble and more radio-opaque than subsurface enamel. It is richer in some trace elements (especially fluoride) but contains less carbonate. The enamel surface presents a variable appearance, exhibiting features such as aprismatic enamel, perikymata, prism-end markings, cracks, pits and elevations.

The surface enamel, if unabraded, is in most areas aprismatic and thus more highly mineralized and resistant to caries (Fig. 7.26). This may help explain why acid etching, unless sufficient to penetrate to the prismatic enamel, may not always enhance adhesion. Although the surface enamel is aprismatic, the incremental striae of Retzius reach the surface and appear as perikymata grooves, wave-like concentric surface rings parallel to the cementum–enamel junction. The perikymata grooves are separated from each other by the wave-like perikymata ridges (Fig. 7.40, see also Figs 7.35–7.37). Attrition and abrasion remove these features after eruption but they may persist in protected cervical areas. In some areas, particularly cervically where the reduced enamel epithelium persists for some time after eruption, small pits are seen within the perikymata. These are the impressions of the ends of the ameloblasts and are 1–1.5 µm in depth (Fig. 7.41).

Small cracks are frequently found in surface enamel (Fig. 7.42), although it is difficult to know whether many of these were present in vivo or were induced by the procedures necessary to examine the tissue. They represent potential areas of weakness. The orientation of the enamel prisms as they reach the surface may determine whether small cracks extend easily. In areas were the prisms make an acute angle with the surface, such as in the intercuspal region, enamel will resist fracture best. Small elevations 10–15 µm across (enamel caps, Fig. 7.43) or depressions (focal holes, Fig. 7.44) are also found, particularly on lateral surfaces. The caps are thought to result from enamel deposition on top of small deposits of non-mineralizable debris late in development. The focal holes result from loss of the cap and underlying material by abrasion or attrition.

Larger surface elevations, enamel brochs, 30–50 µm in diameter, also occur occasionally and consist of radiating groups of crystals (Fig. 7.45). They seem to be more common in premolars but are of unknown origin.

The loss of tooth structure can occur by three different mechanisms: attrition, abrasion and erosion.

- **Attrition** is tooth loss involving tooth to tooth contact. Attrition occurs both occlusally and interproximally. In molars, occlusal attrition is most commonly seen on the palatal surfaces of maxillary molars

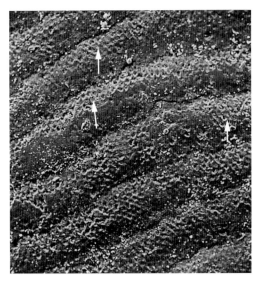

**Fig. 7.41** SEM showing prism-end markings (arrows) on surface of enamel. Compare with Fig. 7.40, which lacks this feature (×300). Courtesy of Professor H.N. Newman.

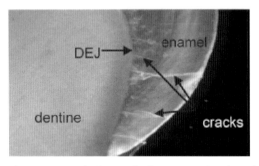

**Fig. 7.42** Optical micrograph of a cross-section through a tooth, showing cracks that have propagated through the enamel but stop at the dentine–enamel junction (DEJ), without penetrating into the dentine. Marshall SJ et al 2003 *Journal of the European Ceramic Society* 23: 2897–2904, with permission.

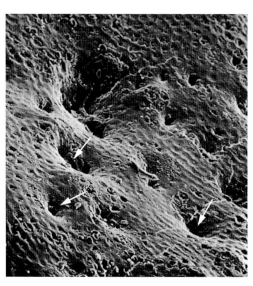

**Fig. 7.44** SEM of enamel surface showing focal holes (arrows) (×400). Courtesy of Professor H.N. Newman.

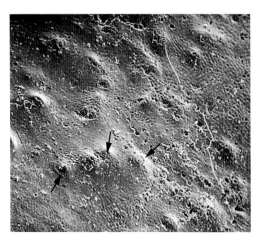

**Fig. 7.43** SEM of enamel surface showing enamel caps (arrows) (×150). Courtesy of Professor H.N. Newman.

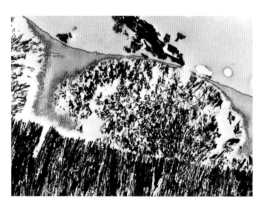

**Fig. 7.45** TEM showing an enamel broch (×10000). Courtesy of Professor H.N. Newman.

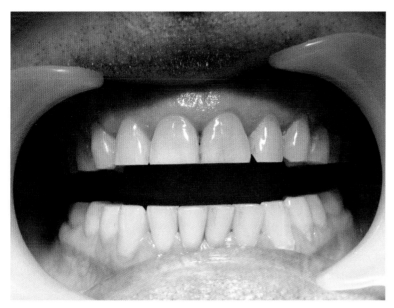

**Fig. 7.46** Attrition in patient suffering from bruxism (tooth grinding). Note the flattened occlusal plane. Courtesy of Professor T.J. Watson.

and the buccal surface of mandibular molars. The potential space to be expected during interproximal wear is generally closed up by mesial drift (see pages 373, 374). Thus, although initial tooth contact areas are small, these become broader with age. In people who habitually clench their teeth (bruxists) attrition may be severe and the occlusal plane flat (Fig. 7.46). There may also be exposure of sensitive dentine.

- **Abrasion** is tooth loss involving friction between the tooth and outside material. A common cause is tooth brush abrasion seen on the labial and buccal surfaces (Fig. 7.47).
- **Erosion** is tooth loss involving contact with acidic agents that may be extrinsic (e.g. soft drinks, citrus fruit – Fig. 7.48) or intrinsic (gastric acids following chronic regurgitation). In cases of bulimia, the erosion characteristically affects the palatal surfaces of the upper anterior teeth (Fig. 7.49).

While non-carious loss of cervical enamel is usually attributed to toothbrush abrasion and/or erosion, it has been suggested that such loss may also be the result of occlusal loading causing flexure and ultimate material fatigue. Such a process has been termed abfraction. If true, this may have to be taken into account when restoring non-carious cervical lesions, in that any evidence of excessive loading should also be treated.

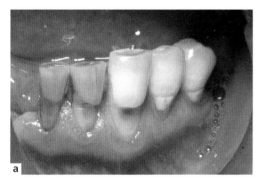
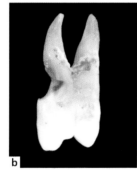

**Fig. 7.47** (a) Toothbrush abrasion in the cervical region of the labial surfaces of the anterior teeth. Courtesy of Professor T.J. Watson. (b) Side view of abrasion. Although this appearance is usually attributed to frictional contact with an outside material such as dental floss or a toothbrush, other factors such as occlusal stress or corrosion from bacterial plaque may also be involved. The term 'abfraction' is used to describe this kind of lesion with a multifactorial basis. Courtesy of Dr J. Grippo.

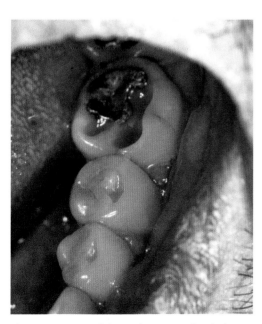

**Fig. 7.48** Erosion of the teeth associated with the consumption of grapefruit, producing irregular concavities on the occlusal surfaces. Courtesy of Professor T.J. Watson.

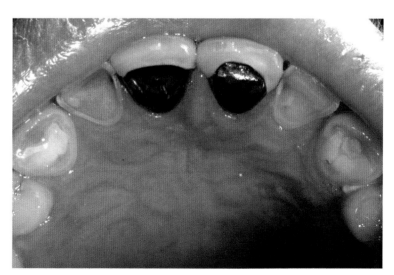

**Fig. 7.49** Erosion of the upper anterior teeth in a patient suffering from bulimia. The central incisors have already been restored. Courtesy of Professor T.J. Watson.

## ENAMEL–DENTINE JUNCTION

The boundary between enamel and dentine is known as the enamel–dentine junction. In permitting the strong union of two such dissimilar mineralized tissues, the enamel–dentine junction must exhibit some unique features, particularly that associated with retardation of crack propagation (Fig. 7.42). Structurally, there are three levels of features. The largest is the characteristic scalloping pattern, varying between 25 μm and 100 μm. This is particularly evident beneath cusps and incisal edges (Figs 7.50, 7.51), areas where shearing forces would be high; the enamel–dentine junction is smoother on the lateral surfaces of the crown. The convexities of the scallops are on the enamel surface (Fig. 7.52), with the concavities on the dentinal surface (Fig. 7.53). With increased magnification, a second order of structure is the presence of smaller, micro-scallops 2–5 μm in size. A third, nanostructural level of organization, yet to be fully determined also

exists, perhaps with the ends of fine collagen fibrils from the dentine mingling with the initial crystals of enamel. Dentine crystals are much smaller than those of enamel and the transition from one to the other at the junction of the tissues is generally clear (Fig. 7.54). The enamel–dentine junction is less mineralized than either the enamel or dentine.

A number of features can be seen at the enamel–dentine junction (amelodentinal junction), extending from the dentine surface into the enamel including enamel spindles and tufts.

## ENAMEL SPINDLES

Narrow (up to 8 μm in diameter), round, sometimes club-shaped tubules – the enamel spindles – extend up to 25 μm into the enamel (Fig. 7.56). They are not aligned with the prisms and are thought to be the result of some odontoblast processes that, during the early stages of enamel devel-

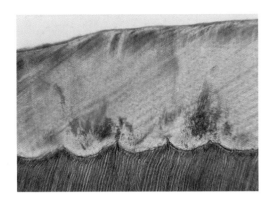

**Fig. 7.50** Scalloped appearance of the enamel–dentine junction beneath the cusp of a tooth (×60).

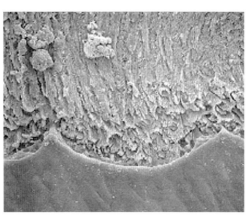

**Fig. 7.51** SEM showing scallop structure in the enamel–dentine junction, with enamel on the top and dentine on the bottom. Marshall SJ et al 2003 *Journal of the European Ceramic Society* 23: 2897–2904, with permission.

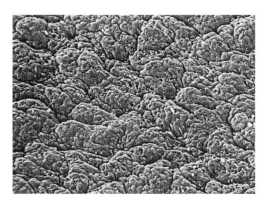

**Fig. 7.52** SEM of the enamel surface that lies in contact with the dentine, separation having been achieved following dehydration and fracture. The enamel surface is convex at this site (×250). Courtesy of Dr D.K. Whittaker.

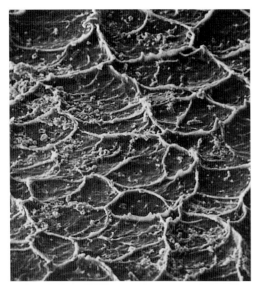

**Fig. 7.53** SEM of dentine surface at the enamel–dentine junction, following removal of enamel by demineralization. The dentine at this site shows a series of concavities (×400). Courtesy of Dr B.G.H. Levers.

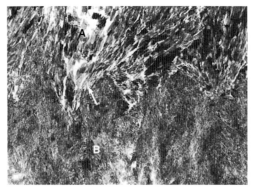

**Fig. 7.54** TEM showing enamel (A) and dentine (B) crystallites at the enamel–dentine junction (arrow). Note the larger size of the enamel crystallites (×18000). Courtesy of Professor H.N. Newman.

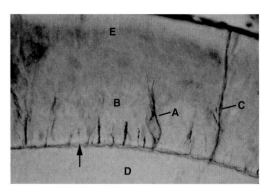

**Fig. 7.55** Transverse section showing the enamel dentine junction. A = enamel tuft; B = enamel spindle; C = enamel lamella; D = dentine; E = enamel (×60). Courtesy of Dr R. Sprinz.

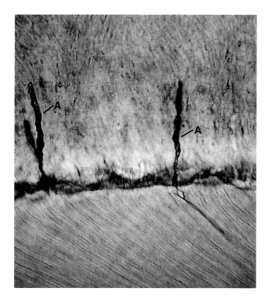

**Fig. 7.56** Longitudinal section of enamel showing enamel spindles (A) (×250). Courtesy of Dr R. Sprinz.

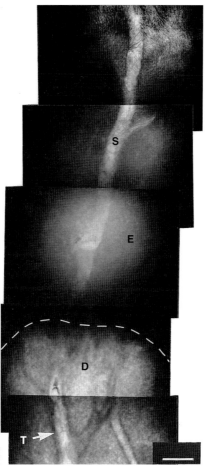

**Fig. 7.57** TEM showing an enamel spindle (S) appearing as the continuation of a dentinal tubule (T) from dentine (D) into enamel (E) (×6500). Courtesy of J. Palamara, P.P. Phakey, W.A. Rachinger and H.J. Orams, and the editor of *Advances in Dental Science*.

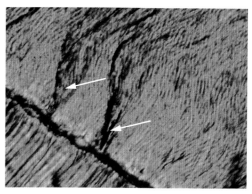

**Fig. 7.58** Transverse section of enamel showing enamel tufts (arrows) (×200).

opment, insinuated themselves between the ameloblasts. The size of some would exceed the usual dimension of dentinal tubules. It has also been suggested that they may be dentinal collagen or the remnants of dead odontoblasts (Fig. 7.57). Enamel spindles are most common beneath cusps where most crowding of odontoblasts would have occurred. In the erupted tooth these tubules do not contain cell processes. Because of their alignment, they are best seen in longitudinal sections of enamel.

## ENAMEL TUFTS

Enamel tuft is the term given to junctional structures in the inner third of the enamel that, in ground sections, resemble tufts of grass (Fig. 7.58). They appear to travel in the same direction as the prisms and, in thick sections, undulate with sheets of prisms. They are hypomineralized and recur at approximately 100 µm intervals along the junction. Each tuft is several prisms wide. It has been suggested that this appearance results from protein, presumed to be residual organic enamel matrix, at the prism boundaries of hypomineralized prisms (Fig. 7.59). Owing to their alignment, tufts are best visualized in transverse sections of enamel. Tufts contain 'tuftelin', a member of the non-amelogenin group of proteins. The protein content of enamel is highest in region of the enamel tufts.

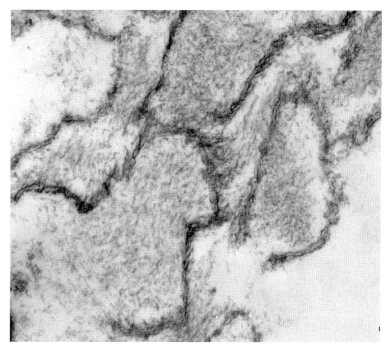

**Fig. 7.59** TEM of an enamel tuft separated from the dentine surface after demineralization of the enamel. The dense staining areas are presumptive prism boundaries representing organic matrix (×11000). Courtesy of Dr R.C. Shore and the CRC Press.

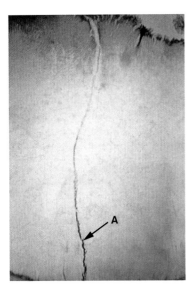

**Fig. 7.60** Demineralized section of enamel sectioned transversely to show an enamel lamella (A) (Light blue stain; ×150).

## ENAMEL LAMELLAE

Enamel lamellae are sheet-like, apparent structural faults that run through the entire thickness of the enamel (Fig. 7.60). They are hypomineralized and narrower, longer and less common than enamel tufts but, like tufts, are best visualized in transverse sections of enamel. In routine ground sections, many lamella-like structures are simply cracks produced during section preparation. This can be confirmed by demineralizing the section, when cracks (but not true lamellae) will disappear.

Lamellae may arise developmentally due to incomplete maturation of groups of prisms (in which case they would contain enamel proteins) or after eruption as cracks produced during loading of enamel and containing saliva and oral debris.

## MICROPOROSITY OF ENAMEL

In vivo, the pores in enamel are water-filled spaces between the crystallites. Figures as high as 10–12% have been quoted for pore volume based on thermogravimetric analysis. These values, however, may be inflated because of the release of water that is normally a structural part of the enamel crystallites. From studies based on water absorption techniques, enamel appears to have a porosity of about 3–5% by volume, but even this figure may not be a true reflection of the porosity as it may incorporate a factor related to water that is bound to the organic material. Within the prisms most pores exist as very narrow gaps between closely packed crystallites but some, although they are still small, appear elongated and tube-like. Most of the pores are accessible only to small molecules such as water. Polarized light studies, internal surface area measurements and etching studies suggest that most, if not all, of the pores that are accessible to molecules larger than water are distributed in the prism boundaries, while the pores that are accessible only to small molecules are found throughout the rest of the enamel. The prism boundaries may thus be thought of as main highways through the enamel, while the rest of the porosity may be thought of as a fine network of footpaths connecting occasionally with the main highways so that access through them is slow and restricted. The pathways for diffusion and, to a lesser extent, electrochemical effects arising from the charge on the pore walls have an important influence on the formation of a carious lesion. Putative micropores are shown in Figures 7.6 and 7.7.

## TOOTH WHITENING

Whether agents – food, drinks, tobacco, etc. – stain the enamel surface or not depends on the attraction of the materials to the tooth surface by such mechanisms as electrostatic charge, van de Waals forces and short-range interactions such as hydration and hydrogen bonds). These forces bring the chromogenic materials or their precursors to the tooth surface and determine if adhesion will occur. The chromogens may then penetrate the enamel fill pores and bind to the organic matrix. Whitening agents such as hydrogen or carbamide peroxide produce reactive molecules (free radicals) that penetrate the enamel pores and act as both an oxygenator and an oxidant, reducing the large chromogenic organic molecules in the enamel matrix to smaller, less noticeable molecules that may diffuse out from the enamel, or will absorb less light and hence give a lighter appearance. These agents are effective (Fig. 7.61). Their degree of effectiveness depends on the concentration of the whitening agent, the duration and number of applications and the ability of the agent to reach the stain. They may, initially, cause a small reduction in the microhardness of enamel, but this soon returns to normal after the treatment.

## AGE CHANGES IN ENAMEL

Enamel wears away slowly with age, the amount lost being dependent on diet and masticatory habits. It seems to darken in colour, which may be in part due to the reduced translucency of the tooth as secondary dentine forms and enamel thins and in part to the accumulation of surface coatings (see Ch. 8) and stains. The composition of the surface enamel alters as a result of additions and exchanges with the oral fluids. Fluoride can beneficially be incorporated into surface enamel. This reduces its porosity and susceptibility to caries. The older patient may have had more time for dental caries to develop.

**Fig. 7.61** Intra-oral photographs of anterior teeth before (a) and after (b) whitening.

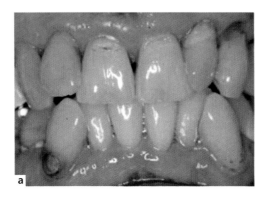
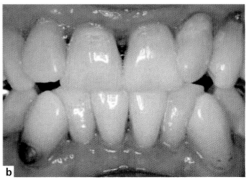

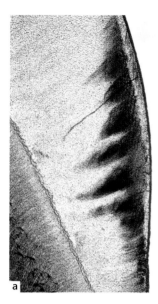
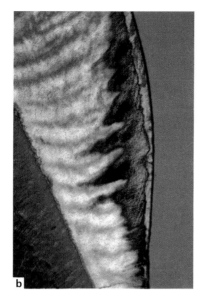
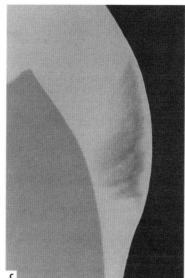

**Fig. 7.62** An early carious lesion, which clinically would appear as a 'white spot' without cavitation. (a) A ground section showing an apparently intact surface zone but darker regions beneath it where mineral has been lost. (b) The same section seen in polarizing light. (c) The same section as a microradiograph with a darker (less radiodense) subsurface zone (×24). Courtesy of Dr B.H. Clarkson.

## CEMENTUM–ENAMEL JUNCTION

This feature is discussed with cementum on page 176.

## CLINICAL CONSIDERATIONS

### ENAMEL STRUCTURE AND DENTAL CARIES

In tooth decay (dental caries), acids produced by plaque dissolve enamel mineral. As there is very little matrix, the histologically observable changes are due to demineralization. The basic description of the structure of the carious lesion is based on the observation of ground sections in polarized light (Fig. 7.62), as this approach gives an appearance related to crystallite content. In early lesions before cavitation occurs the surface enamel shows relatively little change but beneath it, in the 'body' of the lesion, 20–50% of the mineral is lost. When mineral is dissolved the loss begins at the periphery of the prism. The mineral is not necessarily lost permanently, as remineralization does occur (saliva is saturated with mineral). During carious attack a repeating cycle of demineralization and remineralization occurs: clearly, if demineralization dominates the caries progresses. That the possession of a relatively intact surface layer (despite considerable subsurface demineralization) in the carious lesion does not reflect unique features of the surface enamel (but more a process of reprecipitation of mineral) is evident from in vitro studies, in which the surface layer of enamel was ground away to a considerable depth and carious-like lesions induced artificially. In such lesions, an intact surface lesion still appeared as a characteristic feature of the carious lesion.

The basis of the treatment of early caries and the prevention of caries is to tip the balance in favour of remineralization and away from demineralization. Thus, caries is prevented by procedures that minimize plaque formation (diet and oral hygiene), starve such plaque biofilm as is present of acid-producing substrates (diet), render the enamel mineral less soluble (fluoride) and encourage remineralization (diet, fluoride mouthwash and toothpaste).

### ENAMEL STRUCTURE AND RESTORATIVE DENTISTRY

Many of the structural features of enamel are acutely relevant to restorative dentistry. The understanding of the initiation and progress of

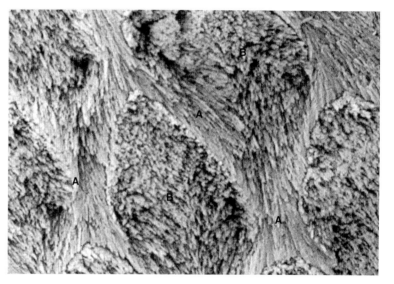

**Fig. 7.63** SEM of enamel prisms etched end-on with an acid (maleic acid), showing a differential etch pattern between the prism boundary region (A) and the prism core region (B). This produces a microscopically rough surface suitable for the retention of a resin-based adhesive (×6000). Courtesy of Professor B. Van

dental caries has been based on knowledge of enamel composition and morphology. This has led to a much more conservative approach by utilizing the phenomenon of remineralization and reducing the need for the removal of sound tissue. This reduced sacrifice of sound tooth structure has also been brought about by the development of adhesives that will bond to enamel, a development that is based on an understanding of the prismatic structure of enamel and the controllable effects of acids on it. Different acids at different concentrations can produce a variety of patterns of partial prism dissolution to provide a roughened surface suitable for adherence of restorative materials (acid conditioning). This reduces or eliminates the need for mechanical retention cut into sound tissue. For agents mechanically binding to enamel, it is necessary to produce microporosities in the surface by acid-etch techniques (Fig. 7.63). Thus, when bonding agents are applied to such a

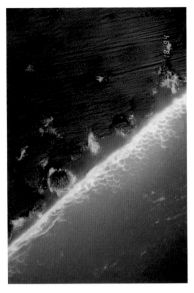

Meerbeek.

**Fig. 7.64** Confocal microscope image showing the penetration of a (yellow) dye-labelled bonding agent into acid-etched enamel. Note tags of resin around the prism boundaries made porous by acid etching (×450). Courtesy of Professor

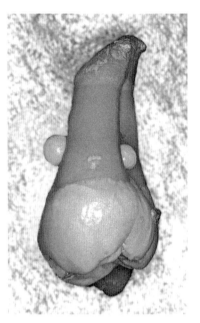

cross-section (×450). Courtesy of Professor T. Watson.

**Fig. 7.66** Palatal view of a maxillary third molar with large pearls on the mesial and distal surfaces. Risnes S et al 2000 *Oral Surgery Oral Medicine Oral Pathology*

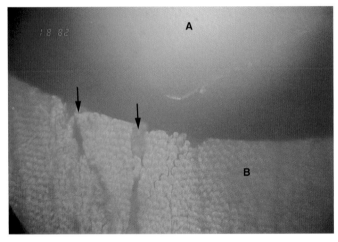

T. Watson.

**Fig. 7.65** Confocal microscope image of the interface between a dental bur (A) and the enamel wall (B) taken during the actual cutting of a cavity. Note the fracture lines (arrows), the prism boundaries, the enamel prisms being viewed in

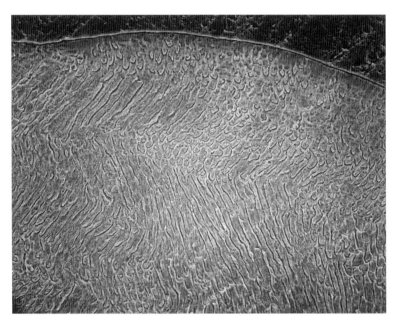

*Radiology & Endodontics* 89: 493–497.

**Fig. 7.67** Enamel from the central part of the pearl showing the irregular course of prisms (Original magnification ×312). Risnes S et al 2000 *Oral Surgery Oral*

surface, microscopic tags can be seen invaginating into the roughened surface (Fig. 7.64).

When cavities are prepared, knowledge of the microanatomy of enamel, particularly in terms of prism orientation, is essential to conserve as much as possible of the original strength of the tissue. Cutting cavities into enamel with rotary instruments will inevitably lead to subsurface cracking. Fortunately, some of the adhesive materials are capable of reinforcing this weakened substrate (Fig. 7.65).

## ENAMEL PEARLS

These are small isolated spheres of enamel that are occasionally found on the root, generally towards the cervical margin (Fig. 7.66). The enamel is

prismatic with the prisms following an irregular course (Fig 7.67). They are particularly common in the root bifurcation region where they may predispose to plaque accretion following gingival recession.

## DEVELOPMENTAL DEFECTS IN ENAMEL

These are considered with the development of enamel in Chapter 22.

Throughout its life, the crown of a tooth is covered by an organic layer or integument. Before the tooth erupts into the oral cavity the crown is covered by the overlying oral mucosa, the coronal part of the dental follicle, and the vestiges of the enamel organ (plus its associated primary enamel cuticle). For information concerning the origins of the enamel organ and the dental follicle during early tooth development, see Chapter 21. After emerging into the mouth, parts of the integument of enamel organ origin are lost by degeneration of its epithelial component and by attrition or abrasion of the underlying cuticular component. In the region of the gingival crevice or sulcus the primary (or pre-eruptive) enamel cuticle acquires additional matter from the lining epithelium and, coronal to the gingival margin, from saliva. The salivary layer is known as the acquired pellicle. Oral bacteria adhere initially to the enamel cuticle, and later to the acquired pellicle, to form the dental plaque.

## INVESTING LAYERS ASSOCIATED WITH THE CROWNS OF UNERUPTED TEETH

The soft tissues covering an erupting tooth comprise the oral mucosa and the subjacent connective tissue of the dental follicle. Between the dental follicle and the enamel is an epithelial layer that is the remains of the enamel organ – the reduced enamel epithelium (Fig. 8.1). The appearance of this epithelium varies from a thin, flattened layer of cells to a more organized layer of recognizable cuboidal or columnar reduced amelo-blasts, deep to which may be additional cell layers (Fig. 8.2). Although it is not evident at the light microscope level, a basal lamina (primary enamel cuticle) is interposed between the enamel surface and the reduced enamel epithelium. The reduced enamel epithelium and the basal lamina comprise **Nasmyth's membrane**. The enamel organ associated with an occlusal fissure appears to be the last to change to a reduced enamel epithelium and the cells adjacent to the enamel in this region may retain a columnar appearance for some considerable time (Fig. 8.3). The reduced enamel epithelium covering the crown of unerupted teeth can be demonstrated with special staining (Fig. 8.4).

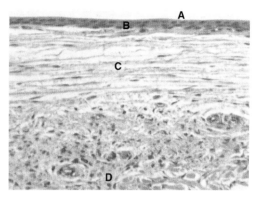

**Fig. 8.2** Immediately adjacent to the enamel space (A) is the reduced enamel epithelium (B). In this section, the reduced enamel epithelium appears flattened. Superficial to the reduced enamel epithelium is the fibrous connective tissue of the dental follicle (C) and superficial to this is the oral submucosa (D) (Demineralized section, H & E; ×160).

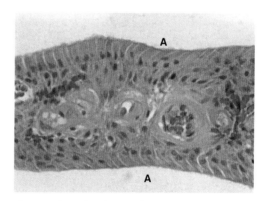

**Fig. 8.3** The reduced enamel epithelium in an occlusal fissure. Although the reduced enamel epithelium covering the rest of the crown comprises cells with a flattened morphology, the cells immediately adjacent to the enamel space (A) still retain a columnar appearance. Note the vascularity of the tissue in this region (Demineralized section, Mallory's trichrome; ×80). Courtesy of Professor H.N. Newman.

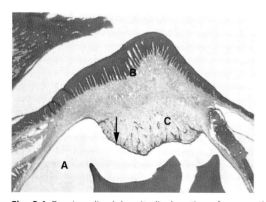

**Fig. 8.1** Demineralized, longitudinal section of an erupting tooth in situ. A = enamel space; B = oral epithelium, immediately beneath which is its associated lamina propria and submucosa; C = dental follicle associated with the underlying erupting tooth. Reduced enamel epithelium (arrow). (H & E; ×10).

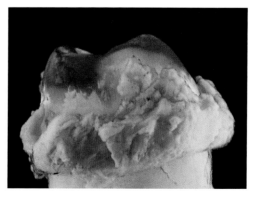

**Fig. 8.4** This unerupted permanent third molar has been stained to show the remains of the dental follicle (yellow) and the vestigial enamel organ (blue). Note that part of the follicle has been lost during the surgical removal of the tooth and that the underlying vestigial enamel organ covers the entire crown (Alcian blue after fixation in Bouin's solution; ×4). Courtesy of Professor H.N. Newman.

## INVESTING LAYERS ASSOCIATED WITH THE CROWNS OF ERUPTED TEETH

The organic layers covering the erupted healthy tooth can be revealed by special stains (Fig. 8.5). That part of the crown well exposed in the mouth is covered by loosely adherent reduced enamel epithelium, which is soon lost, leaving the primary enamel cuticle, which immediately acquires an organic element of salivary origin, the acquired pellicle. Passing towards the gingiva but above the gingival margin, the tooth is likely to be covered by plaque. In the region of the gingival crevice the tooth will be covered only by the primary enamel cuticle. Below this layer the tooth will be covered by the junctional epithelium, its extent being related to the stage of tooth development. Using careful demineralizing techniques it is possible to lift off the organic integument; consequently the plaque, primary enamel cuticle and junctional epithelium appear as a single continuous entity (Figs 8.6, 8.7). The surface of this organic film adjacent to the enamel may even show prism-end markings in the region of the gingival

crevice where it is formed only by the primary enamel cuticle, indicating its intimate association with the enamel surface (Fig. 8.8).

The three distinct zones forming the enamel integument as seen in Figures 8.5 and 8.6 are clearly distinguishable at the ultrastructural level. Beneath the gingival crevice in the region of the junctional epithelium the enamel integument covering the enamel surface consists of the junctional epithelial cells and the primary enamel cuticle (Fig. 8.9). The junctional epithelium is described further on pages 238–240. Immediately coronal to this, in the region of the gingival crevice, the enamel surface is covered only by the primary enamel cuticle, the junctional epithelium having been lost (Fig. 8.10). Above the gingival crest, the primary enamel cuticle exposed in the mouth will become coated with an acquired pellicle derived from saliva and this will become colonized by bacteria to form dental plaque (Fig. 8.11). In health, the firm apposition of the gingiva to the tooth limits the plaque to the gingival margin (Fig. 8.12). Excessive plaque accumulation is associated with both dental caries and chronic inflammatory periodontal disease.

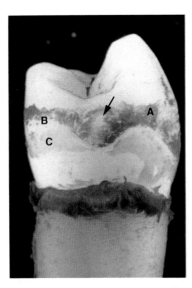

**Fig. 8.5** Approximal view of a partially erupted premolar, showing the zones of its organic integument. Two zones are stained. The dark blue layer (A) is the plaque. The light blue layer (C) is the attachment or junctional epithelium, which in life links the tooth to the gingiva coronal to the periodontal ligament. The unstained zone between them (B) comprises the primary (or pre-eruptive) enamel cuticle. Note that the plaque corresponds to a position above the crest of the gingival margin and around the contact point (arrowed) where adjacent teeth meet, and that the cuticle lies in the region of the gingival crevice. Apical to the junctional epithelium, the enamel was covered in vivo by loosely adherent reduced enamel epithelial cells, which were lost during extraction. Coronal to the plaque the crown is covered by the primary enamel cuticle together with an organic element of salivary origin (the acquired pellicle) (Alcian blue–aldehyde fuchsin; ×4). Courtesy of Professor H.N. Newman.

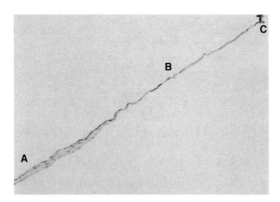

**Fig. 8.6** The organic integument removed from the enamel surface of an erupted tooth following careful demineralization. A = epithelium; B = primary enamel cuticle; C = plaque (Ollett's modification of Twort; ×100). Courtesy of Professor H.N. Newman.

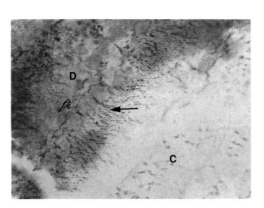

**Fig. 8.8** Deep enamel-related surface of organic integument removed from enamel by careful demineralization, revealing a zone of prism-end markings (arrowed) in the primary enamel cuticle (C) just beneath the plaque (D) (Alcian blue and erythrosin; ×20). Courtesy of Professor H.N. Newman.

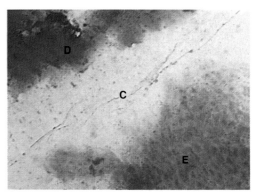

**Fig. 8.7** High-power view of the external surface of part of organic integument removed from enamel by careful demineralization. D = plaque; C = primary (pre-eruptive) enamel cuticle; E = junctional epithelium (Toluidine blue and erythrosin; ×20). Courtesy of Professor H.N. Newman.

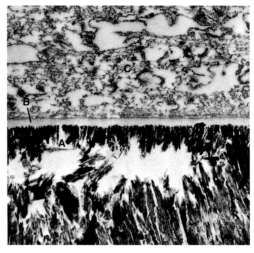

**Fig. 8.9** The enamel integument at the level of the junctional epithelium. This micrograph is taken from a region at the coronal limit of the gingival crevice. The enamel surface (A) is covered by the primary enamel cuticle (B) and the remaining vestige of an attachment or junctional epithelial cell (C) (TEM; ×13 000). Courtesy of Professor H.N. Newman.

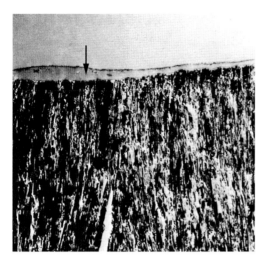

**Fig. 8.10** The enamel integument immediately coronal to the junctional epithelium showing the primary enamel cuticle (arrowed) on the enamel surface. This section is in the region of the gingival crevice coronal to that illustrated in Fig. 8.9 and therefore lacks a junctional epithelial cell. Note that the cuticle usually has an electron-dense outer border (TEM; ×10 000). Courtesy of Professor H.N. Newman.

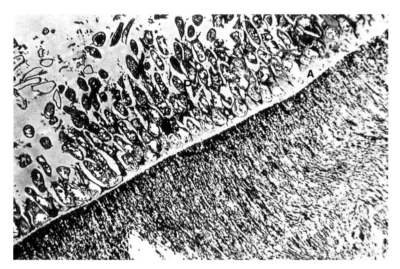

**Fig. 8.11** The enamel integument above the gingival crest showing bacterial colonization forming dental plaque. This micrograph shows early approximal surface plaque on a clear layer (A), which is probably combined primary enamel cuticle and pellicle, above which is a layer of plaque (P) (TEM; ×1250). Courtesy of Professor H.N. Newman.

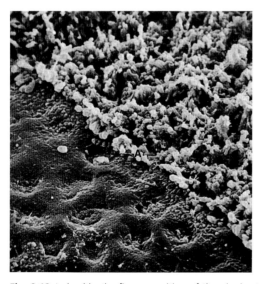

**Fig. 8.12** In health, the firm apposition of the gingiva to the tooth limits the plaque to the gingival margin. There is a sharp boundary to the dental plaque (A), below which lies the plaque-free surface of enamel in the region of the gingival sulcus (SEM; ×1500). Courtesy of Professor H.N. Newman.

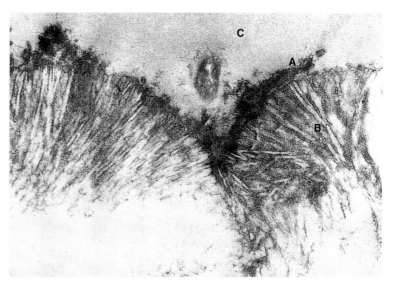

**Fig. 8.13** The thin primary enamel cuticle (A) is in intimate contact with the underlying organic enamel matrix (B). Note the lathe-like spaces occupied in vivo by enamel crystals. In the region of the gingival crevice, the cuticle acquires accretions (C) and appears thicker (Demineralized section, TEM ×30 000). Courtesy of Professor H.N. Newman.

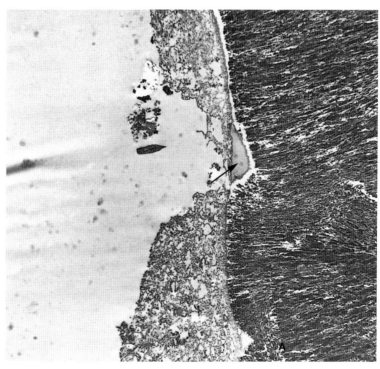

**Fig. 8.14** Localized thickening of the primary enamel cuticle at the enamel surface in relation to an enamel stria reaching the surface (arrow) (TEM micrograph; ×5100). Courtesy of Professor H.N. Newman.

The primary enamel cuticle is in intimate contact with the underlying organic enamel matrix. Generally approximately 30 nm thick, the cuticle acquires accretions in the region of the gingival crevice, which derive from crevicular epithelium and from plasma and may increase the cuticle to about 5 μm thick (Fig. 8.13). Localized thickening of the primary enamel cuticle may also occur on its deep aspect, where enamel maturation is incomplete because of the presence at this site of striae of Retzius reaching the surface (Fig. 8.14). The primary enamel cuticle is thought to be composed of protein. Its accretions are mainly proteoglycan and glycoprotein elements from the contiguous soft tissues. Plasma contributions

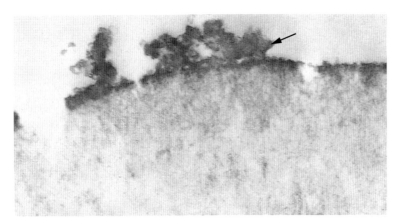

**Fig. 8.15** The primary enamel cuticle at the enamel surface showing positive staining for the immunoglobulin IgG (arrow). This forms part of the host defence system against plaque (TEM with antibody to human IgG; peroxidase method for localization of IgG; ×34 500). Courtesy of Professors H.N. Newman and S.J. Challacombe.

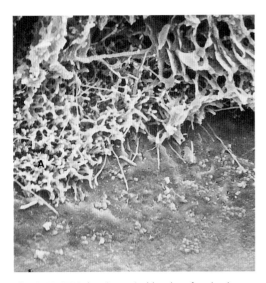

**Fig. 8.16** SEM showing apical border of early plaque composed mainly of cocci (A) and filaments (×1300). Courtesy of Professor H.N. Newman and the editors of the *British Dental Journal*.

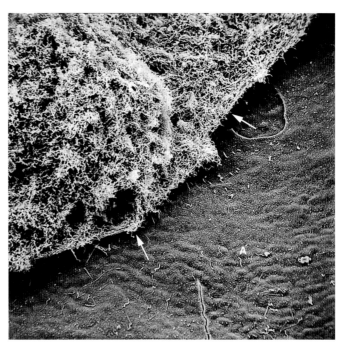

**Fig. 8.17** SEM showing apical border of subgingival plaque (arrows) associated with advanced chronic inflammatory periodontal disease. The predominant organisms are spirochaetes. The details of cementum (A) are obscured by a dental cuticle on which isolated spirochaetes are seen (×430). Newman HN 1977 Ultrastructure of the apical border of dental plaque. In: Lehner T (ed) *The borderland between caries and periodontal disease*, Vol. 1, Academic Press, London, pp 73–103.

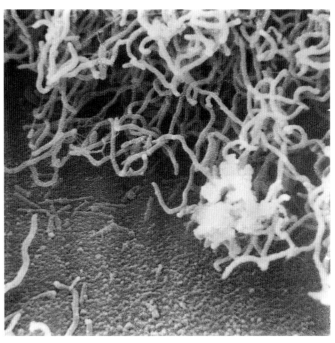

**Fig. 8.18** SEM showing high power of the apical border seen in Fig. 8.17. The subgingival plaque is composed mainly of spirochaetes (×4000). Newman HN 1977 Ultrastructure of the apical border of dental plaque. In: Lehner T (ed) *The borderland between caries and periodontal disease*, Vol. 1, Academic Press, London, pp 73–103.

include immunoglobulins (Fig. 8.15), which form part of the host defence system against plaque.

Where the enamel surface is exposed to wear, either by attrition or abrasion, the vestigial enamel organ is worn away, but the enamel rapidly acquires a layer of acquired pellicle. Indeed, this pellicle always forms a protective coat following any wear. This acellular layer is derived mainly from salivary proteins but includes elements from crevicular fluid and bacteria.

## DENTAL PLAQUE

Dental plaque is the combination of bacteria embedded in a matrix of salivary proteins and bacterial products superimposed on the acquired pellicle (Fig. 8.11). Dental plaque is an example of a biofilm, a term used to describe communities of microbes attached to surfaces. Early plaque is composed of mainly Gram-positive, facultative, anaerobic cocci and filaments (Fig. 8.16). With time, the deposit will thicken, although in non-pathological, supragingival situations its microfloral composition is unlikely to vary greatly (Fig. 8.12).

Where the plaque is associated with chronic inflammatory periodontal disease and becomes subgingival, a more complex flora develops with anaerobic Gram-negative organisms predominating, to include cocci, rods, filaments and many motile forms (particularly spirochaetes) (Figs 8.17, 8.18). The microbial composition of dental plaque will vary, not only with the stages of maturity of the deposit but also from individual to individual, from tooth to tooth, from site to site and from surface to surface. Plaque can be seen on all tooth surfaces that are not subject to constant abrasion, especially in areas that are difficult to clean (such as occlusal pits and fissures, interproximal regions and at the gingival margin). Its presence may be more readily visualized clinically by the use of disclosing solutions (Fig. 8.19). Many plaque bacteria metabolize dietary carbohydrates, often producing polysaccharides, which may be stored intracellularly, on the cell surface and extracellularly in the matrix.

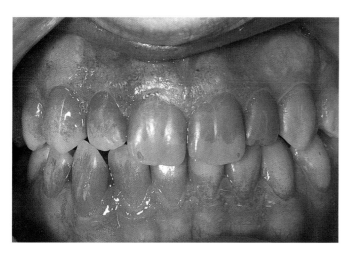

**Fig. 8.19** Plaque stained red and exposed by the use of a disclosing solution. Courtesy of Professor R. Palmer.

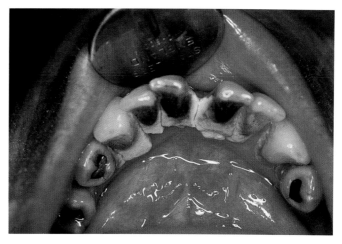

**Fig. 8.21** View of mouth showing the presence of supragingival calculus associated with the lingual surfaces of heavily stained anterior mandibular teeth. Courtesy of Dr M. Ide.

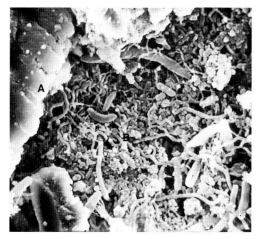

**Fig. 8.20** SEM of calculus showing mineralized (A) and unmineralized areas of plaque composed of a mixed flora (B) (×3000). Newman HN 1977 Ultrastructure of the apical border of dental plaque. In: Lehner T (ed) *The borderland between caries and periodontal disease*, Vol. 1, Academic Press, London, pp 73–103.

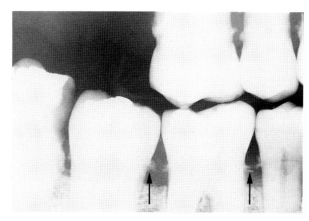

**Fig. 8.22** Subgingival calculus (arrowed) evident in a bitewing radiograph. Courtesy of Dr M. Ide.

## DENTAL CALCULUS

Dental calculus is mineralized plaque (Figs 8.20, 8.21) and may become attached to the enamel of the crown or the cementum (or dentine) of the root. Saliva is supersaturated with minerals (such as calcium and phosphate) that have the potential to mature newly erupted enamel, protect exposed tooth surfaces from acid action and remineralize areas in the early stages of demineralization. Salivary inhibitors prevent precipitation and crystallization of minerals in saliva, but bacterial enzymes can degrade these inhibitors. Thus, under suitable conditions (e.g. with high concentrations of minerals derived from saliva), precipitation and crystallization may occur within dental plaque. Whereas the mineral in enamel consists of carbonated hydroxyapatite, that in dental plaque consists of a number of different mineral forms due to the variety of local factors associated with its formation. There is thus regional variation in the Ca:P ratio of dental calculus. Early calculus formation includes deposition in the matrix of poorly crystalline calcium phosphate types, including dicalcium phosphate dehydrate (brushite) and octacalcium phosphate, together with dying bacterial cells. With time, more structured crystalline elements, including carbonated hydroxyapatite and whitlockite, are formed. In supragingival calculus, hydroxyapatite and octacalcium phosphate are most abundant, while in subgingival calculus whitlockite is most abundant, with little brushite being present. Supragingival plaque is less mineralized than subgingival plaque (approximately 40% v 60%).

The organic component of dental calculus, being derived from plaque, will therefore be derived from saliva, gingival crevicular fluid, desquamated epithelial cells, blood cells, food debris, bacteria and their products.

Dental calculus can be classified into supragingival (above the free gingival margin and attached to enamel) and subgingival (below the free gingival margin and therefore attached to cementum). Supragingival dental calculus is cream-coloured and found adjacent to the opening of the major salivary glands. Thus it is seen predominantly on the lingual surfaces of the anterior mandibular teeth, near the opening of the submandibular and sublingual glands (Fig. 8.21) as well as on the buccal surfaces of the maxillary molars (near the openings of the parotid glands). Subgingival calculus is darker in colour and can occur throughout the dentition from minerals in the inflammatory exudate associated with periodontal disease.

The different distribution of supragingival and subgingival calculus deposits relates to the causes of mineralization: supragingivally, a rise in salivary pH, due to evaporation of dissolved $CO_2$ on entering the mouth (together with the greater viscosity and higher Ca:P ratio of the saliva coming out from the submandibular duct) promotes calculus formation, whereas subgingival calculus formation, promoted by formation of alkaline bacterial waste products within periodontal pockets, may occur anywhere in the mouth.

Large deposits of subgingival calculus are sometimes identified on interproximal surfaces in dental radiographs (Fig. 8.22). Subgingival calculus

**Fig. 8.23** Subgingival calculus exposed following gingival recession associated with chronic inflammatory periodontal disease. Courtesy of Professor R. Palmer.

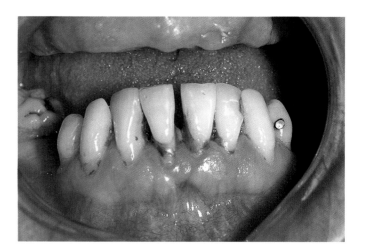

may also be exposed when the gingiva recedes from the teeth following chronic inflammatory periodontal disease (Fig. 8.23). Dental calculus is always covered with a biofilm of living organisms (Fig. 8.21).

## CLINICAL CONSIDERATIONS

The presence of dental plaque predisposes to the onset of the two main dental pathologies: dental caries and periodontal disease. However, different microorganisms are thought to be involved in the two diseases. Dental caries is associated with the metabolism of dietary sugar to acid by predominantly Gram-positive organisms (e.g. *Streptococcus mutans*) in supragingival plaque. Frequent intake of sugar induces a cariogenic plaque in which organisms capable of surviving at low pH are favoured. Periodontal disease is associated with the persistent presence of mature plaque at the gingival margin and exacerbated by an increase in Gram-negative organisms and obligate anaerobes, which are favoured by the environment of periodontal pockets. Gingival inflammation and periodontal destruction are the result of direct action of bacterial products (such as proteases) and indirect promotion of potentially damaging immune responses. The challenge of dental plaque can be limited by reducing dietary sugar intake, mechanical removal of the plaque and modifying the pathogenic potential. Toothbrushing, flossing or professional scaling and root planing may achieve mechanical removal. However, because of the intimate contact of its crystals with those of the tooth surface, calculus may be difficult to remove completely. In this context, plaque control agents should encourage the formation of calcium phosphates that are most easily removed, being either more soluble or less strongly attached to the tooth surface. Pathogenic potential may be modified by the use of personal oral hygiene products such as toothpastes, mouth rinses and gels containing antimicrobials, or delivery of antibiotics as local or systemic treatments by the dental practitioner.

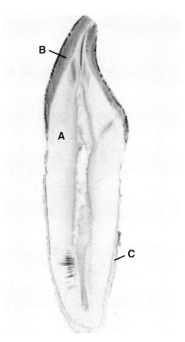

**Fig. 9.1** Ground longitudinal section of a tooth showing dentine (A) forming the bulk of the tooth, covered in the crown by enamel (B) and in the root by cementum (C). The dental pulp has been lost during preparation and the pulp chamber and root canal are empty (×4).

Dentine is the mineralized tissue that forms the bulk of the tooth. In the crown it is covered by enamel, in the root by cementum (Fig. 9.1). It is a rigid but elastic tissue consisting of large numbers of small, parallel tubules in a mineralized collagen matrix. The tubules contain the long processes of the cells responsible for forming the tissue, the odontoblasts, as well as a small volume of extracellular (dentinal) fluid. The cell bodies of the odontoblasts line the deep surface of the dentine defining the outer border of the dental pulp. The combination of enamel and dentine provides a rigid, hard structure suitable for tearing and chewing that resists both abrasion and fracture. The cementum covering the dentine of the root anchors the tooth to the bone of the socket via the periodontal ligament. The junctions of the dentine with these two other hard tissues are biologically unique as is the tissue itself. Two major properties distinguish dentine from enamel. Firstly, dentine is sensitive. Secondly, dentine is formed throughout life, increasing in thickness at the expense of the dental pulp. This is reflected in the presence of an unmineralized layer of dentine matrix at the pulpal surface known as predentine. The physical properties of enamel and dentine are complementary. Thus, although enamel is extremely hard, it is unyielding and may fracture during mastication if the underlying dentine did not provide a degree of deformability.

## PHYSICAL PROPERTIES

Fresh dentine is pale yellow in colour and contributes to the appearance of the tooth through the translucent enamel. Dentine is harder than bone and cementum but softer than enamel. Its organic matrix and tubular architecture provide it with greater compressive, tensile and flexural strength than enamel. Dentine is permeable, the permeability depending on the size and patency of the tubules, which will decline with age. Cracking occurs in dentine when it has been weakened by caries or cavity preparation and can result in an unrestorable tooth. The development of cracks is more likely in older teeth and in teeth in which the dentine has become dehydrated by root canal therapy. Stresses parallel to the direction of the dentinal tubules are more likely to result in fracture than those at right angles to them. Some of the physical properties of dentine (compared with those of enamel) are listed in Table 7.1, page 106.

## CHEMICAL PROPERTIES

The gross composition of dentine approximates to 70% inorganic, 20% organic and 10% water by weight; and 50% inorganic, 30% organic and 20% water by volume.

The inorganic, mineral component is in the form of calcium hydroxyapatite crystals. The percentage dry weight of some of the important elements is shown in Table 9.1. The crystallites are calcium-poor and carbonate-rich in comparison to pure hydroxyapatite and, although similar in shape, are very much smaller (approx. $35 \times 10$ and of indeterminate length) than those in enamel (see Fig. 7.4). The crystallites contain other trace elements including fluoride. The hydroxyapatite crystallites in the mineralized dentine are found on and between the collagen fibrils.

## ORGANIC MATRIX

The organic matrix of dentine in which the crystallites are embedded has a composition similar to that of bone. The organic matrix consists of fibrils embedded in an amorphous ground substance. The fibrils are collagen and comprise over 90% of the organic matrix.

The principal collagen fibril is the ubiquitous type I collagen. Traces of type III and type V collagen, which are present in sizeable amounts in the pulp, have also been detected. Most of the collagen fibrils in dentine run

**Table 9.1** *The major inorganic components of dentine*

| Constituent | % of dry weight |
| --- | --- |
| Calcium | 26.9 |
| Phosphorus | 13.2 |
| Carbonate | 4.6 |
| Sodium | 0.6 |
| Magnesium | 0.8 |

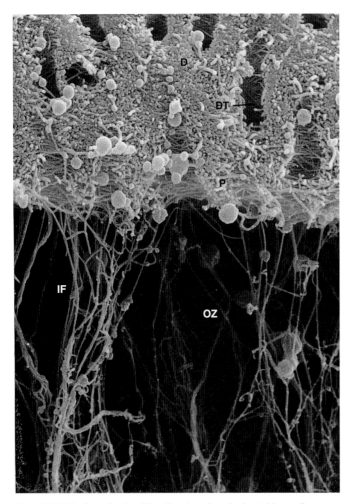

**Fig. 9.2** SEM of predentine (P) with mineral and odontoblast cells removed revealing the pattern of collagen fibrils. In predentine most of the dentinal collagen fibres run parallel to the pulpal surface. Collagen fibrils in the odontoblast layer parallel the long axis of the cell bodies; OZ = odontoblast zone; D = dentine; DT = dentinal tubule; IF = intercellular fibres (×3500). Courtesy of B. Sogaard-Pedersen, H. Boye, M. Matthiessen, and the editor of the *Scandinavian Journal of Dental Research*.

parallel to the pulpal surface (Fig. 9.2). In mineralized dentine the collagen fibrils are of larger diameter (100 nm) and are more closely packed than in predentine. Collagen fibrils in dentine are not assembled into bundles as they are in many non-mineralized connective tissues such as tendons or the periodontal ligament.

## PROTEINS

Though comprising only a relatively small percentage of the organic matrix compared with collagen, the non-collagenous proteins of dentine have important, but as yet poorly understood, biological functions. They include dentine phosphoproteins, proteoglycans, Gla-proteins, other acid proteins and growth factors. Amino acids undergo changes with age, in which they convert from one racemic form to another. This can be measured very accurately by gas chromatography. Measuring these changes in aspartate in dentine is an accurate way of determining the age of human remains (see page 381).

### Dentine phosphoproteins

These represent the main non-collagenous protein. There are several types, but the term dentine phosphoprotein (phosphophorin or PP-H) relates to the highly phosphorylated protein species. Owing to its very high phosphate content it represents the most acidic protein known. Indeed, about 80% of the amino acid residues carry negatively charged phosphate or carboxyl groups. Its high calcium ion binding properties have implicated PP-H in the process of mineralization.

### Proteoglycans

These also form a significant component of the non-collagenous proteins. In dentine, they are represented by the smaller-molecular-weight types known as biglycan and decorin. The glycosaminoglycans are primarily chondroitin-4-sulphate and chondroitin-6-sulphate. Among the important functions of proteoglycans in general are their role in collagen fibril assembly and their cell-mediated effects such as cell adhesion, migration, proliferation and differentiation. As significant biochemical changes occur at the mineralizing front, it can be assumed that proteoglycans have an important but as yet incompletely understood role in mineralization. They appear to bind calcium non-specifically. They may be inhibitors of calcifications that need to undergo some degree of degradation before mineralization will occur.

### Gamma-carboxyglutamate-containing proteins (Gla-proteins)

Little is known about the function of these small proteins, present in low amounts in dentine. They bind strongly, but reversibly, to hydroxyapatite crystallites and may play some role in mineralization.

### Other acidic proteins

Osteonectin, a protein containing high levels of glutamic and aspartic acid, is found in dentine at levels of about 5% of total protein. Osteopontin, a phosphorylated glycoprotein has been identified in predentine and contains the receptor binding sequence Arg–Gly–Asp (RGD). The precise role of osteonectin and osteopontin in dentine (as in bone) is not known.

### Growth factors

Several growth factors can be isolated from the dentine matrix as they can from bone matrix and are presumably absorbed from circulating tissue fluid. These include insulin growth factor (IGF)-II, bone morphogenetic protein (BMP)-2, and transforming growth factor (TGF)-beta. As dentine does not turnover like bone it is unlikely that these factors play an everyday role in the tissue's metabolism, but they could be released during the progress of dental caries and induce the production of reactionary or reparative dentine. They are, apparently, very stable, having been found in teeth from Neolithic times.

## LIPIDS

These comprise about 2% of the organic content of dentine and, as they are conspicuous at the mineralizing front, are thought to play a role in mineralization. Phospholipids have been detected in both predentine and mineralized dentine. They occupy the spaces between collagen fibrils along with the proteoglycans. In the predentine, they are most heavily concentrated near the mineralizing front. In dentine, phospholipids are needle-like 'crystal ghosts' and may be involved in the formation and growth of crystals. They seem to be absent from the centres of calcospherites but present in interglobular dentine.

## DENTINE TUBULES

Dentine is permeated by tubules, the dentine tubules, that run from the pulpal surface to the enamel–dentine and cementum–dentine junctions

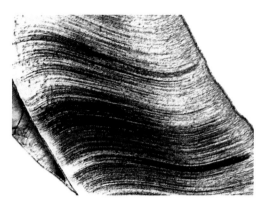

**Fig. 9.3** Ground section showing dentinal tubules cut longitudinally and demonstrating the sinusoidal primary curvatures (×25).

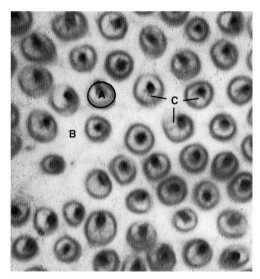

**Fig. 9.4** Ground, partially demineralized section of dentinal tubules cut transversely. A = perimeter of a tubule as initially laid down; B = intertubular dentine; C = peritubular/intratubular dentine (Eosin stain; ×1500). Courtesy of Dr R. Sprinz.

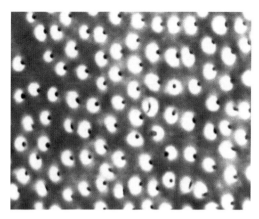

**Fig. 9.5** A demineralized section of dentinal tubules cut transversely. This treatment results in the loss of the peritubular/intratubular dentine, which has little organic matrix. The dark-staining odontoblast processes occupy only a small proportion of the resulting lumen (Haematoxylin; ×1000). Courtesy of Professor E.W. Bradford.

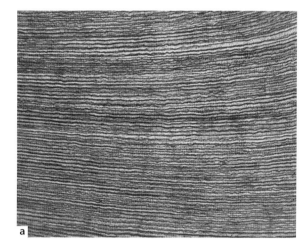

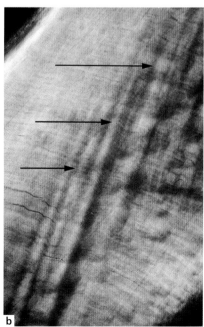

**Fig. 9.6** (a) Decalcified section showing dentinal tubules cut longitudinally. The lumens of the tubules have been stained with picrothionin and demonstrate secondary curvatures (×200). Courtesy of Professor M.M. Smith. (b) Ground section showing dentinal tubules cut longitudinally and exhibiting contour lines (arrows) due to coincidence of secondary curvatures (×150). Courtesy of Dr R.P. Shellis.

(Fig. 9.3). The dentine tubules follow a curved, sigmoid course – the primary curvatures. The convexity of the primary curvatures nearest the pulp chamber faces rootward. In the root and beneath the cusps, the primary curvatures are less pronounced, the tubules running a straighter course. In transverse section the tubules are approximately circular although their appearance is obviously dependent on the plane in which the tissue is sectioned (Figs 9.4, 9.5). The dentine between the tubules is termed intertubular dentine.

The tubules taper from approximately 2.5 μm in diameter at their pulpal ends to 1 μm or less peripherally. During the formation of dentine tubules by the odontoblasts the cells migrate inwards and occupy a smaller surface area. Hence, the tubules are more widely separated at their peripheries. Approximately 22% of the cross-sectional area of the dentine near the pulp is composed of tubules, while near the enamel–dentine junction the tubules comprise only about 2.5%. Estimates of the number of tubules vary somewhat between reports because of differences in tooth age and type and the thickness of the dentine. A reasonable rounding of the numbers suggests 20 000/mm$^2$ in outer dentine, 50 000/mm$^2$ in inner dentine and 40 000/mm$^2$ in the middle.

The tubules also show changes in direction of much smaller (a few μm) amplitude. These are known as the secondary curvatures (Fig. 9.6). In some regions the secondary curvatures may coincide in adjacent tubules. At low magnification, this gives the appearance of a line crossing the dentine, a contour line (of Owen) (Fig. 9.6). These are not commonly seen in most of the dentine, but one such line is usually evident at the junction

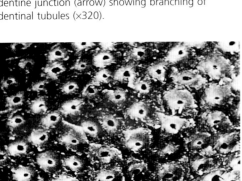

**Fig. 9.7** Ground section of dentine near the enamel–dentine junction (arrow) showing branching of dentinal tubules (×320).

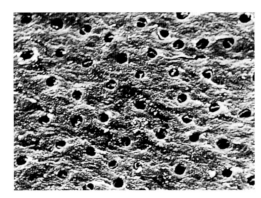

**Fig. 9.8** SEM of transversely sectioned dentinal tubules close to the pulp and lacking peritubular dentine (×540). Courtesy of Professor B.R.R.N. Mendis.

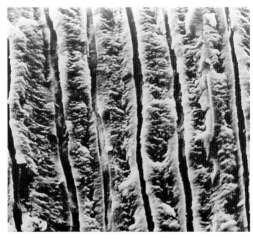

**Fig. 9.9** SEM of longitudinally sectioned dentinal tubules close to the pulp showing little evidence of peritubular dentine (×540). Courtesy of Professor B.R.R.N. Mendis.

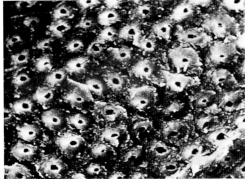

**Fig. 9.10** SEM of dentine tubules cut in cross-section in the middle of the dentine. They reveal a distinctive zone of peritubular dentine, narrowing the original tubule (×1200). Courtesy of Professor B.R.R.N. Mendis.

of primary and secondary dentine where, during deposition, all the odontoblasts seem to take a simultaneous and similar change in direction (see Fig. 9.48).

Dentinal tubules branch. The most profuse branching is in the periphery near the enamel–dentine junction (Fig. 9.7), presumably a reflection of the numerous processes the early odontoblast has. Many small side branches appear to end blindly but some may unite with branches of other tubules. In the root, the terminal tubule branches and the branches loop. This looping is thought by some to be responsible for the appearance of the granular layer of Tomes seen in this region in ground section (see page 140). Branching is not obvious in much of the dentine beneath the periphery but becomes notable in the uncalcified predentine near the pulp. Presumably during mineralization many of the odontoblastic branches retract or atrophy and the small canals they occupied fill in.

## PERITUBULAR DENTINE

The walls of the dentinal tubules in recently formed intertubular dentine at the pulp surface are composed of mineralized type I collagen. With maturation, another type of dentine is deposited on the walls of the dentinal tubule, narrowing the lumen (Figs 9.8–9.11). This type of dentine is known as peritubular dentine (more properly, but not more popularly, also known as intratubular dentine), and its formation gradually leads to obliteration of the tubule (Fig. 9.12). Peritubular dentine differs from intertubular dentine in lacking a collagenous fibrous matrix.

Peritubular dentine can also be distinguished from intertubular dentine as a zone of increased radiographic (Fig. 9.13) and electron (Fig. 9.14) density lining the internal surface of the dentinal tubule. It can be clearly distinguished in specially prepared sections that have been prepared by ion beam milling and have thus not undergone destructive chemical processing (Figs 9.15, 9.16). Peritubular dentine is about 5–12% more mineralized

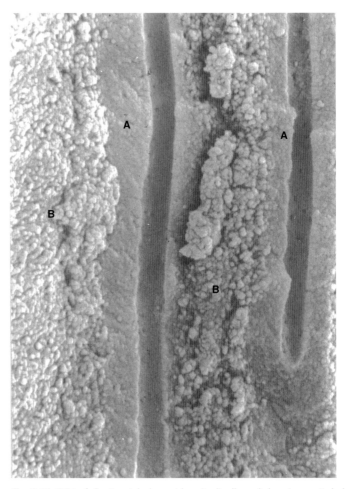

**Fig. 9.11** SEM of dentine tubules cut longitudinally and showing peritubular dentine (A) deposited on the tubule wall. B = intertubular dentine (×7000). Courtesy of Professor M.M. Smith.

than intertubular dentine. When dentine is routinely demineralized, the peritubular dentine will be lost as it lacks the stabilizing feature of collagen. The dimensions of the dentine tubules will thus be increased to their initial dimensions (compare Figs 9.4 and 9.5). Peritubular dentine is found in unerupted teeth. This with its predominant distribution in apical dentine indicates that it is an age change rather than a response tissue.

The main protein of peritubular dentine has a higher molecular weight and an amino acid composition quite different from the phosphophorin

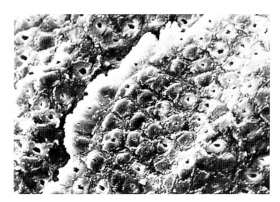

**Fig. 9.12** Dentine tubules sectioned transversely close to the enamel–dentine junction showing peritubular dentine formation obliterating the lumen (×1200). Courtesy of Professor B.R.R.N. Mendis.

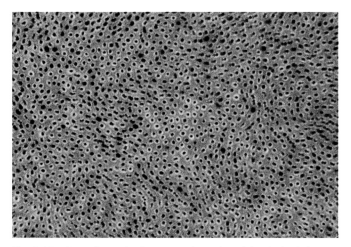

**Fig. 9.13** Microradiograph of transversely sectioned dentinal tubules surrounded by a more radio-opaque (and therefore denser) zone of peritubular dentine (×650). Courtesy of Dr G. McKay.

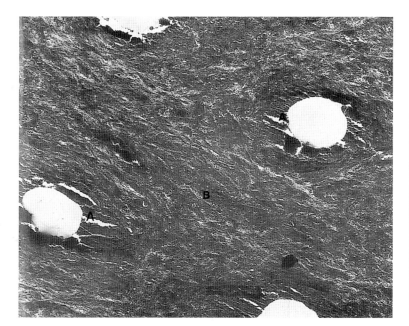

**Fig. 9.14** TEM of peritubular dentine (A) seen in an ultrathin undecalcified section. The peritubular dentine appears non-fibrillar and more electron opaque. It is more fragile than intertubular dentine (B) and shatters during sectioning (×6000). Courtesy of Professor N.W. Johnson.

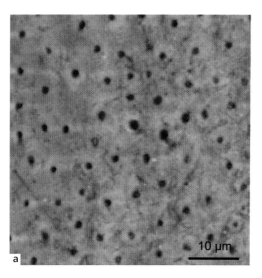

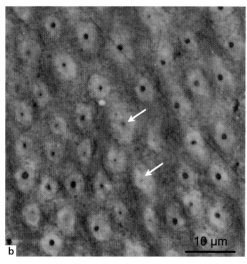

**Fig. 9.15** Atomic force microscopic images of (a) normal (donor age 25 years) and (b) translucent (donor age 67 years) dentine. The dark contrast indicates the tubule sites and the white arrows in (b) show representative tubule lumens occluded with intratubular mineral. Atomic force microscopy is a technique that scans a sample and builds up an image of resolution much higher than that achieved by scanning electron microscopy. Porter AE 2006 *Micron* 37: 681–688, with permission.

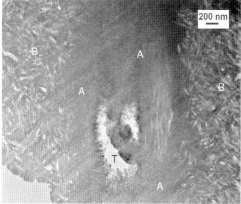

**Fig. 9.16** A partially filled dentinal tubule in a section thinned by less damaging ion beam milling. The very different structure of the peritubular dentine can be clearly seen. T = tubule, A = peritubular dentine, B = intertubular dentine. Porter AE 2006 *Micron* 37: 681–688, with permission.

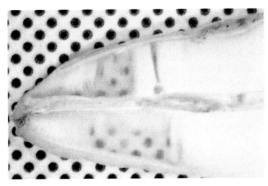

**Fig. 9.17** Old tooth root sectioned longitudinally and placed in water. The presence of peritubular dentine completely occluding the tubules in much of the apical tissue results in this part appearing translucent as water is excluded. Towards the cervical margin (right side), patent tubules become filled with water, which has a refractive index that differs from that of the intertubular dentine. This results in the tissue appearing opaque (×5). Courtesy of Professor A.G.S. Lumsden.

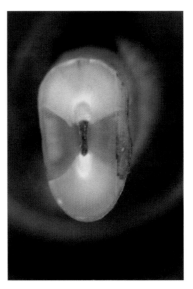

**Fig. 9.18** Transverse section of mandibular premolar showing butterfly-shaped outline of translucent dentine. Courtesy of Dr R. O'Sullivan.

found in intertubular dentine. In demineralized sections at the electron microscope level the matrix appears as an amorphous material. The mineral component of peritubular dentine is mainly carbonated apatite but its crystalline form is distinct from that of intertubular dentine. Some crystallites have a hexagonal shape and appear as compact platelets slightly smaller than (but similar to) those of intertubular dentine. Other crystalline species may also be present. In tubules exposed by attrition, some occluding components may be derived from saliva. Although the bulk of peritubular dentine is hypercalcified relative to the intertubular dentine, hypocalcified areas bound its inner and outer surfaces. Peritubular dentine is formed at about the same time as (or soon after) intertubular dentine. By the time primary dentine formation is complete, all peripheral tubules have a lining of peritubular dentine that extends from the enamel–dentine junction to within 100–50 μm of the predentine. In outer dentine, peritubular dentine occupies two-thirds of the cross-sectional area of the tissue; near to the predentine it occupies only approximately 3% (Fig. 9.8).

Associated with physiological ageing, especially in root dentine, the dentinal tubules become completely occluded by peritubular dentine formation. The contents of the tubule acquire the same refractive index as the intertubular dentine. When a ground section of a root is placed in water (which has a refractive index different from that of dentine), regions blocked by peritubular dentine will appear translucent ('translucent dentine'), while regions with patent tubules will fill with water and appear opaque (Fig. 9.17). Dentine tubules become infilled at the root apex adjacent to the cementum and extend cervically and towards the root canal with age. In cross-section, translucent zones have a butterfly shape owing to the convergence of the tubules pulpally, being wider at the mesial and distal margins (Fig. 9.18). The amount of translucent dentine increases linearly with age and is not affected by function or external irritation. This feature is used in forensic dentistry to age teeth. Translucent dentine is also referred to on page 144; sclerotic dentine, which has features similar to translucent dentine, is discussed on pages 145–147.

## CONTENTS OF THE DENTINAL TUBULES

The dentinal tubules contain the processes of the odontoblasts that are responsible for their formation. In some parts of the tissue they also contain afferent nerve terminals (Fig. 9.19). It is also possible that processes from antigen-presenting cells in the peripheral pulp may extend for a short distance into the tubules. Technical limitations prevent a definitive figure being given for what proportion of the tubule is occupied by cell processes and how far along the tubule the processes extend. It seems likely, however, that there is a periodontoblastic space, and possibly a postodontoblastic

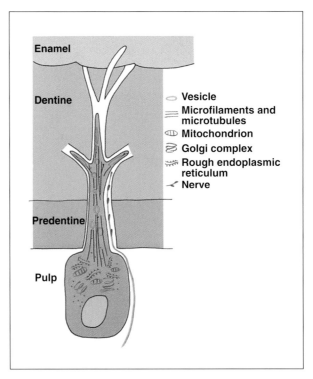

**Fig. 9.19** Diagram of an odontoblast and its main process extending into the dentine. The true extent of the process is controversial, as is the existence of the periodontoblastic space.

space, from which the process has receded. These spaces are thought to be filled with extracellular 'dentinal' fluid, the precise composition of which is unknown. Some studies have suggested a composition that differs from extracellular fluids elsewhere in having a relatively higher concentration of potassium ions and a relatively lower concentration of sodium ions. Such a balance could affect the membrane properties of the nerve endings and odontoblast processes in the tubules. If dentine is fractured, fluid exudes from the tubules and forms droplets on the surface of the dentine. This suggests that there is a positive force, presumably pulpal tissue pressure, that is exerted outwards (page 147). This could help limit the progress of chemicals or toxins on, or in, dentine towards the dental pulp.

The cell body of the odontoblast is described in detail in the section on the dental pulp (pages 156, 157). The process of the odontoblast that

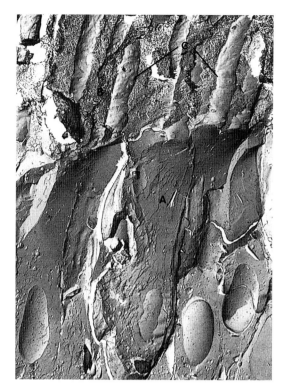

**Fig. 9.20** TEM of a surface replica of the pulp–predentine junction. The odonto-blasts (A) form a continuous layer on the surface of the predentine (B) and their processes (C) completely fill the dentinal tubules with no evidence of a peri-odontoblastic space. The technique involves fracturing the frozen tissue, coating the surface with vaporized metal and then separating the ultrathin coating for examination in the microscope. This complex technique is thought to cause minimal, if any, shrinkage (×2000). Courtesy of Drs A. Riske-Anderson and A. Koling, and the editors of *Acta Scandinavica Odontologica*.

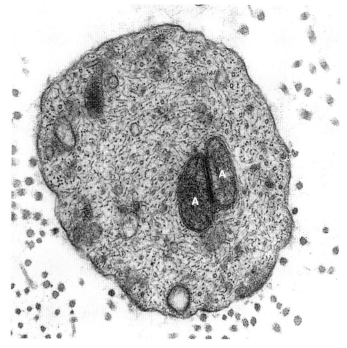

**Fig. 9.21** TEM of an odontoblast process from the predentine in cross-section, A = mitochondrion (×80 000).

extends into the dentine varies in structure at different levels in the tissue, organelles being most numerous in the predentine (Fig. 9.20) whereas, in mineralized dentine, few are present.

There are two technical problems that limit our interpretation of avail-able histological data on the contents of the dentinal tubules. One is the difficulty of fixing small amounts of tissue deep in mineralized tissue. Fixation tends to shrink tissue, and even when this can be minimized the slowness with which most fixatives penetrate means that post-mortem changes will often occur. The second problem is that, in extracting a tooth, it is often compressed by forceps. Releasing the compression often draws tissue up into the tubules (e.g. 'aspiration' of odontoblast nuclei) that is not normally there. Thus, the interpretation of images of tubule contents should be approached with caution. More indirect approaches, such as labelling the tissue in vivo with, for example, a radioactive tag or using immunohistochemical techniques that mark the presence of cell components, can add considerably to our understanding.

Microtubules and intermediate filaments run longitudinally throughout the odontoblast process. Mitochondria are sometimes present in the process in the predentine; strands of rough endoplasmic reticulum are also occa-sionally seen. Vesicles of a variety of sizes are present, being more dense near the cell membrane. Their incidence declines in the more distal parts of the process.

In the predentine and very innermost mineralized circumpulpal dentine the odontoblast process seems to occupy the full width of the dentinal tubule with no discernible periodontoblast space (Figs 9.21, 9.22). At these levels afferent nerve axons are also seen within the tubule and in close apposition to the odontoblast process. The axons contain several mitochon-dria and an occasional vesicle. They do not contain large accumulations of vesicles as are found in synapses although proteins associated elsewhere

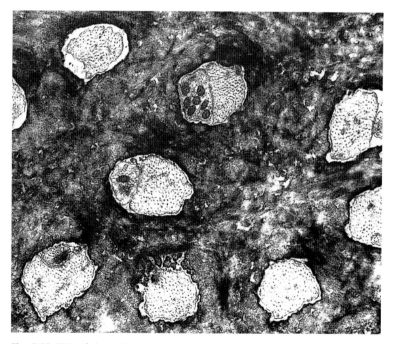

**Fig. 9.22** TEM of dentinal tubules in inner calcified dentine in cross-section. Three of the tubules contain naked nerve endings as well as odontoblast processes. The periodontoblastic space is either small or absent (×10 000).

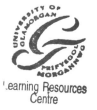

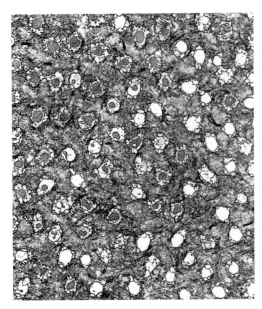

**Fig. 9.23** TEM of dentinal tubules from the middle region of coronal circumpulpal dentine. Some tubules appear to contain cell processes, some contain non-cellular material and some are empty (×3000).

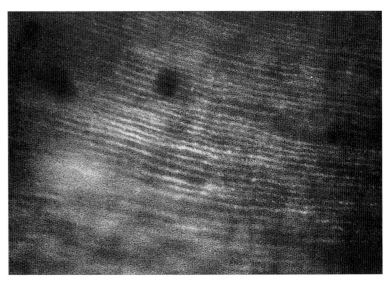

**Fig. 9.25** Components of the cytoskeleton in peripheral dentine. A fluorescent label marks the presence of tubulin, a component of intracellular microtubules (×4200). Courtesy of Drs M. Sigal, S. Pitaru, J. Aubin and A.R. Ten Cate, and the editor of the *Anatomical Record*.

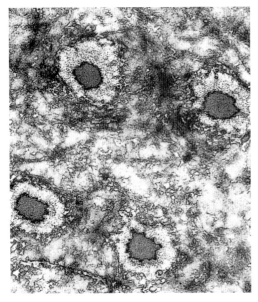

**Fig. 9.24** TEM of dentinal tubules in peripheral dentine. The tubules contain amorphous, non-cellular material (×8000).

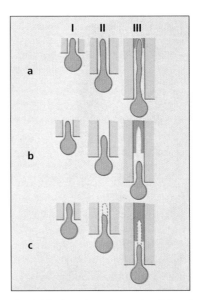

**Fig. 9.26** Three hypotheses describing the pulpward migration of the odontoblast as dentine is deposited (see text for details).

with synaptic vesicle exocytosis have been demonstrated in dentinal tubules. It is not possible by electron microscopy to recognize cell processes in the dentine tubules of peripheral dentine (Figs 9.23, 9.24).

Although the structural characteristics of cells may be lost due to poor fixation, remnants characteristic of cells may still be found (e.g. tubulin – Fig. 9.25). The microtubule and intermediate filament systems are characteristic of cell processes and made up of proteins such as actin, tubulin and vimentin. Some of these proteins can be demonstrated in peripheral dentinal tubules even though no structurally recognizable process can be seen. One possible interpretation for this finding might be that the odontoblast process has degenerated, leaving remnants containing tubulin or microfilamentous material behind. Some studies using this approach suggest that the process extends furthest in the dentine below the cusps.

Clearly, the odontoblast process must occupy the entire dentinal tubule it forms in the early stages of development when the dentine is thin. There are three hypotheses for what might happen later and these are illustrated in Figure 9.26. In Figure 9.26a, the process grows in length as dentine is deposited and its peripheral termination remains at the outer end of the

tubule. This would result in a metabolically unsupported cell process several millimetres long, an arrangement unknown elsewhere in the body where axons (except at their terminations) are supported by Schwann cells. In Figure 9.26b, the process reaches a predetermined length and then moves pulpally as dentine is formed, leaving behind an empty tubule in which peritubular dentine forms. Perhaps peritubular dentine differs from intertubular dentine in being formed by a process that does not directly involve the odontoblast. In Figure 9.26c, the peripheral end of the processes degrades sequentially and its remains form part of the matrix for the peritubular dentine.

The possible existence of an odontoblast process in outer dentine is also complicated by the presence of a very thin, apparently proteinaceous membrane termed the lamina limitans lining the wall of the dentinal tubule. Its composition is unknown but, in certain preparations, it may give rise to the erroneous impression of an odontoblast process (Figs 9.27, 9.28).

In some parts of the dentine, most commonly beneath cusps, the tubules in inner dentine can contain additional small processes (Fig. 9.29). Some

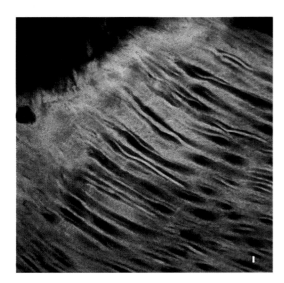

**Fig. 9.27** Dentinal tubules from peripheral to tertiary dentine showing the presence of tubular structures in an area from which the odontoblasts have been lost and which probably represent the lamina limitans (Confocal microscopy of a demineralized section ×1700). Courtesy of Drs G. Goracci, G. Mori, F. Marci and M. Baldi, and the editor of *Minerva Stomatologica*.

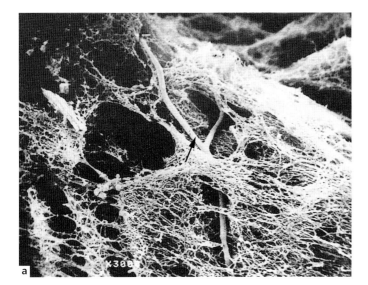

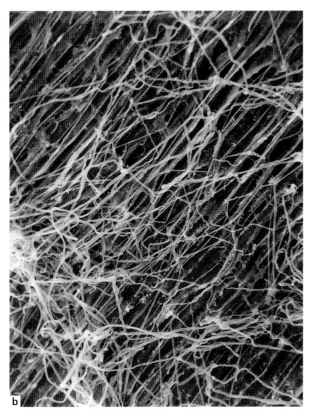

**Fig. 9.28** (a) SEM of a tubular branching structure in peripheral dentine (arrowed) following collagenase treatment. It is difficult to establish whether this is a true odontoblast process or the lamina limitans (×3000). Courtesy of Drs M. Sigal, S. Pitaru, J. Aubin and A.R. Ten Cate, and the editor of the *Anatomical Record*. (b) SEM of demineralized dentine also treated with collagenase to remove the bulk of the organic matrix. The remaining tubular structures seen in this micrograph are thought to represent the lamina limitans as complementary TEM studies show them to possess no cellular characteristics (×1000). Courtesy of Dr H.F. Thomas.

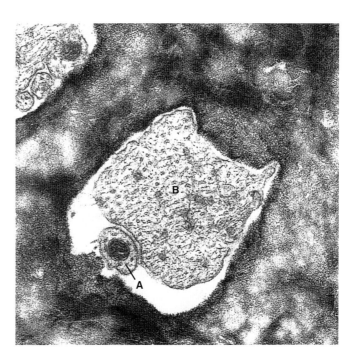

**Fig. 9.29** TEM showing multiple processes within a single dentinal tubule. The larger process (B) is the odontoblast process, the smaller one (A) presumptive nerve terminals (×65 000).

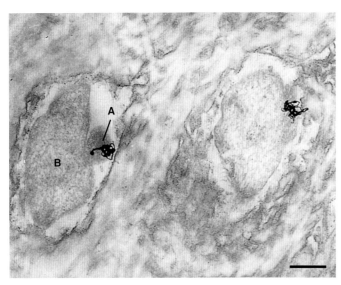

**Fig. 9.30** TEM showing autoradiographically labelled nerve (A) adjacent to an odontoblast process (B). The labelled amino acid was originally injected into the trigeminal ganglion (×20000). Courtesy of Dr M.R. Byers.

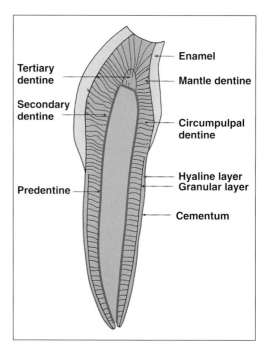

**Fig. 9.31** The regions of varying dentine structure.

of these could be smaller odontoblastic processes that are lost during later deposition; others will be the processes of the immunocompetent antigen-presenting cells that are found in several areas of the pulp, particularly in the periphery within and beneath the odontoblast layer (see page 160). These, and their extensions into the dentinal tubules, are found even in unerupted teeth in small numbers, with intratubular processes limited to the predentine in the coronal pulp. In intact erupted teeth, these processes are present over a much wider area although still limited to predentine. In dentine beneath dental caries, the processes of the immunocompetent cells extend much deeper into the tubules of the circumpulpal dentine. However, in all tubules there is one large odontoblast process.

Sensory terminals have been firmly identified within the dentinal tubule, but special techniques are needed to distinguish them from smaller branches of the odontoblast process. Like the odontoblast process, their extent into dentine is not known for certain. Nerve terminals are limited mainly to the dentine of the crown beneath the cusps (where they may be found in up to 80% of the tubules) and are sparse in cervical and root dentine. The axon in an innervated tubule is narrower than the odontoblast process and contains microtubules, a few microfilaments and often mitochondria. Vesicles are rare in nerve terminals (or in the odontoblast process adjacent to them) and structurally specialized contacts between the nerve terminal and the odontoblast process seem to be absent (Fig. 9.29).

The sensory nature of intratubular axons can be demonstrated by tracer techniques. Radioactive amino acids (e.g. tritium-labelled proline) injected into the trigeminal ganglion are converted into proteins and transported down the axons to the peripheral terminations (Fig. 9.30).

## REGIONAL VARIATIONS IN DENTINE STRUCTURE AND COMPOSITION

The properties and composition of mineralized dentine vary with distance from the predentine to the enamel–dentine junction. The mineral content of dentine decreases and the thickness of mineral crystals increase towards the enamel–dentine junction. Hardness and elastic modulus both decrease towards the junction. Several different regions can be recognized in dentine (Fig. 9.31). The most peripheral region beneath the enamel and dentine has a number of special characteristics bestowed on it by being the earliest formed part of the tissue. In the crown this first-formed layer is known as mantle dentine. In the root there are two morphologically recognizable outer zones: the hyaline layer and the granular layer (of Tomes). There is

some controversy (discussed below) as to whether the hyaline layer is properly a component of dentine or cementum or is a mingling of components of both tissues. Predentine is the innermost unmineralized layer, where new dentine is being deposited throughout life. Just peripheral to the predentine is a zone of mineralization, which is recognizable even in decalcified tissue samples as, simultaneously with mineral deposition, the matrix undergoes considerable modification that results in different staining properties. This region has sometimes been called intermediate dentine. The bulk of the dentine between the mantle layer and the zone of mineralization is the circumpulpal dentine. The outer part of the circumpulpal dentine beneath the mantle layer is often incompletely mineralized and has a characteristic appearance when seen in ground sections, referred to as 'interglobular dentine'. A peripheral region in root dentine, the granular layer (of Tomes) is also hypomineralized but to a lesser extent than the interglobular dentine. In older teeth the inner, pulpal part of the circumpulpal dentine differs somewhat in structure from the bulk of the tissue. This secondary dentine is laid down as an age-related change in the rate of dentine formation once a (presumably) genetically predetermined thickness of primary circumpulpal dentine has been deposited and root development (at least in terms of length) is complete. The rate and amount of secondary dentine laid down varies with tooth type, between crown and root (higher) and, of course, with age. Very approximately in the tooth of an older individual the dentine thickness might be 2.5 mm of which 0.5 mm would be secondary dentine. In teeth that have been subject to external stimuli (such as attrition, dental caries and cavity preparation), another layer of dentine is found pulpal to the circumpulpal (and in older teeth secondary) dentine and restricted to the region beneath the irritation. This tertiary dentine is not formed by the original odontoblasts but by odontoblast-like cells that have differentiated from the dental pulp. It is much more irregular than circumpulpal dentine and has been given a variety of names such as reactionary dentine, reparative dentine, response dentine and irregular secondary dentine. There has been acceptance of the term tertiary dentine in preference to other terms (see pages 143–145).

## MANTLE DENTINE

The outer layer of dentine in the crown differs from the bulk of the circumpulpal dentine in four features:

- It is slightly (approx. 5%) less mineralized.
- The collagen fibres are largely oriented perpendicular to the enamel–dentine junction (see also pages 130, 331). For this reason, it can be distinguished from the circumpulpal dentine beneath using polarized light (Fig. 9.32).
- The dentinal tubules branch profusely in this region (Fig. 9.33).
- It undergoes mineralization in the presence of matrix vesicles (see page 334).

These features give the mantle region an appearance distinct from that of the circumpulpal dentine when seen in polarizing light microscopy of ground, undermineralized sections.

The mantle layer varies in width from 20 μm to 150 μm. The special properties of mantle dentine prevent small cracks developing in the enamel near the junction from spreading into the dentine. The three-dimensional scalloped architecture of the enamel–dentine junction and the extension of some dentinal tubules into the enamel as enamel spindles have been described in Chapter 7.

## INTERGLOBULAR DENTINE

Much of the mineral in dentine is deposited as globules or calcospherites. These, in most areas, fuse to form a uniformly calcified tissue. However, in some areas, usually beneath the mantle layer in the crown and beneath the granular layer in the root, the fusion may be incomplete. When ground sections are viewed in transmitted light, internal reflection of the light makes the uncalcified, interglobular areas appear dark (Fig. 9.34). Dentinal tubules pass without deviation through interglobular areas (Fig. 9.35). As interglobular areas remain uncalcified, peritubular dentine is also absent from the tubules as they pass through interglobular dentine.

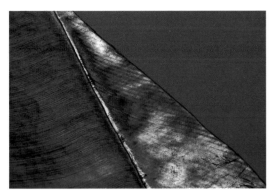

**Fig. 9.32** Ground longitudinal section of the crown of a tooth viewed in polarized light (with a quartz filter). Due to the different orientation of the collagen fibres, the mantle layer immediately beneath the enamel–dentine junction appears red, in contrast to the blue appearance of the rest of the circumpulpal dentine (×50).

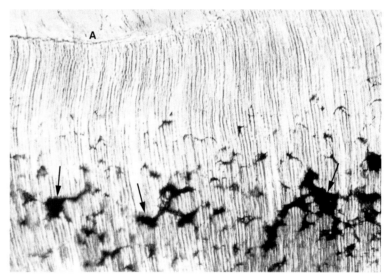

**Fig. 9.34** Ground section of outer dentine showing areas of interglobular dentine (arrowed). A = Enamel (×300). Courtesy of R.V. Hawkins.

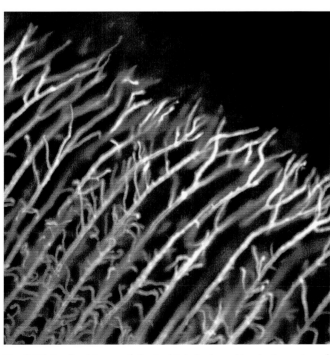

**Fig. 9.33** Confocal image of dentinal tubules branching in the region of the mantle dentine (Alizarin red; ×1200). Courtesy of Drs M. Kagayama, Y. Sasao, S. Kamakura, K. Motegi and I. Mizoguchi, and the editor of *Anatomy and Embryology*.

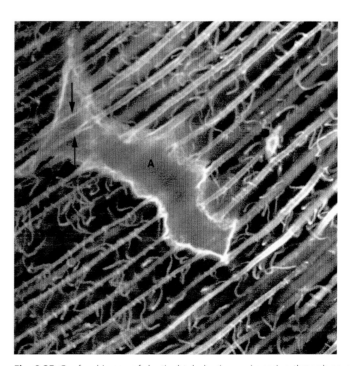

**Fig. 9.35** Confocal image of dentinal tubules (arrows) passing through an area of interglobular dentine (A) (Alizarin red; ×1200). Courtesy of Drs S. M. Kagayama, Y. Sasao, S. Kamakura, K. Motegi and I. Mizoguchi, and the editor of *Anatomy and Embryology*.

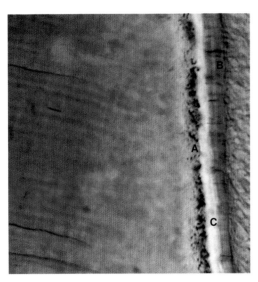

**Fig. 9.36** Ground longitudinal section of a root showing the granular (A) and hyaline (C) layers beneath a layer of acellular cementum (B) (×160).

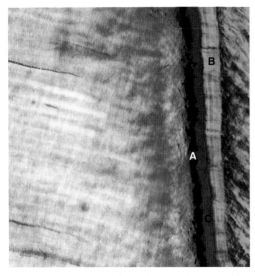

**Fig. 9.37** The same section as in Fig. 9.36 viewed in polarized light with a quartz tint. The hyaline layer can be distinguished from the rest of the underlying dentine and the cementum suggesting a difference in the orientation of its collagen fibres. A = granular layer; B = acellular cementum; C = hyaline layer (×160).

## GRANULAR LAYER

In ground sections the periphery of the dentine in the root is marked by the presence of a dark granular zone, the granular layer (Figs 9.36, 9.37). Various explanations for this appearance have been suggested. That currently most accepted is that the dentinal tubules in this area branch more profusely and loop back on themselves, creating air spaces in ground sections that result in internal reflection of transmitted light. Differences in the rate of formation of coronal and radicular dentine could explain why this appearance is seen in the root but not the crown. Stain-filled tubules viewed in thick sections have a 'tree-top' appearance somewhat supporting this idea (Fig. 9.38). The granular layer is hypomineralized in comparison to circumpulpal dentine, but this may be the result of the presence of more tubular branches. An alternative explanation for the granular appearance is that it is due to the incomplete fusion of calcospherites.

## HYALINE LAYER

Outside the granular layer is a clear hyaline layer usually included as a component of the dentine but whose origin is obscure. This narrow band (up to 20 μm wide) appears to be non-tubular and relatively structureless (Figs 9.36, 9.37). The hyaline layer may serve to bond cementum to

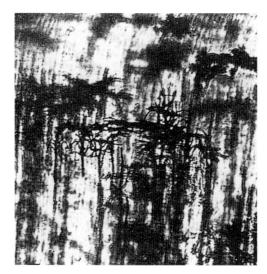

**Fig. 9.38** Ground thick section of root impregnated with silver stain in region of granular layer showing peripheral terminations of tubules exhibiting profuse branching in three dimensions (×490).

dentine and may be of considerable clinical significance when considering periodontal regeneration. It is discussed further on pages 171–173.

## CIRCUMPULPAL DENTINE

The basic structure of dentine as described throughout this chapter is that of circumpulpal dentine. It forms the bulk of the dentine and is uniform in structure except at its edges where, peripherally, interglobular dentine marks incomplete initial mineralization and, centrally, the mineralizing front represents ongoing mineralization. In older teeth its tubular pattern is modified on the pulpal surface due to the age-related deposition of secondary dentine.

## PREDENTINE

In demineralized sections stained with haematoxylin and eosin, the innermost layer of dentine, the predentine, has a distinct pale-staining appearance (Fig. 9.39). This reflects a difference in the composition of its matrix from that of the matrix of the mineralized circumpulpal dentine. The mineralizing front may show a globular (Fig. 9.39) or a linear outline, reflecting the mineralization process (see page 334). The predentine is the initially laid down dentine matrix before its mineralization. During mineralization, the matrix undergoes considerable modification. The principal role of the odontoblast process in predentine is the secretion of matrix components. In mineralizing dentine the role of the odontoblast process is to participate in the modification of that matrix and, perhaps, also in its mineralization (see pages 331, 332). The width of the predentine can vary from 10 μm to 40 μm, depending on the rate at which dentine is being deposited: it is, for example, thicker in young teeth.

## STRUCTURAL LINES IN DENTINE

In sections of dentine viewed by different techniques, a variety of lines approximately perpendicular to the dentinal tubules can be seen. The descriptions and explanations of these lines vary considerably. Some have had the name of the individual who first described them attached to them, causing confusion when later investigators use those names to include somewhat different structures. The description given here will rely on the functional origin of the lines as best understood but will include the eponym to retain the historical flavour these lines have acquired.

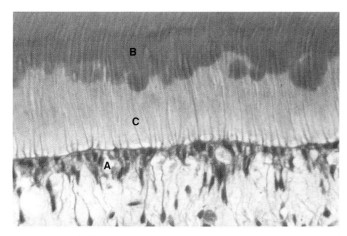

**Fig. 9.39** Decalcified section of the pulpodentinal region showing the odontoblast layer (A) and predentine (C). Note the different staining reaction of the predentine to that of the mineralized dentine matrix (B). The mineralizing front at B is globular (H & E; ×500).

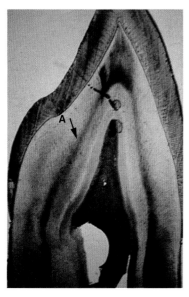

**Fig. 9.40** Ground longitudinal section of a crown showing a broad Schreger line (A), coincident with the apex of one of the primary curvatures of the dentinal tubules. Only one is visible although, hypothetically, two are possible (×5).

There are two related groups of lines: those originating from curvatures in the dentinal tubules and those arising from the incremental deposition of dentine and its subsequent mineralization.

## LINES ASSOCIATED WITH THE PRIMARY CURVATURES OF THE DENTINAL TUBULES

In some longitudinal sections the peaks of the sigmoid primary curvatures coincide to form broad bands in the dentine. These are not apparent in many sections, and rarely can two be seen. They are more difficult to see in horizontal sections where they would be seen as broad concentric bands in the circumpulpal dentine. These lines are known as Schreger lines (Fig. 9.40).

## LINES ASSOCIATED WITH THE SECONDARY CURVATURES OF THE DENTINAL TUBULES

When the secondary curvatures coincide they also give rise to an optical effect, resulting in the appearance of lines, the contour lines of Owen (Fig. 9.41). They are unusual in primary dentine but are sometimes seen. An exaggerated line is found at the border of primary and secondary dentine (see page 143) and between dentine formed before and that formed after

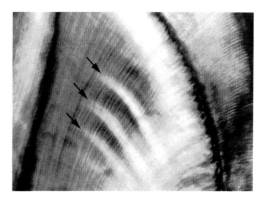

**Fig. 9.41** Ground longitudinal section viewed in polarized light of a crown showing contour lines associated with the coincidence of secondary curvatures (arrows) of the dentinal tubules (×120).

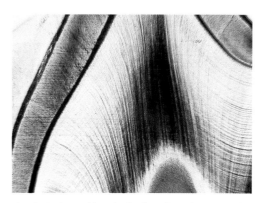

**Fig. 9.42** Ground longitudinal section of a crown showing, on the right side, horizontally running long-period incremental lines (×12). Courtesy of Dr B.A.W. Brown.

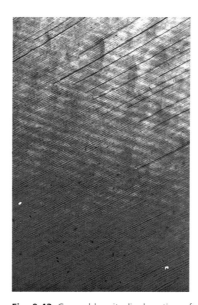

**Fig. 9.43** Ground longitudinal section of dentine viewed in polarized light showing alternate light and dark bands representing long-period incremental lines. The bands are approximately orientated at right angles to the direction of the dentinal tubules (×250).

birth. This latter neonatal line may include compositional variations in the matrix and mineralization.

## INCREMENTAL LINES ASSOCIATED WITH MATRIX DEPOSITION AND MINERALIZATION

Dentine has regular, incremental, short-period and long-period markings. The lines may be seen in normal ground sections (Fig. 9.42), demineralized sections, under polarized light (Fig. 9.43) and in microradiographs.

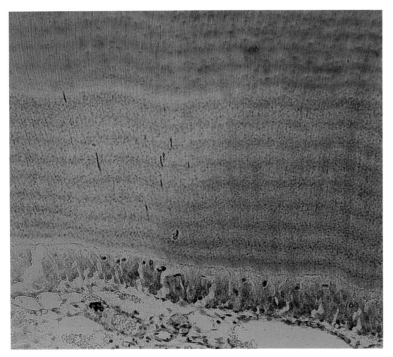

**Fig. 9.44** This decalcified section is taken from a rat injected with tritiated proline. The amino acid is incorporated rhythmically into the collagen of the dentine matrix, as shown by the periodic presence of silver grains developed by the radioactivity from the photographic emulsion layered onto the section. The section is also lightly stained to show incremental lines and how these coincide with the incorporation of proline (H & E; ×350). Courtesy of Drs M. Ohtsuka, S. Saeki, K. Igarashi, H. Shinoda, and the editor of the *Journal of Dental Research*.

They can be attributed to circadian fluctuations in acid–base balance that affect both the mineral content and the refractive index of forming hard tissues. The long-period lines, at least, are greatly enhanced when viewed in polarized light (Fig. 9.43), suggesting that they are associated with changes in collagen fibril orientation.

Short-period markings may be seen as alternating dark and light bands, each pair reflecting the diurnal rhythm of dentine formation (Fig. 9.44). These fine lines are sometimes referred to as von Ebner's lines. In cuspal dentine, where deposition is most rapid, the amount of dentine formed each day and the distance between adjacent dark bands is approximately 4 µm (Fig. 9.45). In the root peripherally near the granular layer, where the dentine has a calcospheritic pattern, the distance between lines is nearer 2 µm (Fig. 9.46). In demineralized sections the values are smaller, presumably because of shrinkage caused by processing of the tissue.

The coarser, long-period lines (Andresen lines) are approximately 16–20 µm apart (Figs 9.42, 9.43, 9.47). Between each long-period line there are six to 10 pairs of short-period lines (Fig. 9.47). The cause for the 6–10-day periodicity is unknown. The same periodicity exists between the long-period striae of Retzius in enamel and the long-period Andresen lines in dentine, making it likely that a common mechanism exists.

As with enamel, an exaggerated line, the neonatal line (Fig. 9.48), can be seen in teeth mineralizing at birth.

## AGE-RELATED AND POSTERUPTIVE CHANGES

Once the tooth is erupted and fully formed, dentine can undergo a number of changes that are either related to age or occur as a response to a stimulus applied to the tooth, such as caries or attrition. With regard to physiological age changes, secondary dentine and translucent dentine will be considered. Concerning the response of dentine to stimuli, tertiary dentine, sclerotic dentine and dead tracts will be discussed.

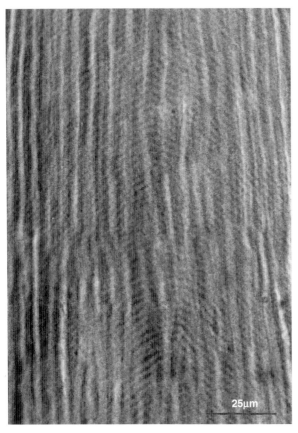

25µm

**Fig. 9.45** Anorganic ground section of dentine high over the cuspal region of a premolar showing short-period incremental lines running across the field approximately 4 µm apart (×720). Courtesy of Professor M.C. Dean and the editor of the *Archives of Oral Biology*.

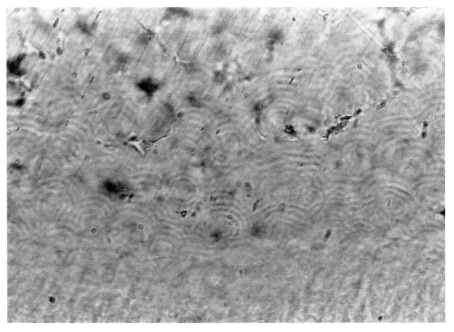

**Fig. 9.46** Anorganic preparation of root dentine near the granular layer (at the lower part of the field) showing short-period incremental lines about 2 µm apart and having a calcospheritic outline (×800). Courtesy of Professor M.C. Dean and the editor of the *Archives of Oral Biology*.

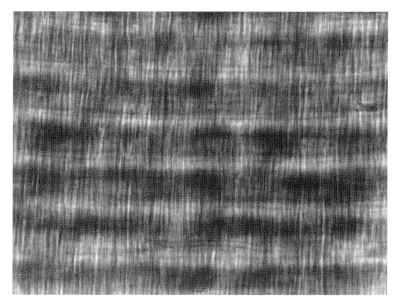

**Fig. 9.47** Ground section of dentine viewed in polarized light. The long period (horizontal) lines are about 20 μm apart and between them are seven or eight short-period incremental lines (×900). Courtesy of Professor M.C. Dean and the editor of the *Archives of Oral Biology*.

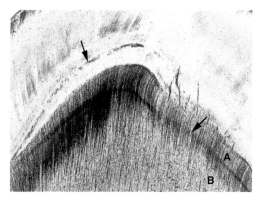

**Fig. 9.48** Ground longitudinal section of a deciduous tooth showing neonatal lines (arrows) in enamel and dentine. These are exaggerated in this example as the tooth came from a patient who suffered from icterus neonatorium (newborn jaundice) (×25). A = dentine formed prenatally; B = dentine formed postnatally.

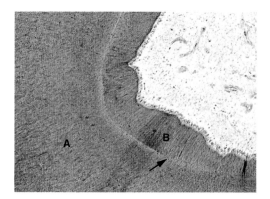

**Fig. 9.49** A decalcified cross-section of dentine showing a pronounced contour line (arrow) separating primary dentine (A) from secondary dentine (B) (Silver staining, ×32).

## SECONDARY DENTINE

The most conspicuous age-associated change in dentine is the formation of secondary dentine. Its structure is very similar to that of primary dentine and it may be difficult to distinguish between the two. However, primary and secondary dentine are often delineated as a result of a change in direc-

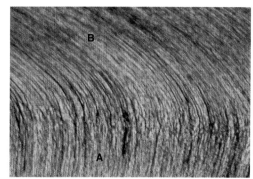

**Fig. 9.50** Ground longitudinal section of dentine illustrating the change in direction of dentinal tubules as they pass from primary (A) to secondary (B) dentine (×125).

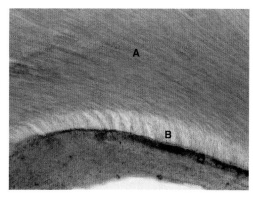

**Fig. 9.51** Ground longitudinal section showing primary (A) and secondary (B) dentine (×80).

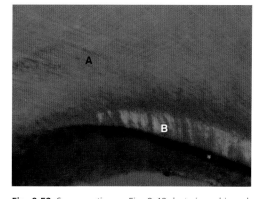

**Fig. 9.52** Same section as Fig. 9.49, but viewed in polarized light with a quartz tint. The difference in colour between primary (A) and secondary (B) dentine is presumably due to the difference in orientation of collagen fibres and/or crystals (×80).

tion of the dentinal tubules with coincidence of secondary curvatures. This produces a particularly pronounced contour line (of Owen) (Figs 9.49–9.52). The same odontoblasts continue to lay down similar dentine and the tubules of primary and secondary dentine are continuous. The increased crowding of odontoblasts as secondary dentine formation continues throughout life, and the slower rate of deposition make the tubular pattern of secondary dentine a little less regular than that of primary dentine and the incremental markings somewhat closer together. Secondary dentine formation begins at the completion of root formation as the tooth comes into occlusion. The main coincidence would seem to be the apparent completion of root formation as secondary dentine still forms in unerupted,

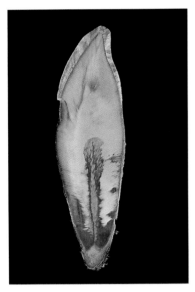

**Fig. 9.53** A section of a whole tooth showing the translucent dentine predominantly in the apical part of the root (Ground section). Courtesy of Drs A.M. Sengupta, D.K. Whittaker and P.R. Shellis, and the editor of the *Archives of Oral Biology*.

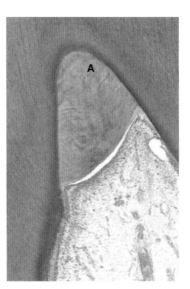

**Fig. 9.55** Demineralized section showing tertiary dentine (A) having an irregular appearance in a pulp horn (H & E; ×50).

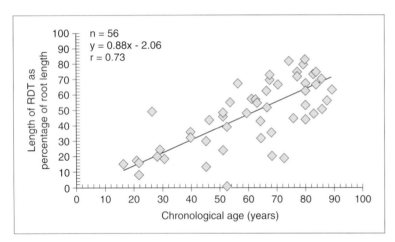

**Fig. 9.54** The relationship between age and the area of translucent dentine (RDT). Courtesy of Drs A.M. Sengupta, D.K. Whittaker and P.R. Shellis, and the editor of the *Archives of Oral Biology*.

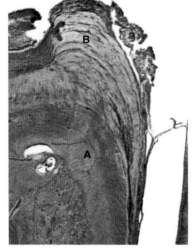

**Fig. 9.56** Tertiary dentine (B) overlying primary dentine (A) on the floor of a pulp chamber extending around the orifice of a root canal (demineralized section stained with Weigerts and van Gieson) (×20).

impacted teeth. Secondary dentine forms most rapidly on the pulpal floor. Its continuing deposition leads to smaller pulp chambers and narrower root canals in older patients.

In physiological ageing, especially in root dentine, the tubules can become completely occluded with peritubular dentine to form translucent dentine. With age, translucent dentine is particularly pronounced at the root apex and increases linearly with age (Figs 9.53, 9.54). For this reason it is used in forensic dentistry to help determine the age of a person from the teeth. Translucent dentine is discussed further on page 134.

## TERTIARY DENTINE

The dental pulp may be induced to produce calcified material in addition to its 'usual' primary and secondary dentine by a variety of outside stimuli including caries, attrition, cavity preparation, microleakage around restorations and trauma. Stimuli of different types and extent may be applied to

teeth at different stages of development or ageing, resulting in a response tissue that may vary considerably in appearance and composition: it may resemble secondary dentine in having a regular tubular structure; it may have few and/or irregularly arranged tubules; or it may be relatively atubular (Figs 9.55–9.57). Continuity of dentinal tubules between normal dentine and tertiary dentine will therefore be lost in many instances (Fig. 9.58).

Because of this wide range of presentations, this response tissue has been given a variety of names, including irregular secondary dentine, reparative dentine, reactionary dentine, response dentine and osteodentine.

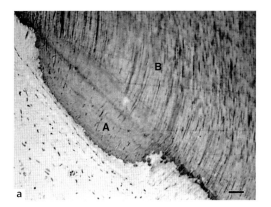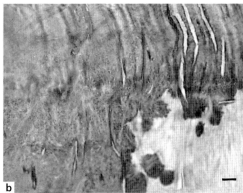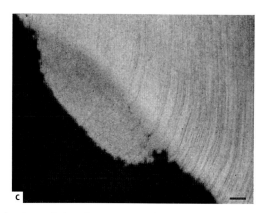

**Fig. 9.57** Tertiary dentine formation in response to deep caries. (a) Zone of tertiary dentine (adjacent to A) at the dentine–pulp interface projecting from normal dentine (B) (H & E; ×300). (b) Higher-power view, showing calcospherites in tertiary dentine (H & E; ×1500). (c) Microradiograph of undemineralized lesion similar to that seen in (a), revealing a difference in mineralization levels between normal and tertiary dentine, there being less mineral in tertiary dentine (×300). Courtesy of Drs L. Bjorndal and T. Darvann, and the editor of *Caries Research*.

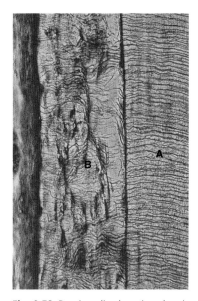

**Fig. 9.58** Demineralized section showing loss of continuity of many dentinal tubules between normal dentine (A) and tertiary dentine (B) (Picrothionin stain; ×100). Courtesy of Professor M.M. Smith.

It seems sensible to rationalize this nomenclature and use the term 'tertiary dentine' for all hard tissue deposited on the pulpal surface in response to an external stimulus.

The pulp does not seem to respond to stimuli by increasing the rate of deposition of secondary dentine but by inducing previously quiescent odontoblast-like cells to produce mineralized tissue. The different appearances of tertiary dentine are thus probably due to its production by newly differentiated mesenchymal cells rather than by the odontoblasts that have produced primary and secondary dentine (although recent studies suggest that, at least on some occasions, primary odontoblasts may be involved in the initial stages of tertiary dentine formation). The newly differentiated cells responsible for tertiary dentine formation are very similar to odontoblasts in that they produce type I collagen and dentine sialoprotein, a dentine-specific protein.

The term reactionary dentine refers to the dentine forming in response to an insult in which, although some damage has been sustained and some odontoblasts die, the existing odontoblasts recover and continue to form dentine. There will be some irregularity in dentine structure depending on the strength of the stimulus and the dentine will have an irregular appearance with fewer tubules.

The term reparative dentine relates to dentine forming after a stimulus in which the original odontoblasts in the associated region have been destroyed and new calcified tissue (reparative dentine) has been formed by newly differentiated cells referred to here as 'odontoblast-like' cells. In considering the origin of odontoblasts during normal tooth formation (see pages 329, 330), reciprocal epithelial/mesenchymal interactions are an essential feature. However, it is clear that odontoblast-like cells arising from the adult pulp after a suitable stimulus do so in the absence of epithelial cells. There are two possible explanations for this. It might be that during initial dentine formation epithelial/mesenchymal interactions guide some cells on the path to becoming odontoblasts but that these cells remain dormant in the pulp awaiting a later stimulus for them to complete their lifecycle and form reparative dentine. A more likely explanation, however, is that odontoblast-like cells are differentiated from a stem cell population in the absence of any epithelial contribution. It is envisaged that the appropriate bioactive molecules necessary for such differentiation (e.g. cytokines, growth factors) are locally synthesized and released during the inflammatory process accompanying the stimulus (such as dental caries). To this effect, a number of factors have been shown to induce the formation of repair dentine in the pulp of experimental animals, such as pieces of native dentine, pieces of demineralized dentine, crude extracts of dentine matrix, fibronectin products and bone morphogenetic protein. It might be envisaged that the addition of suitable activating substances to the region of pulp exposures might aid and speed up clinically the formation of repair dentine over pulp exposures. Recent work, however, also suggests that healing can occur naturally providing that the cavity is completely sealed at its margins.

## SCLEROTIC DENTINE

In addition to infilling with peritubular dentine as a physiological response to ageing (eventually forming translucent dentine – see pages 134, 144), dentinal tubules commonly fill in as a response to an external stimulus such as under slowly advancing caries or beneath areas of severe attrition

(Figs 9.59, 9.60). This type of dentine is termed sclerotic dentine and, like translucent dentine, will present as areas of dentine that lack structure and appear transparent (Fig. 9.61). Little is known about the precipitated material but it appears to differ from peritubular dentine and is thus thought not to be formed by the odontoblast. The mineral is crystalline and possibly an apatite, although plate-like crystals of octocalcium phosphate have also been reported. The mineral concentration, as measured by X-ray computed microtomography, is significantly higher in sclerotic than in young dentine, consistent with the closure of the tubule lumens. Crystallite size, as measured by small angle X-ray scattering, is slightly smaller in sclerotic dentine. The elastic properties of dentine are unchanged by transparency; however, sclerotic dentine, unlike normal dentine, exhibits almost no yielding before failure. In addition, the fracture toughness is lowered by roughly 20%. In tubules exposed by attrition or caries some occluding components may be derived from saliva.

## DEAD TRACTS

If the primary odontoblasts are killed by an external stimulus, or retract before peritubular dentine occludes the tubules, empty tubules will be left. They may be sealed at their pulpal end by tertiary dentine. When ground sections are prepared and mounted, the mounting medium will not enter these sealed off tubules and they will remain air-filled. Under the microscope transmitted light will be totally internally reflected and these tubules will appear dark (Figs 9.62, 9.63). This appearance, which is due partly to the pulpal response and partly to the preparatory procedure, has been termed a 'dead tract'.

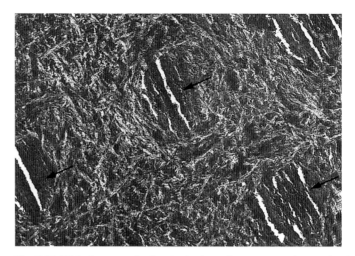

**Fig. 9.59** TEM of a zone of sclerotic dentine adjacent to a carious cavity showing transversely sectioned tubules completely occluded (arrows), forming a zone of sclerotic dentine (×7000). Courtesy of Professor N.W. Johnson.

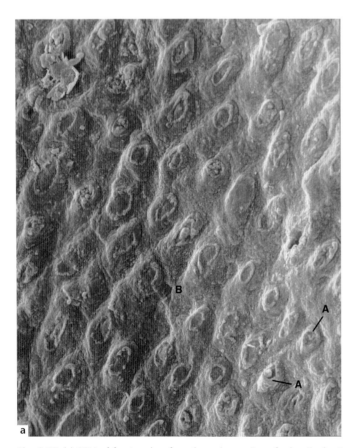

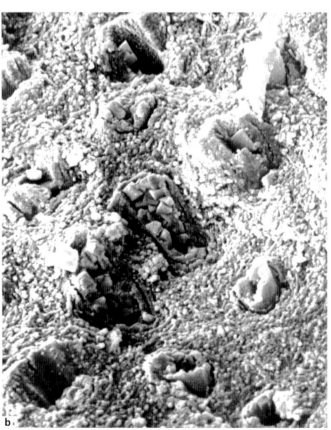

**Fig. 9.60** (a) SEM of fractured surface through a region of sclerotic dentine. In the lower part of the micrograph, within an initial layer of peritubular dentine (A), an additional central plug of mineral has been deposited to occlude the tubule. B = Intertubular dentine. In the upper part of the micrograph, the dentinal tubules remain patent (×1500). (b) High-power view of sclerotic dentine from (a), showing central plug of dentinal tubules containing large rhombohedral crystals (probably whitlockite) (×5000). Courtesy of Professor M.M. Smith.

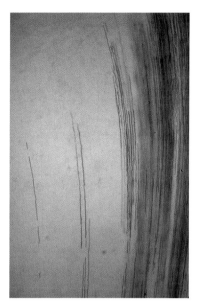

**Fig. 9.61** A longitudinal ground section (mounted in water) of sclerotic dentine on the left of the micrograph showing a loss of tubular structure and appearing transparent as the dentinal tubules have been completely occluded by mineral. The unaffected right edge of the micrograph shows a more normal tubular morphology (×20).

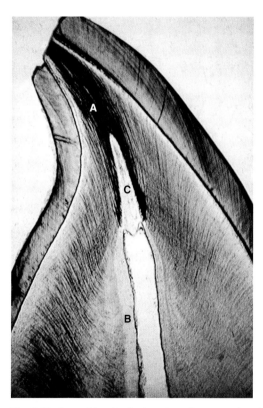

**Fig. 9.62** Ground longitudinal section of a crown showing a dead tract (A) beneath a region of attrition that is sealed pulpally by tertiary dentine (C). Secondary dentine (B) lines the rest of the pulp chamber (×15).

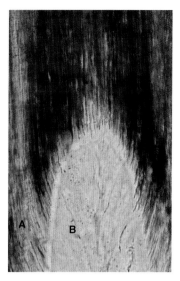

**Fig. 9.63** Ground longitudinal section of coronal dentine showing secondary dentine (A) and tertiary dentine (B) beneath a dead tract (×50).

## CLINICAL CONSIDERATIONS

### PERMEABILITY OF DENTINE

The tubular structure of dentine allows for the possibility of substances applied to its outer surface being able to reach and affect the dental pulp. This depends on a number of factors:

- that the dentine surface is exposed by caries, attrition, abrasion or trauma
- that the tubules are patent. Tubules may be occluded physiologically by peritubular (intratubular) dentine or by exogenous material precipitated in them peripherally. They may also be sealed off from the pulp by tertiary dentine
- that the outward movement of interstitial 'dentinal' fluid does not wash them out of the tubule
- that they are able to pass through the odontoblast layer, which presents a barrier to molecules of higher molecular weight.

Given that these factors are overcome, the most significant materials to travel down the tubules are the bacteria of dental caries and, more importantly, the toxins they produce. It is possible, but unproven, that molecules capable of exciting sensory nerves in the pulp may follow this route and induce pain. Components of dental materials, or etchants used to prepare for their placement, may pass through the dentine and kill or damage the dental pulp. This does not seem to be as large a concern as it may seem. The poor pulpal response to some restorative materials is more likely to be due to the poor marginal seal the material provides, allowing microleakage and the presence of bacteria on the surface of the dentine, whose toxins affect the pulp. Although in vitro some components of dental materials pass through dentine, in vivo the outward flow of dentinal fluid opposes this.

### RESPONSE TO EXTERNAL STIMULI (FOR EXAMPLE CARIES, ATTRITION)

The response to outside stimuli comes from the dental pulp but is manifest in the structure of the dentine it produces. The deposition of tertiary dentine provides a barrier to the progress of caries and toxins. The presence of secondary dentine and its continuing deposition throughout life, although not a response to external stimuli, contributes to the barrier function of the dentine.

## ADHESION OF DENTAL MATERIALS TO DENTINE

Many of the advances in restorative dentistry are a result of the development of materials that will adhere to enamel and dentine. This allows more conservative cavity preparations, less pulpal injury and improved aesthetic results. Adhesion to dentine is more complex than that to enamel because of the high organic content of the tissue and its tubular architecture. In addition, when dentine is cut with a dental bur a smear layer (Fig. 9.64) forms on its surface, consisting of dentine that has been melted and reset; it may also contain embedded in it bacteria from caries that was being removed. Smearing has an advantage in that it occludes the dentinal tubules but a disadvantage in that it may harbour bacteria and provides a difficult surface to adhere to. Removing the smear layer is therefore a prerequisite before applying bonding agents. Like enamel, dentine is first etched with strong acids to remove the smear layer and to provide a porous surface that can be infiltrated by the bonding agent (Fig. 9.65). The bonding agent will then penetrate the dentinal tubules and the exposed collagen in the intertubular dentine (Figs 9.66, 9.67).

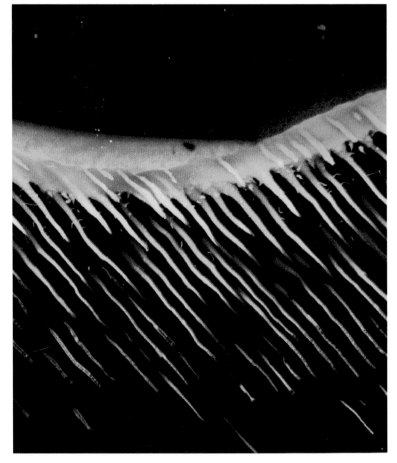

**Fig. 9.66** Confocal image of acid-etched dentine infiltrated with a multiple dye-labelled bonding agent. Notice the penetration of the bonding agent into the tubules and the intertubular region at the surface forming a 'hybrid zone' (×1000). Courtesy of Professor T. Watson.

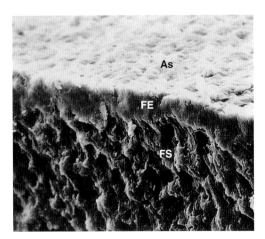

**Fig. 9.64** SEM showing a smear layer on the surface of dentine cut with a high-speed bur; As = abraded surface; FE = smear layer on fractured edge; FS = fractured surface (×35). Courtesy of Dr J. Dennison.

**Fig. 9.65** SEM of a fractured surface of dentine after etching with 37% phosphoric acid. Notice the exposed collagen fibrils in the superficial layers (A) and loss of peritubular dentine (seen in deeper layers, B). Open lateral tubules (C) are visible. Mineralized collagen fibrils (arrow) are evident in the intertubular dentine (×6500). Courtesy of Professor B. Van Meerbeek.

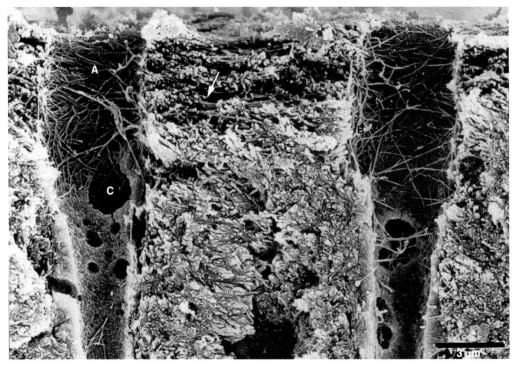

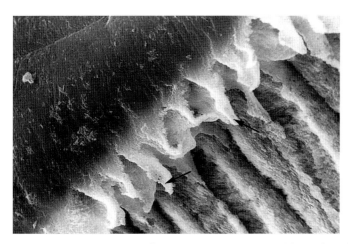

**Fig. 9.67** SEM showing tags of resin in a restorative material (arrows) conforming to the dentinal tubules in etched dentine and enhancing retention of the restoration (×35). Courtesy of Dr J. Dennison.

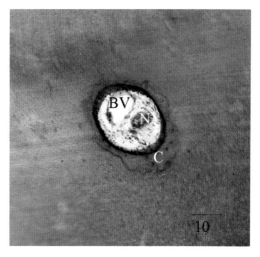

**Fig. 9.69** A small (lateral) canal of the root canal system containing a blood vessel (BV), nerve bundle (N) and lined by cementum (C).

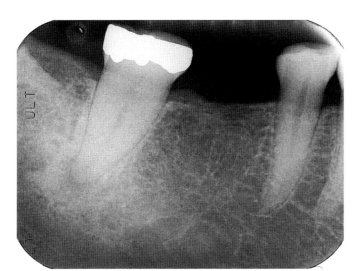

**Fig. 9.68** Clinical radiograph of a molar tooth in which the root canals have been obliterated by mineralization.

## ENDODONTICS

The continuing deposition of secondary dentine throughout life and the development of tertiary dentine in response to caries and restorative procedures can lead to a reduction in size – even, effectively, obliteration of the pulp chamber and root canals (Fig. 9.68). Root canal therapy (endodontics) consists of cleaning, shaping and filling the root canal system. There are a number of smaller, lateral canals (Fig. 9.69) entering the main canal that may not be cleaned during treatment.

## SENSITIVITY

Exposed dentine is often (but not always) sensitive. Three main hypotheses have been put forward to account for its sensitivity, implicating:

- nerves in dentine
- the odontoblast processes
- fluid movements in the dentinal tubules (Fig. 9.70).

Arguments against the view that pain is due to direct stimulation of nerves in the dentine relate to their relative scarcity and to the fact that they appear to be absent in the outer parts of dentine. In addition, the application of local anaesthetics to the surface of dentine does not abolish the sensitivity.

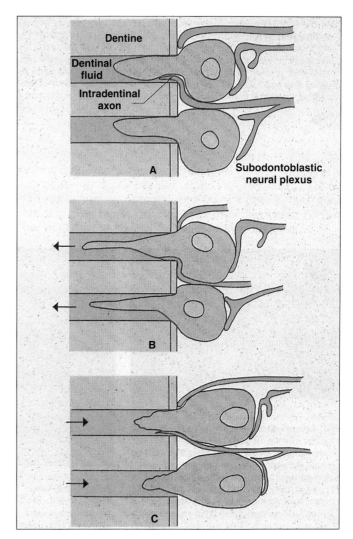

**Fig. 9.70** The effects of outward (B) and inward (C) fluid movement in the dentinal tubules.

Referring to the second hypothesis, there is no physiological evidence to date that indicates that the odontoblast process is analogous to a nerve fibre and can similarly conduct impulses pulpwards. Furthermore, the process may not extend to the enamel–dentine junction, nor is the application of substances designed to prevent transmission of such impulses effective. Odontoblasts have not been shown to be synaptically connected to nerve fibres.

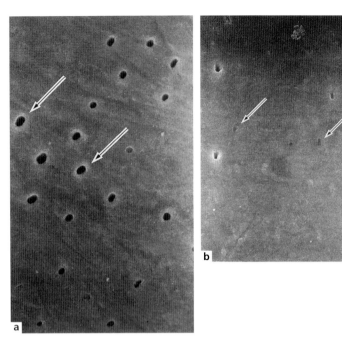

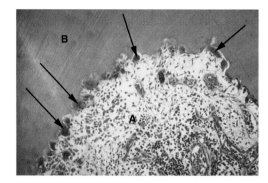

**Fig. 9.72** Section of tooth undergoing internal dentine resorption. The pulp (A) has lost its peripheral odontoblast layer and is replaced by a vascular granulation tissue. The dentine (B) is undergoing resorption by large multinucleated odonto-clast-like cells (arrows) (H & E stain; ×200). Courtesy of Dr H. Trowbridge.

**Fig. 9.71** (a) SEM of an exposed dentine surface of a hypersensitive area. A large proportion of dentinal tubules (arrows) are seen to be open. (b) SEM of exposed dentine from a non-sensitive area. The tubules are occluded (arrows) (×2400). Courtesy of Dr M. Yoshiyama and the editor of the *Journal of Dental Research*.

The most plausible hypothesis to explain the transmission of sensory stimuli suggests that all effective stimuli applied to dentine cause fluid movement through the dentinal tubules, and that this movement is sufficient to depolarize nerve endings in the inner parts of tubules, at the pulp–predentine junction and in the subodontoblastic neural plexus. Some stimuli, such as heat, osmotic pressure and drying, would tend to cause fluid movement outwards while others, such as cold, would cause movement inwards (Fig. 9.70). Movement in either direction would mechanically distort the terminals. These stimuli have been shown to cause such fluid movement in vitro. Chemicals (in strong solution) and thermal stimuli induce a response much more quickly than can be explained by conduction or diffusion. This, too, is consistent with the hydrodynamic hypothesis. In animal experiments, however, the response of intradental nerves to chemical stimuli is often slow and may be more readily explained by diffusion. It may be that both 'direct' and 'hydrodynamic' mechanisms operate, but that the hydrodynamic force predominates whenever there is pulpal inflammation and a lowering in threshold of intrapulpal nerves to the small mechanical forces generated by fluid flow.

Exposed dentine that is sensitive is sometimes described as 'hypersensitive'. Such dentine has tubules that are patent (Fig. 9.71a). Exposed dentine in which the tubules are not patent is not sensitive (Fig. 9.71b).

Eliminating or reducing the sensitivity of exposed dentine is not always easy. The most effective approach is to occlude the dentinal tubules either by smearing or by the precipitation of crystalline fluorides or oxalates.

## DENTINE RESORPTION

Apart from the dentine that is resorbed during the shedding of deciduous teeth, dentine in permanent teeth is normally stable throughout adult life. However, it can be resorbed in permanent teeth. This resorption is usually

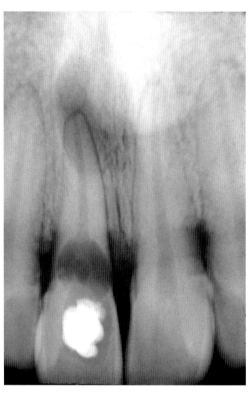

**Fig. 9.73** Radiograph showing a large central radiolucent area thought to be related to internal dentine resorption. Courtesy of Dr H. Trowbridge.

associated with inflammation. However, rarely the cause is unknown and this condition is termed idiopathic resorption. Dentine resorption may be initiated from two sites: from the pulpal surface, when it is known as internal dentine resorption, or from the from the root surface, when it is known as external dentine resorption.

## Internal dentine resorption

In the case of internal resorption, the pulp contains at the pulp–dentine surface multinucleated cells known as odontoclasts that are responsible for resorbing the dentine (Fig. 9.72). This will be evident radiologically as an enlarged radiolucency in the pulp (Fig. 9.73).

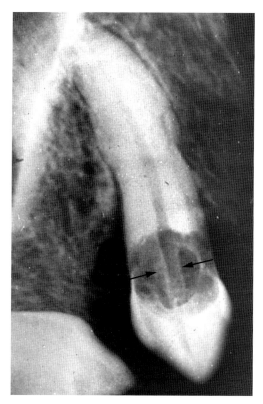

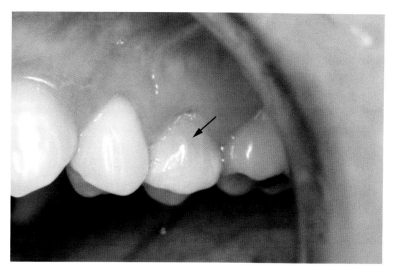

**Fig. 9.75** Patient with underlying dentine resorption involving a second maxillary premolar (arrow). The crown shows a pinkish colouration compared with the normal adjacent teeth. The cause may be either internal or external resorption. Courtesy of Dr N. McDonald.

**Fig. 9.74** Radiograph of tooth showing external dentine resorption. The presence of a radiopaque layer of dentine internally (arrows) helps distinguish this case from one of internal dentine resorption (compare with Fig. 9.73). Courtesy of Dr J.D Harrison.

## External dentine resorption

External resorption of the dentine begins on the external surface of the root and penetrates through the cementum into dentine. It does not normally penetrate the pulp and, radiologically, is difficult to distinguish from internal resorption. However, a thin shell of dentine may be visible on a radiograph (Fig. 9.74). If resorption proceeds far enough, the crown may have a pinkish coloration as the vascular granulation tissue is seen beneath the translucent enamel (Fig. 9.75).

Root resorption may be seen following periapical inflammation (Fig. 9.73), orthodontic treatment and tooth implantation.

# 10 Dental pulp

The dental pulp is the tissue derived from the dental papilla responsible for the formation of dentine. It is contained within the pulp chamber and root canals of the tooth (see pages 28–33). At the apical constriction of the root canal it becomes continuous with the periodontal ligament (see Fig. 26.6). Although the pulp is most obviously active during development and eruption of the tooth, it remains productive throughout life, forming secondary dentine slowly but regularly. It is able to respond (within certain important limits) to stimuli such as caries, trauma, tooth movement and restorative procedures by producing tertiary dentine (see pages 144, 145).

## ORGANIZATION

The dental pulp is a specialized connective tissue with a unique anatomical arrangement determined by its position inside a rigid chamber and by its role in forming hard tissue on the walls of that chamber (Fig. 10.1). The cells responsible for dentine deposition, the odontoblasts, lie at the periphery of the tissue. Also in the periphery are two elements capable of detecting external stimuli and initiating a response to them. These are the nerve terminals of trigeminal afferents and specialized dendritic antigen-presenting cells. The odontoblasts themselves may also be able to detect the presence of foreign antigens. The rest of the dental pulp acts as a support system for these three components. Blood vessels and nerves enter and leave the root canals through an apical foramen at the root end. Each root has at least one main canal and apical foramen; many have two. Smaller accessory canals branch from the main canal and have their own foramina. They are found most commonly in the apical third of the root (Fig. 10.2). In multirooted teeth some small vascular canals enter the pulp chamber from the bone between the roots.

## COMPOSITION

The composition of any connective tissues varies during development and with ageing. It changes when the tissue is injured or challenged with a bacterial toxin. Different cells may be activated, migrate to the tissue or develop from stem cells. It is impossible to study all the elements of a tissue at the same time. Each cell type may contribute different products to the extracellular matrix at different times. Often cells are observed in culture separated from all other components. In this situation they may produce extracellular materials that they do not create in the intact tissue. Larger molecules are built up from smaller components and, conversely, some smaller molecules may be breakdown products from larger molecules. The end result is that the composition is dynamic and will vary depending when and how it is studied. What follows is a static description some of which may be correct all the time but some of which will only be correct some of the time!

The dental pulp is a loose connective tissue and made up of a combination of cells embedded in an extracellular matrix of fibres in a semi-fluid gel. It contains 75% water and 25% organic material by weight. As with most connective tissues the matrix is more plentiful than the cells. The extracellular matrix is made up of a versatile group of polysaccharides and proteins secreted by the cells of the tissue and assembled into a complex framework closely associated with the cells. The extracellular matrix forms a scaffold that stabilizes the structure of the tissue, but it is far from inert: indeed, in the dental pulp, where there is a rigid supporting and protecting hard shell, the skeletal function is minimal. The matrix plays a very active role in controlling the activity of the cells within it. It affects their development, migration, division, shape and function. Collagen is the predominant extracellular matrix component, comprising 25–32% of the dry weight. The composition of the dental papilla and dental pulp changes during development and can vary between tooth types. Much of the data that are available derives from animal tissues, which may differ somewhat from human. In addition much of the published work is on the products

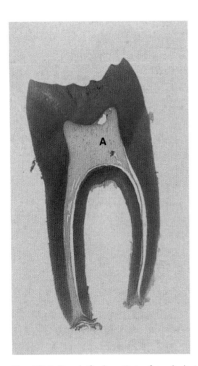

**Fig. 10.1** Decalcified section of a whole tooth showing the general disposition of the dental pulp (A) (H & E).

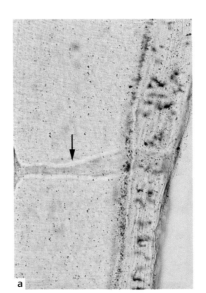 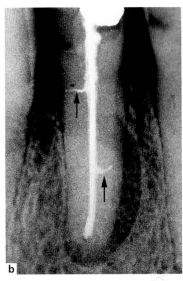

**Fig. 10.2** (a) Ground section of root showing a lateral branch from the main root canal (arrow) (×12). Courtesy of Dr M.E. Atkinson. (b) Radiograph of a root-filled tooth showing accessory canals (arrows). Courtesy of Dr J. Souyave.

of isolated cell types maintained *in vitro*. Their output may differ in the intact tissue.

## FIBRES

The principal fibrous component of the dental pulp is a combination of collagen types I (60%) and III (40%) (Figs 10.3, 10.4) present as fibrils 50 nm in diameter grouped into fibres thinly and irregularly scattered throughout the tissue (see Fig. 10.13). The arrangement becomes more organized in the periphery with the fibres aligned parallel to the forming predentine surface. Type III collagen has a similar 67 nm banding pattern to type I but differs from it by having only α1 chains rather than α1 and α2. The functional significance of the high levels of type III collagen is not known. In other sites it has been associated with rapid remodelling. Overall, collagen forms 3–5% of the wet weight of the pulp, a low proportion in comparison to other loose connective tissues. Small amounts of type V and type VI collagen are also present as a meshwork of fine microfibrils. Type IV is non-fibrous and present in the basement membrane of blood vessels.

Fibronectin is a glycoprotein found in several forms one of which is fibrous and found throughout the pulp. It anchors cells and may be important in determining their shape.

Non-collagenous beaded microfibrils 10–14 nm in diameter are also present. These are formed from fibrillin, a large glycoprotein which, in other tissues, is associated with elastic fibres. There has been no convincing demonstration of elastic fibres in the pulp.

## NON-FIBROUS MATRIX

The macromolecules that make up the bulk of the non-fibrous component of the extracellular matrix are proteoglycans, glycoproteins and unbound glycosaminoglycans.

### Glycosaminoglycans

Glycosaminoglycans (GAGs) are unbranched polysaccharide chains composed of repeating disaccharide units. There are four GAGs: chondroitin sulphate, dermatan sulphate, heparan sulphate and hyaluronic acid. All are present in the dental pulp. Most of the GAGs are covalently bound to a protein core to form proteoglycans. These are bulky hydrophilic molecules that swell when hydrated and form gels that fill most of the extracellular space. They readily allow the movement of water and ions and probably act as a reservoir for holding growth factors and other bioactive molecules. Hyaluronic acid is the only GAG found in any quantity unbound to protein. As well as having a mechanical function it is thought to facilitate cell migration particularly during development.

In mature pulp 60% of the GAG content is hyaluronic acid, 20% dermatan sulphate, 12% chondroitin sulphate (Fig. 10.5) and the remainder heparin sulphate. In the developing pulp chondroitin sulphate is the major GAG, with hyaluronic acid only a minor component.

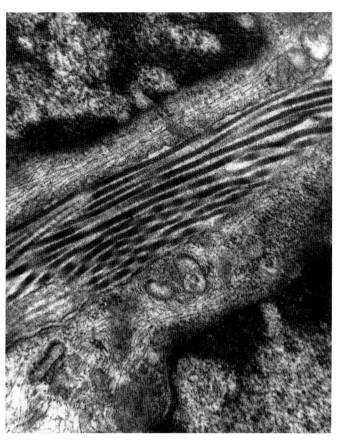

**Fig. 10.3** TEM showing collagen fibrils (A) within the pulp (×134 000).

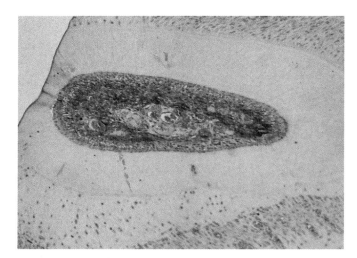

**Fig. 10.4** Section of developing mouse molar root showing type III collagen stained brown by immunohistochemical methods (×30). Courtesy of Dr Y. Ohsaki and the editor of the *Anatomical Record*.

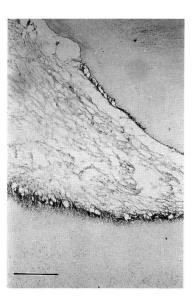

**Fig. 10.5** Adult human dental pulp stained by immunohistochemical methods for chondroitin sulphate (staining black at the pulp–dentine junction), showing widespread presence but a greater concentration peripherally in the odontoblast layer, suggesting (circumstantially) a role for this molecule in the development of dentine (×40). Courtesy of Drs P.M. Bartold and U. Schlagenhauf, and the editor of the *International Endodontic Journal*.

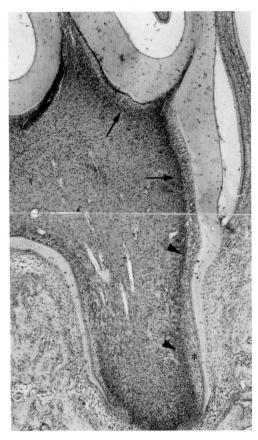

**Fig. 10.6** A section of rat pulp stained immunohistochemically for the proteo-glycan versican (dark stain). Staining is most intense in the sub-odontoblastic zone of the coronal pulp (arrow). The staining moves centrally in the cervical region (arrowheads) and is weak in the sub-odontoblastic zone of the root (*) (×1000). Courtesy of Dr S. Shibata and the editor of the *International Journal of Endodontics.*

## Proteoglycans

Proteoglycans (glycosaminoglycans attached to a protein core) are functionally diverse molecules. Some, such as versican (Fig. 10.6), contribute to the bulk of the matrix, others may bind to fibres, to other non-fibrous components of the tissue or contribute (e.g. syndecan) to the basement membranes of epithelially derived cells such as Schwann cells and endothelial cells. They cement the various components of the tissue together and are largely responsible for limiting its permeability. Table 10.1 summarizes the proteoglycans present in the pulp and their possible functions.

## Glycoprotein

Collagen is a glycoprotein (saccharides attached to a protein core). Two other glycoproteins, fibronectin (Figs 10.7, 10.8c) (which also occurs in fibrous form – see above) and tenascin (Fig. 10.8d), have been described in the pulp and are at their highest concentration near the odontoblast layer leading to the suggestion that they may be involved in the deposition of dentine.

An important group of molecules described by function as cell adhesion molecules are predominantly glycoproteins. Four groups of cell adhesion molecules are generally recognized, the immunoglobulin superfamily, the selectins, the cadherins and the integrins (Fig. 10.9). They are responsible (along with structurally specialized cell junctions) for cell to cell adhesion. The selectins have a very special role in guiding the diapedesis of leukocytes during inflammation. The large family of integrins anchor cells to the matrix.

The basement membrane of the epithelial cells in the pulp, the Schwann cells and the endothelial cells, consist of a meshwork created from collagen IV in which many adhesion and bioactive molecules are embedded.

Molecules more intimately associated with dentine, dentine sialoprotein and dentine phosphoprotein are produced by the odontoblasts and can be detected in the periphery of the pulp.

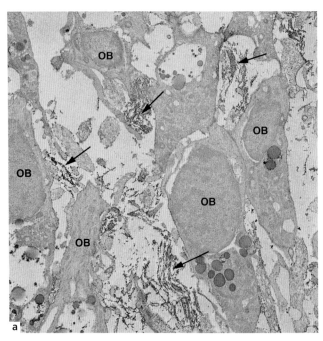
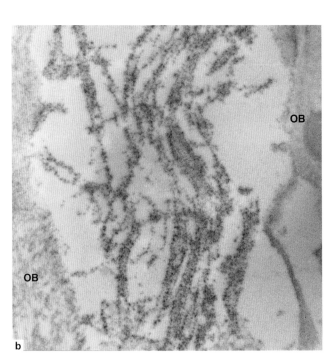

**Fig. 10.7** (a) Light micrograph showing immunolabelling for fibronectin (dark staining, arrows) on surface of collagen fibres of the odontoblast layer (OB). There is little staining in the predentine (×170). (b) Immunoelectron micrograph showing presence of fibronectin as dark-staining fibrillar fascicles between odontoblasts (OB) (×3600). Courtesy of Dr N. Yoshiba et al and the editor of the *Archives of Oral Biology.*

**Table 10.1** *Proteoglycans of the dental pulp*

| | |
|---|---|
| Versican<br>Syndecan | Form large hydrated aggregates creating a gel |
| Decorin | Binds to type I collagen |
| Biglycan | May help regulate collagen fibrillogenesis |
| Integrins | Cell surface adhesion receptors |
| Fibronectin | Concentrated near the odontoblast layer. Binds cells to extracellular matrix |
| Tenascin | Associated with cell movement. Concentrated near the odontoblast layer |
| Osteoadherin | Associated with mineralization |

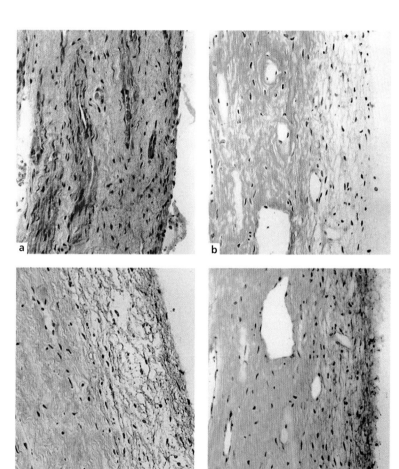

**Fig. 10.8** (a) H & E staining. (b) Immunostaining for collagen III. The periphery of the pulp is unstained. (c) Immunostaining for fibronectin. There is strong staining in the cell-free zone. (d) Immunostaining for tenascin. The peripheral tissue is negative (×250). Courtesy of Dr E.F. Martinez and the editor of the *Journal of Endodontics*.

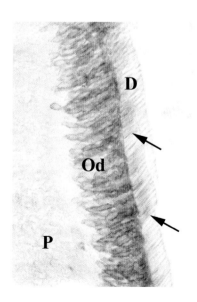

**Fig. 10.9** Immunolocalization of an integrin in human dental pulp. An intense membrane staining with an anti-integrin antibody in mature odontoblasts (Od) of the pulp horn, including processes in dentine tubules (arrows). P = pulp; D = dentine (×1000). Courtesy of Dr J.-C. Farges and the editor of the *Journal of Dental Research*.

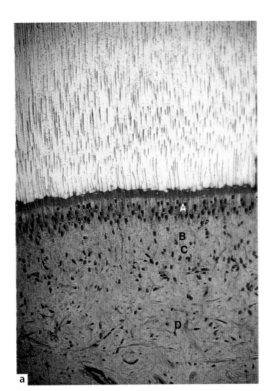

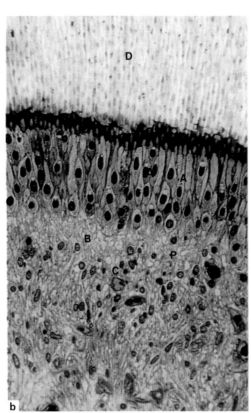

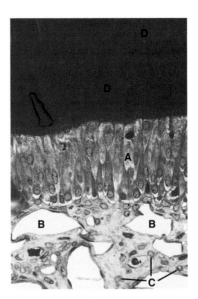

**Fig. 10.11** Semithin section showing pseudostratified odontoblast layer (A). B = subodontoblastic capillary plexus; C = pulp fibroblasts; D = dentine (Toluidine blue; ×450).

**Fig. 10.10** (a) Low-power micrograph showing some cell types and their distribution in the pulp. A = odontoblast layer adjacent to dentine; B = cell-free zone; C = cell-rich zone; D = central pulp showing principally fibroblasts (Toluidine blue; ×200). (b) Higher-power view showing pseudostratified odontoblast layer (A). B = Cell-free zone; C = cell-rich zone; D = dentine (Toluidine blue; ×650).

## CELLS

### Odontoblasts

The odontoblast (Figs 10.10–10.13) is responsible for the formation of dentine. The origin and differentiation of these cells are described on pages 329–331. In the fully developed tooth the odontoblasts continue to lay down secondary dentine throughout life and survive for as long as the tooth remains vital. If the tooth is subjected to a severe insult, such as dental caries, the odontoblast is able to respond by laying down tertiary reactionary dentine, which is essentially an accelerated deposition of secondary dentine. The odontoblast is a postmitotic cell and cannot divide: insult or injury will result in the death of odontoblasts. However, subodontoblastic stem cells can, in these circumstances, divide and differentiate and lay down a protective barrier of reactive tertiary dentine. Growth factors, especially members of the transforming growth factor (TGF)-β family, play an important role in controlling the synthetic activity of odontoblasts during development. They may also be significant in initiating the production of tertiary dentine in response to dental caries as they seem to be sequestered within mature dentine and may be released during carious breakdown. Odontoblasts in both healthy and diseased teeth express membrane receptors for the TGF-β family well above the level of other cells in the pulp.

The fully differentiated odontoblast (Figs 10.10–10.13) is a polarized columnar cell with a long cell process that extends into the predentine and dentine within a dentinal tubule. It also has numerous smaller processes that link it to adjacent odontoblasts and other pulp cells.

The cell body is approximately 50 µm long and 5–10 µm in width. The nucleus sits in the basal (pulpal) half of the cell with the other organelles involved in dentine synthesis, the rough endoplasmic reticulum, Golgi complex and mitochondria, above it. These organelles are much more pronounced in an actively secreting cell (Fig. 10.13).

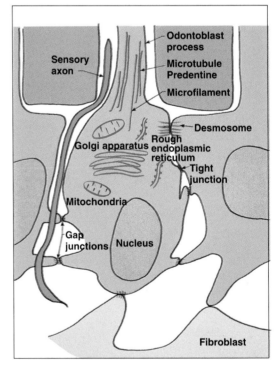

**Fig. 10.12** The ultrastructure of the odontoblast in a mature tooth is typical of a polarized protein-synthesizing cell of low activity containing all the organelles associated with this process (mitochondria, rough endoplasmic reticulum, Golgi apparatus) in the supranuclear region. One large process enters a dentinal tubule but many smaller ones link the odontoblasts to its neighbouring odontoblasts and fibroblasts.

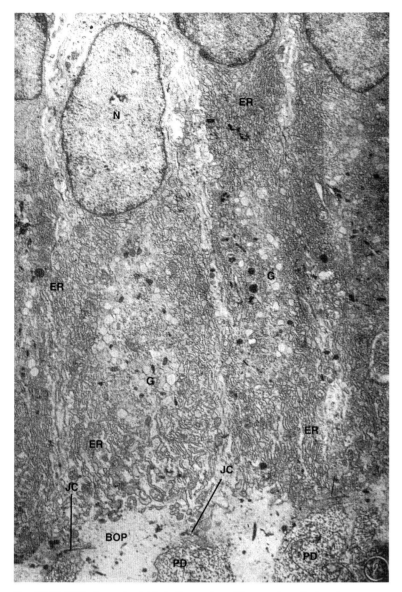

**Fig. 10.13** TEM of an odontoblast. N = nucleus; ER = rough endoplasmic reticulum; G = Golgi complex; JC = junctional complex; PD = predentine; BOP = base of odontoblast process (×12 000). Courtesy of Professor M.M. Smith.

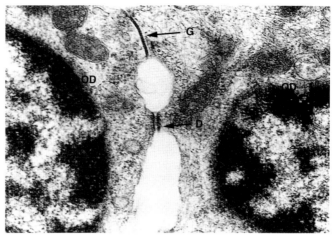

**Fig. 10.14** TEM illustrating cell junctions between two odontoblast cell bodies (OD). G = gap junction; D = desmosome (×45 000).

tubules. There is a potential outward pressure of this 'dentinal fluid' that, should the dentine lose its enamel or cementum covering, would lead to an outward fluid flow that would dilute and wash away toxins diffusing along the tubules from the surface. The dentinal fluid differs in composition from the tissue fluid within the pulp, suggesting that the odontoblasts have a role in controlling its composition.

Odontoblasts are capable of producing proinflammatory mediators in response to bacterial toxins such lipopolysaccharides and may produce cytokines such as interleukin (IL)-8, which participates in the recruitment of neutrophils.

It has been suggested that the odontoblast could act as a sensory receptor passing on information from the outer dentine to nerve fibres in the peripheral pulp. Odontoblast cell membranes contain numerous potassium channels in their apical end. These channels may have a role not only in mineralization but also in the transduction of mechanical displacement into an electrical signal. There is no convincing evidence of synaptic junctions between odontoblasts and nerves but as, at least in the crown, axons and odontoblast processes occupy the same narrow dentinal tubule it is possible that the odontoblast could affect the excitability of the axon by modifying the ionic environment.

### Cell junctions on odontoblasts

The odontoblast layer provides a controlled barrier between the pulp and the dentine. The integrity of the odontoblast layer and its limited permeability are maintained by numerous cell-to-cell junctions (Fig. 10.14). These are of three types.

- The macula adherens junctions (**desmosomes**) have a clear inter-cellular component as well as an intracellular system of anchoring fibrils and are largely responsible for mechanical union. Junctions that completely encircle the cells (zonula type) are not present.
- **Tight junctions** appear as a near fusion of apposing cell membranes and limit the permeability of the cell layer. The more tight junctions are and the closer they are together the lower the permeability. These junctions do not completely encircle the odontoblasts and so limit rather than eliminate permeability. The tight junctions also add to the mechanical integrity of the layer. An arrangement like the 'terminal bar' apparatus found in epithelia (in which a regular pattern of both tight and adherens type junctions is arranged uniformly at the outer

In the mature tooth the odontoblasts form a single layer of cells attached to the predentine surface. Coronal odontoblasts are columnar in outline; in the root they are commonly more cuboidal. The nuclei of adjacent cells in the layer lie at different levels and when the layer is sectioned obliquely this gives the false appearance of multiple layers ('pseudostratification' – Figs 10.10 and 10.11).

Dentine is formed almost exclusively by the odontoblasts except possibly during the initial dentine formation that results in the mantle layer, when some products from other cells are included (see pages 138–140). The odontoblast continues to lay down secondary dentine at a slow rate throughout life. As it does so the pulp chamber becomes smaller and root canals narrower. The odontoblast layer becomes a flatter layer of cells and the number of cells declines by apoptosis. It has been estimated that in a premolar half the odontoblasts will die in the 4 years following the completion of root formation. Though the odontoblast layer's prime role is dentinogenesis it has other significant properties that help preserve the well-being of the pulp. It acts as a selective barrier reducing the speed with which toxins can reach the pulp while at the same time allowing tissue fluid from the pulp to enter and perhaps circulate within the dentinal

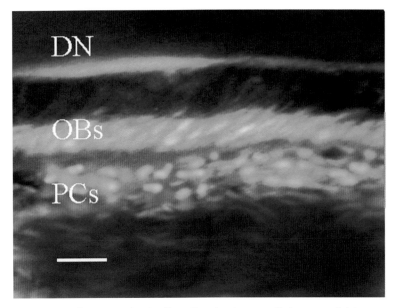

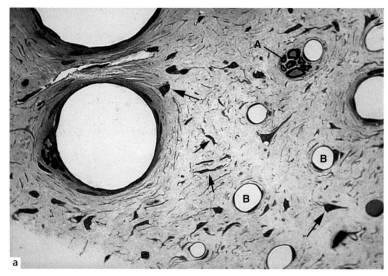

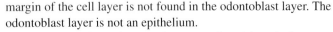

**Fig. 10.15** A fluorescent dye, Lucifer yellow, has been applied to enamel. It is taken up by underlying odontoblasts (OBs) and passed on to other odontoblasts and other pulpal cells (PCs). DN = dentine (×50). Ikeda H et al 1995 *Archives of Oral Biology* 40: 895–904, with permission.

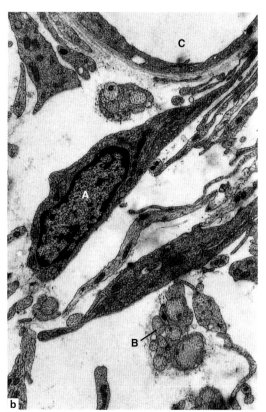

margin of the cell layer is not found in the odontoblast layer. The odontoblast layer is not an epithelium.

- The third type of junction seen between odontoblasts is the **gap junction**. This allows the movement of small molecules directly between adjacent cells. It is important in cell-to-cell communication and would presumably have a role in synchronizing the activity of all the odontoblasts in the layer.

As well as forming junctions with themselves, odontoblasts are also linked to other pulpal cells. In histological sections it is difficult to recognize the origin of most of the cell processes. Small processes from an odontoblast, fibroblast, stem cell and possibly even a defence cell or an unsheathed axon have a superficially similar appearance. Odontoblasts do have a close relationship with dendritic antigen-presenting cells (see page 160), although the functional nature of this relationship has not been demonstrated. Figure 10.15 shows that the odontoblast layer and the underlying pulpal cells form a kind of syncytium. A low-molecular-weight fluorescent dye, Lucifer yellow, was placed on the enamel surface of a tooth for 30 minutes. The tooth was then sectioned and examined under ultraviolet light. The dye fluoresces with a green colour. This is present within the cells of the odontoblast layer and the underlying pulpal cells, demonstrating that they are linked by junctions permitting the passage of small molecules.

During tooth development the activity of the odontoblasts is affected by a number of signalling and growth factors. In mature odontoblasts the genes for several growth factors including TGF-β and bone morphogenetic protein are expressed, suggesting perhaps that these cells are primed to activate other cells. Odontoblasts do not produce nerve growth factor (NGF) but may have it transferred to them as the odontoblast cell membrane contains NGF receptors. Injured odontoblasts produce heat shock proteins, metalloproteinases and the enzymes responsible for nitric oxide production.

The odontoblast process found in the dentinal tubules is described on pages 134–137.

**Fig. 10.16** (a) Semithin section of the central portion of the pulp showing the appearance of pulpal fibroblasts, which may vary from spindle-shaped (small arrows) to a more rounded and stellate shape (large arrow). A = myelinated fibres; B = capillary (Toluidine blue; ×450). (b) TEM illustrating spindle-shaped pulpal fibroblasts (A). B = unmyelinated nerve axons; C = capillary. Note the absence of collagen fibrils in the extracellular matrix (×20 000).

## Fibroblasts

The fibroblast is the ubiquitous cell of non-mineralized connective tissues. In the dental pulp fibroblasts form a loose network throughout the tissue linked by adherens type junctions and gap junctions. Their morphology is highly variable but is most aptly described as stellate, with the arms of the stars linking fibroblast to fibroblast or fibroblast to odontoblast (Fig. 10.16). Their most obvious role in the development of the tissue is the production of extracellular fibres and ground substance for the dental pulp. As this production (and presumably turnover) is relatively slow, pulpal fibroblasts show only moderate amounts of associated intracellular organelles such as endoplasmic reticulum, Golgi complex or mitochondria. They make little or no contribution to the production of dentine.

Much of what is known about pulpal fibroblasts has been obtained from experiments in which they have been maintained in cell culture. These studies show that the pulpal fibroblast, as well as being able to secrete the components that form the extracellular matrix, can participate in their degradation. It thus seems likely that, in the mature tooth, the fibroblasts slowly turn over the matrix. Cultured pulpal fibroblasts do undergo cell division, although mitotic figures are rarely encountered in the normal, uninjured dental pulp. Apoptosis (programmed cell death) has been demonstrated in the continuously growing incisor of the rat. It seems reasonable to expect cell turnover in the pulps of mature teeth of limited eruption.

## Stem cells

In routinely stained sections the connective tissue cells in the pulp below the odontoblast layer all have a similar morphology. There are, in fact, significant functional differences in that subsets of this population are stem cells (Fig. 10.17). Many of the cell types in the dental pulp, including the odontoblasts, defence cells and possibly many fibroblasts, are terminally differentiated and, although able to respond to stimuli in a predetermined manner, are unable to differentiate into another cell type. It has long been known that there is a population of cells in the dental pulp that can, in response to a severe challenge, produce tertiary dentine. These have, in the past, been given a number of names, including 'pluripotential mesenchymal' and 'ectomesenchymal' cells, but are now recognized as stem cells. They are defined by a similarity in gene expression to odontoblasts and by their ability to differentiate and form dentine under appropriate stimulation. *In vivo* they are 'tissue-specific' stem cells, meaning that they will only differentiate into cell types present in the tissue in which they are found. 'Embryonic' stem cells can, at least in theory, differentiate into any cell type. Dental pulp stem cells differentiate into odontoblast-like cells when the original odontoblasts are killed by toxin or injury. Following molecular signals released during injury they will form tertiary reparative dentine. Their significance is considerable, as they may be harnessed in treatment using known signalling molecules to initiate or enhance the regenerative process.

## Defence cells

T lymphocytes are present in small numbers in the normal dental pulp (Fig. 10.18).

Their numbers increase enormously when the pulp is injured or subjected to toxins.

***Macrophages*** (Fig. 10.19) are a substantial presence. In their resting form (sometimes termed histiocytes or periocytes) they can appear in a variety of morphological forms and are difficult to distinguish from fibroblasts in routine histological preparations. Immunohistochemical techniques, however, show that they are widely distributed in considerable numbers.

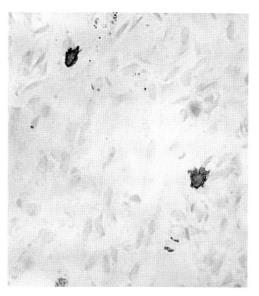

**Fig. 10.18** Antibody staining (black) to identify T lymphocytes in the dental pulp (×500). Courtesy of Dr T. Okiji and the editor of the *Journal of Dental Research*.

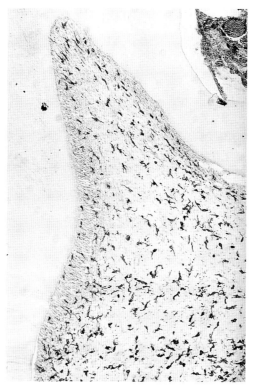

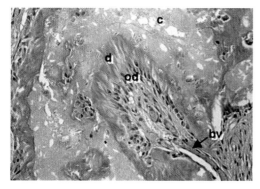

**Fig. 10.17** Stem cells that were isolated and then grown in culture were placed subcutaneously in mice in contact with a ceramic powder. The stem cells (od) lay down a dentine-like tissue (d) in contact with the ceramic (c). bv = blood vessel. (Polarised image.) Courtesy of Dr S. Gronthos et al and the editor of the *Proceedings of the National Academy of Sciences of the USA*.

**Fig. 10.19** Antibody staining (black) to demonstrate the wide distribution of macrophages in healthy rat dental pulp (×50). Courtesy of Dr T. Okiji and the editor of the *Journal of Dental Research*.

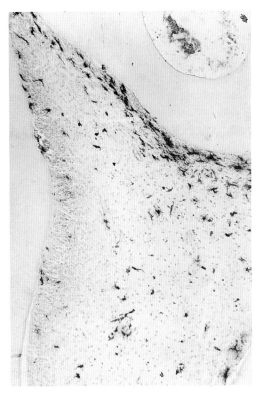

**Fig. 10.20** Immunohistochemical stain (black) identifying antigen-presenting cells particularly prominent at the periphery of rat molar pulp (×70). Courtesy of Dr T. Okiji and the editor of the *Journal of Dental Research*.

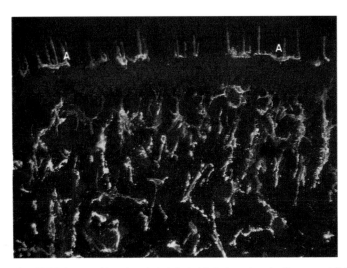

**Fig. 10.21** Immunohistochemical stain (white) viewed under fluorescent light showing the distribution of antigen-presenting cells. Note the cells (A) in the periphery of the odontoblast layer have processes extending into the dentine (×200). Courtesy of Dr N. Yoshiba and the editor of the *Journal of Dental Research*.

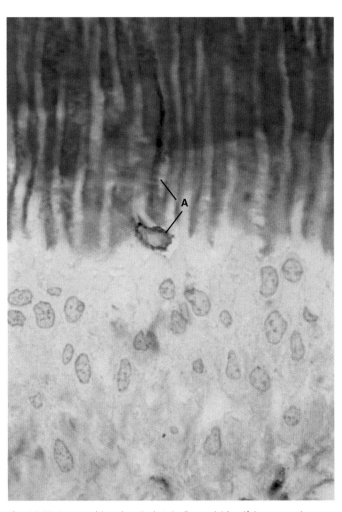

**Fig. 10.22** Immunohistochemical stain (brown) identifying an antigen-presenting cell (A) in the outer odontoblast layer and extending a process into the inner dentine (Methylene blue; ×500). Courtesy of Dr N. Yoshiba and the editor of the *Journal of Dental Research*.

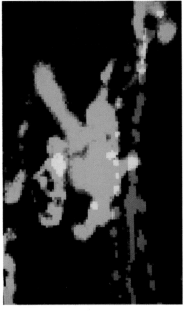

**Fig. 10.23** Confocal laser scanning micrograph of a section of dental pulp from the pulp horn of a rat. It is double stained with two fluorescent dyes staining macrophages (green) and substance-P-containing nerve fibres (red). This technique allows great depth of focus and, in this case, shows areas (in yellow) where the nerve and macrophage are in close contact (×1000). Courtesy of Dr T. Okiji and the editor of the *Journal of Dental Research*.

**Dendritic antigen-presenting cells** (Figs 10.20–10.23) are also an important component of the normal dental pulp. They are at least 50 µm long and have three or more main dendritic processes which branch. Like the macrophages, they are distributed throughout the pulp but most densely around in the periphery and around nerves and blood vessels (Figs 10.20, 10.21). Some dendritic cells extend processes into the dentinal tubules (Figs 10.21, 10.22).

The dendritic cells act, at least primarily, as antigen-presenting cells stimulating the division and activity of naive T lymphocytes. They initiate the primary immune response and migrate, with trapped antigen, to regional lymph nodes and induce T lymphocyte division and differentiation there.

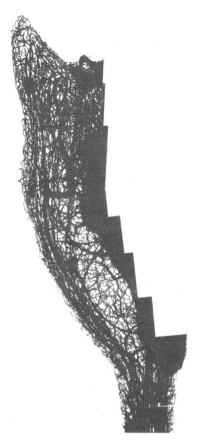

**Fig. 10.24** India ink has been drawn into the vessels of the pulp in a human premolar, which has subsequently been cleared. This image is a montage of a number of micrographs. A large vessel, an arteriole, is seen running through much of the pulp with a network of branches arising from it. Ikeda H et al 1995 *Archives of Oral Biology* 40: 895–904, with permission.

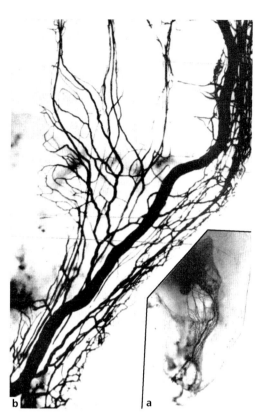

**Fig. 10.25** (a) A molar root prepared as for Fig. 10.24. Note that the apex has two tips with one apical foramen in one and two in the other. (b) An enlargement of part of Fig. 10.25a showing a large central vessel and to the right a capillary plexus that would be below the odontoblast layer. Ikeda H et al 1995 *Archives of Oral Biology* 40: 895–904, with permission.

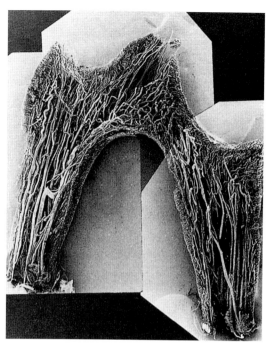

**Fig. 10.26** SEM of a vascular cast of a dog mandibular molar. Arterioles run coronally along the sides of the root canal; venules drain in the centre. Larger vessels follow relatively straight pathways. Side branches subdivide to form a capillary network beneath the dentine (×8). Courtesy of Drs Y. Kishi, K. Takahashi and K. Kanagawa, and the editor of the *Journal of Dental Research*.

Mast cells are difficult to demonstrate in the dental pulp as they are fragile and destroyed during processing for histology.

There is an intimate relationship between the immune and neural systems. Following pulp injury, nerves release a number of neuropeptides and other molecules that participate in the immune response. In animal experiments removing the sympathetic innervation to the pulp increases the number of lymphocytes present even in the uninjured tissue. Many of the signalling molecules released by cells of the immune system have an effect on nerves, either increasing their excitability or in some cases reducing it. There is a close structural relationship between nerve fibres and immunocompetent cells (Fig. 10.23).

## BLOOD VESSELS OF THE DENTAL PULP

The architectural arrangement of the blood vessels of the dental pulp closely parallels that of the nerves. The arrangement is clearly seen in pulps perfused with India ink and cleared (Figs 10.24, 10.25). Arterioles and venules enter the dental pulp via the apical foramina (Fig. 10.25b) and lateral canals as components of neurovascular bundles. The largest of the arterioles are approximately 150 mm in diameter. They run longitudinally through the root canals (Fig. 10.24). Within the root canals, they send off side branches to the periphery (Figs 10.24, 10.25). The vessels divide and narrow to some degree in the root canal but branch profusely once they are within the coronal pulp. Capillary loops extend towards the dentine.

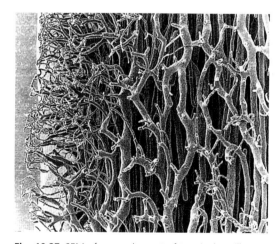

**Fig. 10.27** SEM of a vascular cast of terminal capillary network in pulp. There are three layers of the terminal supply to the odontoblast layers: most superficially the flat-ended capillary loops, beneath these the capillary network and under these the venular network. Deep to all these layers are straight arterioles (×11). Courtesy of Drs K. Takahashi, Y. Kishi and S. Kim, and the editor of the *Journal of Endodontics*.

This looping is most easily demonstrated in animal preparations as plastic resins can be perfused through the vascular system and casts prepared (Figs 10.26, 10.27).

A network of vessels beneath the odontoblasts (the subodontoblastic capillary plexus) is more evident in sectioned histological material than it is in three-dimensional casts. These capillaries are 6–8 mm in diameter.

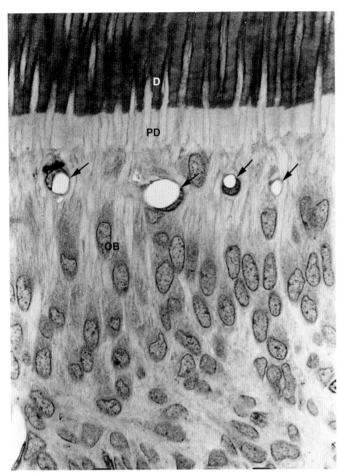

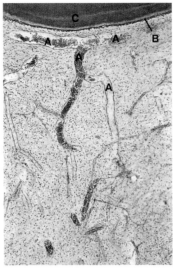

**Fig. 10.29** Section of the dental pulp showing branching capillaries (A) below the odontoblast layer (B). C = Dentine (H & E; ×100). Courtesy of Professor L. Fonzi.

**Fig. 10.28** TEM showing capillaries (arrows) in the odontoblast layer (OB). D = Dentine; PD = predentine (×1200). Courtesy of Drs S. Yoshida and H. Oshima, and the editor of the *Anatomical Record*.

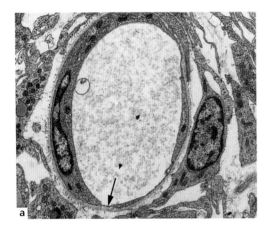

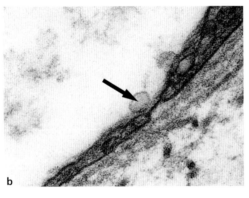

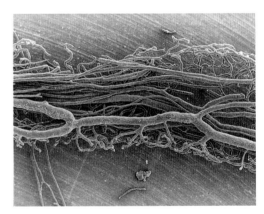

**Fig. 10.31** SEM of a vascular cast showing a venous–venous anastomosis (×160). Courtesy of Drs Y. Kishi and K. Takahashi.

**Fig. 10.30** (a) TEM of a subodontoblastic capillary with fenestration (arrowed) (×12 600). (b) TEM showing a fenestration (arrow) in a capillary wall (×31 500).

Capillaries are present both within (Fig. 10.28) and below the odontoblast layer (Fig. 10.29) and between the odontoblasts and the predentine. Capillaries do not enter the dentinal tubules. The fluid that is present in the dentine is probably an ultrafiltrate of the pulpal interstitial fluid. The arrangement of the blood vessels supplies oxygen and nutrients where they are most needed during dentinogenesis. The capillary network beneath the odontoblasts is dense enough to be known as the subodontoblastic capillary plexus. Approximately 4–5% of the capillaries in the subodontoblastic zone are fenestrated (Fig. 10.30). Fenestrations are 60–80 nm in diameter. Only basement membrane is present at the fenestrations, presumably allowing rapid movement of materials out of the capillary.

Numerous arteriovenous and venous-venous anastomoses (Fig. 10.31) are found between peripheral pulpal vessels presumably to allow rapid changes in blood perfusion.

It is difficult to differentiate lymphatic vessels in the dental pulp. Structures consistent with their known structure elsewhere (like capillaries but with less completely linked endothelial cells and a less well developed basement membrane) have been found (Fig. 10.32). Vessels whose basement membranes have immunohistochemical characteristics in common with lymphatic vessels elsewhere have also been reported (Fig. 10.33). The presence of lymphatics in the pulp has been established by tracing particulate material kept within the pulp from the pulp to regional lymph nodes. Retrograde lymphography deposits material into pulpal vessels.

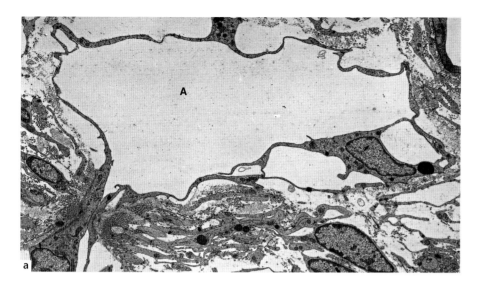

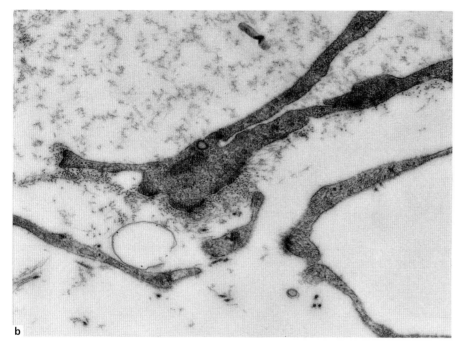

**Fig. 10.32** (a) TEM of a lymphatic vessel (A) in the central dental pulp (×400). (b) Higher-power TEM of part of the wall of the lymphatic vessel, showing incomplete junctions between the cells and absence of a basement membrane (×3000). Courtesy of Dr M. Bishop.

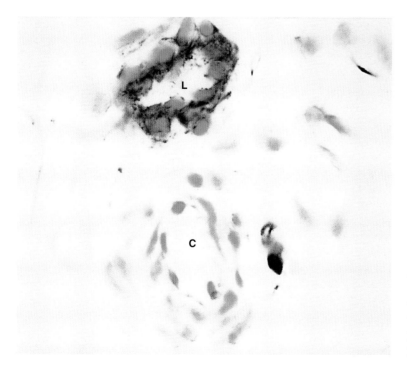

**Fig. 10.33** A lymphatic vessel (L) from human dental pulp stained with an antibody against human thoracic duct. The dark-blue stain attaches to the endothelium. Another vessel, presumably a blood capillary (C), nearby remains unstained (×1000). Courtesy of Drs Y. Sawa, S. Yoshida, Y. Ashikaga, T. Kim, Y. Yanaoka and M. Suzuki, and the editor of *Tissue and Cell*.

In the healthy pulp blood flow is under nervous control. The smooth muscle of the arterioles (present in the central radicular pulp) is innervated by terminals of sympathetic nerves, which maintain a vasoconstrictor tone as they do in most other sites. The neurotransmitters are noradrenaline (norepinephrine) and neuropeptide Y. There is little evidence for parasympathetic innervation of the pulp. Vasoconstrictor tone probably accounts for most of the vascular control but afferent (sensory) nerves also have effects not only on vessel dilatation but also on capillary permeability. The vasoactive contribution of the afferent nerves is largely in the peripheral pulp and becomes significant when there is inflammation. The most prominent neuropeptides in these nerves are calcitonin-gene-related

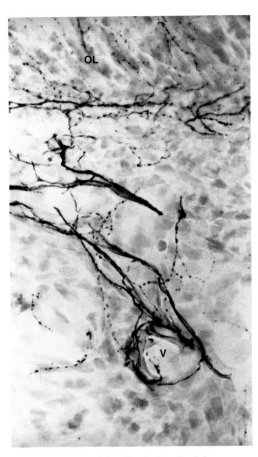

**Fig. 10.34** Immunohistochemical method demonstrating varicose CGRP-immunoreactive nerve fibres (black) around a blood vessel (V) and in the odontoblast layer (OL) (×1600). Courtesy of Drs J.-Q. Zhang, K. Nagata and T. Iijima, and the editor of the *Anatomical Record.*

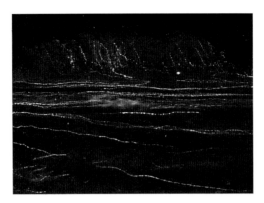

**Fig. 10.35** Immunohistochemical staining demonstrating substance-P-containing nerve fibres (white) in the odontoblast layer (top) and in the subodontoblastic plexus (Dark field illumination; ×300).

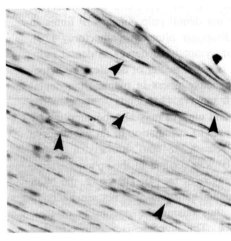

**Fig. 10.36** Immunohistochemical staining to show nerve fibres (arrrowed) staining for nitric oxide synthetase in dog coronal pulp (×16000). Courtesy of Dr Z. Lohinai et al and the editor of *Neuroscience Letters.*

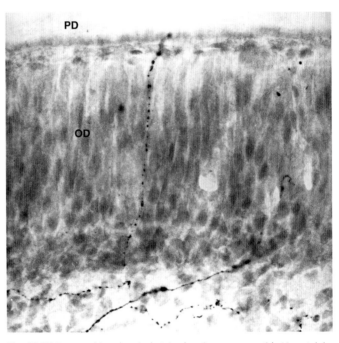

**Fig. 10.37** Immunohistochemical stain showing neuropeptide-Y-containing nerve fibres in and below the odontoblast layer (OD). PD = predentine (×1600). Courtesy of Drs J.-Q. Zhang, K. Nagata and T. Iijima, and the editor of the *Anatomical Record.*

peptide (CGRP) (Fig. 10.34) and substance P (Fig. 10.35), both of which induce vasodilatation and increased capillary permeability. Nitric oxide also acts as a vasodilator. It is too volatile to demonstrate directly but the presence of the enzyme responsible for forming it, nitric oxide synthetase, has been found in nerve fibres in the coronal pulp (Fig. 10.36). Neuropeptide Y has also been demonstrated in peripheral axons (Fig. 10.37), including some within the odontoblast layer. Their role in this position is unknown.

Pulpal blood flow has been estimated to be 20–60 ml/min per 100 g of tissue. The pulp has a high, pulsatile interstitial tissue fluid pressure. This pressure would allow dentinal fluid to move outwards whenever the dentinal tubules were patent peripherally. It may also slow the inward movement of toxins during the progression of dental caries.

## NERVES OF THE DENTAL PULP

The dental pulp is heavily innervated. For example, approximately 2500 axons enter the apical foramen of a mature premolar; 25% of these are myelinated afferents whose cell bodies lie in the trigeminal ganglion. Of these 90% are narrow Aδ fibres (1–6 mm in diameter), with the rest belonging to the wider Aβ group (6–12 mm in diameter). The unmyelinated C fibres are either afferent or autonomic. Although the nerve fibres enter the dental pulp in bundles, there is only a scant perineurium or epineurium.

The nerve bundles run centrally in the pulp of the root in close association with the blood vessels. A few fibres leave the central bundles in the root and travel to the periphery. Most continue to the coronal pulp where they spread apart and branch profusely (Fig. 10.38). Most of the branches end in the odontoblastic or subodontoblastic regions (Fig. 10.39). In the crown there is a pronounced plexus of nerves beneath the odontoblasts, known as the plexus of Raschkow. This plexus is not evident until after the tooth has erupted. Branches from the plexus pass into the odontoblast layer and form the marginal plexus between the odontoblast layer and the predentine; others continue into the dentine to accompany odontoblast processes in the dentinal tubules. This subodontoblastic plexus may be one of the sites of sensory activation in the pulp. Many of the axons are devoid of a Schwann cell covering, either completely or partially, rendering them susceptible to changes in the extracellular environment (Fig. 10.40). The axons branch profusely, providing a broad surface area for activation. Within the Schwann cell, there are often many axons in a single pocket and the spread of signals from axon to axon is possible.

## NERVE FIBRE TYPES

The myelinated nerves (Fig. 10.16a) are trigeminal afferents. They carry sensations of sharp pain centrally. The larger diameter Aβ afferents in some

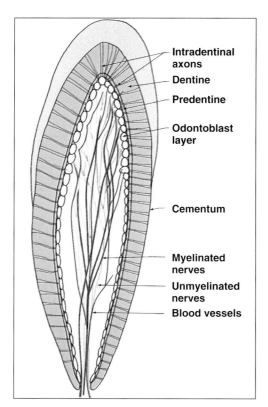

Fig. 10.38 General distribution of myelinated nerves (dark green), non-myelinated nerves (light green) and blood vessels (red) in the pulp.

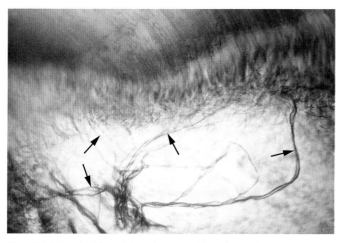

Fig. 10.39 Terminal branching of sensory fibres (arrows) in the dental pulp. This very thick section allows the axons at several levels to be seen, including the subodontoblastic nerve plexus of Raschkow (Silver stain; ×140).

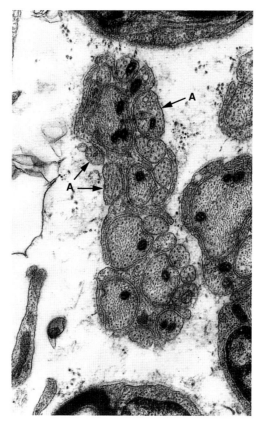

Fig. 10.40 TEM showing nerve fibres in the subodontoblastic plexus. Many of the axons are incompletely sheathed by Schwann cells (A), perhaps making them more susceptible to changes in the local environment (×40000).

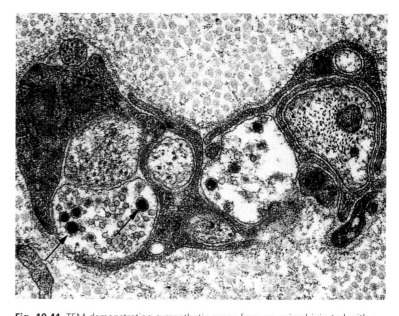

Fig. 10.41 TEM demonstrating sympathetic axons from an animal injected with a false neurotransmitter, 6-hydroxydopamine, which is taken up but not released by noradrenergic axons. The false neurotransmitter accumulates as dense-cored vesicles (arrowed) identifying the sympathetic axons. In this nerve fibre the sympathetic axons are contained in the same Schwann cell pocket as unlabelled, presumably sensory, axons. Simultaneous activation of sympathetic axons amplifies the activity in sensory nerves. The close approximation of sensory and sympathetic axons may explain this interaction (×31000).

regions carry other non-noxious sensations but there is no clear evidence that any sensation other than pain can be experienced from the pulp with physiological stimuli. Most of the non-myelinated C fibres (Fig. 10.16b) are also afferent and involved in the conduction of noxious information centrally. At least as important as the sensory functions of both these afferent nerve groups is their role in axon reflexes. In these reflexes, action potentials generated in one terminal branch travel centrally and then pass anterogradely (central to peripheral) down other branches, resulting in the release of neuropeptides important in the local control of blood flow (but perhaps with other functions as well). It has been suggested that some pulpal nerves may have direct trophic effects, perhaps controlling, in part, the activity of odontoblasts. There is, however, no convincing evidence of an effect other than one that might be mediated by blood flow changes.

Some of the C fibres are sympathetic efferents and supply arteriolar smooth muscle. As there are only a few arterioles within the dental pulp

sympathetic fibres are scarce (Fig. 10.41). They seem to mediate their vasoconstrictive effect by the release of noradrenaline (norepinephrine) and neuropeptide Y. Evidence for parasympathetic innervation of the dental pulp is weak. Acetylcholine, the principal mediator for the parasympathetic system, is rarely detected in the dental pulp. Vasodilatation seems to be effected by axon reflexes involving afferent nerves as well as (presumably as in other tissues) by the build-up of metabolites locally. Nitric oxide produced following hypoxia and tissue injury in the dental pulp is the signalling molecule most likely to induce vasodilatation under these conditions.

## NERVE ENDINGS

It is difficult to determine where all nerve fibres end. Autonomic nerves end on the smooth muscle of the arterioles and special neuromuscular junctions are present. Some of the afferent fibres (probably a proportion of the Aδ fibres) enter the tubules largely in the coronal dentine and predentine. Others may end at the pulp–predentine junction in what is sometimes known as the marginal plexus (Fig. 10.42). Both of these groups would be in an ideal position to detect stimuli applied to the outside of the dentine.

Many axons end in close proximity to odontoblasts. It has been suggested that there are specialized junctions between odontoblasts and nerves but confirmatory evidence is lacking, although recent studies describe the proteins synapsin and synaptotagmin, characteristic of neural junctions, in the dentinal tubules. Whilst odontoblasts participate in many gap junctions (which elsewhere can act as electrical synapses), the cell processes involved in these junctions seem to come from other odontoblasts or from fibroblasts. The nerve–odontoblast relationship may be functionally if not structurally significant as the odontoblast or its process would dominate the local environment in which naked axons were present, especially in the dentinal tubules.

The nerves in the dentinal tubules, at the pulp–predentine border and among the odontoblast cell body have all lost their ensheathing Schwann cells and their axolemmas are exposed directly to the extracellular environment (Fig. 10.42). Changes in the composition of, or movement within, the extracellular fluid could readily affect the membrane properties of these terminals. Most activity in these terminals probably does not reach the level of sensation but presumably results locally in the release of neuropeptides by axon reflexes. The variety of neuropeptides found in the dental pulp is considerable. The most widely distributed and possibly the most significant functionally is CGRP (Fig. 10.43a), whose name derives

from its first discovery and does not represent the widespread role it is now known to have.

CGRP is a potent vasodilator and quite possibly the principal agent controlling blood flow locally in the periphery of the dental pulp. CGRP is synthesized in the cell bodies of the nerves in the trigeminal ganglion and moved peripherally by axonal transport. Clearly a message, presumably a signalling molecule such as nerve growth factor (NGF), is carried from the periphery of the dental pulp to the ganglion cell body to modulate the production of CGRP. As well as having a role in pulpal blood flow CGRP may participate in initiating or controlling hard-tissue production. Dental pulp cells, when maintained *in vitro*, respond to the application of CGRP with increased production of bone morphogenetic protein-2, a signalling molecule known to be involved in dentine formation. NGF and NGF receptors have been detected in the peripheral dental pulp. Both NGF and receptors for it are found on odontoblasts as well as pulpal nerves. NGF appears not to be produced by odontoblasts but donated by neighbouring fibroblasts. The expression of both NGF and its receptors increases in the injured pulp. Apart from a direct neural role, NGF may be a chemoattractant for leukocytes in the damaged pulp.

Though something of a paradigm shift from the original division of sensory and motor functions between different components of the nervous system, it seems reasonable to suggest that the major role of the trigeminal afferents in the dental pulp is in controlling the local environment rather than in carrying sensory information centrally. Some neuropeptides may function to control the flow of sensory activity centrally. The experience of toothache makes one realize that the balance of activities is flexible.

Several other neuropeptides and transmitters have been found in the normal dental pulp and it is possible, based on their known activities in other sites, to speculate on their role in the pulp (Table 10.2). We are a long way from understanding what such a large number of agents contributes in the intact pulp and how they interact. In the injured pulp the number of biologically active molecules present increases substantially and many of those detectable in normal pulps increase in quantity and distribution. It is likely that the continuous release of such peptides plays a role in the homeostasis of the dental pulp (Fig. 10.43b).

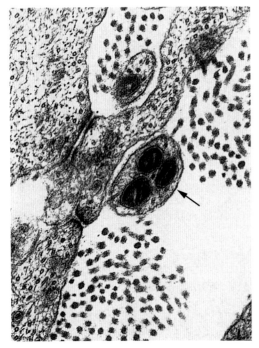

**Fig. 10.42** Unsheathed, unmyelinated axons (arrowed) at the pulp (left) predentine border. Such axons may be activated by stimuli applied to dentine that cause fluid movement through the dentinal tubules (TEM; ×85000).

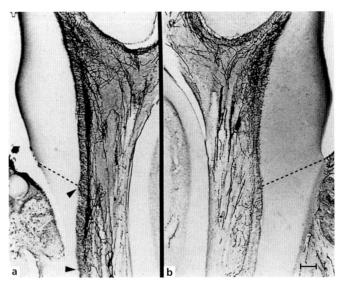

**Fig. 10.43** Pulpal nerves stained immunohistochemically (black) for CGRP. (a) A tooth in which a cervical cavity was cut 12 days earlier; (b) a normal control tooth. The broken line approximates the boundary between coronal and radicular dentine. There are many more CGRP-staining nerves after cavity preparation (×650). Courtesy of Drs R. Taylor and M. Byers and the editor of *Brain Research*.

**Table 10.2** *Neuropeptides and neurotransmitters identified in the dental pulp with possible roles (largely interpolated from actions in other tissues)*

| Neuropeptide/small molecule transmitter | Possible role |
| --- | --- |
| Calcitonin-gene-related peptide | Vasodilatation, stimulates cell division in pulpal fibroblasts |
| Substance P | Vasodilatation, ?nociceptive transmitter, stimulates cell division in pulpal fibroblasts |
| Neuropeptide Y | Sympathetic vasoconstrictor |
| Noradrenaline (norepinephrine) | Sympathetic vasoconstrictor |
| Enkephalin | Silencer of nociceptors |
| Somatostatin | Silencer of nociceptors |
| Endorphin | Silencer of nociceptors |
| Dopamine | Vasoactive or a precursor of adrenaline (epinephrine) |
| Adrenaline (epinephrine) | Vasoconstrictive via smooth muscle in arterioles |
| Cholecystokinin | Unknown |
| Vasoactive intestinal polypeptide | ?Parasympathetic |
| Secretoneurin | Axon reflexes |
| Neurokinin A | Vasodilatation, ?nociceptive transmitter, stimulates cell division in pulpal fibroblasts |
| Peptide histidine isoleucine amide | ?Parasympathetic |
| ?Acetylcholine | ?Parasympathetic |

## REGIONS

The structure of the dental pulp can be described on a regional basis (Fig. 10.11). Beginning from the outside the potential space between the odontoblast layer and the predentine could be described as the *supraodontoblast region*. In most histological preparations there is shrinkage of the soft pulp away from the dentine, creating a space in this region that is not present in the vital tissue. However, such preparations are useful in demonstrating the presence of odontoblast processes (Fig. 10.44). Two important structures are located in this region.

- Unsheathed axons, found almost exclusively in the crown. These have been described as the predentinal plexus (of Bradlaw). They are not a true plexus (network) but an area where a number of axons congregate. It is not clear whether many axons end in this plexus. Most, presumably, continue to enter and end within dentinal tubules. These axons are in an ideal position to sense changes in fluid

movement through the dentinal tubules as well as changes in the extracellular fluid composition, which, because of the barrier properties of the odontoblast layer, will be delayed in reaching the core of the pulp.

- Dendritic antigen-presenting cells (described above).

This region thus deserves some special recognition as (after the odontoblast process) the first level at which external stimuli can be detected in the pulp.

*The odontoblast layer* (Figs 10.11 and 10.12) is, self-evidently, the effector system of the pulp. All other elements of the pulp are supportive or protective of the cells forming dentine or programmed to replace them should they be killed.

*The subodontoblastic zone* (Fig. 10.11) has several terms associated with it. Immediately beneath the odontoblast layer a *cell-free zone* (of Weil) is commonly described in which, in standard paraffin-embedded sections, no cells are apparent. Many routine stains such as haematoxylin and eosin stain principally nuclei and areas that lack nuclei appear empty: this is the case with the area immediately beneath the odontoblasts. Electron microscopy reveals that many cell processes of fibroblasts, odontoblasts, axons and capillaries cross this region. More correctly this area could be described as anuclear. The cell-free zone is usually absent from the radicular pulp and usually appears in the coronal pulp once the tooth has erupted. There is no apparent reason for this feature and it has been suggested that it is an artefact of histological processing produced by differential shrinkage of the odontoblast and the deeper pulp.

Immediately deep to the 'cell-free' zone is another region in which there are, apparently, many cells – the so-called *cell-rich zone* (Fig. 10.13). This too may be an artefact induced by contrast to the cell-free zone. In this region there is a high concentration of both capillaries (the subodontoblastic capillary plexus) and axons (the subodontoblastic neural plexus). The Schwann cells, endothelial cells, etc. associated with these 'plexi' could result in the 'cell-rich' appearance.

Central to the subodontoblastic region is the bulk of the dental pulp, which, devoid of its peripheral structures and its central neurovascular core, would be similar to loose connective tissue in many other sites although having a richer nerve and blood supply. The central core itself is most evident in the root canal. Once it enters the crown repeated branching of both nerves and blood vessels renders the neurovascular bundle less obvious.

## ROLE OF THE DENTAL PULP

Once differentiated from the dental papilla the dental pulp is a single industry organ dedicated to the production of dentine rapidly during development, slowly during adult life or suddenly in response to insult. The presence of a soft-tissue core in a tooth affects its physical properties. A young tooth with a large vital pulp is more elastic than a tooth in which most of the pulp has been replaced with secondary dentine or all of the pulp with a filling material as occurs during root canal therapy.

## AGE-RELATED CHANGES IN THE DENTAL PULP

The dental pulp gets smaller with age because secondary dentine deposition continues, albeit at a slow rate, throughout life. The older pulp is less vascular and, apparently, more fibrous than the young pulp. The innervation is reduced. The pulp often mineralizes in the form of pulp stones. Many older human teeth show some degree of mineralization, which can occur as many tiny spicules of mineralized tissue throughout the pulp ('snow storm' calcification) or as discrete pulp stones either singly or in small groups. Pulp stones may resemble dentine in being, at least partially,

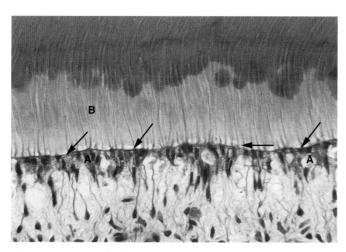

**Fig. 10.44** Micrograph of the pulp–dentine boundary exhibiting slight shrinkage and showing continuity of odontoblast processes (arrow) with odontoblast cell bodies (A). B = predentine (H & E; ×400).

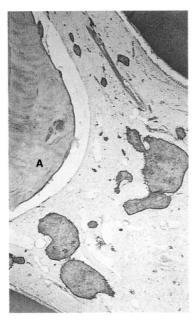

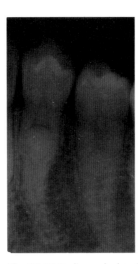

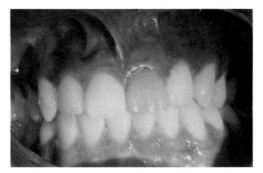

**Fig. 10.47** Patient with a maxillary left permanent central incisor, the dental pulp of which necrosed following trauma. It is darker than the adjacent tooth.

**Fig. 10.46** Radiograph showing large calcifications in the pulp chambers of lower premolars in a young individual. Courtesy of Dr S. Parekh and the editor of *Oral Surgery, Oral Medicine, Oral Pathology, Oral Radiology, and Endodontics.*

**Fig. 10.45** Multiple free pulp stones present in the dental pulp and lacking dentine structure (false denticles). A = dentine (H & E; ×40).

tubular ('true' denticles) or resemble bone by having cells embedded within them ('false' denticles; Fig. 10.45). In some (lamellated pulp stones), accretion by layers is evident. Some larger pulp stones may be attached to the dentine. The incidence of pulpal calcifications increases with age and they are generally regarded as an age-related change rather than being pathological. Pulp stones can usually be detected on radiographs (Fig. 10.46). If detected in the absence of symptoms or pathological change pulp stones are not an indication for root canal therapy. The pre-sence of pulp stones can complicate root canal therapy when it is indicated for other reasons. The factors determining why some individuals and not others produce pulp stones are not known – nor why, when present, one form or another occurs. If an individual has pulp stones in one tooth it is likely that they have pulp stones in other teeth. Widespread mineralization of the pulp may be associated with genetically determined dentine dysplasias.

## CLINICAL CONSIDERATIONS

Genetic, congenital, nutritional and traumatic factors that affect dentinogenesis exert that effect via the dental pulp. In the mature tooth, the pulp is the sense organ that mandates the use of anaesthesia during cavity preparation. It is the tissue that defends (or at least tries to defend) the integrity of the tooth in response to dental caries, attrition and trauma. Following pulp exposures and restorations it will, under the right conditions, form tertiary dentine and maintain tooth vitality. When dental caries begins the pulp responds at a very early stage. Pulpal inflammation can often be detected when caries is limited to the enamel. On some occasions pulpal inflammation (pulpitis) is painful and induces a memorable experience for the patient, and sometimes a therapeutic challenge for the dentist.

Pain from the dental pulp is difficult to localize and is commonly referred to other sites, either teeth or elsewhere. Sometimes pain in other sites is referred to the dental pulp (even angina). On many occasions pulpitis is painless and the dental pulp necroses. Necrotic pulp tissue can induce inflammation and sepsis in the supporting tissues around the tooth with possibly serious sequelae. It is not known why pulpal inflammation on some occasions results in severe pain and on other occasions is silent.

The lack of sensitivity associated with older teeth, whether due to the increased thickness of dentine or the reduced innervation of the pulp, may allow, on some occasions, for the restorative treatment of teeth without anaesthesia.

Gingival recession may expose the opening of a lateral root canal, especially in the furcation area of cheek teeth, causing pain and the possible spread of infection into the pulp. Infection associated with periodontal disease may also affect the pulp and vice versa. The successful treatment of these endodontic–periodontic lesions is dependent on determining in which of the tissues the disease process originated.

If an uninfected pulp is exposed during cavity preparation in a tooth it can, if treated appropriately, repair and form a bridge of dentine over the exposure. New odontoblasts differentiate and lay down tertiary (reparative) dentine. Some materials, such as calcium hydroxide, seem to facilitate dentine bridge formation. Their effect may be more by their ability to protect the pulp and their biocompatibility rather than any direct stimulation of dentine-producing cells. Other, more biologically active molecules, such as bone morphogenetic protein, TGF-β and some of the components of dentine matrix, may have a direct effect on the differentiation and activation of hard-tissue-forming cells. These have not, as yet, been widely applied clinically. If the exposed pulp is infected or contaminated the likelihood of successful bridge formation is much reduced. It may, in the future, be possible to control infection and inflammation in the pulp. It may also be possible to replace or regenerate all or part of a diseased pulp that has been removed using biological matrices carrying growth factors and/or cultures of pulpal cells. Currently, the definitive treatment of the irreversibly diseased or necrotic pulp is to remove it and replace it with an inert root canal filling material.

If the dental pulp undergoes death and necrosis, degradative products may pass along the dental tubules, giving the crown a darker appearance (Fig. 10.47).

Cementum is the thin layer of calcified tissue covering the dentine of the root (Fig. 11.1). It is one of the four tissues that support the tooth in the jaw (the periodontium), the others being the alveolar bone, the periodontal ligament and the gingivae. Although many of these periodontal tissues have been extensively studied, cementum remains the least known. Indeed, it is the least known of all the mineralized tissues in the body. For example, very little is known about the origin, differentiation and cell dynamics of the cementum-forming cell (the cementoblast) and it has been questioned whether these cells are a subpopulation of osteoblasts or have a unique phenotype. It is known that both cementoblasts and osteoblasts have receptors for parathormone (PTH) and parathormone receptor protein (PTHrP). Furthermore, they respond similarly to many of the factors that regulate cell activity. This, however, does not mean that the cells are of the same lineage.

Although restricted to the root in humans, cementum is present on the crowns of some mammals as an adaptation to a herbivorous diet. Cementum varies in thickness at different levels of the root. It is thickest at the root apex and in the interradicular areas of multirooted teeth and thinnest cervically. The thickness cervically is 10–15 μm, and apically 50–200 μm (although it may exceed 600 μm).

Cementum is contiguous with the periodontal ligament on its outer surface and is firmly adherent to dentine on its deep surface. Its prime function is to give attachment to collagen fibres of the periodontal ligament.

It therefore is a highly responsive mineralized tissue, maintaining the integrity of the root, helping to maintain the tooth in its functional position in the mouth, and being involved in tooth repair and regeneration.

Cementum is slowly formed throughout life and this allows for continual reattachment of the periodontal ligament fibres – some regard cementum as a calcified component of the ligament. Developmentally, cementum is said to be derived from the investing layer of the dental follicle. Like dentine, there is always a thin layer (3–5 μm) of uncalcified matrix on the surface of the cellular variety of cementum (see page 174). This layer of uncalcified matrix is called precementum (Fig. 11.2). Similar in chemical composition and physical properties to bone, cementum is, however, avascular and has no innervation. It is also less readily resorbed, a feature that is important for permitting orthodontic tooth movements. The reason for this feature is unknown but it may be related to:

- differences in physicochemical or biological properties between bone and cementum
- the properties of the precementum
- the increased density of Sharpey fibres (particularly in acellular cementum)
- the proximity of epithelial cell rests to the root surface.

Unlike bone, cementum does not have a lamellar appearance and has no marrow spaces.

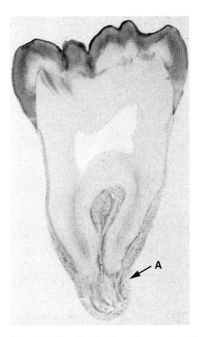

**Fig. 11.1** The distribution of cementum (A) along the root of a tooth (Ground longitudinal section of a tooth; ×4).

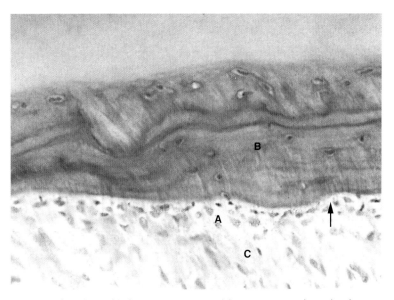

**Fig. 11.2** The relationship between cementum (B), precementum (arrow), a layer of cementoblasts (A) and the periodontal ligament (C) (Decalcified section; H & E; ×200).

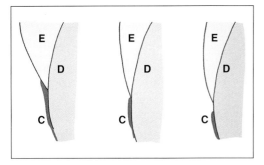

**Fig. 11.3** Three patterns for the arrangement of the cement-enamel junction. C = cementum; E = enamel; D = dentine. See text for further details.

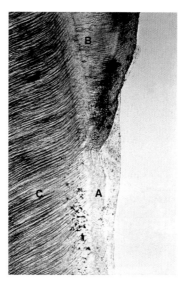

**Fig. 11.5** Ground longitudinal section through a tooth to show cementum (A) overlapping enamel (B). C = dentine (Ground section; ×80). Courtesy of Professor A.G.S. Lumsden.

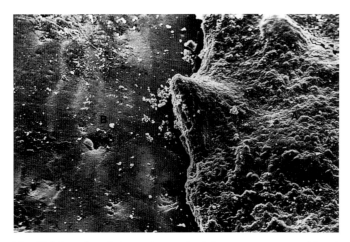

**Fig. 11.4** Scanning electron micrograph of the cementum–enamel junction where the cementum overlaps the enamel. A = cementum; B = enamel (SEM; ×250).

The arrangement of tissues at the cementum–enamel junction is shown in Figures 11.3–11.5. In any single section of a tooth, three arrangements of the junction between cementum and enamel may be seen. Pattern 1, where the cementum overlaps the enamel for a short distance, is the predominant arrangement in 60% of sections. Pattern 2, where the cementum and enamel meet at a butt joint, occurs in 30% of sections. Pattern 3, where the cementum and enamel fail to meet and the dentine between them is exposed, occurs in 10% of sections. Although one of these patterns may predominate in any individual tooth, all three patterns can be present.

## PHYSICAL PROPERTIES

Cementum is pale yellow with a dull surface. It is softer than dentine. Permeability varies with age and the type of cementum, the cellular variety being more permeable. In general, cementum is more permeable than dentine. Like the other dental tissues, permeability decreases with age. The relative softness of cementum, combined with its thinness cervically, means that it is readily removed by abrasion when gingival recession exposes the root surface to the oral environment. Loss of cementum in such cases will expose dentine.

## CHEMICAL PROPERTIES

Cementum contains on a wet-weight basis 65% inorganic material, 23% organic material and 12% water. By volume, the inorganic material comprises approximately 45%, organic material 33% and water 22%. The degree of mineralization varies in different parts of the tissue; some

acellular zones may be more highly calcified than dentine. The principal inorganic component is hydroxyapatite, although other forms of calcium are present at higher levels than in enamel and dentine. The hydroxyapatite crystals are thin and plate-like and similar to those in bone. They are on average 55 nm wide and 8 nm thick. Their length varies, but values derived from sections cut with a diamond knife are underestimates due to shattering of the crystals along their length. As with enamel, the concentration of trace elements tends to be higher at the external surface. This, for example, is true of fluoride levels, which are also higher in acellular than in cellular cementum. Indeed, the fluoride content of cementum is greater than that of bone. The organic matrix is primarily collagen. The collagen is virtually all type I (although types III, V, VI and XII have been found in small quantities). In addition, the non-collagenous elements are assumed to be similar to those found in bone (see pages 206, 207). However, because of the difficulties of obtaining sufficient material for analysis, less information is available. Nevertheless, among the important molecules known to be present are bone sialoprotein, dentine sialoprotein, fibronectin, tenascin and osteopontin and possibly other cementum-specific elements that are conjectured to be involved in periodontal reattachment and/or remineralization. Sialoproteins are located in the cementum matrix and osteopontin in the incremental lines. Cementum-derived attachment protein (CAP) is a 56 kDa or 65 kDa collagenous protein in cementum that promotes the attachment of mesenchymal cells to the extracellular matrix. It is located in the matrix of mature cementum and in cementoblasts (but not in bone). Thus, CAP may be a marker to differentiate bone and cementum. Cementum is rich in glycosaminoglycans, predominantly chondroitin sulphate. This glycosaminoglycan is primarily located around the lacunae of cementum. In addition, dermatan sulphate and hyaluronan can be found. Among the proteoglycans found in cementum are lumican, versican, decorin, biglycan and fibromodulin. These are also found in bone and, for both tissues, are located especially at the peripheries of lacunae and canaliculi. It appears that fibromodulin and lumican are more abundant in cementum.

## CLASSIFICATION OF CEMENTUM

The various types of cementum encountered may be classified in three different ways: the presence or absence of cells, the nature and origin of the organic matrix, and a combination of both.

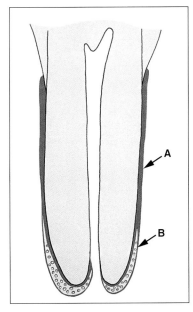

**Fig. 11.6** The distribution of acellular (A) and cellular (B) cementum.

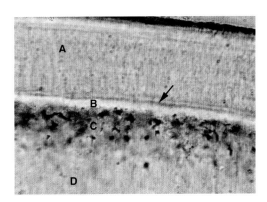

**Fig. 11.7** The appearance of acellular cementum (A). B = hyaline layer (of Hopewell-Smith); C = granular layer (of Tomes); D = root dentine. Note that the dark layer arrowed between the hyaline layer and the acellular cementum may be related to the afibrillar cementum patchily present at this position (Ground section; ×200).

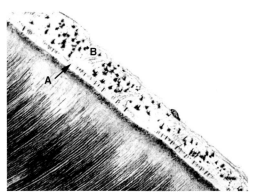

**Fig. 11.8** Cellular cementum (B) overlying acellular cementum (A). Note the greater thickness of the cellular layer (Ground section; ×50).

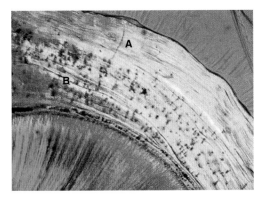

**Fig. 11.9** Acellular cementum (A) overlying cellular cementum (B) (Ground section of the root; ×50).

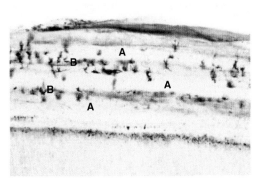

**Fig. 11.10** Alternating acellular (A) and cellular cementum (B) (Ground section; ×60).

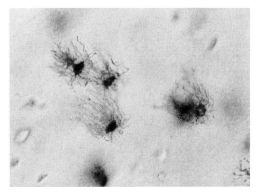

**Fig. 11.11** Lacunae and canaliculi in cellular cementum. In this section, the preferential orientation of the lacunae indicates that the external surface is above and to the left (Ground section; ×500).

## CLASSIFICATION BASED ON THE PRESENCE OR ABSENCE OF CELLS: CELLULAR AND ACELLULAR CEMENTUM

Cellular cementum, as its name indicates, contains cells (cementocytes); acellular cementum does not. In the most common arrangement, acellular cementum covers the root adjacent to the dentine, whereas cellular cementum is found mainly in the apical area and overlying the acellular cementum (Fig. 11.6). Deviations from this arrangement are common and sometimes several layers of each variant alternate. Being formed first, the acellular cementum is sometimes termed primary cementum and the subsequently formed cellular variety secondary cementum. Cellular cementum is especially common in interradicular areas.

Acellular cementum appears relatively structureless (Fig. 11.7). In the outer region of the radicular dentine, the granular layer (of Tomes) can be seen and outside this the hyaline layer (of Hopewell-Smith). These layers are also described on page 140. A dark line may be discerned between the hyaline layer and the acellular cementum; this may be related to the afibrillar cementum that is patchily present at this position. The usual arrangement at the apical region of the root is of a layer of cellular cementum overlying acellular cementum (Fig. 11.8). Many of the structural differences between cellular and acellular cementum are thought to be related to the faster rate of matrix formation for cellular cementum. Indeed, a major difference is that, as cellular cementum develops, the formative

cells (the cementoblasts) become embedded in the tissue as cementocytes. The different rates of cementum formation are also reflected in the presence of a precementum layer and in the more widely spaced incremental lines in cellular cementum.

Although the usual relationship between acellular and cellular cementum is for the cellular variety to overlie the acellular, the reverse may occur (Fig. 11.9). Furthermore, it is also common for the two variants of cementum to alternate (Fig. 11.10), probably representing variations in the rate of deposition.

The spaces that the cementocytes occupy in cellular cementum are called lacunae and the channels that their processes extend along are the canaliculi (Fig. 11.11; see also Fig. 11.2). Adjacent canaliculi are often connected and the processes within them exhibit gap junctions. In ground sections (Fig. 11.11), the cellular contents are lost, air and debris filling the voids to give the dark appearance. In thicker layers of cellular cementum, it is highly probable that many of the lacunae do not contain vital cells. This contrasts with the situation in bone. Furthermore, compared with osteocytes in bone, cementocytes are more widely dispersed and more randomly arranged. In addition, their canaliculi are preferentially oriented towards the periodontal ligament, their chief source of nutrition. Unlike bone, the cementocytes are not arranged circumferentially around blood vessels in the form of osteons (Haversian systems). In decalcified sections (Fig. 11.2), the cellular contents of the lacunae are retained, albeit in a shrunken condition.

Figure 11.12 illustrates the ultrastructural appearance of a cementocyte within a lacuna. Although derived from active cementoblasts, once they become embedded within the cementum matrix, cementocytes become relatively inactive. This is reflected in their ultrastructural appearance. Their cytoplasmic/nuclear ratio is low and they have sparse, if any, representation of the organelles responsible for energy production and for synthesis. Some unmineralized matrix may be seen in the perilacunar space. The cementocyte processes can extend for distances several times longer than the diameter of the cell body. There is presently no evidence that cementocytes have a function in tissue homeostasis.

Cementum is deposited in an irregular rhythm, resulting in unevenly spaced incremental lines (of Salter; Fig. 11.13). Unlike enamel and dentine, the precise periodicity between the incremental lines is unknown, although there have been unsuccessful attempts to relate it to an annual cycle. In acellular cementum, incremental lines tend to be close together, thin and even. In the more rapidly formed cellular cementum, the lines are further apart, thicker and more irregular. The appearance of incremental lines in cementum is mainly due to differences in the degree of mineralization but these must also reflect differences in composition of the underlying matrix since, as shown in Figure 11.13, the lines are readily visible in decalcified sections. Recent evidence suggests that the incremental lines are rich in osteopontin and that this might aid the cohesion of the matrix molecules at these sites.

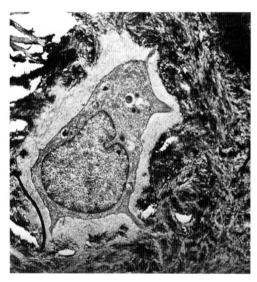

**Fig. 11.12** TEM of a cementocyte within a lacuna. Note that the cementocyte processes here appear short only because they extend out of the plane of section (×4500).

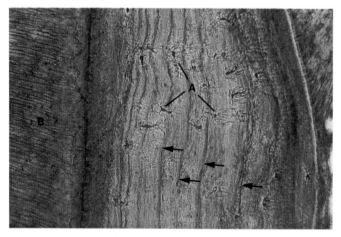

**Fig. 11.13** Incremental lines of Salter (arrowed) in cementum. A = cementocytes; B = dentine (Decalcified section; picrothionin; ×75). Courtesy of Professor M.M. Smith.

Table 11.1 summarizes differences between acellular and cellular cementum.

## CLASSIFICATION BASED ON THE NATURE AND ORIGIN OF THE ORGANIC MATRIX

Cementum derives its organic matrix from two sources: from the inserting Sharpey fibres of the periodontal ligament and from the cementoblasts. It is therefore possible to classify cementum according to the nature and origin of the fibrous matrix. When derived from the periodontal ligament, the fibres are referred to as the *extrinsic fibres*. These Sharpey fibres continue into the cementum in the same direction as the principal fibres of the ligament (i.e. perpendicular or oblique to the root surface; see page 182). When derived from the cementoblasts, the fibres are referred to as *intrinsic fibres*. These run parallel to the root surface and approximately at right angles to the extrinsic fibres. Where both extrinsic and intrinsic fibres are present, the tissue may be termed *mixed fibre cementum*.

## CLASSIFICATION BASED ON THE PRESENCE OR ABSENCE OF CELLS AND ON THE NATURE AND ORIGIN OF THE ORGANIC MATRIX

This classification, which is becoming more widely used, contains a number of types of cementum. For human teeth, two main varieties of cementum are found – *acellular extrinsic fibre cementum* (AEFC) and *cellular intrinsic fibre cementum* (CIFC). AEFC is located mainly over the cervical half of the root and constitutes the bulk of cementum in some teeth (e.g. in premolars). AEFC is the first formed cementum (see pages 347–352) and layers attain a thickness of approximately 15 μm.

### Acellular extrinsic fibre cementum (AEFC) (Fig. 11.14)

For this type of cementum all the collagen is derived as Sharpey fibres from the periodontal ligament (the ground substance itself may be produced by the cementoblasts). This type of cementum corresponds with primary acellular cementum and therefore covers the cervical two-thirds of the root (Fig. 11.7). It is therefore formed slowly and the root surface is smooth (Fig. 11.4). The fibres are generally well mineralized. As shown in Figure 11.15, however, the extrinsic fibres seen in ground sections may have unmineralized cores. These may be lost during preparation of a ground section and replaced with air or debris. This results in the total internal reflection of transmitted light, giving the appearance of thin black lines.

### Cellular intrinsic fibre cementum (CIFC) (Figs 11.16, 11.17)

This type of cementum is composed only of intrinsic fibres running parallel to the root surface. The absence of Sharpey fibres means that intrinsic fibre cementum has no role in tooth attachment. It may be found in patches

**Table 11.1** *Summary of differences between acellular and cellular cementum*

| Acellular cementum | Cellular cementum |
| --- | --- |
| No cells | Lacunae and canaliculi containing cementocytes and their processes |
| Border with dentine not clearly demarcated | Border with dentine clearly demarcated |
| Rate of development relatively slow | Rate of development relatively fast |
| Incremental lines relatively close together | Incremental lines relatively wide apart |
| Precementum layer virtually absent | Precementum layer present |

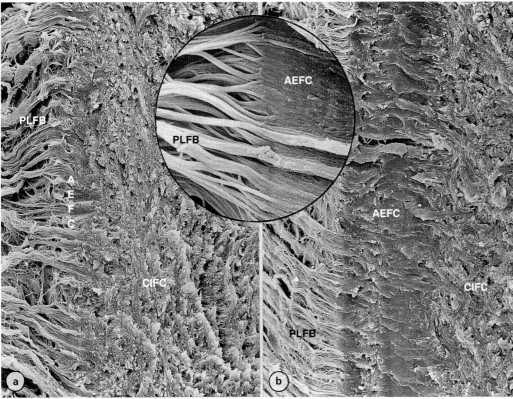

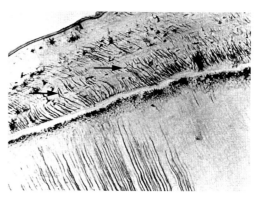

**Fig. 11.15** Extrinsic fibres in ground sections. The arrows indicate that the core of the extrinsic fibre bundle has been lost during preparation of the ground section and replaced with air or debris (Ground section; ×100). Courtesy of Dr P.D.A. Owens.

**Fig. 11.14** SEMs of fractured surface of root illustrating acellular extrinsic fibre cementum (AEFC). PLFB = inserting periodontal ligament fibre bundles; CIFC = underlying cellular intrinsic fibre cementum (a and b ×630; inset ×1650). From Schroeder HE 1993 Human cellular mixed stratified cementum: a tissue with alternating layers of acellular extrinsic and cellular intrinsic fiber cementum. *Schweizer Monatsschrift fur Zahnmedizin* 103: 550–560.

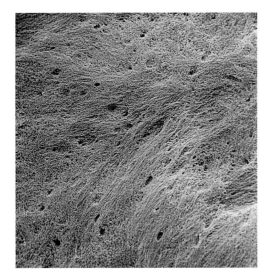

**Fig. 11.16** SEM showing the appearance of intrinsic fibre cementum at the surface of the root apex. Note the absence of Sharpey fibres and the parallel distribution of the bundles of mineralized intrinsic fibres (Anorganic preparation; ×150). Courtesy of Professor S.J. Jones.

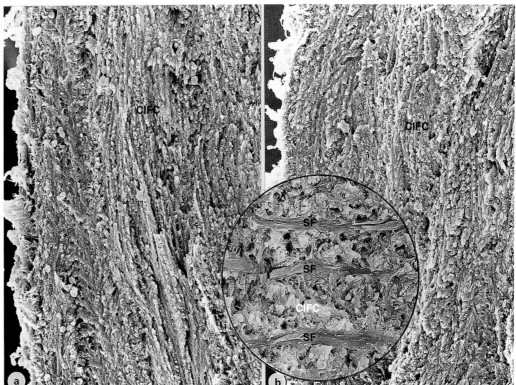

**Fig. 11.17** SEMs of fractured surface of root showing the appearance of cellular intrinsic fibre cementum (CIFC). Note the absence of Sharpey fibres and the parallel distribution of the bundles of mineralized intrinsic fibres (a and b ×470; inset shows that Sharpey fibres (SF) can occasionally be seen inserting into CIFC ×1650). From Schroeder HE 1993 Human cellular mixed stratified cementum: a tissue with alternating layers of acellular extrinsic and cellular intrinsic fiber cementum. *Schweizer Monatsschrift fur Zahnmedizin* 103: 550–560.

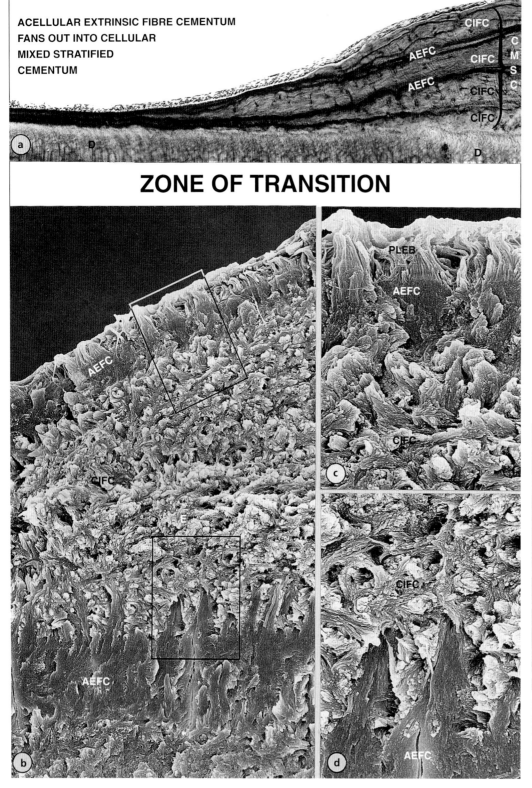

**Fig. 11.18** (a) The appearance of mixed fibre cementum. A light micrograph to show the alternating distribution of acellular extrinsic fibre cementum (AEFC) and cellular intrinsic fibre cementum (CIFC), forming cellular mixed stratified cementum (CMSC) (Ground section; ×80). (b–d) SEMs illustrating mixed fibre cementum; (c) and (d) are highlighted areas provided by the boxes in (b). (SEM; (b) ×900; c, d ×2450). From Schroeder HE 1993 Human cellular mixed stratified cementum: a tissue with alternating layers of acellular extrinsic and cellular intrinsic fiber cementum. *Schweizer Monatsschrift fur Zahnmedizin* 103: 550–560.

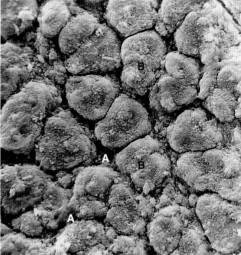

**Fig. 11.19** SEM of the surface of a root showing the appearance of mixed fibre cementum. A = mineralized intrinsic fibres (present here in small amounts); B = mineralized extrinsic fibres. Note the smaller dimensions of the intrinsic fibre bundles (Anorganic preparation; ×3000). Courtesy of Professor S.J. Jones.

in the apical region. It may be a temporary phase, with extrinsic fibres subsequently gaining a reattachment, or may represent a permanent region without attaching fibres. It generally corresponds to secondary cellular cementum and is found in the apical third of the root and in the interradicular areas. Although intrinsic fibre cementum is generally cellular because of the rapid speed of formation, sometimes intrinsic fibre cementum is formed more slowly and cells are not incorporated (acellular intrinsic fibre cementum). Cellular intrinsic fibre cementum is less cellular than bone and has a cementoid seam on its outer surface (see Fig. 11.2). This cementoid seam is similar to the osteoid seam seen for bone. Note that a cementoid seam is not present on the surface of acellular extrinsic fibre cementum.

Towards the root apex, and in the furcation areas of multirooted teeth, the acellular extrinsic fibre cementum and the cellular intrinsic fibre cementum are commonly present in alternating layers known as cellular mixed stratified cementum (Fig. 11.18).

## Mixed fibre cementum (Fig. 11.19)

For this third variety of cementum, the collagen fibres of the organic matrix are derived from both extrinsic fibres (from the periodontal ligament) and intrinsic fibres (from cementoblasts). The extrinsic and intrinsic fibres can be readily distinguished. First, the intrinsic fibres run between the

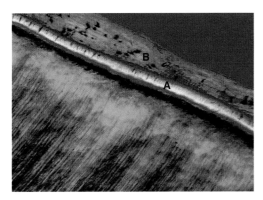

**Fig. 11.20** Fibre orientation in acellular and cellular cementum. The root surface is seen in polarized light, the different colours reflecting different orientations of the collagen fibres. A = acellular cementum; B = cellular cementum (Ground, longitudinal section; polarized light; ×50).

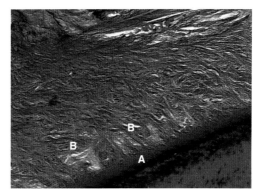

**Fig. 11.21** Attachment of the periodontal ligament fibres to cementum. The fibres of the periodontal ligament (B) are seen to run into the organic matrix of precementum (A) (Decalcified section; Masson's blue trichrome; ×200).

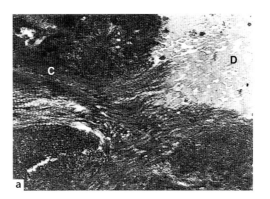

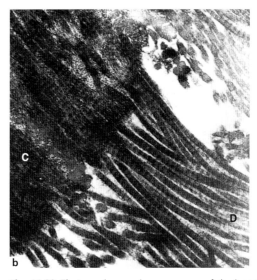

**Fig. 11.22** Electronmicroscopic appearance of the insertion of Sharpey fibres into cementum. (a) Ground section showing that the inserting collagen fibres darken as they enter the cementum due to their partial mineralization. (b) Decalcified section showing the grouping of collagen into a bundle and collagen cross banding. C = cementum; D = periodontal ligament (TEM; (a) ×8000; (b) ×15000). Courtesy of Dr D.K. Whittaker.

extrinsic fibres with a different orientation. Indeed, the fewer the number of intrinsic fibres in mixed fibre cementum, the closer the extrinsic fibre bundles (Fig. 11.19). Second, the fibre bundles are of different sizes: the extrinsic fibres are ovoid or round bundles about 5–7 μm in diameter; the intrinsic fibres are 1–2 μm in diameter (Fig. 11.19).

If the formation rate is slow, the cementum may be termed acellular mixed-fibre cementum and is generally well mineralized. If the formation rate is fast, the cementum may be called cellular mixed-fibre cementum and the fibres are less well mineralized (especially their cores).

Figure 11.20 shows the fibre orientation in acellular and cellular cementum as seen in polarized light, the different colours reflecting different orientations of the collagen fibres. The acellular cementum contains primarily extrinsic fibres arranged perpendicular to the root surface. The overlying cellular cementum contains mainly intrinsic fibres running parallel to the root surface. Thus, there is a colour difference between the two layers.

Finally, a variety of acellular intrinsic fibre cementum has been characterized and this, like cellular intrinsic fibre cementum, displays a cementoid seam.

Chemical differences exist between the different forms of cementum. Dentine sialoprotein, fibronectin and tenascin are not present in acellular extrinsic fibre cementum but are found in cellular intrinsic fibre cementum. Furthermore, acellular extrinsic fibre cementum is deficient in lumican, versican, decorin, biglycan and fibromodulin. These differences probably reflect differences in the secretory activities of the cells involved in the development of these two varieties of cementum. It has also been reported that enamel matrix components, possibly secreted by epithelial root sheath cells and their derivatives, can result in cells synthesizing acellular extrinsic fibre cementum.

### Afibrillar cementum

The extrinsic, intrinsic and mixed fibre cementum types all contain collagen fibres. However, there is a further type of cementum that contains no collagen fibres. This afibrillar cementum is sparsely distributed and consists of a well-mineralized ground substance that may be of epithelial origin. Afibrillar cementum is a thin, acellular layer (difficult to identify at the light microscope level), which covers cervical enamel or intervenes between fibrillar cementum and dentine. Afibrillar cementum is thought to be formed at this site following the loss of the reduced enamel epithelium (see page 123).

## ATTACHMENT OF THE PERIODONTAL LIGAMENT FIBRES TO CEMENTUM

The fibres of the periodontal ligament run into the organic matrix of pre-cementum that is secreted by cementoblasts. Subsequent mineralization of precementum will incorporate the extrinsic fibres as Sharpey fibres into cementum (Figs 11.21, 11.22). It has been estimated that, for acellular extrinsic fibre cementum, there are approximately 30,000 principal fibres of the periodontal ligament attached into the cemental tissue per square millimetre.

## CEMENTUM–DENTINE JUNCTION

The nature of the cementum–dentine junction is of particular importance, being of interest biologically because it forms an interface (a 'fit') between two very different mineralized tissues that are developing contemporarily. It is also of clinical importance because of the processes involved in maintaining tooth function while repairing a diseased root surface. The cementum–dentine junction appears to have a lower mineral content and is a composite of inorganic and organic components (including dermatan sulphate and collagen fibrils).

It is often reported that an 'intermediate layer' (Fig. 11.23) exists between cementum and dentine and that this layer is involved in 'anchoring' the periodontal fibres to the dentine. A variety of names has been given to the 'intermediate layer' (including 'innermost cementum layer', 'superficial layer of root dentine' and 'intermediate cementum'). Indeed, it appears that the term has even been used to describe the hyaline layer of dentine (see page 140).

The intermediate layer is said to be characterized by wide, irregular, branching spaces (Fig. 11.24) and is most commonly found in the apical region of cheek teeth. The spaces may interconnect with dentinal tubules. The nature and origin of the spaces is controversial; they may be related to entrapped epithelial cells (cell remnants containing filaments characteristic of epithelial cells have been described in this region). Alternatively, they may be enlarged terminals of dentinal tubules.

There appears to be marked species differences with respect to the intermediate layer. In rat molars, a distinct intermediate layer exists that is rich in the glycoproteins sialoprotein and osteopontin (both these glycoproteins being normally bone related), although the role of these glycoproteins remains unclear. The origin of this layer in rat molars is also unclear, some believing that it is derived from the epithelial root sheath that lines the developing root (see pages 342–343), while others claim that it is cementoblast-derived. Indeed, there are reports suggesting that, in humans, the region between the cementum and the root dentine contains enamel matrix protein and is a product of the epithelial root sheath. However, it has been claimed that, for many human teeth, the collagen within the AEFC layer intermingles with the dentine matrix, there is no sialoprotein and osteopontin, and there is no obvious zone between dentine and cementum.

Where an intermediate layer exists, it has been suggested that this functions as a permeability barrier, that it may be a precursor for cementogenesis, and that it is a precursor for cementogenesis in wound healing. These potential functions remain speculative. If, however, there is doubt about the very presence of an intermediate zone in human teeth then either human teeth do not require such functions (which is highly unlikely) or too much is being conjectured with too little experimental evidence.

The clinical significance of the interface between cementum and dentine relates to regeneration of the periodontium following periodontal surgery. Although a layer of cementum may regenerate, subsequent histological examination may show a 'space' between regenerated cementum and surface dentine, perhaps indicating an absence of a true union.

## ULTRASTRUCTURAL APPEARANCE OF CEMENTUM

This varies with the level of the tissue examined. Near the periodontal surface (Fig. 11.25), cementum is not homogeneous because of ongoing calcification and the presence of Sharpey fibres. The calcification of precementum is probably initiated in the early phases by the presence of the underlying root dentine mineral and continues on, and around, the collagen fibres (both those formed by the cementoblasts and those included as attachment fibres from the periodontal ligament). The outer part of the cementum, where Sharpey fibres predominate, may be considered as calcified periodontal ligament. Unlike dentine, no calcospherites are present within precementum. At deeper levels (Fig. 11.26), closer to the cementum–dentine junction, acellular cementum resembles peripheral dentine and a demarcation is often difficult to see. The small channels seen at this level may be canaliculi derived from more superficial cementocytes, but some may be the terminals of dentinal tubules that traverse the border between the two tissues.

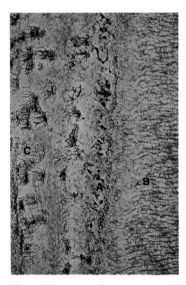

**Fig. 11.23** Intermediate cementum (A). B = root dentine. C = cellular cementum (Demineralized section; picrothionin; ×75). Courtesy of Professor M.M. Smith.

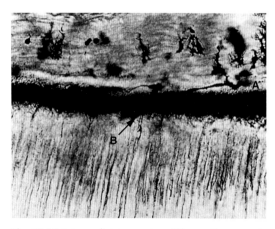

**Fig. 11.24** Intermediate cementum (A) near the cementum–dentine junction. B = granular layer (Ground section; ×250). Courtesy of Dr P.D.A. Owens.

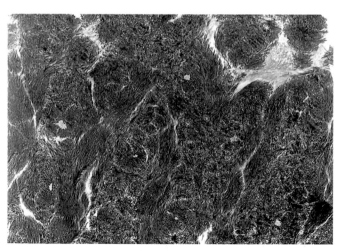

**Fig. 11.25** Appearance of cementum near the periodontal surface (TEM; ×2000).

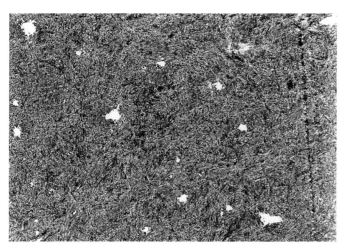

**Fig. 11.26** Appearance of cementum near the cementum–dentine junction (TEM; ×2000).

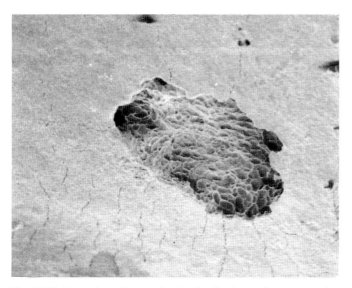

**Fig. 11.27** The surface of a root showing localized area of resorption of cementum (SEM; ×250). Courtesy of Professor S.J. Jones.

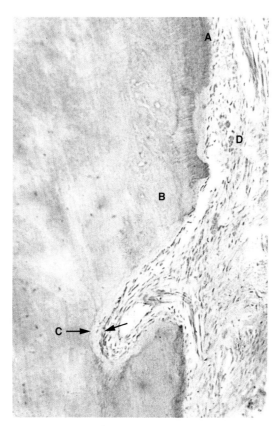

**Fig. 11.28** Repair of cementum following a localized region of root resorption. A = acellular cementum; B = root dentine; C = reversal line separating repair tissue from underlying dental tissues; D = periodontal ligament; arrows indicate cementoblasts depositing layer of precementum in resorption deficiency (Decalcified section of a root; H & E; ×90).

## RESORPTION AND REPAIR OF CEMENTUM

Although cementum is less susceptible to resorption than bone under the same pressures (e.g. with orthodontic loading), most roots of permanent teeth still show small, localized areas of resorption (Figs 11.27–11.29). The cause of this is not known but may be associated with microtrauma. The resorption is carried out by multinucleated odontoclasts (see page 361) and may continue into the root dentine. It has been suggested that the different levels of fluoride in cementum and bone (higher in cementum) may explain why cementum is less susceptible to resorption. Alternatively, the greater resistance to resorption might relate to the fact that the surface of the cementum is covered by a layer of tightly packed collagen and therefore the mineralized surface is relatively inaccessible. The unmineralized surface layer of collagen thus protects against the action of odontoclasts. It has also been suggested that cementoblasts lining the root surface do not retract from this surface in response to parathormone and that therefore the surface is not exposed to odontoclasts.

Resorption deficiencies may be filled by deposition of mineralized tissue. Indeed, a line known as a reversal line may be seen separating the repair tissue from the normal underlying dental tissues (repair of cementum following a localized region of root resorption is illustrated in Fig. 11.28). In this section, odontoclasts have resorbed through the thin layer of acellular cementum and penetrated into the root dentine. Repair is occurring and a layer of formative cells (cementoblasts) have deposited a thin layer of matrix (precementum) in the deficiency. An irregular, and

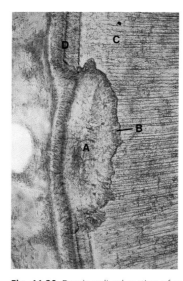

**Fig. 11.29** Demineralized section of root showing infilled area of repair cementum (A). B = reversal line; C = dentine; D = cementum (Picrothionin; ×75). Courtesy of Professor M.M. Smith.

dark-staining, reversal line separates the repair tissue from the underlying dental tissues. Figure 11.29 shows an infilled area where dentine has been resorbed.

The repair tissue resembles cellular cementum. The formative cells have a similar ultrastructure to cementoblasts. Lines resembling incremental lines may be seen and there is a zone of uncalcified repair tissue homologous to precementum. However, differences can be noted between the repair tissue and cementum: the width of the uncalcified zone of reparative cementum (15 μm) is greater than that for precementum (5–10 μm); its degree of mineralization is less (as judged by electron density); its crystals are smaller; and calcific globules are present, suggesting that mineralization is not proceeding evenly.

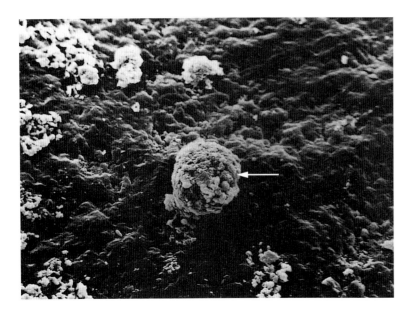

**Fig. 11.30** SEM appearance of a cementicle (arrowed). This cementicle is attached to the root surface (×1000).

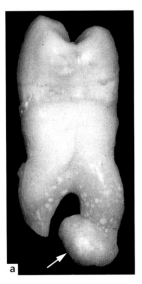

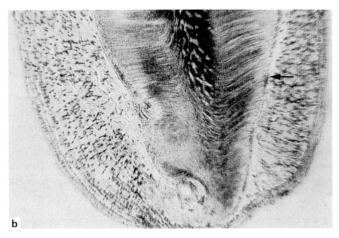

**Fig. 11.31** (a) Hypercementosis at root apex (arrow). Courtesy of Dr J. Potts. (b) Ground section near the root apex showing hypercementosis. Arrow shows cementum–dentine junction (×25).

These differences may be related to the speed of formation of the repair tissue. Where this is very slow, the repair tissue cannot be distinguished histologically, or in its mineralization pattern, from primary cementum. However, where the repair tissue is formed rapidly (as in resorbing deciduous teeth), it closely resembles woven bone.

Acellular extrinsic fibre cementum grows throughout the life of a tooth, with a rate of between 0.005 μm and 0.01 μm per day. During its formation, cellular intrinsic fibre cementum grows about 50 times as fast. In comparison, bone grows by 1 μm to 2 μm per day (faster for woven bone).

## CLINICAL CONSIDERATIONS

Root fractures may, on some occasions, repair by the formation of a cemental callus. Unlike the callus that forms around fractured bone, the cemental callus does not usually remodel to the original dimensions of the tooth.

Cementicles (Fig. 11.30) are small, globular masses of cementum found in approximately 35% of human roots. They are not always attached to the cementum surface but may be located free in the periodontal ligament. Cementicles may result from microtrauma, when extra stress on the Sharpey fibres causes a tear in the cementum. They are more common in the apical and middle third of the root and in root furcation areas.

Cementum continues to be deposited slowly throughout life, its thickness increasing about threefold between the ages of 16 and 70, although whether this proceeds in a linear manner is not known. Cementum may be formed at the root apex in much greater amounts as a result of compensatory tooth eruption in response to attrition (wear) at the occlusal surface. Where there has been a history of chronic periapical inflammation, cementum formation may be substantial, giving rise to local hypercementosis (Fig. 11.31). This may cause problems during tooth extraction. If interdental bone is lost, continued cementum formation may result in fusion of the roots of adjacent teeth. Such a condition is known as concrescence (see Fig. 2.176b) and will lead to difficulties during tooth extraction. Hypercementosis affecting all the teeth may be associated with Paget's disease.

Hypophosphatasia is a rare condition in which there is a reduction in the activity of tissue non-specific alkaline phosphatase. The gene for this enzyme is located on chromosome 1. The condition is characterized by a significant reduction in the amount of cementum formed and affects both acellular and cellular cementum. As a result, the attachment of the principal fibres of the periodontal ligament is compromised, with premature loss of the deciduous teeth. Permanent teeth are similarly affected.

Where the root canal exits at the apex of the tooth, cementum is deposited not only over the apex but also for a short distance (usually 0.5–1.5 mm) from the anatomical apex. This results in a narrowing of the canal at this point, the apical constriction (see Fig. 26.9). This represents the junction of the pulp and periodontal tissue (although there is no visible demarcation in the soft tissue). In clinical procedures of root canal therapy that call for the removal of a diseased or decayed pulp, this is the point to which the cleansing should be extended.

The periodontal ligament is the dense fibrous connective tissue that occupies the periodontal space between the root of the tooth and the alveolus (Fig. 12.1). It is derived from the dental follicle (see page 301). Above the alveolar crest, the periodontal ligament is continuous with the connective tissues of the gingiva; at the apical foramen, it is continuous with the dental pulp. The continuity with the gingiva is important when considering the progression of periodontitis from gingivitis. The continuity with the pulp explains why inflammation from this dental tissue (often related to dental caries) spreads to involve the periodontal ligament and the other apical supporting tissues.

Although the average width of the periodontal space is said to be 0.25 mm, there is considerable variation both between teeth and within an individual tooth. The space has been described as hourglass in shape, being narrowest in the mid-root region, near the fulcrum about which the tooth moves when an orthodontic load (tipping load) is applied to the crown. The width of the periodontal space also varies according to the functional state of the periodontal tissues. The space is reduced in non-functional and unerupted teeth and is increased in teeth subjected to heavy occlusal stress. With age, the periodontal space narrows slightly. The periodontal spaces of the permanent teeth are said to be narrower than those of the deciduous teeth.

Much research has been conducted in recent times into the structure, function and composition of the periodontal ligament, because the tissue is associated with important dental functions (in particular the mechanisms of tooth support and tooth eruption; see pages 362–365 and 201–203

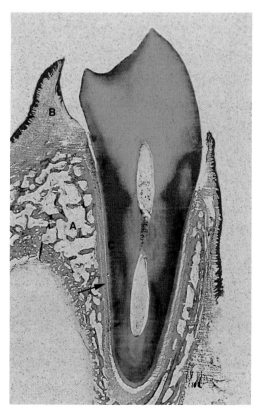

**Fig. 12.1** The relationship of the periodontal ligament and the periodontal space (arrow) to the other tissues of the periodontium. A = alveolar bone; B = gingiva; C = root of tooth lined by cementum (Decalcified, longitudinal section of a tooth in situ; H & E; ×4). Courtesy of Dr D.A. Lunt.

respectively) and for clinical reasons. The tissue is involved with inflammatory periodontal disease (a common cause of tooth loss) and there is considerable interest in tissue reattachment following such disease. Furthermore, with the application of orthodontic loads, the periodontal tissues must adjust to permit tooth relocation. Despite the amount of research undertaken, many of the important features of the periodontal ligament are not well understood and consequently there is much controversy.

Although we are only now beginning to understand the extent of specialization of the tissue (see pages 200, 201), we still do not know why the periodontal ligament remains a soft connective tissue and does not calcify, even though it is enclosed by bone externally and cementum internally. Indeed, the periodontal ligament width is preserved over time and the alveolar bone rarely 'colonizes' the periodontal space. It is evident that there must be some 'signalling systems' to accurately 'measure' and maintain the periodontal space. Failure of such a system is implicated in tooth ankylosis: that heat killing of periodontal cells induces ankylosis provides some crude evidence that periodontal fibroblasts may regulate periodontal ligament width. More convincingly, periodontal cells can inhibit mineralized bone nodule formation by bone stromal cells and there is evidence to suggest that the block exerted by periodontal cells may be due to prostaglandin production. Recent work also indicates that bradykinin and thrombin can stimulate prostanoid synthesis by periodontal ligament cells. Contrariwise, periodontal ligament cells are capable of producing bone-like tissue in vitro, can form mineralized nodules and can express alkaline phosphatase. Indeed, alkaline phosphatase, an enzyme expressed by mineralized tissue forming cells, is expressed constitutively by periodontal ligament cells. That the ground substance may be implicated in preventing mineralization may be deduced from in vitro experiments in which, following the administration of hyaluronidase, mineralization can be produced in the remaining periodontal ligament connective tissue.

The periodontal ligament has the following functions:

- It is the tissue of attachment between the tooth and alveolar bone. It is thus responsible for resisting displacing forces (the tooth support mechanism) and for protecting the dental tissues from damage caused by excessive occlusal loads (especially at the root apex).
- It is responsible for the mechanisms whereby a tooth attains, and then maintains, its functional position. This includes the mechanisms of tooth eruption, tooth support (particularly the recovery response after loading) and drift.
- Its cells form, maintain and repair alveolar bone and cementum.
- Its mechanoreceptors are involved in the neurological control of mastication (see pages 98, 99 for reflex jaw activities).

The periodontal ligament has been likened to a fibrous joint (a gomphosis) and to periosteum. As will become apparent, however, such comparisons are not accurate (either from a structural or a functional point of view). In common with other dense fibrous connective tissues, the periodontal ligament consists of a stroma of fibres and ground substance containing cells, blood vessels and nerves.

## FIBRES

The connective tissue fibres are mainly collagenous (comprising well over 90% of the periodontal ligament fibres) but there may also be small amounts of oxytalan and reticulin fibres and, in some species, elastin fibres.

## COLLAGEN

The main types of collagen in the periodontal ligament are types I and III, and these are categorized as fibrous collagens. Most (approximately 80%) of the periodontal collagen is type I collagen. This variety of collagen is the major protein component of most connective tissues (including bone and skin) and contains two identical $\alpha_1$ chains and a chemically different $\alpha_2$ chain. It is low in hydroxylysine and glycosylated hydroxylysine. Unusually, however, the periodontal ligament is relatively rich in type III collagen (about 15%). This variety consists of three identical $\alpha_1$ III chains. It is high in hydroxyproline, low in hydroxylysine and contains cysteine. The function of type III collagen is not properly understood, although it is associated in other sites of the body with rapid turnover (e.g. granulation tissues and fetal connective tissue). Type III collagen is not localized to any specific region of the periodontal ligament but is covalently linked to type I collagen throughout the tissue. It is found in the periphery of Sharpey fibre attachments into alveolar bone (see Fig. 13.37) and around nerves and blood vessels. In vitro studies have shown that there is clonal heterogeneity for expression of type I and type III collagens and for fibronectin in periodontal ligament cell populations.

Small amounts of types V and VI collagens have been found in the periodontal ligament as well as traces of basement membrane collagens (types IV and VII) associated with epithelial cell rests (see pages 193, 194) and blood vessels. Type V collagen coats cell surfaces and other types of collagen. This collagen may increase in amount with periodontal inflammatory periodontal disease. Although evident in all zones of the periodontal ligament in fully erupted teeth, type VI collagen is absent from the middle zone of erupting molars and from the tooth-related portion of the ligament of continuously growing incisors of rats (Fig. 12.2). This type of collagen forms part of the oxytalan fibre system and can promote proliferation of fibroblasts.

Recently, it has been proposed that periodontal cells regulate the periodontal ligament's connective tissue architecture through expression of type XII collagen (Fig. 12.3). Type XII collagen is a non-fibrous collagen (known as a fibril-associated collagen) with interrupted helices. It may

function by linking together other collagens. There is evidence to suggest that type XII collagen occurs within the periodontal ligament only when the ligament is fully erupted and functional. Furthermore, it appears on the pressure side of the periodontal ligament following orthodontic loading and remodelling of the tissue. Transgenic mice with a mutation of collagen type XII show disruption of the normal architecture of the collagen fibre system within the periodontal ligament. Type XIV collagen can also be expressed in the periodontal ligament.

Much of the collagen is gathered together to form bundles approximately 5 μm in diameter. These bundles are termed the principal fibres. They appear to be more numerous (but smaller) at their attachments to cementum than at the alveolar bone (see Fig. 12.19). Figure 12.4 shows principal collagen fibres passing across the periodontal space from the root to the alveolar bone. The close association between the principal fibres and

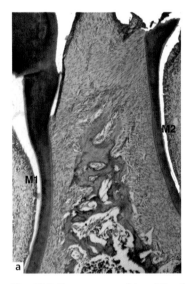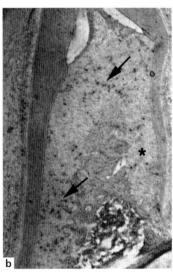

**Fig. 12.3** The presence of type XII collagen within the periodontal ligament. (a) Developing periodontal ligament of maxillary first molar (MI) and second molar (M2) in a 25-day-old rat. In this specimen, the first molar has completed eruption and its periodontal ligament is more organized, whereas the second molar has not yet erupted. (b) In situ hybridization of the S35-labelled type XII collagen cDNA probe. The type XII collagen probe hybridized to fibroblasts in the periodontal ligament of the first molar (arrows). Fibroblasts in the second molar periodontal ligament (*) were less active in type XII collagen synthesis. It has been postulated that type XII collagen may contribute to the organization of the mature and functional ligament collagen fibre architecture, which serves to resist unidirectional force. Courtesy of Dr Ichiro Nishimura and the UCLA Weintraub Center for Reconstructive Biotechnology.

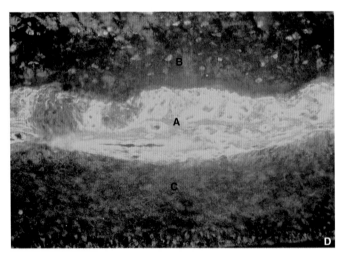

**Fig. 12.2** Longitudinal cryosection of rat incisor periodontal ligament with immunofluorescent staining for type VI collagen showing strong positive yellow staining (A) towards the alveolar bone surface (B) with an absence of staining (C) in the ligament towards the tooth surface (D) (×80). From Sloan P, Carter DH 1995 Structural organisation of the fibres of the periodontal ligament. In: Berkovitz BKB, Moxham BJ, Newman H (eds) *The periodontal ligament in health and disease*, 2nd edn. Mosby–Wolfe, London, pp 35–53.

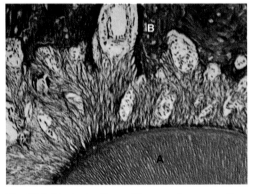

**Fig. 12.4** Principal collagen fibres passing across the periodontal space from the root (A) to the alveolar bone (B). Note also the vascular nature of the periodontal ligament (Decalcified, transverse section through the periodontal ligament; Gomori's silver stain; ×250).

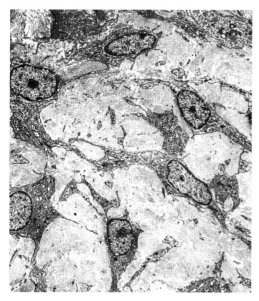

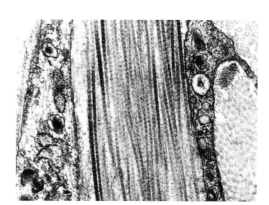

**Fig. 12.6** High-power view of a fibroblast process enveloping a principal fibre. Note the individual collagen fibrils within the principal bundle sectioned longitudinally (TEM; ×10 000).

**Fig. 12.5** TEM showing the close association between the principal fibres and the fibroblasts of the periodontal ligament (×3000).

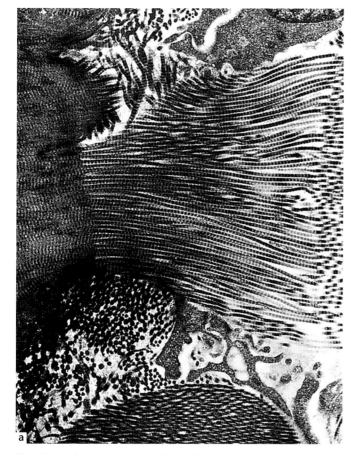

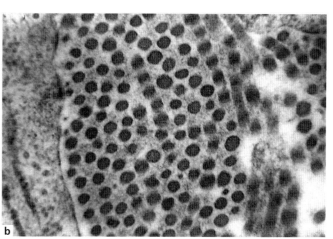

**Fig. 12.7** High-power view of collagen fibrils within a principal fibre of the periodontal ligament. (a) Fibrils sectioned longitudinally. (b) Fibrils sectioned transversely. The fibrils in longitudinal section display the banding characteristic of collagen. The fibrils in transverse section appear to be small and of uniform diameter (TEM; (a) ×16 000; (b) ×100 000).

the fibroblasts of the periodontal ligament is shown in Figures 12.5 and 12.6. The fibroblasts are responsible for the synthesis and degradation of collagen. Cellular processes surround, or envelop, the fibre bundles; indeed, processes from adjacent cells are joined by intercellular contacts (see page 190) to form a cellular network. Many of the isolated islands of cytoplasm present in the section in Figure 12.5 are cell processes from fibroblasts whose cell bodies are beyond the plane of section.

Within each collagen bundle, subunits of structure called collagen fibrils can be seen. The individual collagen fibrils illustrated in Figure 12.7a are sectioned longitudinally and show the classical banding characteristic of collagen. The collagen fibrils are formed by the packing together of individual tropocollagen molecules. The diameters of the collagen fibrils reflect the mechanical demands put upon the connective tissue. The collagen fibrils of the periodontal ligament are small and of uniform diameter

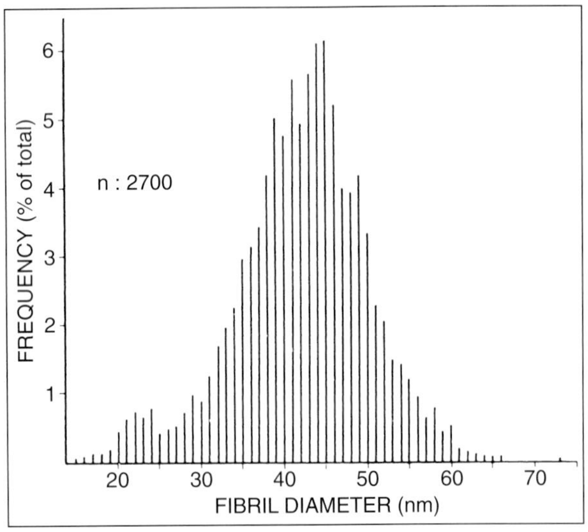

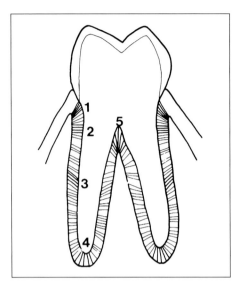

**Fig. 12.8** Histogram showing the range of collagen fibril diameters in the periodontal ligament.

**Fig. 12.9** The orientation of the principal fibres of the periodontal ligament seen in longitudinal section of a multirooted tooth: 1 = dentoalveolar crest fibres; 2 = horizontal fibres; 3 = oblique fibres; 4 = apical fibres; 5 = interradicular fibres.

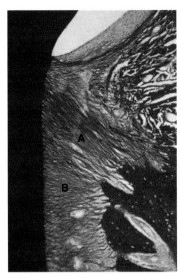

**Fig. 12.10** The dentoalveolar crest fibres (A) and the horizontal fibres (B) of the periodontal ligament (Decalcified, longitudinal section through the ligament in the region of the alveolar crest; aldehyde fuchsin and van Gieson; ×80).

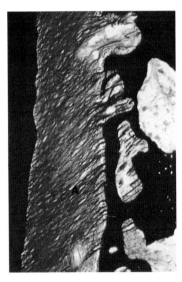

**Fig. 12.11** The oblique fibres (A) of the periodontal ligament (Decalcified, longitudinal section; aldehyde fuchsin and van Gieson; ×80).

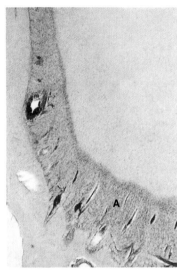

**Fig. 12.12** The apical fibres (A) of the periodontal ligament (Decalcified, longitudinal section through the ligament in the region of the root apex; aldehyde fuchsin and van Gieson; ×30).

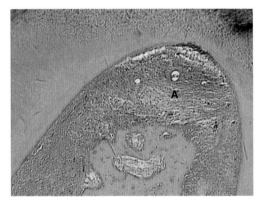

**Fig. 12.13** Interradicular fibres (A) of the periodontal ligament (Decalcified, longitudinal section of the ligament in the region of a root bifurcation; orange green and light green; ×40). Courtesy of Dr R. O'Sullivan.

(Fig. 12.7b). The histogram provided as Figure 12.8 shows that, for the rat periodontal ligament, there is a sharply unimodal distribution of collagen fibrils (range ≈20–70 nm) with a mode of approximately 42 nm. For humans, the mean is only slightly larger (50 nm). This confirms that the periodontal fibrils are small and of essentially uniform diameter. The pattern of distribution is reminiscent of collagen in connective tissues placed under compression and differs markedly from the bimodal distribution with large fibrils usually associated with tissues under tension (e.g. tendon). Research indicates that the distribution of periodontal collagen alters neither with changes in periodontal function nor with age. The lack of change with age differs from many other fibrous connective tissues.

The principal collagen fibres show different orientations in different regions of the periodontal ligament (Figs 12.9–12.13). They comprise: dentoalveolar crest fibres, horizontal fibres, oblique fibres, apical fibres and interradicular fibres. It has been usual to ascribe specific functions to each of the groups of principal fibres. For example, it has been suggested that the orientation of the oblique fibres shows that they form a suspensory

ligament, which translates pressure on the tooth into tensional forces on the alveolar wall. However, no physiological evidence exists to support such a concept and many of the structural features of the periodontal ligament (e.g. the collagen fibril diameters) suggest compression (see pages 201–203).

Controversy exists concerning the extent of individual fibres across the width of the periodontal ligament. One view holds that there are distinct tooth-related and bone-related fibres, and that these intercalate near the middle of the ligament at an intermediate plexus (Fig. 12.14). However, recent evidence suggests that the fibres cross the entire width of the periodontal space but branch en route and join neighbouring fibres to form a complex three-dimensional network. While remodelling of fibres in the intermediate plexus provides a convenient model to explain how such axial tooth movements as eruption may be sustained, the plexus is usually seen only in longitudinal sections of continuously growing incisors (of rodents and lagomorphs): it is not seen in cross-sections. Thus, the plexus is an artefact, probably related to the fact that the collagen fibres in the periodontal ligaments of continuously growing incisors are arranged mainly in the

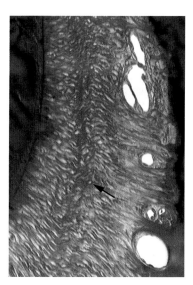

**Fig. 12.14** Longitudinal section through the periodontal ligament producing an appearance of an intermediate plexus (arrowed) (Decalcified, longitudinal section; Alcian blue; ×200).

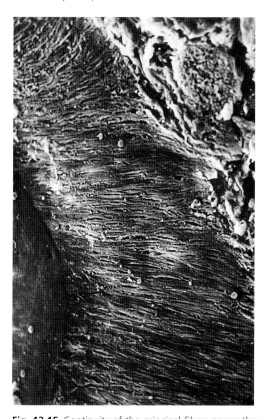

**Fig. 12.15** Continuity of the principal fibres across the periodontal space seen in a periodontal ligament cut transversely (SEM; ×500). Courtesy of Professor P. Sloan.

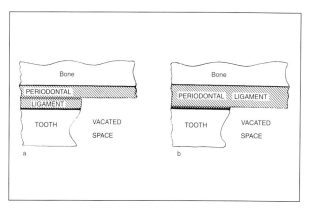

**Fig. 12.16** The effects of root resection on the periodontal ligament and its significance to the 'zone of shear' and tissue remodelling. (a) The situation that would pertain if the zone of shear occurs centrally within the periodontal ligament – the tooth-related part of the ligament should move with the tooth, leaving behind the bone-related tissue only. (b) The whole width of the ligament is left behind the erupting tooth, indicating that the zone of shear is close to the tooth surface.

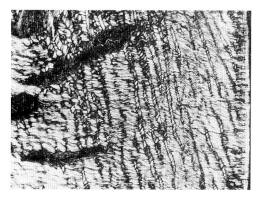

**Fig. 12.17** Crimping of collagen in the periodontal ligament as viewed under polarized light. The fibres are seen to be banded between crossed polars, reflecting an underlying periodicity along the fibre (Transverse section of the central region of the rabbit incisor periodontal ligament; polarizing optical micrograph; ×200). Courtesy of Professor P. Sloan.

form of sheets rather than bundles. The continuity of the principal fibres across the periodontal space in teeth of non-continuous growth is displayed in Figure 12.15. Here, no intermediate plexus can be seen, the fibres branching and joining with each other.

Despite the lack of histological evidence for an intermediate fibre plexus, it has been proposed that there is a 'zone of shear' – a site of remodelling during eruption. However, the location of this zone is in dispute. Some believe that it lies near the centre of the periodontal ligament, the relatively avascular, tooth-related part of the ligament moving with the erupting tooth. Studies using tritium-labelled proline have claimed that there is increased uptake in a zone in the mid-region of the periodontal ligament. However, other studies have been unable to support this, demonstrating uniform uptake of various labels over the whole width of the ligament. In contrast, counts of the number of intracellular collagen profiles in the periodontal fibroblasts (which indicate degenerating colla-

gen: see pages 188, 189) indicate that greater remodelling occurs in the centre of the tissue. The physiological significance of a central location for the zone of shear is thrown into doubt by experiments on the resected rodent incisor, which indicate that the zone of shear is close to the root surface (Fig. 12.16). Root resection involves surgical removal of the growing base of the incisor. Because this tooth continues to erupt, it passes up the socket, leaving a space below its base. Accordingly, if the zone of shear occurs centrally within the periodontal ligament, the tooth-related part of the ligament should move with the tooth, leaving behind the bone-related tissue only. In fact, the whole width of the ligament is left behind the erupting tooth, indicating that the zone of shear is close to the tooth surface. This is further supported by experiments where lathyrogens – drugs that inhibit the formation of collagen crosslinks – are administered in the rodent diet: the lathyritic rat periodontal ligament is characterized by a longitudinal cleft down the ligament adjacent to the tooth surface.

The principal fibres of the periodontal ligament do not necessarily run a straight course as they pass from the region of the alveolar bone to the tooth. Indeed, they are said to be wavy, although it is not known whether the waviness is real or is an artefact of histological preparation. If real, it could have important implications for the biomechanical properties of the ligament and consequently the mechanism of tooth support (see pages 201–203). A specific type of waviness seen in collagenous tissues (including the periodontal ligament) is crimping. Collagen crimps are best seen under the polarizing microscope (Fig. 12.17). The fibres are banded in polarized light, reflecting an underlying periodicity along the fibre. The

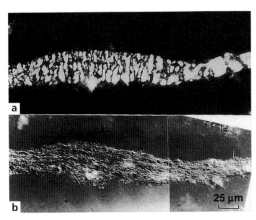

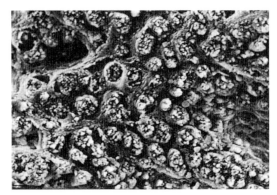

**Fig. 12.20** SEM of Sharpey fibres in the alveolar bone showing 'stub-like' appearance (×300). Courtesy of Professor P. Sloan.

**Fig. 12.18** Crimping displayed in a single teased-out collagen fibre from the periodontal ligament. (a) Polarizing optical micrograph. (b) Nomarski differential interference contrast of same field as (a) (×200). Courtesy of Dr L.J. Gathercole.

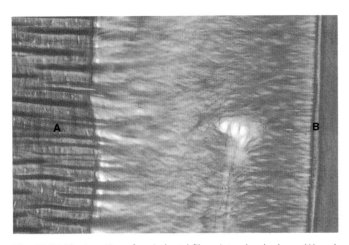

**Fig. 12.19** The insertion of periodontal fibres into alveolar bone (A) and cementum (B). The horizontal lines in the bone and cementum represent the Sharpey fibres (Decalcified section; aldehyde fuchsin and van Gieson; ×250).

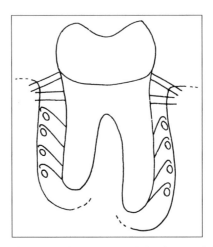

**Fig. 12.21** The location and distribution of Sharpey fibres from the periodontal collagen along the tooth socket.

period is about 16 μm and the angular deflection from the fibre axis in excess of 20°. It is important to realize that the banding does not rely on seeing shapes (waves in particular); the alternating dark and bright bands are evident in otherwise straight and smooth cylindrical fibres. Indeed, crimping can be displayed in a single, teased-out collagen fibre from the periodontal ligament (Fig. 12.18) and the banding relates to the wavy course of the fibrils in the bundle. In functional terms, it has been proposed that the crimp is gradually pulled out when the ligament is subjected to mechanical tension, until it eventually disappears.

The principal fibres of the periodontal ligament that are embedded into cementum and the bone lining the tooth socket are termed Sharpey fibres (Fig. 12.19). The principal fibres are more numerous, but smaller, at their attachments into cementum than at the alveolar bone. Under the electron microscope, the mineralized parts of the Sharpey fibres in alveolar bone (Fig. 12.20) appear as projecting stubs covered with mineral clusters. The occurrence of mineralization at approximately right angles to the long axes of the fibres may indicate that, in function, the fibres are subjected to tensional forces. The location and distribution of Sharpey fibres from the periodontal collagen along the tooth socket is illustrated in Figure 12.21. This diagram is conjectured from data obtained from a variety of species and suggests that the fibres near the alveolar crest show pronounced Sharpey fibre insertions. Elsewhere, however, many of the principal fibres in the periodontal ligament do not insert into bone but appear to terminate around the blood vessels of the ligament.

The rate of turnover of collagen within the periodontal ligament is faster than virtually all other connective tissues (half-life of collagen 3–23 days). The rate appears to vary in different parts of the same tooth, being highest towards the root apex. However, turnover seems to be relatively even across the width of the periodontal ligament, perhaps providing evidence against the existence of separate tooth-related and bone-related parts to the tissue (see page 183). The explanation for the high rate of turnover is not known, but it is reasonable to suppose that the high rate may relate to the considerable functional demands placed upon the tooth in terms of remodelling as a reaction to occlusal stress and to tooth movements. However, the ligaments of teeth subjected to greatly reduced masticatory loads do not show different rates of turnover from teeth subjected to normal loads. Furthermore, the turnover rate in teeth erupting very rapidly is no different from that in the ligaments of fully erupted teeth.

Recent studies indicate that measuring rates may not reflect total protein turnover and that there may be several protein pools having different turnover rates, each contributing to a different extent to overall protein turnover in the periodontal ligament. Indeed, control of matrix morphostasis may be more dependent on extracellular processing (e.g. fibrillogenesis, proteolysis) than upon initial rate of protein secretion. For example, far more collagen may be synthesized than is eventually secreted, the excess being degraded intracellularly without ever leaving the cell.

The high rate of turnover may also be reflected in the type of reducible crosslink found in the periodontal collagen (i.e. dehydrodihydroxylysinonorleucine).

The possible role of the periodontal collagen in tooth support and tooth eruption is considered further on pages 201–203 and 362–365 respectively.

## OXYTALAN

Depending upon species, the periodontal ligament contains either oxytalan fibres or elastin fibres: in humans, it contains oxytalan fibres. In order to demonstrate periodontal oxytalan fibres at the light microscope level it is necessary to oxidize tissue sections strongly before staining with certain elastin stains. Unlike collagen, oxytalan fibres are not susceptible to acid hydrolysis. Although little is known about their composition, their ultrastructural characteristics suggest that they are immature elastin fibres (pre-elastin) and they appear to have elastin and type VI collagen components.

Oxytalan fibres are attached into the cementum of the tooth and course out into the periodontal ligament in various directions (Fig. 12.22), rarely being incorporated into bone. In the cervical region, they follow the course of gingival and transseptal collagen fibres but within the periodontal ligament proper they tend to be more longitudinally oriented, crossing the oblique fibre bundles more or less perpendicularly. In the outer part of the ligament, they are said to often terminate around blood vessels and nerves. Oxytalan fibres vary from 0.5 μm to 2.5 μm in diameter (as assessed with the light microscope) and constitute no more than about 3% of the extracellular fibre composition. The oxytalan fibre can be recognized at the ultrastructural level (Fig. 12.23) as a collection of unbanded fibrils arranged parallel to the long axis of the fibre. Each fibril is approximately 15 nm in diameter and an interfibrillar amorphous material is present in variable amounts. In cross-section, the oxytalan fibre is oval and its dimensions are smaller than reported using the light microscope. They are thought to resemble pre-elastin in that, unlike mature elastin, there is no central amorphous core.

The functions of the oxytalan fibres remain unknown and there is a paucity of experimental data. They are said to be thicker and more numerous in teeth that carry abnormally high loads, including abutment teeth for bridges and teeth being moved for orthodontic reasons. Thus, it appears that oxytalan may have a role in tooth support (perhaps also indicated by the relationship with the periodontal vasculature). However, experimental evidence shows that oxytalan fibres do not change with age or reduction in masticatory loading. Elastin fibres are restricted to the walls of the blood vessels, although in some animals (e.g. herbivores) they replace the oxytalan fibres. Reticulin fibres are related to basement membranes within the periodontal ligament (i.e. associated with blood vessels and epithelial cell rests) and are a variety of collagen.

Oxytalan microfibrils have a similar ultrastructure to the fibrils of fibronectin. In addition, they are stained strongly by immunohistochemical stains for fibronectin (Fig. 12.24). As fibronectin is important in fibroblast adhesion and migration, this would support the suggestion that oxytalan fibres aid fibroblast migration in the periodontal ligament.

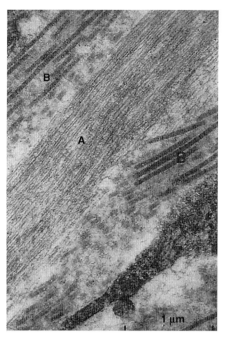

**Fig. 12.23** TEM of an oxytalan fibre (A). B = collagen fibres (×25 000).

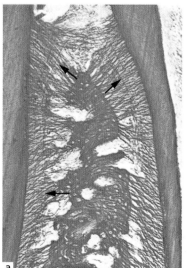
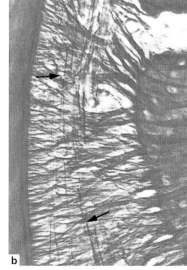

**Fig 12.22** The course of oxytalan fibres (arrowed) (Decalcified, longitudinal section through the periodontal ligament; potassium monopersulphate, aldehyde fuchsin counterstained with van Gieson; (a) ×40; (b) ×120). Courtesy of Dr A.D. Beynon.

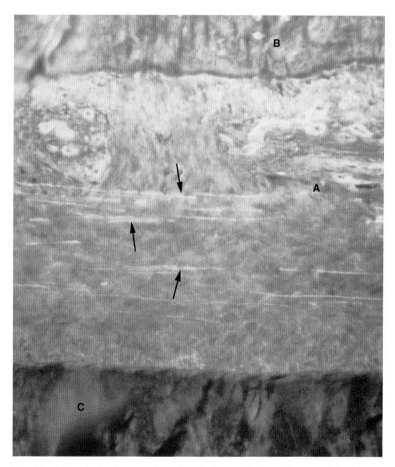

**Fig. 12.24** Longitudinal cryosection of rat incisor periodontal ligament (A) with immunofluorescent staining for fibronectin showing positive staining (arrows) with the same longitudinal orientation as for oxytalan fibres. B = alveolar bone; C = tooth (×55). From Sloan P, Carter DH 1995 Structural organisation of the fibres of the periodontal ligament. In: Berkovitz BKB, Moxham BJ, Newman H (eds) *The periodontal ligament in health and disease*, 2nd edn. Mosby–Wolfe, London, pp 35–53.

## GROUND SUBSTANCE

Because of its relative inaccessibility and complex biochemical nature, little detailed information concerning this important component of the periodontal ligament is available. Although we are used to thinking of the ligament as a collagen-rich tissue, in reality it is a tissue rich in ground substance. Indeed, even the collagen fibre bundles are composed of about 60% ground substance by volume (Fig. 12.25). Furthermore, 70% of the ground substance comprises bound water. The turnover rate of the components of the periodontal ligament ground substance is more rapid than that for the collagens.

The ground substance of the periodontal ligament consists mainly of glycosaminoglycans, proteoglycans and glycoproteins. All components of the periodontal ligament ground substance are presumed to be secreted by fibroblasts. The main type of glycosaminoglycan is hyaluronan, although dermatan, chondroitin and heparin sulphates are also found. Much of the glycosaminoglycan is located near the surfaces of the collagen fibrils. Hyaluronan is a highly charged molecule and this type of glycosaminoglycan occupies a large volume of the periodontal ligament. Consequently,

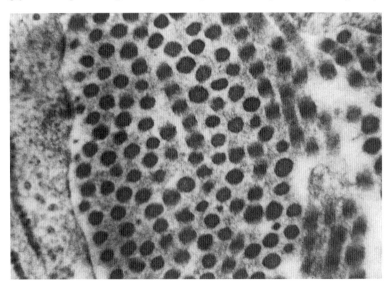

**Fig. 12.25** Electron micrograph of the extracellular matrix of the periodontal ligament. About 60% by volume is ground substance (TEM; ×100 000).

it has a major influence upon the permeability of the tissue. It can also influence cell motility.

The proteoglycans are compounds containing anionic polysaccharides (glycosaminoglycans) covalently attached to a protein core. Two main proteoglycans have been isolated in the periodontal ligament: proteodermatan sulphate and a proteoglycan containing chondroitin sulphate/dermatan sulphate hybrids. Proteodermatan sulphate proteoglycan is related to decorin in skin whereas the other proteoglycans are akin to biglycan. Decorin proteoglycans are known to assist collagen fibrillogenesis and increases the strength of collagen fibrils. Biglycan is thought to control the hydration of the extracellular matrix of a connective tissue.

The ground substance is thought to have many important functions (ion and water binding and exchange, control of collagen fibrillogenesis and fibre orientation, binding of growth factors). Tissue fluid pressure is high in the periodontal ligament, about 10 mmHg above atmospheric pressure, and the tissue fluid has been implicated in the tooth support and eruptive mechanisms (see pages 201–203, 362–365). Furthermore, the composition of the ground substance in the periodontal ligament varies according to the developmental state of the tissue (Fig. 12.26) and according to location (Fig. 12.27). The data suggest that there is a marked change in the amount of hyaluronan as development proceeds from the dental follicle to the initial periodontal ligament, a trend that occurs during embryonic development of other connective tissues. Furthermore, a significant increase in the amount of proteoglycans occurs during eruption.

The nature of the ground substance may also explain why the periodontal ligament rarely mineralizes, as it may act as an inhibitor of this process. This is suggested by in vitro experiments whereby enzymes that degrade elements of the ground substance (hyaluronidase and chondroitinase) have been applied and, following the addition of mineralizing solutions, mineral crystals appear within the periodontal ligament (but do not appear within the normal ligament). Calcium-binding proteins such as S100A4 in the extracellular matrix have also been implicated in inhibiting mineralization in the periodontal ligament. In cases of ankylosis, the homeostasis controlling the width of the ligament is disrupted. Experimentally, ankylosis can be produced by the administration of a bisphosphonate (which may act by reducing cell numbers and by inducing the expression of the osteogenic factors in the body of the periodontal ligament).

Much interest has been shown in a complex glycoprotein called fibronectin. This protein is thought to promote attachment of cells to the

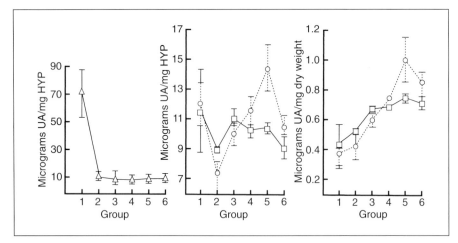

**Fig. 12.26** Glycosaminoglycans in the periodontal ligament at different stages of development (from bovine incisors). △ = Hyaluronate; □ = proteodermatan sulphate; ○ = PG1 proteoglycan. Group 1 specimens are of dental follicle. Group 2 is the initial stage of formation of the periodontal ligament. Sharpey fibre attachments were discernible in group 3. Groups 4 and 5 were for erupting teeth (the typical orientation of collagen fibres being first observed in group 5). Group 6 specimens were from fully erupted teeth. HYP = hydroxyproline, enabling determinations of ground substance components relative to collagen content. From Pearson CH 1982 The ground substance of the periodontal ligament. In: Berkovitz BKB, Moxham BJ, Newman HJ (eds) *The periodontal ligament in health and disease*, 1st edn. Pergamon Press, Oxford, pp 119–149.

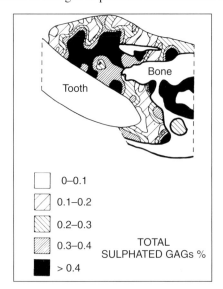

**Fig. 12.27** Glycosaminoglycans (sulphated GAGs) at different sites in the periodontal connective tissues (from sheep incisors). From Kirkham J, Robinson C, Spence J 1989 Site specific variations in the biochemical composition of healthy sheep periodontium. *Archives of Oral Biology* 34: 405–411.

substratum, especially to collagen fibrils. Furthermore, as cells preferentially adhere to fibronectin, it may be involved in cell migration and orientation. Considering these functions together with the high rate of turnover in the periodontal ligament, it is not surprising that fibronectin may have considerable biological significance within the periodontal ligament. Immunofluorescent techniques at the light microscope level have revealed that fibronectin is uniformly distributed throughout the periodontal ligament in both erupting and fully erupted teeth. Ultrastructural studies have localized the glycoprotein over collagen fibres and at certain sites on the cell–collagen interface. As loss of fibronectin has been observed during the terminal maturation of many connective matrices, its continued presence within the periodontal ligament may be indicative of the ligament retaining immature, fetal-like characteristics. Clinically, fibronectin has been employed to 'condition' the roots of teeth in expectation of improving periodontal wound healing. Tenascin and vitronectin are other glycoproteins that have been identified in the periodontal ligament. Like fibronectin, tenascin is more characteristic of a fetal-like connective tissue than a fully 'mature' connective tissue. Unlike fibronectin, tenascin is not uniformly localized throughout the ligament but is concentrated adjacent to the alveolar bone and the cementum. Vitronectin is associated with elastin fibres. The role of these glycoproteins in the functions of the periodontal ligament still awaits clarification. However, they may play a role in tissue remodelling since there are important reactions between the matrix and fibroblast surface receptors that can change cell secretion of collagen to secretion of extracellular matrix degradative enzymes.

Analysis of the ground substance following the onset of periodontal disease indicates that there may be a change in the content of the ground substance of the periodontal ligament, with a decrease in the dermatan sulphate content and an increase in chondroitin sulphate. Occlusal hypofunction results in remodelling of the ligament with a significant decrease of chondroitin sulphate, decorin and heparin sulphate. That there are differences in the ground substance (as well as in the nature of collagen) between the periodontal ligament and adjacent alveolar bone may provide a clinical diagnostic tool when analysing gingival crevicular fluid to assess, and predict, patient susceptibility to further progress of the disease.

## CELLS

Although the predominant connective tissue cell within the periodontal ligament is the fibroblast, the tissue presents a heterogeneous population (Fig. 12.28). Formative cells covering the surface of both cementum and alveolar bone (i.e. cementoblasts and osteoblasts) are considered part of the ligament and have a similar mesenchymal origin. Resorbing cells on the surface of bone and cementum are osteoclasts and cementoclasts; these are derived from a monocyte/macrophage lineage from the blood. In addition, the periodontal ligament contains undifferentiated mesenchymal cells (stem cells and precursors such as preosteoblasts and precementoblasts), defence cells and epithelial cells (rests of Malassez). The type and number of cells varies according to the functional state of the ligament.

## FIBROBLASTS

The fibroblasts in the periodontal ligament are responsible for regeneration of the tooth support apparatus and have an essential role in the adaptive responses to mechanical loading of the tooth (including orthodontic loading). The periodontal ligament fibroblasts (Figs 12.29, 12.30) seem to

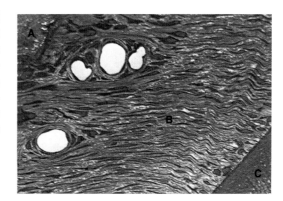

**Fig. 12.29** A periodontal ligament (B) comprising numerous fibroblasts. A = alveolar bone; C = cementum (Decalcified, longitudinal section through the periodontal ligament; toluidine blue; ×300).

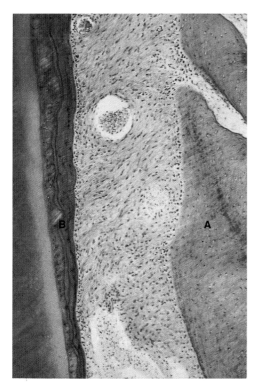

**Fig. 12.28** The distribution of cells in the periodontal ligament. In addition to the numerous fibroblasts within the ligament, the surfaces of the alveolar bone (A) and cementum (B) are lined with osteoblasts and cementoblasts, indicating active deposition of bone and cementum in this specimen (Decalcified, longitudinal section through the periodontal ligament; H & E; ×80).

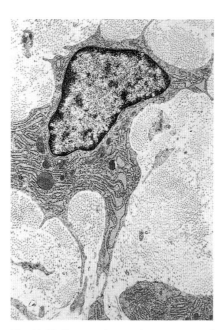

**Fig. 12.30** Electronmicroscopic appearance of a periodontal fibroblast in vivo (TEM; ×4000).

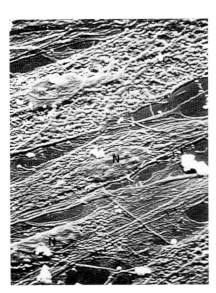

**Fig. 12.31** The appearance of motile periodontal fibroblasts cultured on plastic. N = nucleus (SEM; ×1200).

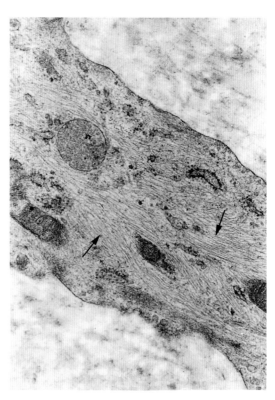

**Fig. 12.32** The appearance of contractile periodontal fibroblasts cultured on collagen gels. Note the numerous microfilaments (arrows) (TEM; ×30 000). Courtesy of Dr C.A. Shuttleworth.

have a variety of shapes with many fine cytoplasmic processes, although they are usually described as being fusiform. However, the overall shape can only be determined by consideration of the cell outlines in different planes. When this is done, the periodontal fibroblasts often appear as flattened, disc-shaped cells. However, in vitro studies (see below) have led to the suggestion that the periodontal ligament fibroblasts are polarized with respect to the site of secretion of collagen, which appears to take place preferentially at one end of the cell.

Periodontal fibroblasts, being very active cells, have low nuclear:cytoplasmic ratios, and each nucleus contains one or more prominent nucleoli. The typical periodontal fibroblast is rich in the intracytoplasmic organelles associated with the synthesis and export of proteins: rough endoplasmic reticulum, Golgi material and mitochondria (Fig. 12.30). Indeed, the high rate of protein synthesis in the periodontal ligament is shown by autoradiographic studies involving tritiated proline or glycine. The findings indicate that, within 30 minutes of the injection of the tritiated amino acids, labelled collagen appeared in the extracellular matrix of the periodontal ligament. Progenitor fibroblasts are said to be smaller than the mature fibroblasts in the periodontal ligament and have less distinct Golgi apparatus and rough endoplasmic reticulum.

Periodontal ligament fibroblasts differ in several respects from gingival fibroblasts. First, they are derived from different sources. Periodontal ligament fibroblasts are ectomesenchymal, being derived from the neural crest (see page 299), whereas gingival fibroblasts are mesodermal in origin. Second, the gingival fibroblasts are less proliferative. Third, the expression of alkaline phosphatase and cAMP is greater in periodontal ligament fibroblasts. Other features distinguishing fibroblasts from the periodontal ligament and the gingiva are shown in Table 25.2 on page 355.

Much has been made of the possibility that the periodontal fibroblasts are motile–contractile cells and that they are thereby capable of generating a force responsible for tooth eruption. Much of the evidence for migratory or contractile activities comes from research on the behaviour and appearance of periodontal fibroblasts in vitro. In vitro, periodontal fibroblasts can organize a fibrous network and can generate significant forces. However, the behaviour and appearance depends upon the method of culture. For example, cells cultured on plastic (Fig. 12.31) assume the properties of motile cells, are thin and highly polarized with respect to both shape and location of organelles. In particular, there are numerous microtubules and microfilaments (as stress fibres) that run along the length of the cell. Cells with these characteristics have not been seen in the periodontal ligament in vivo. Periodontal fibroblasts cultured on collagen gels (Fig. 12.32),

during contraction of the gel, assume the appearance of myofibroblasts (see also pages 363, 364), cells that have the properties of both fibroblasts and smooth muscle cells, and are found in contracting wounds. Myofibroblasts are characterized ultrastructurally by having polarity of shape, crenulated (folded) nuclei and numerous microfilaments (as shown in Fig. 12.32). Adjacent cells contact by means of gap junctions. While periodontal fibroblasts in vivo may show occasional gap junctions (see Fig. 12.36b), they show no other features characteristic of myofibroblasts. Thus, although the evidence from in vitro studies suggests that the periodontal fibroblasts have the potential to be migratory or contractile cells, under normal functional conditions the cells are primarily involved in protein synthesis and secretion.

There is sufficient evidence, however, to show that there may be some localized movement of cells in the periodontal ligament in vivo and that the migration may be directed along the collagen fibres in an apicocoronal direction. Such migration is likely to be dependent on appropriate chemotactic stimuli. Evidence suggests that extracts from both bone and cementum have a potent chemotactic influence upon periodontal fibroblasts. The dependence of migratory behaviours upon the cytoskeleton and upon surface integrins has also been suggested. New populations of periodontal fibroblasts, osteoblasts and cementoblasts appear to arise from stem cells in the vicinity of blood vessels and then migrate to other regions of the ligament. However, how much the change in position of periodontal cells is due to active, rather than passive, movements (i.e. being carried with tooth movements) awaits clarification.

There is evidence that, in addition to synthesizing and secreting proteins, the cells are responsible for collagen degradation. This contrasts with earlier views that degradation was essentially an extracellular event involving the activity of proteolytic enzymes such as collagenases. The main evidence indicating that the periodontal fibroblasts are also 'fibroclastic' is the presence of organelles termed intracellular collagen profiles (Figs 12.33, 12.34). These profiles show banded collagen fibrils within an elongated membrane-bound vacuole. It is thought that the intracellular collagen vacuoles are associated with the degradation of collagen that has been

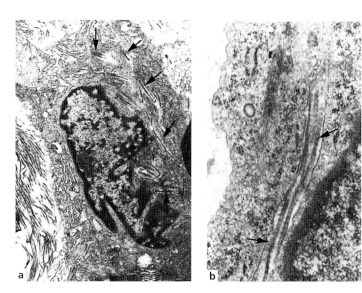

**Fig. 12.33** (a) Periodontal fibroblast showing intracellular collagen profiles (arrowed) (TEM; ×5000) (b) Banded collagen fibrils (arrowed) seen within an elongated membrane-bound vacuole (TEM; ×25 000).

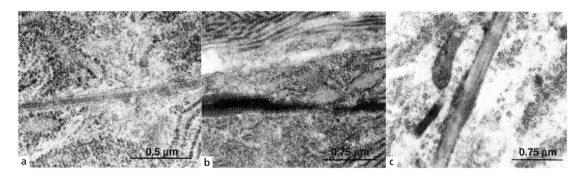

**Fig. 12.34** The temporal sequence for intracellular digestion of collagen in the periodontal ligament. (a) Banded fibril surrounded by an electron-lucent zone. (b) Banded fibrils surrounded by an electron-dense zone. (c) Fibrils with indistinct banding surrounded by an electron-dense zone (TEM). From Berkovitz BKB, Shore RC 1995 Cells of the periodontal ligament. In: Berkovitz BKB, Moxham BJ, Newman HJ (eds) *The periodontal ligament in health and disease*, 2nd edn. Mosby–Wolfe, London, pp 9–33.

'ingested' from the extracellular environment. The temporal sequence for intracellular digestion of collagen in the periodontal ligament is illustrated in Figure 12.34. When a collagen fibril is first phagocytosed by the fibroblast, a banded fibril surrounded by an electron-lucent zone is seen. Subsequently, the banded fibrils are surrounded by an electron-dense zone. At this stage, the phagosome fuses with primary lysosomes to form a phagolysosome in which there is a gradual increase in electron density of the matrix. At the terminal stage, the fibrils show indistinct banding and are surrounded by an electron-dense zone: enzymic degeneration of the fibril has proceeded to the point where the fibril loses its characteristic structure. The time taken to degrade collagen intracellularly is not known, although about 30 minutes has been suggested (a time similar to that required for synthesis). Evidence suggests that biochemically the internal degradation of collagen involves not matrix metalloproteinase (MMP)-1 but acid phosphatase and cathepsins. In addition, cell surface located alkaline phosphatase and MMPs may be involved in the process of internalizing a collagen fibril from the extracellular matrix.

It has been argued that the collagen profiles within periodontal fibroblasts are not truly intracellular and that the collagen merely lies in surface invaginations. If this were so, the degradation would still be an extracellular phenomenon. It has also been suggested that, because the periodontal fibroblasts may be synthesizing collagen in excess of requirements, the profiles contain collagen that is being degraded without ever having been secreted extracellularly. Overall, however, the evidence suggests that the collagen is ingested from the extracellular compartment of the periodontal ligament and that the profiles are intracellular. Nevertheless, it is not known whether all periodontal fibroblasts are capable of phagocytosis.

The degradation of collagen may be expected to include both extracellular and intracellular events. There is, however, little evidence for the presence of the enzyme collagenase within the normal periodontal ligament, and other experimental data suggest that collagenase is not essential for collagen remodelling. If this is correct, then other enzymes (e.g. cysteine proteinase) and other metalloproteinases are involved in collagen remodelling in the normal physiological situation. Fibroblasts in the periodontal ligament secrete matrix metalloproteinase-1 (which degrades extracellular matrix collagen at physiological conditions) and can secrete tissue inhibitors of metalloproteinases (TIMPs). TIMPs are found in high concentrations at healthy periodontal sites.

Collagenase production and phagocytosis can be upregulated after exposure to cytokines such as prostaglandin $E_2$, interleukin (IL)-1 or lectin concanavalin A. Furthermore, because fibroblasts are induced to secrete prostaglandin when mechanical loads are applied, the periodontal fibroblasts may have 'intrinsic' mechanisms for remodelling the matrix. However, the precise role of collagenase in physiological remodelling awaits clarification as inhibition of its activity in vitro does not prevent the ingestion of collagen by fibroblasts.

As the amount of collagen present within the periodontal ligament must represent a balance between the rate of synthesis and the rate of degradation, the loss of collagen (e.g. during periodontal disease) could result from either a more rapid rate of breakdown and/or a slower rate of synthesis, and/or the loss of fibroblasts. Furthermore, the process of collagen loss during periodontal disease probably represents a different process, as in the diseased inflammatory state there is evidence for the activity of collagenase. The presence of TIMPs in the periodontal ligament, some produced by its fibroblasts, provides the rationale for the use of drugs that have a similar activity to combat periodontal disease, such as the designer tetracycline doxycycline.

The fibroblasts of the periodontal ligament have cilia and many intercellular contacts, a feature that is not particularly common in the fibroblasts of other fibrous connective tissues (intercellular contacts are a feature of fibroblasts in fetal-like connective tissues). Figure 12.35 shows a cilium lying within an invagination of the cell membrane of a periodontal ligament fibroblast. The cilium differs from those seen in other cell types in that it contains no more than nine tubule doublets (compared to the usual '9 plus 2' configuration). The significance of the cilia in fibroblasts is unknown, although they may be associated with control of the cell cycle or inhibition of centriolar activity. The intercellular contacts (simplified desmosomes and gap junctions) between the fibroblasts of the periodontal ligament are shown in Figure 12.36. The simplified desmosome is the most frequently seen of the contacts. There is little information concerning the functional significance of these organelles in the periodontal fibroblast.

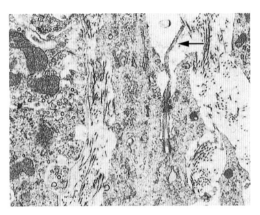

**Fig. 12.35** A cilium (arrowed) lying within an invagination of the cell membrane of a periodontal ligament fibroblast (TEM; ×11 000).

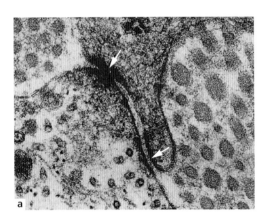

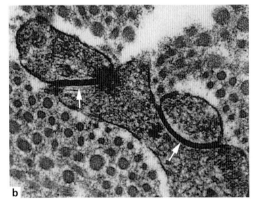

**Fig. 12.36** Intercellular contacts (arrowed) between the fibroblasts of the periodontal ligament. (a) Simplified desmosome. (b) Gap junction. (TEM; ×80 000.)

## Cytoskeleton

As expected for cells of mesenchymal origin, periodontal ligament fibroblasts label for vimentin intermediate cytoskeletal filaments at all stages of development (Fig. 12.37) and there is no labelling for cytokeratins, tubulin or F-actin in the 'mature' periodontal ligament. However, labelling for cytokeratin 19 (an intermediate filament usually associated with epithelial cells) occurs during the active stage of a tooth's eruption (Fig. 12.38). Furthermore, transient expression for cytokeratin 19 can be observed in the aged periodontal ligament (Fig. 12.39). Some changes in labelling for vimentin are also detected in the aged tissues, labelling being weaker in cementoblasts and fibroblasts contained in the cementum-related portion of the periodontal ligament. The coexpression of cytokeratins and vimentin is not unknown for mesenchymal cells, being reported for those of the eye, choroid plexus fibroblasts, chondrocytes and in regenerating organs.

The functions of intermediate filaments are poorly understood but are presumed to be structural. There is some evidence to suggest that cells may increase their intermediate filament content in response to mechanical loading. Where coexpression of different intermediate filaments occurs, these cytoskeletal elements have been associated with the cell environment, cell shape or the possible secretory activity of the cell. The specific distribution of different intermediate filaments indicates particular functions for these elements within tissues. For instance, the presence of cytokeratins could be related to the combined shear and compressive

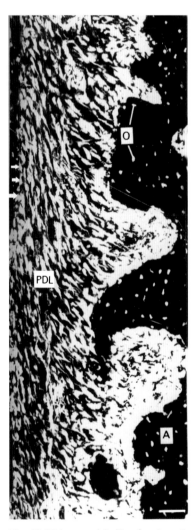

**Fig. 12.37** Immunolabelling for vimentin intermediate cytoskeletal filaments in cells of the mature (non-aged) periodontal ligament. The labelling is observed in the fibroblasts of the periodontal ligament (PDL), osteocytes (O) within alveolar bone (A) and cementoblasts (arrows) lining the root surface. Bar = 100 μm.

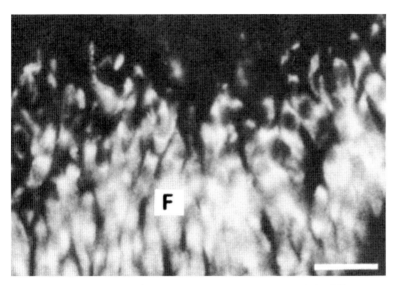

**Fig. 12.38** Immunolabelling for cytokeratin-19 intermediate cytoskeletal filaments in periodontal ligament fibroblasts (F) during an active stage of eruption. Bar = 25 μm.

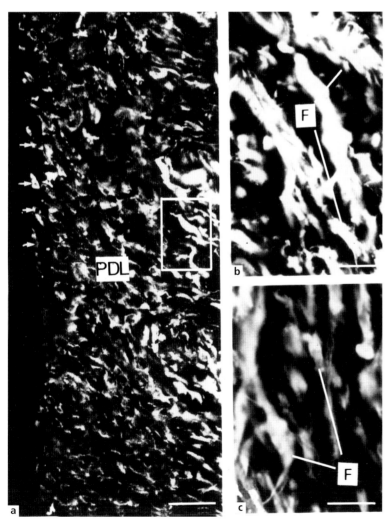

**Fig. 12.39** Immunolabelling for immediate filaments in cells of the aged periodontal ligament. (a) Vimentin labelling in the periodontal ligament (PDL) and cementoblasts (arrows) was reduced in comparison with earlier stages (see Fig. 12.37). Bar = 100 μm. (b) Higher-power view of the region enclosed by the rectangle in (a) showing labelling for vimentin in fibroblasts (F) of the periodontal ligament. Bar = 10 μm. (c) Cytokeratin-19 labelling in periodontal ligament fibroblasts (F). Bar = 15 μm.

forces to which they are subjected. The accumulation of vimentin may also be related to mechanical loading.

That periodontal fibroblasts transiently express cytokeratin 19 during the active phase of tooth eruption could relate to the fact that the periodontal ligament must undergo major structural reorganization of its extracellular matrix. It has been suggested that intermediate filaments could form part of a mechanotransduction system that enables the cells to respond to external forces and sense changes in the extracellular matrix. Thus, the expression of an additional type of filament could be related to the effects of periodontal ligament remodelling and the changing conditions during tooth eruption. In epithelia, cytokeratin 19 commonly occurs at sites of rapid cell proliferation. This may also be the case in the periodontal ligament at the time of eruption. However, this explanation for the expression of cytokeratin 19 in the aged periodontal tissue is difficult to sustain. To understand the processes involved, we need to know much more about the biomechanical properties and remodelling characteristics of the periodontal ligament with age. However, despite the obvious importance (both biologically and clinically) of investigating the effects of ageing on the oral fibrous connective tissues, our understanding of this subject is at present poor. There have been, for example, remarkably few studies concerned with the changing composition and functions of the periodontal ligament, and the effects of ageing upon the turnover rates of the extracellular matrices have yet to be assessed.

## Growth Factors and Cytokines

The activities of periodontal ligament fibroblasts are modulated by numerous bioactive molecules. These molecules may be produced by the cells themselves, be produced by local inflammatory cells or be present within the extracellular matrix of the periodontal ligament or of bone and cementum. They include growth factors and cytokines. The cell membrane also contains a multitude of receptors to bioactive molecules. At the cell–matrix interface are found a group of adhesion molecules, the integrins, that regulate many cellular activities, including those relating to cell spreading, cytoskeletal reorganization and apoptosis. Through the activities of bioactive molecules and receptors, the fibroblast is involved in maintaining homeostasis. There may be rapid up- or down-regulation of activities following, for example, the application of mechanical stress associated with orthodontic tooth movement or the onset of periodontal inflammation. Periodontal ligament fibroblasts produce numerous growth factors and cytokines, such as insulin-like growth factor (IGF)-I, bone morphogenetic proteins (BMPs), platelet-derived growth factor (PDGF) and IL-1. Transforming grown factor (TGF)β, for example, stimulates the synthesis of collagen and inhibits the synthesis of metalloproteinases such as collagenase. It is not surprising, therefore, that increased production of cytokines is related to the onset of tissue damage. Fibroblasts may release factors that inhibit osteoclastic differentiation and function (e.g. osteoprotegerin), while supporting it by expressing RANKL (receptor activator nuclear factor kappa B ligand) on its surface. The cells also release prostaglandins, which may influence bone cell activity. Periodontal ligament fibroblasts are rich in substances such as alkaline phosphatase (that might be related to the formation of acellular cementum) cellular retinoic acid-binding protein, and in receptors to epidermal growth factor (that may inhibit the fibroblast from differentiating into a cementoblast/osteoblast that lacks such receptors). Presumably, periodontal ligament fibroblasts have the genome to produce any of the proteins in the body, but the majority of these are inactivated. For example, whereas the cell does not normally produce elastin in vivo (or only in negligible amounts), in vitro tropoelastin mRNA is transcribed. This transcription is suppressed by basic fibroblast growth factor, suggesting one possible role for this

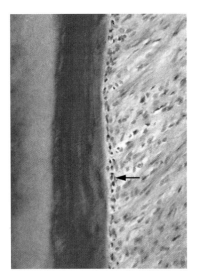

**Fig. 12.40** A layer of cementoblasts (arrowed) lining the cementum (Decalcified, longitudinal section of periodontal ligament; H & E; ×160).

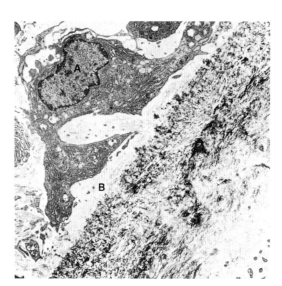

**Fig. 12.41** A cementoblast (A) lining cementum. B = precementum (TEM; ×3700).

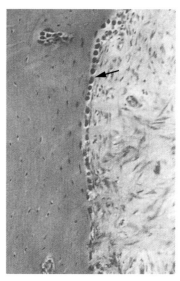

**Fig. 12.42** A layer of osteoblasts (arrowed) lining the alveolar bone (Decalcified, longitudinal section of periodontal ligament, H & E; ×230).

growth factor. Bioactive molecules, such as TGFβ, IGF-I, PDGF, BMP-2, BMP-7 and fibroblast growth factor (FGF-2), that can regulate the proliferation and differentiation of fibroblasts, osteoblasts and cementoblasts, as well as promoting angiogenesis, have been applied in animal models, alone and in combination, in the hope of inducing/improving periodontal regeneration, with varying degrees of success being reported. However, whether any of these growth factors will be found to be suitable for promoting periodontal regeneration in humans remains to be seen (see also pages 355, 356).

## CEMENTOBLASTS

The connective tissue cells of the periodontal ligament also include cementoblasts and cementoclasts, and osteoblasts and osteoclasts. Cementoblasts are the cement-forming cells lining the surface of cementum (Figs 12.40, 12.41). Cementoblasts are not as elongated as periodontal fibroblasts, being squat cuboidal cells. They are rich in cytoplasm and have large nuclei. Like fibroblasts, they contain all the intracytoplasmic organelles necessary for protein synthesis and secretion. The nucleus of a cementoblast is distinctly vesicular, with one or more nucleoli. The appearance of a cementoblast will depend upon its degree of activity. Cells actively depositing acellular cementum do not have prominent cytoplasmic processes. However, cells depositing cellular cementum exhibit abundant basophilic cytoplasm and cytoplasmic processes, and their nuclei tend to be folded and irregularly shaped (see also pages 347–353).

## OSTEOBLASTS

Osteoblasts are the bone-forming cells lining the tooth socket (Fig. 12.42), closely resembling cementoblasts. The layer of osteoblasts is prominent only when there is active bone formation. Each osteoblast appears cuboidal and exhibits a basophilic cytoplasm that is related to the extensive endoplasmic reticulum within the cell. The prominent, round nucleus tends to lie towards the basal end of the cell. A pale, juxtanuclear area indicates the site of the Golgi apparatus. When bone is not forming, its surface is occupied by flattened, inactive, bone-lining cells. Like the periodontal

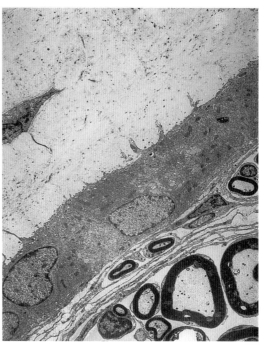

**Fig. 12.43** Ultrastructural features of the osteoblast (TEM; Decalcified section. ×6000).

fibroblasts, active osteoblasts contain an extensive rough endoplasmic reticulum and numerous mitochondria and vesicles (Fig. 12.43) although their Golgi apparatus appears more localized and extensive. Microfilaments are prominent beneath the cell membrane at the secreting surface. The cells contact one another by means of desmosomes and tight junctions. The cell surface adjacent to bone has many fine cytoplasmic processes, some of which contact underlying osteocytes by tight junctions to form part of a transport system throughout the bone (see also page 209).

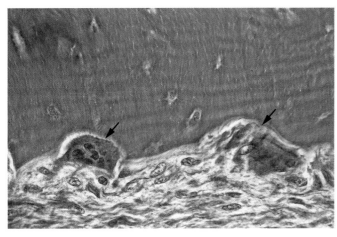

**Fig. 12.44** Resorbing alveolar bone and the osteoclast. Resorption concavities termed Howship's lacunae in which lie osteoclasts are arrowed (Decalcified, longitudinal section of the periodontal ligament; H & E; ×250). Courtesy of Professor M.M. Smith.

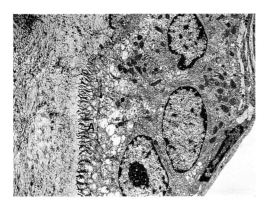

**Fig. 12.45** Ultrastructural features of a multinucleated osteoclast. A = brush border (TEM; ×3000). From Berkovitz BKB, Shore RC 1995 Cells of the periodontal ligament. In: Berkovitz BKB, Moxham BJ, Newman HJ (eds) *The periodontal ligament in health and disease*, 2nd edn. Mosby–Wolfe, London, pp 9–33.

## OSTEOCLASTS AND CEMENTOCLASTS

Osteoclasts and cementoclasts (or odontoclasts) are found in areas where bone and cementum are being resorbed. Recent evidence shows that these cells are actively involved in the resorption process. Osteoclasts and cementoclasts have the same cytoplasmic features. These cells are now known to arise from blood cells of the macrophage type. When osteoclasts resorb alveolar bone (Fig. 12.44) the surface of the alveolar bone shows resorption concavities termed Howship's lacunae, in which lie the osteoclasts. Osteoclasts show considerable variation in size and shape, ranging from small mononuclear cells to large multinuclear cells. The part of the cell that lies adjacent to bone often has a striated appearance, the so-called 'brush border' (Fig. 12.45). The brush border comprises many tightly packed microvilli, which may be coated with fine, bristle-like structures. At the circumference of the brush border the plasma membrane tends to become smooth and the cytoplasm beneath it more dense. This modified annular zone may serve to limit the diffusion of hydrolytic enzymes, thereby creating a microenvironment in which resorption can take place. The osteoclast contains numerous mitochondria distributed throughout the cytoplasm, except for the region immediately beneath the brush border. The rough endoplasmic reticulum is less conspicuous than in osteoblasts, but Golgi material is prominent (especially in juxtanuclear areas). Most of the remaining cytoplasm contains large numbers of vesicles of different sizes and types; some contain acid phosphatase (see Fig. 13.17).

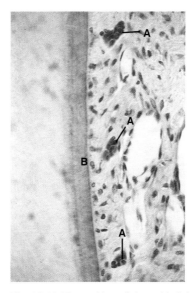

**Fig. 12.46** The position of the epithelial rests (A) close to the cementum (B) (Decalcified section through periodontal ligament; H & E; ×240).

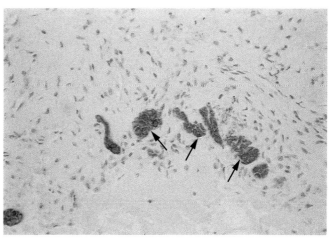

**Fig. 12.47** Decalcified section of the periodontal ligament showing positive brown staining for simple cytokeratins in epithelial cell rests (arrowed) (Immunohistochemistry; ×300). Courtesy of Dr A.E. Barrett.

## EPITHELIAL CELLS

Aggregations of epithelial cell rests, the rests of Malassez (Fig. 12.46), are a normal feature of the periodontal ligament. They are said to be the remains of the developmental epithelial root sheath (of Hertwig) (see pages 342, 343). Epithelial rests can be distinguished from adjacent fibroblasts by the close packing of their cuboidal cells and their tendency to stain more deeply. The rests lie about 25 μm from the cementum surface. Differences have been observed in the distribution of epithelial cells according to site and age: during the first and second decades they are most prevalent in the apical zone; between the third and seventh decades the majority are located cervically in the gingiva above the alveolar crest. This might imply that they have a slow rate of turnover, which might be related to the presence of receptors for epidermal growth factor. That the cell rests are epithelial in origin is indicated by using immunofluorescent techniques for the detection of cytokeratins (Fig. 12.47).

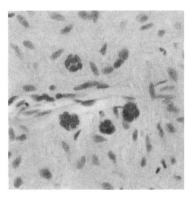

**Fig. 12.48** Cluster-like appearance of epithelial rests (Decalcified section through periodontal ligament; H & E; ×250).

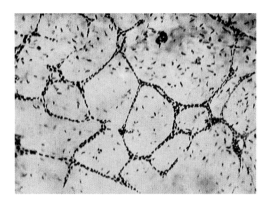

**Fig. 12.49** Tangential section through the epithelial rests showing a network appearance (Iron haematoxylin; ×60).

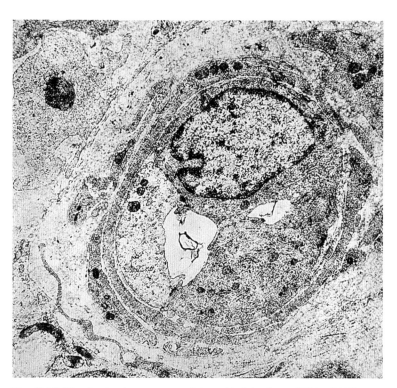

**Fig. 12.50** Ultrastructural appearance of the epithelial cell rest (TEM; ×6100).

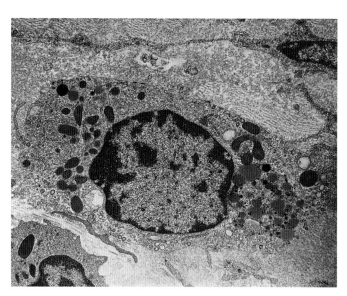

**Fig. 12.51** Ultrastructural features of a macrophage (TEM; ×6000).

In cross-section, the epithelial cells appear cluster-like (Fig. 12.48), although tangential or serial sections show a network of interconnecting strands parallel to the long axis of the root (Fig. 12.49).

The ultrastructural appearance of the epithelial cell rests is illustrated in Figure 12.50. The cluster arrangement of the cells is reminiscent of a duct-like structure. The cells are separated from the surrounding connective tissue by a basal lamina. The nucleus of each cell is prominent and often shows invaginations. The scanty cytoplasm is characterized by the presence of tonofibrils, some of which insert into the desmosomes that are frequently found between adjacent cells, and into hemidesmosomes between the cells and the basal lamina. Tight junctions are also found between the cells. Mitochondria are distributed throughout the cytoplasm, while the rough endoplasmic reticulum and Golgi apparatus are poorly developed. A primary cilium is often present, although its function is not understood. Histochemical and electron microscope studies reveal little activity in the epithelial cells, and cell turnover is slow (they can, however, be readily cultured), although they may proliferate to form cysts or tumours if appropriately stimulated (e.g. by chronic inflammation). Following orthodontic movement, there is no regeneration of the epithelial rests, although there is regeneration of connective tissue on the compression side. There is some evidence that secretory products from the epithelial cell rests could direct cellular events during cementogenesis and might inhibit cementogenesis in the mature tooth. In vitro, the cell rests are capable of phagocytosing collagen and synthesizing metalloproteinases and prostaglandins.

## DEFENCE CELLS

Defence cells within the periodontal ligament include macrophages, mast cells and eosinophils. These are similar to defence cells in other connective tissues.

Monocytes/macrophages make up about 4% of the periodontal ligament cell population (Fig. 12.51) and they are preferentially located near the nerves and blood vessels and not in the dense connective tissue of the periodontal ligament. Indeed, monocytes are blood-borne cells that enter the periodontal ligament from the blood vessels. Monocytes are oval cells with a ruffled border produced by numerous microvilli. They have prominent Golgi apparatus and rough endoplasmic reticulum and they contain many vesicles and lysosomes. There is some evidence that fibroblasts produce a chemoattractant protein that, as its name implies, attracts monocytes into the tissue and is synthesized in response to inflammation. Monocytes contain many enzymes that can degrade connective tissue extracellular matrix. Macrophages are derived from monocytes and are responsible for phagocytosing particulate matter and invading organisms and synthesizing a range of molecules with important functions such as interferon (the antiviral factor), prostaglandins and factors that enhance the growth of fibroblasts and endothelial cells. Their structure depends upon their site of activity. The resting macrophage differs from the

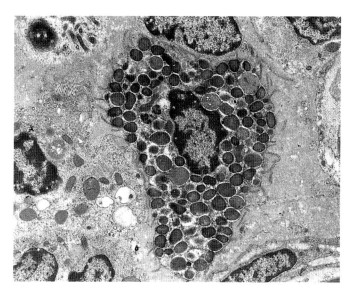

**Fig. 12.52** The ultrastructural appearance of the mast cell. Note the numerous dense membrane-bound vesicles (TEM; ×5000).

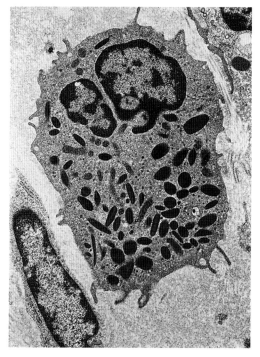

**Fig. 12.53** The ultrastructural features of an eosinophil. Note the characteristic granules (peroxisomes) (TEM; ×2500).

fibroblast in that there is a paucity of rough endoplasmic reticulum, there are thin, finger-like projections from the cell surface, and many lysosomes and other membrane-bound vesicles of varying density. When active, macrophages have many mitochondria and vesicles and may possess many branching processes. It has been speculated that the 'looser' arrangement of the periodontal connective tissues near the alveolar bone and the blood vessels relates to the presence there of monocytes/macrophages.

Mast cells (Fig. 12.52) are often associated with blood vessels. They show a large number of intracytoplasmic granules (which explains the intense staining reaction with basic aniline dyes for light microscopy). The granules are dense, membrane-bound vesicles of varying sizes. Other cytoplasmic organelles are relatively sparse. When the cell is stimulated it degranulates. Numerous functions have been ascribed to the mast cell, including the production of histamine, heparin and factors associated with anaphylaxis.

Eosinophils (Fig. 12.53) are only occasionally seen in the normal periodontal ligament. Characteristically, they possess granules (peroxisomes) that consist of one or more crystalloid structures. The cells are capable of phagocytosis.

The various cells of the periodontal ligament are capable of synthesizing and releasing bioactive molecules such as cytokines, growth factors and cell adhesion molecules. These are important when considering the biology of the tissues. Many of these substances are upregulated during orthodontic tooth movement. Neutrophils and lymphocytes can also be seen within the periodontal ligament in response to inflammation.

## CELL KINETICS

Periodontal ligament fibroblasts need replenishing. Furthermore, as osteoblasts and cementoblasts of the periodontal ligament become incorporated into alveolar bone and cellular cementum, replacement cells must be provided within the ligament to permit osteogenesis and cementogenesis to continue. In contrast to periodontal ligament fibroblasts, gingival fibroblasts belong to two progenitor cell populations: one with limited proliferative capacity, the other having extensive self-renewal capacity. Some of these differences are listed in Table 25.2.

The actual mechanisms that contribute to the development of cellular lineages in the periodontal ligament are largely unknown. During the development of the periodontal ligament, the cells populating the dental follicle (see page 301) are probably ectomesenchymal (neural crest) in origin and migrate from the dental papilla (see page 354). In the mature periodontal ligament, progenitor cell populations of the periodontal ligament are located adjacent to the blood vessels near the surface of the alveolar bone and in the contiguous endosteal spaces. At the blood vessels, some of the cells exhibit the classical features of stem cells – small size, responsiveness to stimulating factors and slow cycle time. Grafting experiments suggest that the tooth-related part of the ligament also contains cementoblast precursors (which have no paravascular association) while the bone-related part contains osteoblast precursors. Tritiated thymidine injections show that mitotic cells appear at paravascular sites and then migrate towards the bone surface. In addition, cells from the vascular channels within alveolar bone migrate towards the periodontal ligament. It has also been reported that there is a significant migration of periodontal cells to the surface of the alveolar bone with orthodontic tooth movement. In the normal periodontal ligament, the rate of cell generation (mitotic index) is modest (0.5–3%); the higher level has been found in the central part of the periodontal ligament where there is the least cell density. Such variation may be related to diurnal periodicity, or to location within the ligament, as well as to individual variation. There is a reduction of the mitotic index with age, although this rate is relatively rapid for a soft connective tissue. Cell mitosis and cell differentiation increase markedly with wounding or after the application of orthodontic loads, while different stimuli may recruit progenitors giving rise to different cell types (e.g. an osteoblastic rather than fibroblastic response following orthodontic loading).

For the fibroblasts, the cellular hierarchies in fibroblast populations of adult mammalian periodontal tissues are poorly understood, in part because of the lack of clear-cut phenotypic markers. Nevertheless, some reports suggest that there is significant morphological heterogeneity among periodontal cells. For example, there are said to be varying nuclear sizes (perhaps related to different capacities for undergoing cell division), a feature that has been claimed to provide a system for identifying the various cells in the osteoblast lineage. Other quantitative electron microscopy studies, however, indicate that the cells are remarkably homogeneous. Furthermore, morphological diversity is not itself indicative of functional heterogeneity. Periodontal fibroblasts comprise a renewal cell system in steady state and the progenitors can generate multiple cell types of more differentiated, specialized cells. Renewal systems are characterized by a balance between newly generated cells and cells lost by apoptosis and migration out of the tissue.

For cementoblasts and osteoblasts, a major question concerns whether periodontal fibroblasts, cementoblasts and osteoblasts all arise from a common precursor or whether each cell type has its own specific precursor cell. Although progenitor cells can be identified by their ability to incorporate tritium-labelled thymidine, little is known about their origin and life cycle. One of the problems of answering this question is the lack of specific markers to distinguish fibroblasts, osteoblasts and cementoblasts (and their precursors). However, progress is being made and the combined use of markers such as type I and III collagens (present in periodontal fibroblasts), bone sialoprotein and osteocalcin (present in cementoblasts and osteoblasts) and receptors for epidermal growth factor (present in periodontal fibroblasts and possibly osteoblasts) may help to alleviate the problem. Table 12.1 summarizes some of the features that help to distinguish fibroblasts, cementoblasts and osteoblasts in the periodontal ligament.

**Table 12.1** *Groups of markers helping to distinguish cementoblasts, fibroblasts and osteoblasts within the periodontal ligament*

|  | Cementoblasts | Periodontal ligament fibroblasts | Osteoblasts |
|---|---|---|---|
| Bone sialoprotein | + | − | + |
| Osteopontin | + | − | + |
| Osteocalcin | + | − | + |
| Osteonectin | ? | + | + |
| Epithelial growth factor receptors | − | + | +/− |
| Parathyroid hormone receptors | + | − | + |
| Vitamin-D-responsive | + | ? | + |
| Alkaline phosphate | +/− | + | + |
| Collagens: |  |  |  |
| Type I | + | + | + |
| Type III | − | + | − |
| Type V | − | + | − |

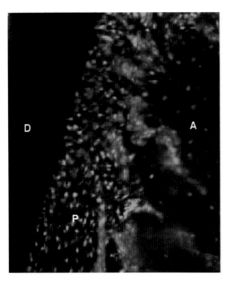

**Fig. 12.54** Labelling for apoptosis within the periodontal ligament using the TUNEL technique. D = root dentine of a rat second molar in an aged animal; P = periodontal ligament showing many positively labelled green apoptotic cells (such cells are absent in the non-aged tissue); A = alveolar bone (TUNEL fluorescent micrograph; ×120). Courtesy of J.M. Pycroft.

The presence of binding sites for EGF on periodontal fibroblasts is said to have an important role in their differentiation. Recently, it has been shown that numerous receptors for EGF (EGFRs) are expressed on the cells of the periodontal ligament, particularly for fibroblasts, paravascular cells and pre-osteoblasts. However, they are not expressed on fully differentiated cementoblasts and osteoblasts. Such observations have led to the hypothesis that the fibroblast phenotype in the periodontal ligament requires the continued expression of EGFRs and that they inhibit their differentiation into mineralized tissue-forming cells. When exposed to EGF, periodontal fibroblasts showed slightly increased mitogenic and chemotactic responses but decreased collagen synthesis. It has also been reported that PDGF-A,B, PDGF-BB and IGF-I have potent mitogenic and chemotactic effects on the cells of the periodontal ligament. Furthermore, PDGF stimulates collagen synthesis. In contrast, TGFβ had only slight chemotactic effects and inhibited mitogenic responses.

Apoptosis (programmed cell death) is not a common feature in the mature connective tissues of the periodontal ligament. In the aged animal, however, many of the cells are apoptotic (Fig. 12.54) and this is supported by immunocytochemical studies, which show a reduced level of focal adhesions in the cells of the aged tissues. Upregulation of the enzyme focal adhesion kinase within the periodontal ligament is seen during a phase of maximum eruption of the tooth (particularly at the root base) and this feature is associated with upregulation of proliferating cell-nuclear antigen.

Knowledge of the basic cell biology of the periodontal ligament is important to clinical practice in enabling a detailed understanding of the principles involved in obtaining periodontal regeneration (as opposed to repair) and in developing successful clinical strategies towards this end. During regeneration, cells such as fibroblasts, cementoblasts and osteoblasts must be induced in appropriate numbers, at the right time and in the right place, and then synthesize their appropriate extracellular matrices. New Sharpey fibres must gain a functional attachment into new bone and cementum. In addition, epithelial downgrowths must be excluded from the cementum surface. Unfortunately, in vitro studies to advance the development of these clinical strategies are often scientifically suspect. For example, when papers describe studies obtained by culturing cells scraped from the roots of extracted teeth (and often calling them periodontal ligament fibroblasts), it is difficult to know precisely what cell types are involved and how homogeneous the population is. Furthermore, as different culture techniques (with different passage numbers and different culture media) are used, it is not surprising that different authors report different results.

A clinical procedure said to be important in the attainment of periodontal regeneration is that of tissue guided regeneration. This is discussed on pages 353 and 354 in relation to the development of the tooth's root.

## BLOOD VESSELS AND NERVES

### BLOOD VESSELS

The rich blood supply to the periodontal ligament is derived from the appropriate superior and inferior alveolar arteries, although arteries from the gingiva (such as the lingual and palatine arteries) may also be involved (Fig. 12.55). The arteries supplying the periodontal ligament are primarily derived not from those entering the pulp at the apex of the tooth but from a series of perforation arteries passing through the alveolar bone. This source of blood supply allows the periodontal ligament to function following removal of the root apex as a result of various endodontic treatments. The coronal part of the periodontal ligament is supplied by vessels from the gingival tissues.

The volume of the periodontal ligament occupied by blood vessels varies between about 10% and more than 30% according to species, tooth

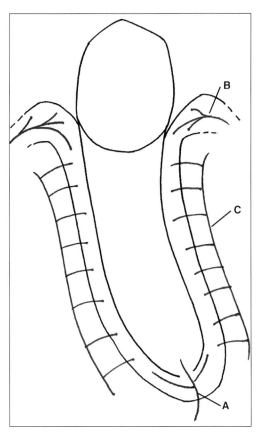

**Fig. 12.55** The blood supply to the periodontal ligament. A = arteries from dental pulp; B = arteries from gingiva; C = arteries from alveolar bone.

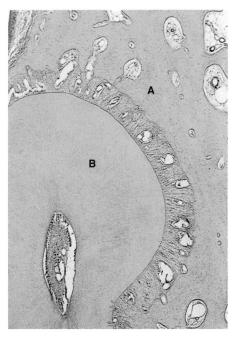

**Fig. 12.56** Transverse section through a periodontal ligament to show blood vessels lying close to alveolar bone. A = alveolar bone; B = dentine (van Gieson; ×30).

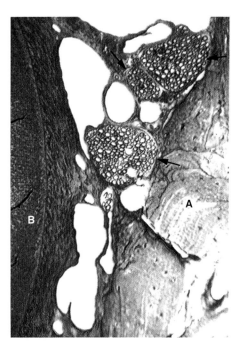

**Fig. 12.57** Semithin section of periodontal ligament showing large blood volume in the periodontal space. Nerve bundles are arrowed. A = alveolar bone; B = dentine (Toluidine blue; ×100).

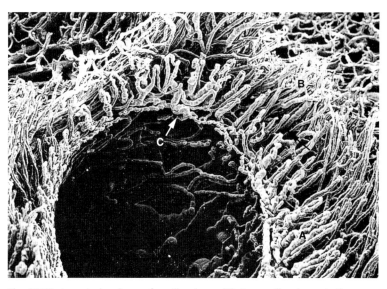

**Fig. 12.58** A crevicular plexus of capillary loops (A). B = capillary loops in the gingival surface; C = circular plexus; arrow indicates a gap between crevicular and circular plexuses (SEM of vascular cast; ×80). Courtesy of Professor M.R. Sims.

type, whether the tooth is erupting or is fully erupted, and site within the periodontal ligament.

The vessels found near the root surface are said to form a capillary plexus. Vessels nearer the bone surface form a postcapillary plexus from which venules pass into the alveolar bone. Many of the vessels of the periodontal ligament lie between the principal fibre bundles and close to the wall of the alveolus (Fig. 12.56). They have an average diameter of about 20 μm. The vessels branch and anastomose to form a capillary

plexus around the teeth. Semithin sections of periodontal ligament show that the blood vessels are seen as large spaces (Fig. 12.57). Indeed, the volume of the periodontal space occupied by blood vessels and by blood may be so great that we should perhaps think of the periodontal ligament as a 'blood space' as much as a 'connective tissue'!

Specialized features of the vasculature of the periodontal ligament vasculature are a crevicular plexus of capillary loops and the presence of large numbers of fenestrations in the capillaries. A crevicular plexus of capillary loops (Fig. 12.58) completely encircles the tooth within the connective tissue beneath the region of the gingival crevice. Each loop consists of one or two thin (8–10 μm in diameter) capillary ascending limbs and one or two postcapillary-sized venules. The crevicular capillary loops are separated from other more marginally situated loops in the gingival surface by a distinct gap and arise from a circular plexus, which is composed of between one and four intercommunicating vessels

(6–30 µm in diameter) lying at the level of the junctional epithelium. The circular plexus anastomoses with both the gingival and periodontal ligament vessels. Species differences may occur in the pattern of the vasculature, which may also be affected by inflammation. More complex glomerular-like structures have also been described. The functional significance of the complex vasculature in this region is not fully understood, although it may be related to the provision of a dentogingival seal. It may provide a means for blood flow reversal and rapid redistribution of the blood under varying occlusal loads and as a reaction to pathological stimuli.

Fenestration of capillaries within the periodontal ligament (Figs 12.59, 12.60) is unusual because fibrous connective tissues usually have continuous capillaries. The presence of fenestrated capillaries in large numbers (up to $40 \times 10^6/mm^3$ of tissue) is therefore a specialized feature of the periodontal ligament. Fenestrated capillary beds differ from continuous capillary beds in that the diffusion and filtration capacities are greatly increased. It is possible that the fenestrations are related to the high metabolic requirements of the periodontal ligament (high rate of turnover). Experimental evidence suggests that the number of fenestrations also relates to the stage of eruption.

The veins within the periodontal ligament do not usually accompany the arteries. Instead, they pass through the alveolar walls into intra-alveolar venous networks. Anastomoses with veins in the gingiva also occur. A dense venous network is particularly prominent around the apex of the alveolus.

The junctions between vascular endothelial cells in the periodontal ligament vary from close to tight to open. Open junctions are more permeable and provide pathways for fluid and molecular transport. These open junctions appear to be characteristic of the venous capillaries in the periodontal ligament.

Very few studies have investigated quantitatively and at the ultrastructural level the nature of vessels comprising the microvascular bed of the human periodontal ligament. One study that provides some data is illustrated in Figure 12.61. The results give a total luminal volume of approximately 9.5%, with significant variation both across the width of the ligament and from coronal to apical parts. Postcapillary venules formed the predominant vessels.

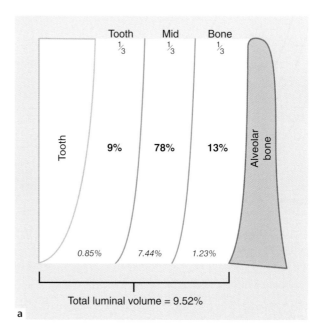

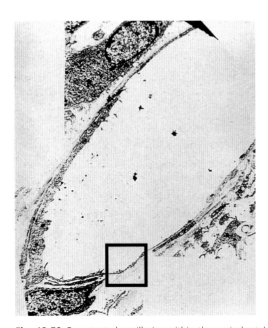

**Fig. 12.59** Fenestrated capillaries within the periodontal ligament. Note the thinning of the endothelium in the boxed area where fenestrations are present (TEM; ×10 000).

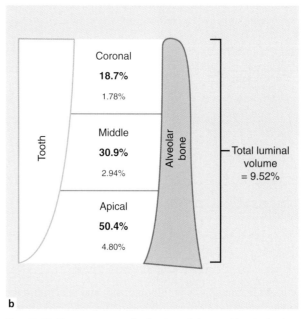

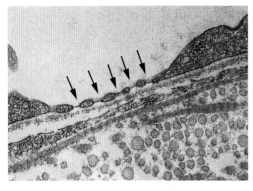

**Fig. 12.60** Fenestrated capillaries within the periodontal ligament. This is a higher-power view of the boxed area shown in Fig. 12.59. Arrows indicate the fenestrations (TEM; ×35 000).

**Fig. 12.61** The percentage distribution of the total luminal volume of the microvascular bed (a) across the circumferential thirds of the periodontal ligament and (b) in each vertical third of the periodontal ligament. The numbers in italics show the distribution of blood volume as a percentage of the total ligament volume. Redrawn from Foong K, Sims MR 1999 Blood volume in human bicuspid periodontal ligament determined by electron microscopy. *Archives of Oral Biology* 44: 465–474.

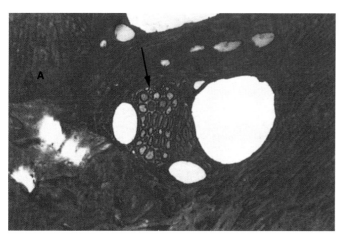

**Fig. 12.62** The rich nerve supply (arrow) to the periodontal ligament. A = alveolar bone. (Decalcified, transverse section through a tooth and its periodontal ligament; toluidine blue; ×150).

## NERVES

The nerve fibres supplying the periodontal ligament are functionally of two types: sensory and autonomic. The sensory fibres are associated with nociception and mechanoreception. The autonomic fibres are associated mainly with the supply of the periodontal blood vessels. Compared with other dense fibrous connective tissues, the periodontal ligament is well innervated (Fig. 12.62).

The nerve fibres entering the periodontal ligament are derived from two sources. Some nerve bundles enter near the root apex and pass up through the periodontal ligament; others enter the middle and cervical portions of the ligament as finer branches through openings in the alveolar walls.

Periodontal nerve fibres are both myelinated and unmyelinated. The myelinated fibres are on average about 5 μm in diameter (although some are as large as 15 μm) and are sensory fibres only. The unmyelinated fibres are about 0.5 μm in diameter and are both sensory and autonomic.

At the light microscope level, a plethora of forms that are assumed to represent nerve endings have been described within the periodontal ligament. These forms vary from simple free endings to more elaborate arborizing structures, although they still only mediate two sensory modalities – pain or pressure.

Most attention has been paid to the periodontal mechanoreceptors. These have a low threshold, being activated with loads as low as 0.01 N. The discharge of afferent impulses from mechanoreceptors has been recorded from single nerve fibres dissected free from the inferior alveolar nerve in animals. The discharge appears to vary according to the direction and amplitude of the displacing force. Periodontal mechanoreceptors exhibit directional sensitivity in that they respond maximally to a force applied to the crown of the tooth in one particular direction. Their conduction velocities (approx. 50 m/s) place them within the Aβ group of fibres. The response characteristics appear to vary from slowly adapting through to rapidly adapting fibres (Fig. 12.63). The question arises as to whether the slowly adapting, intermediate adapting and rapidly adapting mechanoreceptors are truly different types of receptor. Where it has been possible to examine histologically nerve endings that have been physiologically characterized, it seems that the endings of the mechanoreceptors are all similar, being unencapsulated, Ruffini-like terminals. Furthermore, the response characteristics (i.e. whether slowly or rapidly adapting) are dependent upon the position of the ending within the ligament relative to the position of loading. Present evidence suggests that the periodontal mechanoreceptors respond maximally to a force applied to the crown of the tooth in one particular direction and that the size of the response is directly related to the magnitude of the force applied. Evidence is also

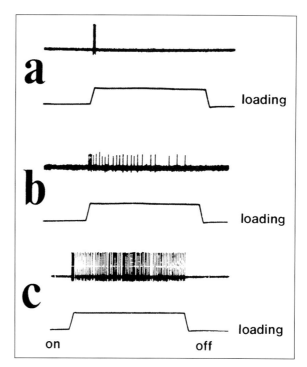

**Fig. 12.63** The responses of three periodontal ligament mechanoreceptors to suprathreshold ramp-plateau stimuli of 1 N (duration 3 s; rise time 50 ms). (a) Rapidly adapting response. (b) Intermediate adapting response. (c) Slowly adapting response. The receptors were located in the same tooth: (a) 1.5 mm, (b) 3.0 mm, (c) 5.5 mm from the fulcrum. Courtesy of Professor R.W.A. Linden.

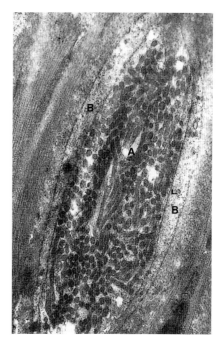

**Fig. 12.64** The putative nerve endings (A) that may represent Ruffini-like mechanoreceptors in the periodontal ligament. B = ensheathing Schwann-type cell. Note the large number of mitochondria (TEM; ×5700).

available to show that the responses of periodontal mechanoreceptors are temperature-dependent, with the activity peaking close to body temperature.

Putative nerve endings, which may represent mechanoreceptors, are characterized by the very large concentrations of mitochondria in the unmyelinated terminations of myelinated nerves (Fig. 12.64). The surrounding process of the ensheathing Schwann-type cell is noteworthy and this type of ending is regarded as being akin to a Ruffini-like nerve terminal. Even more complex putative nerve endings have very occasionally

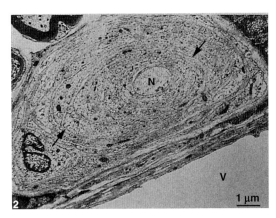

**Fig. 12.65** Complex putative nerve ending in the periodontal ligament. Arrows indicate numerous circularly arranged cell processes. N = nerve terminal; V = blood vessel (TEM; ×4500).

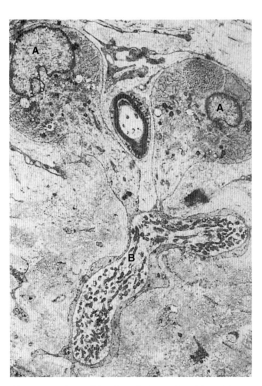

**Fig. 12.66** The cell bodies of the ensheathing Schwann-type cells. A = indented nuclei; B = mitochondria-rich nerve terminal (TEM; ×5000).

been observed within the periodontal ligament (Fig. 12.65). These are characterized by numerous circularly arranged cell processes surrounding a central structure containing microfilaments, microtubules and mitochondria. This central structure is thought to represent a nerve terminal. The morphology of this lamellated structure is reminiscent of cutaneous mechanoreceptors of the Paccinian type. However, because of their rarity, their significance in the periodontal ligament is unknown. Following removal of antagonist teeth, the ultrastructural features of the putative nerve endings are changed, including loss of organelles and changes in the location of the mitochondria. Occlusal loading may therefore be essential for maintaining the integrity of the periodontal mechanoreceptors.

The majority of neurones associated with periodontal mechanoreceptors have a receptive field confined to one tooth. About 75% of mechanoreceptors within the periodontal ligament have their cell bodies in the trigeminal ganglion while the remaining 25% of cell bodies lie in the mesencephalic nucleus. The trigeminal ganglion is associated mainly with touch, pressure and movement of the teeth during mastication, swallowing and speech. Thus, being primarily proprioceptive, the mechanoreceptor afferents relaying to the trigeminal ganglion are involved in unconscious detection of tooth contact for reflex control of mandibular movements during mastication. The evidence indicates that most periodontal mechanoreceptor neurones with their cell bodies in the mesencephalic nucleus have no functional role after tooth extraction. Indeed, the control of precisely directed, low biting forces is markedly disturbed in patients with osseointegrated implants.

There is evidence that afferents from anterior teeth (the incisors and canines) convey information about the state of contact between the food and the teeth and thereby play an important role in the specification of the level of force needed to fold and manipulate the food between the teeth. Not only are the mechanoreceptors involved in masticatory reflexes but there is evidence that they are involved in salivatory reflexes, especially on the ipsilateral side. When the teeth are clenched in the absence of a food bolus, some parotid saliva is secreted. This is reduced if the intra-oral nerves are anaesthetized. The periodontal mechanoreceptors also modulate the activity of the motor neurones of the hypoglossal cranial nerve, helping to control tongue position during mastication. In addition, activity of the neck musculature is probably modulated by periodontal mechanoreceptors, since pain and dysfunction of this musculature is frequently reported by patients suffering from occlusal or temporomandibular joint disorders.

The cell bodies of the ensheathing Schwann-type cells contain rough endoplasmic reticulum and the nucleus may be indented (Fig. 12.66).

Numerous vesicles may be observed within, and forming on, both the inner and outer surfaces of the ensheathing cells. These vesicles may be associated with rapid transport of materials to, and from the nerve terminal. The collagen in the immediate vicinity of the nerve ending appears to be arranged in a lamellar pattern.

Little is known about pain fibres within the periodontal ligament, but it is presumed that, as elsewhere in the body, they are represented by fine, unmyelinated fibres terminating as free nerve endings. A similar lack of information exists concerning the fine (0.2–1 µm diameter) autonomic fibres. These fibres are important in the control of regional blood flow, having vasoconstrictor activity. Thus, experiments affecting the sympathetic system are seen to produce changes in tooth position.

As for the pulp, sensory nerve endings in the periodontal ligament can release neuropeptides such as substance P, vasoactive intestinal peptide and calcitonin-gene-related peptide. These substances can have widespread effects on blood vessels and cells and must have an important, but as yet undetermined, role in the biology of the ligament. Many of them are upregulated during orthodontic tooth movement.

The importance of maintaining the innervation of the periodontal ligament for assuring proper functioning of the teeth has already been alluded to when considering the effects of tooth extraction. Indeed, the presence of osseointegrated implants seems to improve orodental sensation and, even for badly damaged teeth, it could be clinically advantageous to retain tooth fragments/roots. Furthermore, some regeneration of periodontal mechanoreceptors occurs following reimplantation of teeth, although there will still be decreased neural activity.

## THE PERIODONTAL LIGAMENT AS A SPECIALIZED CONNECTIVE TISSUE

Although the periodontal ligament has the same components as other soft, fibrous connective tissues (i.e. it is composed essentially of an unmineralized collagen and proteoglycan stroma in which are found connective tissue cells), it has the following features that, in combination, provide a specialized tissue.

- The principal collagen fibres have a characteristic orientation.
- The types (and amounts) of collagen (types I and III) and the variety of collagen cross-links are unlike those found within most other adult fibrous connective tissues.
- In some species, a pre-elastin-like fibre (oxytalan) is present within the periodontal ligament.
- The rate of turnover of the periodontal ligament is very fast.
- The periodontal ligament is remarkably cellular and rich in ground substance.
- The type of proteoglycan in the periodontal ligament may be specific to this tissue.
- The tissue hydrostatic pressure may be high.
- The periodontal ligament fibroblasts have features unusual for fibroblasts in adult fibrous connective tissues (e.g. many intercellular contacts, cilia).
- The periodontal ligament has cells concerned with the formation of dental tissues.
- The periodontal ligament has a rich vascular and nerve supply.
- The capillaries within the periodontal ligament are fenestrated.

However, the mere listing of these specialized characteristics does not permit inference of the role of these features in the function and pathobiology of the tissue. To do this, we need to discover whether there are structural and/or biochemical analogues for the periodontal ligament elsewhere in the body.

Initially, an analogue for the periodontal ligament was sought in mature (adult) fibrous connective tissues with known mechanical demands (i.e. connective tissue placed under either tension or compression). However, such comparisons showed that the periodontal ligament had some characteristics of a tissue under tension and others suggestive of compression (see Table 12.2). More recently, it has been shown that the periodontal ligament resembles immature, fetal-like connective tissues.

The periodontal ligament and fetal connective tissues (mesenchyme) have the following common features:

- high rates of turnover
- sharp, unimodal size/frequency distributions of small collagen fibrils
- significant amounts of type III collagen
- the major reducible collagen crosslink is dehydrodihydroxylisinonorleucine
- changes in collagen fibrils with lathyrogens
- large volumes of ground substance
- high content of glucoronate-rich proteoglycans
- high content of the glycoproteins tenascin and fibronectin
- presence of pre-elastin fibres (oxytalan in the periodontal ligament)
- high cellularity, the fibroblast-like cells passing numerous intercellular contacts
- similar biomechanical properties.

The functional significance of the periodontal ligament being fetal-like relates to the fact that the structural, ultrastructural and biochemical features of the tissue do not depend primarily upon mechanical demands. Indeed, the high rates of turnover may have a greater role in determining the characteristics of the periodontal ligament.

The fetal-like characteristics of the periodontal ligament also may aid our understanding of inflammatory periodontal disease. First, it is well known that processes involved in wound healing in fetal connective tissues differ markedly from those in adult tissues; consequently, our understand-

ing of repair/periodontal reattachment may benefit from an appreciation of the mode of repair of fetal wounds. Second, it has been proposed that periodontal defects produced by inflammatory periodontal disease may be corrected by grafting of connective tissues. At present, adult-type connective tissues have been tried with varying success. Perhaps grafting of fetal-like connective tissues may be more appropriate.

## TOOTH SUPPORT MECHANISM

The tooth support mechanism describes the manner whereby the periodontal ligament resists the axially directed intrusive loads that occur during biting.

It is still frequently stated that the periodontal ligament behaves as a 'suspensory ligament' during masticatory loading. Accordingly, loads on the tissue are dissipated to the alveolar bone primarily through the oblique principal fibres of the ligament, which, being placed in tension, are analogous to the guyropes of a tent. On release of the load, there is elastic recoil of the tissue, which enables the tooth to recover its resting position. The essentially elastic responses of the periodontal ligament during both loading and recovery imply that the tissue obeys Hooke's law. However, tooth mobility studies, surgical studies and morphological and biochemical studies have provided evidence against the notion that the periodontal ligament is a suspensory ligament.

Physiological tooth mobility studies provide information concerning the basic biomechanical properties of the periodontal ligament. They rely upon analysis of the patterns of mobility when loading teeth whose periodontal tissues have not been altered experimentally. These studies show that the ligament: does not obey Hooke's law during loading and recovery (Fig. 12.67), shows the property of hysteresis (Fig. 12.67) and exhibits responses whose time dependency suggests that the tissue has viscoelastic properties

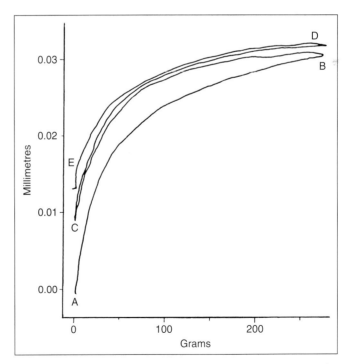

**Fig. 12.67** Axial load/mobility curve for a human maxillary incisor to show hysteresis. A = initial position of tooth; B = position at peak force on the first application of load; C = return point on removal of load; D = position at peak force on second application; E = return point after second removal of load. Note the lack of straight-line relationship between load and displacement (expected for elastic responses) and also that successive loads and recovery cycles pass along different paths (i.e. there are hysteresis loops). From Parfitt GJ 1960 Measurement of the physiological mobility of individual teeth in an axial direction. *Journal of Dental Research* 39: 608–618.

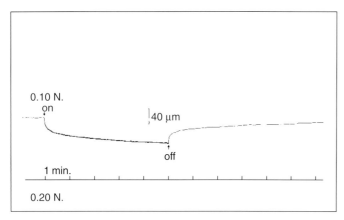

**Fig. 12.68** The viscoelastic responses of a tooth observed with an axially directed intrusive load. This is a pen recorder trace of tooth position which shows the effect of applying a load and then sustaining the load for a period of 5 minutes. Note the time dependency of the response, which is biphasic. The first phase is an elastic phase, the more gradual second phase is indicative of the property of creep (i.e. a viscous phase). The recovery responses are also biphasic and suggestive of viscoelasticity. From Coelho AJ, Moxham BJ 1989 The intrusive mobility of the incisor tooth of the guinea pig. *Archives of Oral Biology* 34: 383–386.

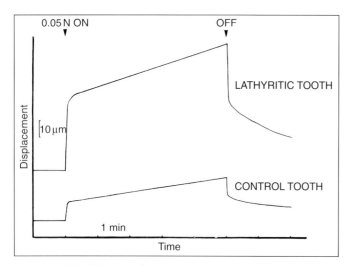

**Fig. 12.69** The effects of lathyrogens on tooth support. This experiment assesses the effects of the drug on axially directed extrusive loads. Note the significant increase in mobility for the tooth in the lathyritic animal, which suggests a role for the periodontal collagen in tooth support. However, the precise mechanism of action remains elusive since the patterns of mobility are the same for normal and lathyritic animals. From Moxham BJ, Berkovitz BKB 1984 The mobility of the lathyritic rabbit mandibular incisor in response to apically directed extrusive loads. *Archives of Oral Biology* 29: 773–778.

(Fig. 12.68). Furthermore, the patterns of loading are not dependent on the direction of the load relative to the orientation of the principal fibres in the periodontal ligament and, for loads of similar magnitude, the amount of displacement for an axially directed intrusive load is greater than for an extrusive load.

Experimental tooth mobility studies rely upon investigating the effects on the patterns of mobility obtained following alterations to a specific component of the periodontal ligament. Experiments with lathyrogens (drugs that specifically inhibit the formation of collagen crosslinks and disrupt the fibrous network of the periodontal ligament; Fig. 12.69), with vasoactive drugs and following surgical disruption of the periodontal ligament indicate that both the periodontal collagen fibres and the periodontal vasculature are involved in tooth support.

**Table 12.2** *Relationship between the ultrastructural features of the periodontal ligament and mechanical properties*

| Features of the periodontal ligament suggesting tension | Features of the periodontal ligament suggesting compression |
|---|---|
| Sharpey fibre structure (Fig. 12.20) | Small collagen fibril diameters (Fig. 12.7) |
| The flattened, disc shape of the fibroblasts | Unimodal collagen size/frequency distribution (Fig. 12.8) |
| Dermatan-sulphate-rich composition of ground substance (page 186) | Distribution of Sharpey fibres to socket (Fig. 12.21) |
| | Smooth surface of fibroblast membrane |
| | Large amounts of ground substance (page 186) |

In experiments where the apical half of the periodontal ligament was removed and the tooth was loaded to assess the effects on its mobility no effects were observed; consequently, it was argued that the ligament did not behave as a compressive structure because it was presumed that only the tissue around the root apex could behave in this manner. Subsequent experiments performed to assess the role of tension in the more cervically situated principal fibres of the ligament have shown that the periodontal ligament around the alveolar crest could also be removed without major changes in tooth mobility. These experiments therefore do not provide definitive evidence for or against tension or compression in the periodontal ligament but do suggest that, even where there is marked trauma to a region of the ligament, the remaining tissue can still perform a supporting function in the short term.

Some morphological evidence suggesting that the periodontal collagen is placed in tension during masticatory loading comes from study of the Sharpey fibre attachments and from the collagen crimps. As mentioned previously (see page 184), the Sharpey fibres appear as mineralized stubs projecting into the periodontal ligament from the wall of the alveolus. The occurrence of mineralization at approximately right angles to the long axes of the fibres has been adduced as evidence that the fibres are under tension. However, even if this were the case, the distribution of Sharpey fibres along the alveolus indicates that they are limited mainly to the region of the alveolar crest (Fig. 12.21). The crimping of collagen in the periodontal ligament was described on pages 183, 184. Evidence from connective tissue elsewhere in the body (particularly from tendons) suggests that the crimps are involved in the initial stages of loading, allowing some degree of movement before the tissue is placed under tension.

Morphological and biochemical comparisons between the periodontal ligament and other connective tissues known to be under tension or compression have been undertaken to throw some light on the role of the periodontal ligament in tooth support. This has been undertaken on the assumption that the structure of a connective tissue is dictated by the mechanical demands placed upon it. Table 12.2 shows the results of such a comparison. Whereas some features of the periodontal ligament suggest a tensional mode of activity, many of the features indicate a compressive mode. Indeed, experiments involving relatively long-term changes in the mechanical demands placed upon the tissue (e.g. pinning a tooth to completely prevent tooth movements) produced no major changes in the structure of the periodontal ligament and provided evidence for the view that the ligament is not as affected by the mechanical demands placed upon it as tissues elsewhere in the body.

Recent biochemical analysis of the proteoglycans within the periodontal ligament and under different loading regimens shows that the degree of aggregation/disaggregation of the ground substance may have a role in

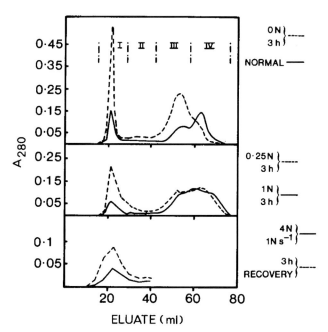

**Fig. 12.70** Molecular size profiles of periodontal ligament proteoglycans following various degrees of intrusive loadings of macaque monkey teeth. (Top) High-molecular-weight fraction (peak I) increased when the periodontal ligament is undisturbed for 3 hours. (Middle) Decrease in peak I size between 0.25 N and 1 N loads. (Bottom) Further decrease in peak I size with 4 N loads followed by an increase during a 3-hour undisturbed recovery phase. From Embery G, Picton DC, Stanbury JB 1987 Biochemical changes in periodontal ligament ground substance associated with short-term intrusive loading in adult monkeys (*Macaca fascicularis*). *Archives of Oral Biology* 32: 545–549.

tooth support (Fig. 12.70). Where teeth are unloaded for a period of 3 hours, a high-molecular-weight fraction within the periodontal ligament is greatly increased. On the other hand, with loads between 0.25 N and 1 N, this fraction is greatly reduced. Loads of 4 N are associated with a further decrease, followed by an increase during a 3-hour undisturbed recovery phase.

There is thus evidence that the collagen fibres, vasculature and ground substance of the periodontal ligament are all involved in tooth support. Consequently, the mechanism of tooth support should not be regarded as a property of a single component of the periodontal ligament but as a function of the tissue as a whole.

## CLINICAL CONSIDERATIONS

The most important clinical condition affecting the periodontal ligament is chronic inflammatory periodontal disease, when toxic products released by dental plaque (and the host's defence mechanisms) result in the destruction and loss of periodontal ligament tissue and adjacent alveolar bone. Such a process results in the formation of a deeper periodontal pocket and the vicious circle continues. The loss of attachment tissue will expose the root of the tooth in the mouth, increasing tooth mobility, and the tooth may eventually be lost. When faced with such a condition, the dental surgeon may have two aims in mind: to repair the existing condition so that the disease process progresses no further (usually involving surgical removal of diseased tissue) and to regenerate the lost tissues, restore the bone and periodontal ligament to their original form, and reattach new periodontal ligament fibres to the tooth and bone. One common problem following surgery is that the junctional epithelium proliferates rapidly downwards to cover the root surface, which will prevent periodontal ligament fibres from attaching to cementum.

Following periodontal surgery (with the removal of diseased tissue and the possible application of various methods of conditioning the root surface to make it more likely to reattach periodontal ligament fibres, such as root planing, citric acid etching), a blood clot will form. It is obvious that the connective tissue of the wound may be repopulated from either the gingiva growing down or the periodontal ligament growing up. There is a body of opinion that believes that the best result is achieved when most of the wound is repopulated by cells of the existing periodontal ligament. Although the tissues may appear to be similar, they differ in a number of features that may be important to the final outcome. For this reason, a particular surgical technique may be adopted to exclude the gingival tissues from the deeper part of the wound by placing some sort of tissue barrier over the alveolar crest to obtain 'guided tissue regeneration'.

Bioactive molecules such as growth factors and cytokines may be important during the induction of periodontal cells (osteoblasts, cementoblasts and fibroblasts) and bone itself. Such bioactive molecules (e.g. bone morphogenetic protein) have been placed in suitable carriers within wounds and have been claimed to help regenerate the periodontal tissues (bone, cementum and periodontal ligament). Periodontal regeneration is discussed further on pages 353–357.

In the process of cementogenesis (see pages 347–354), enamel proteins may have an important role during the early stages. Evidence is accumulating that the application of such proteins to the root surface may be an aid to periodontal regeneration (see page 356).

Important changes take place within the periodontal ligament with orthodontic loading. Should such a load act perpendicularly to the longitudinal axis of the tooth, wide areas or pressure on one side of the root and corresponding areas of tension on the other side are produced. Only if the force is placed near the centre of the root (through its centre of resistance) could a translation (or bodily) movement of the tooth be produced, with essentially uniform distribution of pressures on one side of the root and of tension on the other. However, tipping can easily occur as a result of the application of an orthodontic load, the point of rotation depending on the site of force application, the shape of the tooth, and the nature of the periodontal tissues supporting the tooth. The result is that crown and the root tip in opposite directions, producing pressure and tension zones on either side of the root and a varying distribution of stress such that the load is concentrated in localized areas of the periodontal ligament. In such areas, the fibrous part of the periodontal ligament will differ where the tooth is pressed against the alveolar wall and where it is drawn away from it.

On the side under tension, the periodontal space will become wider where the tooth is drawn away from the alveolar bone following the application of a continuous orthodontic load. Bundles of fibres are stretched and the alveolar crest is pulled in the same direction. There is an increase in connective tissue cell number, particularly near the socket wall. The periodontal fibroblasts appear spindle-shaped, although the cells near the alveolar wall appear more spherical. The blood vessels also appear to be distended. Osteoid tissue is deposited on the socket wall and, where the fibrous bundles are thick, new bone appears to be deposited along them. If the bundles are thin, a more uniform layer is deposited along the root surface. Calcification in the deeper layers of the osteoid starts shortly afterwards, while the superficial part remains uncalcified. New Sharpey fibres are secreted simultaneously with new bone deposition. As the fibroblasts migrate with the bone, they may deposit either entirely new Sharpey fibres or new fibrils, which are incorporated into existing fibres. While part of the newly synthesized collagen will be incorporated into the new osteoid, some will be incorporated into the periodontal ligament, perhaps associated with the increase in width on the tension side. Lengthening of fibres also seems to occur by incorporation of new fibrils into existing fibres (even at some distance from the alveolar bone wall). On the side under pressure, the periodontal space becomes narrower and the crest of the alveolar bone is slightly deformed. Resorption of the alveolar bone surface occurs on the side towards which the tooth is moving by means of osteoclasts. Vascular activity is low and few leukocytes and macrophages are seen. Changes on the pressure side can be categorized broadly into 'direct resorption', where the pressure is relatively light, and 'hyalinization', where the pressure is large enough to produce degenerative changes. With 'direct resorption', osteoclastic activity is evident; with 'hyalinization', osteoclasts are absent: there is oedema and obliteration of the blood vessels within the periodontal ligament. Degenerative changes in the fibroblasts are also seen. The term 'hyalinization' comes from the 'glassy' appearance of the periodontal ligament in routine histological specimens. The necrotic hyalinized tissue is primarily removed by macrophages. In addition, multinucleated, TRAP-positive cells lacking a ruffled border also appear to be involved in removing the necrotic tissue. When these multinucleated cells reach the cement surface, they may continue their resorbing activity and initiate some root resorption.

An unwanted side effect of orthodontic treatment is resorption occurring at the root apex, with resultant loss in tooth length. This particularly affects permanent maxillary central incisors. In severe cases, there may be a 20% loss of root length (see Fig. 13.44 in bone). The factors that predispose teeth to root resorption are unknown, there being considerable individual variation. However, root resorption appears to be correlated with the size of the force and/or the total treatment time. Root morphology may be involved as teeth with blunted roots may show more resorption. The development of new dental materials and designs for orthodontic wire (e.g. superelastic nickel–titanium) and brackets that have shape memory and are able to provide a constant force over the period of treatment (bioefficient therapy) should help reduce the amount of root resorption.

The part of the maxilla or mandible that supports and protects the teeth is known as alveolar bone. An arbitrary boundary at the level of the root apices of the teeth separates the alveolar processes from the body of the mandible (Fig. 13.1) or the maxilla. Like bone in other sites, alveolar bone functions as a mineralized supporting tissue, giving attachment to muscles, providing a framework for bone marrow and acting as a reservoir for ions (especially calcium). Apart from its obvious strength, one of the most important biological properties of bone is its 'plasticity', allowing it to model/remodel according to the functional demands placed upon it. In modelling, bone is formed at a different site from where resorption is occurring, leading to a change in the shape and/or size of a bone (as in growth): in remodelling (internal turnover), bone formation occurs at the same site following resorption and there is no change in the overall shape of the bone (Fig. 13.2).

Bone depends on function (i.e. mechanical stimuli) to maintain its structure and mass, although the period of loading need only be short to trigger an adaptive response. Such loading needs to be intermittent rather than static. Too little function may cause it to atrophy (including bone loss during space flight): increased stimuli, especially high-impact activities such as tennis, may cause it to thicken: excessive stimuli may cause it to fracture. Alveolar bone is dependent on the presence of teeth for its development and maintenance. Where teeth are congenitally absent (as in hypodontia/anodontia), or where a tooth is extracted, alveolar bone is poorly developed.

## CLASSIFICATION OF BONE

Bone may be classified in several ways. Developmentally, there is **endochondral bone** (where bone is preceded by a cartilaginous model that is eventually replaced by bone in a process termed endochondral ossification) and **intramembranous bone** (where bone forms directly within a vascu-lar, fibrous membrane). Histologically, mature bone may be categorized as **compact** (cortical) or **cancellous** (spongy) according to its density. As the names suggest, compact bone forms a dense, solid mass, while in spongy bone there is a lattice arrangement of the individual bony trabeculae that surround soft tissue.

Internally, a thin layer of compact bone lines the tooth socket and gives attachment to the principal fibres of the periodontal ligament. Externally, on the buccal/labial and lingual/palatal surfaces, are thicker layers of compact bone, forming the external and internal alveolar plates. Between these plates of compact bone are variable amounts of spongy bone, depending on site (Fig. 13.1; see also page 12). This combination of compact and cancellous bone aims for maximum strength at minimum weight. In newly formed bone, the collagen fibres have a more variable diameter and lack a preferential orientation, giving the bone a matted (basket-weave) appearance when viewed in polarized light. This immature bone, termed **woven bone**, has larger and more numerous osteocytes that comprise about 30% of the volume of the tissue (compared with about 2% for adult bone). It is formed more rapidly and has a higher turnover rate. Woven bone is also seen initially at sites of fracture repair or in healing tooth sockets. It mineralizes faster than adult bone and is more mineralized. Woven bone is subsequently converted to fine-fibred **adult lamellar bone**.

One of the most important properties of bone concerns its ability to continuously remodel and adapt to changing functional situations. This relates to the different types of bone cell, one type having the property to form bone (osteoblasts), other types the ability to detect the mechanical stresses and strains to which the bone is subjected (osteoblasts and osteocytes), while another type of cell has the capacity to resorb bone (osteoclasts). Although bone under mechanical load will remodel, cementum is less readily resorbed than bone under similar loads. Although the reasons for this difference are unclear, it is a fundamental principle on which the basis of orthodontic tooth movement relies.

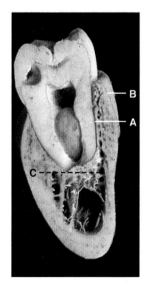

Fig. 13.1

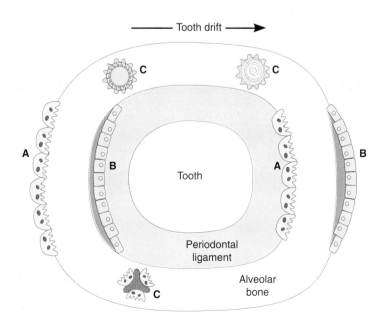

Fig. 13.2

**Fig. 13.1** Ground longitudinal through the mandible showing the alveolar bone. A = inner layer of compact alveolar bone lining the tooth socket wall; B = outer alveolar plate of compact bone (note the spongy bone lying between the two plates of alveolar bone); C = arbitrary boundary between the alveolar bone and the body of the jaw. Courtesy of the Royal College of Surgeons of England.

**Fig. 13.2** Modelling of alveolar bone during physiological tooth drift in which resorption (A) and deposition (B) of bone take place at different sites, resulting in a change in bone morphology. Compare this with remodelling of bone (C), where resorption and deposition occur at the same site without any resulting change in bone morphology.

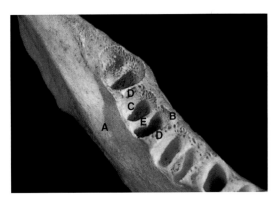

**Fig. 13.3** Mandible with teeth removed to demonstrate the components of alveolar bone. A = outer alveolar plate; B = inner alveolar plate; C = cribriform plate lining the socket wall; D = interdental septum; E = interradicular septum.

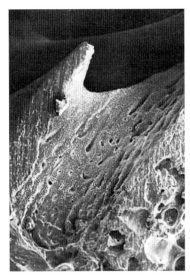

**Fig. 13.4** A tooth socket showing the cribriform nature of the cribriform plate (SEM; ×5). Courtesy of Professor P. Sloan.

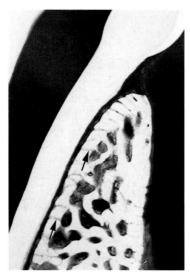

**Fig. 13.5** Microradiograph of vascular canals in the cribriform plate (arrowed). Note the spongy bone lying in the central part of the alveolar bone. (×7).

## CHEMICAL PROPERTIES OF BONE

Bone is a mineralized connective tissue. About 60% of its wet weight is inorganic material, about 25% organic material and about 15% water. By volume, about 36% is inorganic, 36% is organic and 28% is water. The mineral phase provides the hardness and rigidity of bone and consists of hydroxyapatite, much of it carbonated. As with the other mineralized tissues, many trace elements are also present. The mineral is in the form of needle-like crystallites or thin plates about 50 nm wide, up to 8 nm thick and of variable length. The crystallites are distributed both within the spaces between, and on the surfaces of, the collagen fibrils. Although contributing little to the weight of bone, the cells, through their capacity for osteosynthesis and resorption, have a pivotal role in the maintenance of the matrix.

## ORGANIC MATRIX

The organic matrix of bone is about 90% collagen. Most can be regarded as intrinsic collagen secreted by osteoblasts. However, collagen inserted as Sharpey fibres can be considered as extrinsic collagen formed by adjacent fibroblasts. The dominant collagen in bone is type I, although small amounts of other types (e.g. type III and type V) may be present, particularly in immature or healing bone. The collagen contributes towards the important biomechanical properties of the tissue in terms of resisting loads and providing the necessary resilience that prevents fractures. Mutation in the genes encoding the constituent peptides of the collagen type I triple helix are clinically important and may give rise to the inherited conditions of osteogenesis imperfecta, where the strength of bone is much reduced.

## NON-COLLAGENOUS PROTEINS

The non-collagenous proteins, which are a heterogeneous group of about 200 proteins, collectively comprise the bulk of the remaining 10% of the total organic content of bone matrix. Most are endogenous proteins produced by the bone cells, while some, like albumin and immunoglobulins, are derived from other sources (such as the blood) and become incorporated into the bone matrix during bone formation The main non-collagenous proteins comprise the proteoglycans (e.g. decorin, biglycan and versican), the glycoproteins (e.g. osteonectin, osteopontin, bone sialoprotein, thrombospondin and fibronectin), bone Gla-containing proteins (osteocalcin), and serum proteins (e.g. albumin). The biological function

## GROSS MORPHOLOGY OF BONE

The alveolar, tooth-bearing portion of the jaws is composed of outer and inner alveolar plates. The individual sockets are separated by plates of bone termed the interdental septa, while the roots of multirooted teeth are divided by interradicular septa (Fig. 13.3). The compact layer of bone lining the tooth socket has been given various names. It has been referred to as the cribriform plate, reflecting the sieve-like appearance produced by the numerous vascular canals (Volkmann's canals) passing from the alveolar bone into the periodontal ligament (Figs 13.4, 13.5); it has also been called bundle bone because numerous bundles of Sharpey fibres pass into it from the periodontal ligament. In clinical radiographs, the bone lining the alveolus commonly appears as a dense white line and is given the name lamina dura (see page 50). The radio-opaque appearance might give the false impression that it is denser than adjacent bone. However, the radiographic appearance derives from the X-ray beam passing tangentially through the socket wall and relates to the quantity of bone the beam passes through and not to any greater degree of mineralization than adjacent bone. Superimposition also obscures the Volkmann's canals. The cribriform plate varies in thickness from 0.1 mm to 0.5 mm. The external alveolar plate is usually about 1.5–3 mm thick over posterior teeth but is highly variable around anterior teeth, depending on tooth position and inclination. The gross morphology and radiographic appearance of the alveolus and tooth sockets are described on pages 10–12 and page 50.

of individual glycoproteins awaits clarification. Some are presumably involved in the initial, formative aspects of bone, while others may play a role following their release during bone resorption. As the proteoglycans bind to collagen, they may help regulate collagen fibril diameters and/or play a role in mineralization. Osteonectin, for example, has the ability to bind calcium and collagen, suggesting a role in mineralization. The RGD-containing glycoproteins osteopontin, bone sialoprotein and fibronectin contain the specific tripeptide sequence arginine–glycine–aspartic acid (Arg–Gly–Asp). Bone cells have specific cell membrane receptors (e.g. integrins) binding to this sequence, allowing them to adhere to the matrix and, through secondary messengers, to modify their behaviour. If, for example, the tripeptide sequence is not available to the bone cell, this may result in its apoptosis. The bone Gla-containing protein osteocalcin (with the amino acid gamma-carboxyglutamic acid) is a calcium-binding protein synthesized only by osteoblasts and odontoblasts. This specificity means that recognition of osteocalcin in a cell characterizes that cell as being of an osteoblastic or odontoblastic lineage.

Other exogenously derived proteins that may circulate in the blood and become locked up in the bone matrix include cytokines (such as interleukin, tumour necrosis factor and colony-stimulating factor) and growth factors (such as transforming growth factors (TGFs), fibroblast growth factors, platelet-derived growth factors and insulin-like growth factors (IGFs)). Such molecules have important biological activity in the life cycle of bone cells. When present within the bone itself, they are inactive but may become mobilized when bone is resorbed by osteoclasts. They may then play a determining role on the pattern of subsequent bone activity. Bone morphogenetic proteins (BMPs), of which about 16 have so far been identified, are also represented in bone. They are part of the TGFβ super-family and have the ability to induce bone to form by their ability to influence the movement, cell division and differentiation of stem and osteoprogenitor cells. BMPs are currently being assessed for use clinically as a method for inducing bone formation.

form the seeds around which further mineralization can occur by epitaxy. A similar process of initial mineralization via matrix vesicles seems to occur in dentine (see pages 334, 335). However, whereas certain molecules involved in the mineralization process may bypass the predentine by being transported via the odontoblast process directly to the mineralizing front, this would not appear to be possible in osteoid. There is a lag phase before the deeper layer of the osteoid has matured sufficiently to undergo mineralization.

## BONE ORGANIZATION

Bone is deposited in layers, or lamellae, each lamella being 3–5 μm thick. In compact bone the lamellae are arranged in two major patterns. At external (periosteal) and internal (endosteal) surfaces they are arranged in parallel layers completely surrounding the bony surfaces known as circumferential lamellae. Deep to the circumferential lamellae, the lamellae are arranged as small, concentric layers around a central neurovascular canal. The central (haversian) canal (about 50 μm in diameter), together with the concentric lamellae, is known as a **haversian system** or **osteon** (Fig. 13.6). There may be up to about 20 concentric lamellae within each haversian system, the number being limited by the ability of nutrients to diffuse from the central vessel to the cells in the outermost lamella. A cement line of mineralized matrix delineates each haversian system. The collagen fibrils within each lamella are parallel to one another and spiral along the length of the lamella but have a different orientation to those in the adjacent lamella. This change in orientation can be demonstrated by viewing bone in polarized light (Fig. 13.7). The longitudinally running haversian canals are connected by a series of horizontal ones (interconnecting canals). As a consequence of remodelling, fragments of previous

## HISTOLOGY OF BONE

### OSTEOID

Any surface where active bone formation is occurring will be covered by a layer of newly deposited, unmineralized, bone matrix called osteoid (see Fig. 13.9). This layer is analogous to predentine. The molecular ingredients of osteoid are secreted by osteoblasts that form a well-defined layer at its surface. Osteoid has a thickness of approximately 5–10 μm before reaching a level of maturity conducive to mineralization. However, in certain pathological conditions, where there is delayed mineralization (e.g. osteomalacia) or increased bone formation (e.g. Paget's disease), this thickness may be increased (hyperosteoidosis).

The mineralizing front is relatively linear at the light microscope level, unlike that of dentine, which may reveal a calcospheritic pattern. In routine, light microscopic, demineralized sections, osteoid will stain differently from that of the matrix associated with mineralized bone, indicating that biochemical changes take place within the matrix at the mineralizing front to enable mineralization to occur; some molecules may be added, others may be degraded.

Osteoid consists of type I collagen fibrils arranged more or less parallel to the bone surface, embedded in a complex ground substance of proteoglycans, glycoproteins and other protein molecules. The biochemical changes occurring at the mineralizing front are poorly understood. When alveolar bone is first formed, initial mineralization may be controlled by osteoblasts from whose cell membrane matrix vesicles are budded off into the osteoid: the first crystals are formed within the matrix vesicles. The cell membrane of these matrix vesicles breaks down and the first crystals

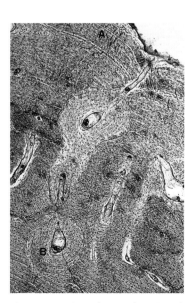

**Fig. 13.6** Horizontal ground section of alveolar bone showing circumferential lamellae (A) and haversian systems (B) where a central vascular canal is surrounded by concentrically arranged bony lamellae (×80).

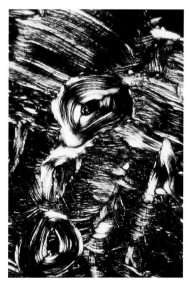

**Fig. 13.7** Same section as Fig. 13.6, viewed in polarized light. The alternating black and white bands indicate the different orientations of collagen in adjacent lamellae. Note the characteristic 'X' superimposed on the haversian system (×80).

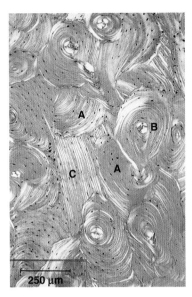

**Fig. 13.8** Horizontal ground section of bone showing interstitial lamella (A), haversian system surrounding a central canal (B) and original circumferential lamella lying deep within the bone following remodelling (C) (×60). Courtesy of Professor M.M. Smith.

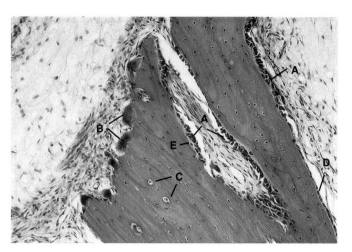

**Fig. 13.9** Horizontal section of bone demonstrating a layer of osteoblasts (A) lining a surface where active bone formation is occurring (as indicated by the presence of a pale staining layer of osteoid), some large multinucleated osteoclasts (B) lying against Howship's lacunae in a region of bone undergoing resorption, and large numbers of osteocytes (C) lying embedded within the bone matrix itself. D = bone-lining cells; E = pale-staining osteoid layer (Decalcified section; H & E; ×80). Courtesy of Dr T.R. Arnett.

haversian systems may be present (the interstitial lamellae; Fig. 13.8) as well as old circumferential lamellae (Fig. 13.8). This may cause confusion to the uninformed, who may misinterpret relocated Sharpey fibres (which originally were in the circumferential lamellar bone but are now embedded deep within the bone in isolated islands among osteones) as 'unusual coarse fibres'. This is a common feature in growth with active cortical drift.

In spongy bone, the lamellae are apposed to each other to form trabeculae up to about 50 μm thick. The trabeculae are not arranged randomly but are aligned along lines of stress so as best to withstand the forces applied to the bone while adding minimally to mass. The trabeculae surround the marrow spaces, from which they derive their nutrition by diffusion: osteones are only occasionally encountered in thicker trabeculae. In young bone, the marrow is red and haemopoietic. It contains stem cells of both the fibroblastic/mesenchymal type (capable of giving rise to fibroblasts, osteoblasts, adipocytes, chondroblasts and myoblasts) and blood cell lineage (capable of giving rise to osteoclasts). In old bone, the marrow is yellow, with loss of haemopoietic potential and increased accumulation of fat cells.

In the body as a whole, about 80% of bone is of the cortical variety while about 20% is spongy. However, these figures are likely to vary according to site and age. Although it only occupies a small percentage of bone volume, spongy bone has a far higher turnover rate than cortical bone: cortical bone is said to remodel about 3% of its mass each year, while spongy bone remodels about 25%. The cortical bone functions mainly in a mechanical/protective role, while the spongy bone has a more metabolic function.

## CELL TYPES IN BONE

Several cell types are responsible for the synthesis, maintenance and resorption of bone (Fig. 13.9). They can be regarded as belonging to two main families, one mesenchymal and the other haemopoietic. The osteoblasts, osteocytes and bone-lining cells are derived from a mesenchymal (or ectomesenchymal) stem cell. These stem cells reside in the bone marrow and in a region of proliferating cells adjacent to the osteoblast layer in the periosteum. In the periodontal ligament and other bone-forming tissues, the osteogenic precursors may be associated with small blood vessels. The osteoclasts, however, belong to a different lineage. They form

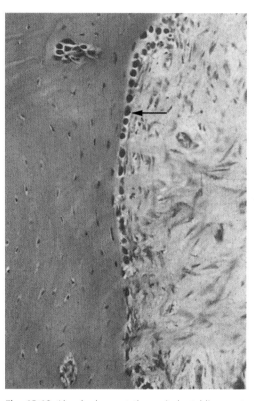

**Fig. 13.10** Alveolar bone at the periodontal ligament surface showing a layer of osteoblasts (arrowed). Sharpey fibres are seen passing into the bone and there is a pale-staining osteoid layer. Within the bone itself are seen osteocytes, which, in routine demineralized sections, do not exhibit obvious canaliculi (Decalcified section; H & E; ×400).

part of the haemopoietic system, being derived from the mononuclear/phagocyte system (including monocytes and macrophages).

## OSTEOBLASTS

Osteoblasts are specialized fibroblast-like cells of mesenchymal origin. A layer of these cells is prominent on bone surfaces where there is active bone formation (Fig. 13.10). Unlike cartilage, which grows interstitially, bone can be deposited (or resorbed) only at surfaces. However, these surfaces are widespread and include the periosteal and endosteal surfaces, the linings of the haversian canals and the surfaces of bony trabeculae in

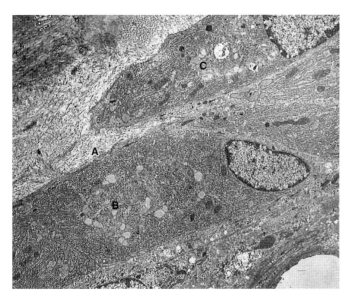

**Fig. 13.11** Electronmicroscopic appearance of an active osteoblast. The cell contains an extensive rough endoplasmic reticulum and a conspicuous and localized Golgi apparatus (B), and is connected to adjacent cells by cell contacts. The cell surface adjacent to the demineralized bone (A) has many fine cytoplasmic processes, some of which contact underlying osteocytes. The flattened cell (C) immediately adjacent to the osteoblasts may represent an osteoprogenitor cell (×6000).

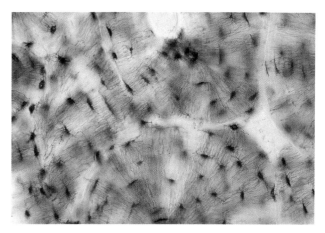

**Fig. 13.12** Ground section of part of a haversian system cut horizontally to show osteocyte lacunae and associated canaliculi (×200).

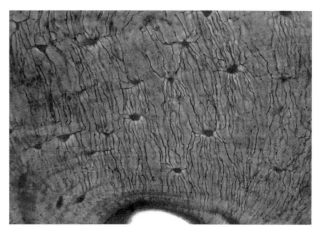

**Fig. 13.13** Demineralized section of bone perfused with picrothionin to visualize the osteocyte lacunae and canaliculi (×280). Courtesy of Professor M.M. Smith.

spongy bone. Active osteoblasts appear cuboidal and exhibit a basophilic cytoplasm that is related to the conspicuous amounts of endoplasmic reticulum within the cells. The cells are polarized and the prominent, round nucleus tends to lie towards the basal end. A pale, juxtanuclear area indicates the site of the Golgi complex. Numerous cell contacts are seen between the cell membranes of adjacent cells. Osteoblasts are also in contact with underlying osteocytes.

Osteoblasts contact one another by means of adherens, gap and tight junctions. These are functionally connected to microfilaments and enzymes (such as protein kinases) associated with intracellular secondary messenger systems. This complex arrangement provides for intercellular adhesion and cell–cell communication, helping to ensure that the osteoblast layer completely covers the osteoid surface and that the osteoblasts function in a coordinated manner. At the ultrastructural level, active osteoblasts can be seen to contain an extensive rough endoplasmic reticulum (arranged in parallel stacks), a localized and extensive Golgi complex and numerous mitochondria and vesicles (Fig. 13.11).

Osteoblasts secrete the organic matrix of bone that initially is represented by an unmineralized layer known as osteoid, about 5–10 μm thick (Figs 13.9, 13.10). Some of the components of osteoid, such as collagen type I, are widely distributed and not unique to osteoblasts. Others are specific to cells of the osteoblast lineage and provide useful markers of the osteoblast phenotype. These include osteocalcin and osteoblast transcription factor, Cbfa-1 (Runx2). Alkaline phosphatase activity, although not entirely specific to bone, is easy to identify and is a reliable indicator of osteoblastic differentiation. Although the precise role of this enzyme in osteoblasts is not known, it is thought to be involved in the mineralization of the matrix. The secreted, intrinsic, collagen fibrils lie parallel to the bone surface. At the surface of alveolar bone adjacent to the periodontal ligament, extrinsic Sharpey fibres pass more or less perpendicularly into the osteoid layer (Fig. 13.10). Osteoblasts have a lifespan of the order of about 1 month. Up to 30% of osteoblasts become embedded in the organic matrix as osteocytes, while the remainder appear to undergo apoptosis.

In addition to secreting the formative components of bone, the osteoblast secretes molecules controlling its own activity (i.e. paracrine secretion), such as growth factors, cytokines and prostaglandins. The cell also possesses surface receptors to bind to such molecules. In addition, the osteoblast releases molecules that have a controlling influence in activating

the bone-resorbing cells, the osteoclasts. This autocrine secretion involves molecules such as macrophage colony-stimulating factor (M-CSF) and RANKL (see pages 213–215). Osteoblasts also possess receptors for a number of hormones (e.g. parathyroid hormone, 1,25 dihydroxyvitamin D, sex steroids) that help regulate bone metabolism.

## OSTEOCYTES

Osteocytes are the postmitotic cells lying within the bone itself and represent 'entrapped' osteoblasts. There are about 25 000 osteocytes per cubic millimetre of bone. In preparing ground sections of bone, the osteocytes themselves are lost, but the spaces or lacunae they occupy are filled with air or cell debris and appear black in routine transmitted light sections (Fig. 13.12). The lacunae are regularly distributed and many narrow canals called canaliculi radiate from them in all directions. Numerous cell processes from the osteocytes run in the canaliculi in all directions, more being directed perpendicularly to the bone surface than parallel to it. The processes of neighbouring osteocytes are linked by cell contacts called gap junctions (see below) and those of superficially situated osteocytes are in contact with cells lining the bone surface. In this manner, osteocytes are in constant communication with both osteoblasts and bone-lining cells. The cell processes in the canaliculi allow the diffusion of substances from adjacent blood vessels through the bone. Cell processes do not appear to cross cement lines and therefore are unlikely to allow osteocytes to make cell contacts with cells in adjacent osteones. Some osteocytes in interstitial lamellae may die and their lacunae may become filled in with mineral. In routine, demineralized sections the osteocytes are retained, but the canaliculi are little in evidence. However, the canaliculi can be visualized in demineralized sections if perfused with a stain such as picrothionin (Fig. 13.13). It is

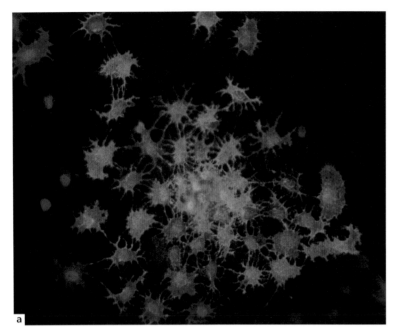

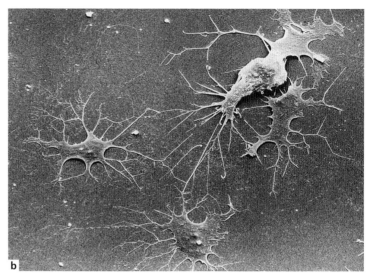

**Fig. 13.14** Osteocytes in tissue culture. (a) A group of osteocytes isolated from bone and maintained for 24 hours in tissue culture on glass. The cytoplasm (green fluorescence) has been stained with an osteocyte-specific monoclonal antibody (OB7.3) while the nuclei have been stained using a blue fluorescence. A small number of osteoblasts (negative for the green osteocyte-specific antibody but with a blue-staining nucleus) can also be seen (×350). (b) SEM of cultured osteocytes. The cells were characterized by their positive staining with an osteocyte-specific antibody (OB7.3). Like osteocytes in vivo, the cells have long, slender, often branched cell processes by which they have contacted those of adjacent cells during culture (×1000). From Van der Plas A, Nijweide PJ 1992 Isolation and purification of osteocytes. *Journal of Bone and Mineral Research* 7: 389–396.

possible to isolate and culture osteocytes, which retain their characteristic morphology (Fig. 13.14).

In comparison with cementocytes (see pages 171, 172), osteocytes are more regularly distributed and do not show the more preferential orientation of cementocyte canaliculi (towards the periodontal ligament). It is not known what becomes of osteocytes that are released following bone resorption activity by osteoclasts, but it is likely that the majority undergo apoptosis and are subsequently phagocytosed.

As they are derived from osteoblasts, it is not surprising that osteocytes share many common markers, such as the presence of osteopontin, osteocalcin, osteonectin, fibronectin and parathyroid hormone and oestrogen receptors. However, osteocytes do not express alkaline phosphatase and also possess specific antigens that should eventually help with their identification, although these have not yet been fully characterized.

At the ultrastructural level, the appearance of osteocytes vary according to their position in relation to the surface layer. Osteocytes newly incorporated into bone matrix from the osteoblast layer have a high organelle content similar to osteoblasts. However, as they become more deeply situated with continued bone formation, they appear to be less active. The cells are then seen to have a nucleus and thin ring of cytoplasm containing few organelles, reflecting the decreased cellular activity (Fig. 13.15). However, some secretion is likely to be necessary for osteocyte function if, for example, the cells are involved in the reception and transduction of mechanosensory information.

Numerous slender processes containing bundles of actin filaments extend from the osteocyte into canaliculi in the matrix. The processes of one cell are joined to those of another by gap junctions, which allow cell-to-cell communication and coordination of activity. In this feature, they differ from chondrocytes, which are said to lack processes and are isolated from one another. A pericellular space (which might represent a shrinkage artefact) is usually seen to intervene between the cell membrane and the surrounding bone and contains unmineralized matrix, consisting of proteoglycans and a few collagen fibrils.

As a result of their widespread distribution in bone and their interconnections, osteocytes are obvious candidates to detect load-induced strains in bone and are therefore regarded as the primary mechanosensors in bone. In support of this view is evidence of rapid changes in metabolism follow-

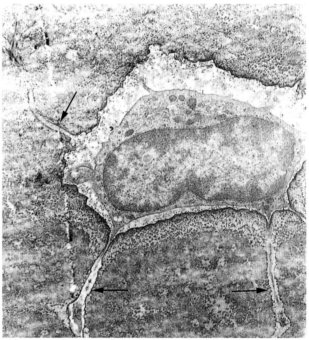

**Fig. 13.15** Electron microscopic appearance of demineralized bone showing an osteocyte. The cell has few organelles and possesses cell processes (arrowed) extending into canaliculi. A pericellular space is seen between the cell membrane and the wall of the lacuna and is probably related to a shrinkage artefact (×5300).

ing intermittent loading of bone. How strain is detected is not known for certain, but fluid flow through canaliculi and/or cell deformation have been suggested. In this context, the presence of cell adhesion molecules such as integrins at the cell membrane may be relevant.

## BONE-LINING CELLS

When bone surfaces are neither in the formative nor resorptive phase, the bone surface is lined by a layer of flattened cells termed bone-lining cells (Fig. 13.9), with little or no osteoid being present. Like osteoblasts, the bone-lining cells are connected to underlying osteocytes. They show little sign of synthetic activity, as evidenced by their reduced organelle content, and may be regarded as postproliferative osteoblasts. By covering the

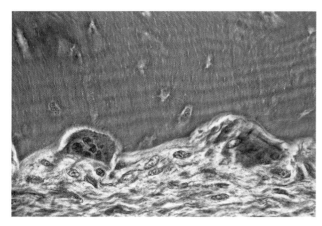

**Fig. 13.16** Demineralized section of a resorbing alveolar bone showing two osteoclasts lying in Howship's lacunae (×350). Courtesy of Professor M.M. Smith.

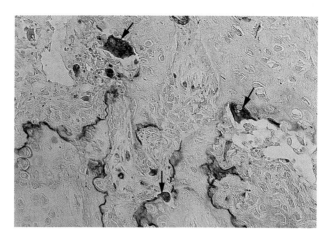

**Fig. 13.17** Demineralized section of bone showing osteoclasts staining positively (red) for tartrate-resistant acid phosphatase (arrows) (×240). Courtesy of Dr A. Grigoriadis.

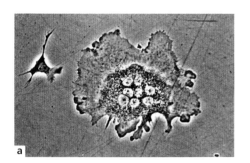

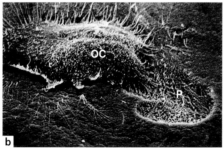

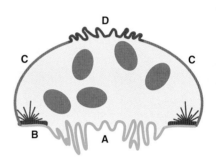

**Fig. 13.18** Osteoclasts in tissue culture: (a) phase contrast; (b) SEM. The osteoclast (OC) has moved away from an area of resorption (P) in which collagen fibrils have been exposed following removal of mineral (×700). Courtesy of Dr T.R. Arnett.

Bone

**Fig. 13.19** Diagram showing four zones on osteoclast. A = ruffled border; B = sealing zone; C = basolateral zone; D = functional secretory domain.

surface of bone, they may 1) play a role in calcium and phosphate metabolism, 2) protect the surface from any resorptive activity by osteoclasts, 3) participate in initiating bone remodelling. Bone-lining cells could also be a source of osteoprogenitor cells and be reactivated to form osteoblasts.

## OSTEOPROGENITOR CELLS

In order to generate osteoblasts throughout life, a stem cell population is required. Stem cells have the ability to maintain their numbers throughout life. When a stem cell divides, one of the daughter cells remains as a stem cell, while the other can differentiate into another cell type. This property of self-renewal is a unique property of stem cells. In the case of alveolar bone, the cells derived from the initial stem cells and that eventually give rise to osteoblasts are termed osteoprogenitor cells. They reside in the layer of cells beneath the osteoblast layer in the periosteal region, in the periodontal ligament or in the marrow spaces. Initially, the osteoprogenitor cells are fibroblast-like cells, with an elongated nucleus and few organelles (Fig. 13.11). Their life cycle may involve up to about eight cell divisions before reaching the osteoblast stage. There is a gradual acquirement of osteoblast-like features associated with an ordered increase in gene expression. Initially, genes related to cell growth are expressed (such as c-*myc*, c-*fos* and *Cbfa1*), followed by genes related to osteoblast products such as type I collagen, fibronectin, some growth factors and alkaline phosphatase. Finally, genes are expressed related to products associated with mineralization (such as osteocalcin, osteopontin and bone sialoprotein).

## OSTEOCLASTS

Osteoclasts are the cells responsible for bone resorption. They are derived from haemopoietic cells of the monocyte/macrophage lineage by fusion of mononuclear precursors, giving rise to multinucleated cells. This cell fusion takes place close to the bone surface, so that multinucleated osteoclasts are rarely seen at any distance from bone. The precise mechanism that guides osteoclasts to their sites of resorption is unknown but may involve chemotaxis. Resorbing surfaces of alveolar bone show typical resorption concavities (Howship's lacunae) in which the osteoclasts lie (Fig. 13.16). An osteoclast appears to undertake a number of resorption cycles before finally disappearing. A useful marker for osteoclasts is the enzyme tartrate-resistant acid phosphatase (Fig. 13.17), the function of which is not fully understood.

Tissue culture studies indicate that osteoclasts are highly motile, although the cells will resorb only when attached to bone (Fig. 13.18). Evidence from the presence of elongated 'snail track' resorption lacunae on bone surfaces (see Fig. 13.32) suggests that osteoclasts also move across the bone in vivo. Osteoclasts are recruited only when required and there is, consequently, no significant reservoir of inactive osteoclasts. The lifespan of osteoclasts is not known with any certainty, although it is thought to be at least 10–14 days, after which the cells finally undergo apoptosis.

Different nuclei within the osteoclast are often of different ages. The possibility exists that additional fusion of new cells may prolong the activity of osteoclasts.

Osteoclasts show considerable variation in size and shape, ranging from small mononuclear cells to very large cells with many nuclei. Characteristically, human osteoclasts may be up to 100 μm in diameter and have on average 10–20 nuclei, but there may be species variation in size. When actively resorbing, osteoclasts are highly polarized cells and exhibit four main different membrane domains (Fig. 13.19): the ruffled border and the sealing zone in contact with bone and the basolateral and functional secretory domains away from the bone.

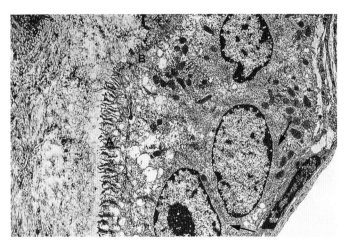

**Fig. 13.20** Electron microscopic appearance of demineralized bone showing part of an osteoclast. The brush border (A) comprises numerous microvilli adjacent to the bone surface. At the circumference of the brush border the annular zone (B) contains numerous microfilaments. There are numerous vesicles and mitochondria and three nuclei are evident (×3600). From Berkovitz BKB, Shore RC 1995 Cells of the periodontal ligament. In: Berkovitz BKB, Moxham BJ, Newman HJ (eds) *The periodontal ligament in health and disease*, 2nd edn. Mosby–Wolfe, London, pp 9–33.

The *ruffled border* is that part of the cell that lies adjacent to bone and where resorption occurs. More than one ruffled border may be present at any one time. At the light microscope level it often has a foamy or striated appearance. At the ultrastructural level, the ruffled border is composed of many tightly packed microvilli adjacent to the bone surface, providing a large surface area for the resorptive process. It has been postulated that products from the osteoclast (such as protons and proteases) are discharged (exocytosed) at the lateral aspects of the ruffled border and the resulting degraded matrix absorbed (endocytosed) in the central region of the ruffled border, thereby allowing for continuous activity.

The *sealing zone* (also referred to as the annular or clear zone) at the periphery of the ruffled border separates the ruffled border from the basolateral membrane. Here, the plasma membrane tends to become smooth and the organelle-free cytoplasm beneath it contains numerous contractile actin microfilaments (surrounded by two vinculin rings) (Fig. 13.20). It has been suggested that this sealing zone may serve to attach the cell very closely to the surface of the bone, thus creating an isolated microenvironment in which resorption of bone can take place without diffusion of the protons and proteases produced by the cell into adjacent soft tissue. This isolated microenvironment can be considered as a specialized 'extracellular' lysosome.

The attachment of the osteoclast cell membrane to the bone matrix at the sealing zone is mainly due to the presence of cell membrane adhesion proteins known as integrins (mainly $\alpha_v\beta_3$, but also $\alpha_v\beta_1$, $\alpha_2\beta_1$) but there are also non-integrin membrane receptors, such as CD44. The integrins bind to specific amino acid sequences present in proteins of the bone matrix, namely Arg–Gly–Asp (RGD). Interference with the formation of such integrins, or the administration of competing synthetic RGD peptides that prevent osteoclasts from attaching to bone, will inhibit bone resorption.

The membrane regions of the osteoclast away from the bone are subdivided into functional secretory and basolateral domains. The *functional secretory domain* opposite the ruffled border is a collection site of vesicles. It is believed that bone matrix, degraded at the ruffled border, passes across the cell in these vesicles to be exocytosed here (transcytosis) (Fig. 13.19). The *basolateral surface* may be a regulatory surface for receiving messages from neighbouring cells.

The osteoclast contains numerous mitochondria distributed throughout the cytoplasm (except for the region immediately beneath the ruffled border). The rough endoplasmic reticulum is less conspicuous than in osteoblasts, but Golgi material is prominent (especially in juxtanuclear

areas). Most of the remaining cytoplasm contains large numbers of vesicles of different sizes and types, some containing lysosomal enzymes such as cathepsins (e.g. cysteine proteinases) and matrix metalloproteinases (such as collagenases) capable of degrading the organic matrix of bone.

The osteoclast has far fewer surface receptors than the osteoblast and is not directly responsive to the majority of hormones or growth factors. This has led to the concept that the osteoblast has a controlling influence in the development and maturation of the osteoclast. However, important receptors that the osteoclast does express are those for calcitonin (a powerful inhibitor of osteoclasis that interferes with the cell attachment mechanism to bone), prostaglandins and RANK (the receptor for RANKL – see pages 213–215). Although not widely mentioned in the literature, osteoclasts, like osteoblasts, also express receptors for parathyroid hormone. This allows for the possibility of a different action for this hormone on the two cell types.

Once the osteoclast has been activated, bone resorption occurs in two stages. Initially, the mineral phase is removed and later the remaining organic matrix. To provide a low pH for dissolving the mineral phase, the osteoclast secretes protons across the ruffled border by means of a V-type ATPase proton pump: the enzyme carbonic anhydrase II is involved in generating protons by catabolizing the reaction of carbon dioxide with water to form carbonic acid. Secretion of anions balances the pumping of protons, accounting for the large number of chloride channels in the ruffled border.

The organic matrix exposed in the resorbing lacuna (Fig. 13.18b) is then degraded by enzymes such as the matrix metalloproteinases (MMPs) and lysosomal and non-lysosomal enzymes (especially cathepsin K). It is not known how much of this organic degradation takes place extracellularly and how much intracellularly. Compared with the fibroblasts of the periodontal ligament (see Fig. 12.34), intracellular collagen profiles have hardly ever been reported as being present within osteoclasts.

## CELL KINETICS

## FORMATION OF OSTEOBLASTS

Much research on the lifecycle of osteoblasts has been undertaken using stromal cells removed from bone marrow, where it has been demonstrated that stem cells are multipotential and can give rise to osteoblasts as well as fibroblasts, chondroblasts, adipoblasts and myofibroblasts. Stem cells for osteoblasts in the periodontal ligament may be derived from perivascular cells in the ligament as well as from the adjacent bone marrow. From a stem cell, intermediate progenitor cell forms have been described leading to postmitotic osteoblasts. These forms include osteoprogenitors (immature and mature forms) and preosteoblasts and involve about eight cell divisions. As cells generally increase in size during differentiation, the size of the cell has been used in an attempt to distinguish osteoblasts and their precursors. The process of bone formation requires 1) cell proliferation, 2) the synthesis and secretion of an extracellular matrix and 3) mineralization of the matrix. The process is characterized by a decreasing proliferative capacity and an increasing degree of differentiation of the cells.

Among the earliest markers to indicate that a stem cell is progressing along an osteogenic phenotype are the expression of the nuclear transcription factor core binding factor 1 (Cbfa1, also called Runx2), which is responsible for regulating the production of a number of important protein products in bone matrix, and specific cell surface markers (e.g. STRO-1). Supporting the importance of Cbfa1 is the observation that knockout mice lacking this gene lack bone. The induction of Cbfa1 involves the action of growth factors such as TGFβ and BMP-2.

Osteoprogenitor cells can be identified by the progressive expression of molecules such as type I collagen, alkaline phosphatase and osteopontin, and by the appearance of specific receptors such as PTH1R. In the pre-

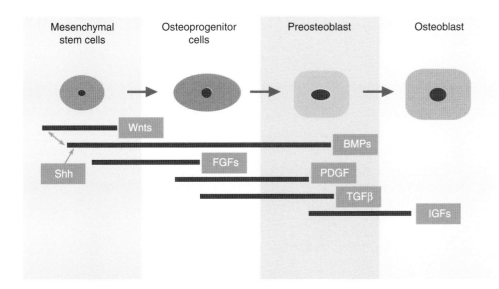

**Fig. 13.21** The main stages of growth factor activity during osteoblast differentiation. BMPs = bone morphogenetic proteins; FGFs = fibroblast growth factors; IGFs = insulin-like growth factors; PDGF = platelet-derived growth factor; Shh = sonic hedgehog; TGFβ = transforming growth factor-β; Wnts = Wnt proteins. Redrawn after Hughes FJ et al 2000 *Periodontology 2000* 41: 48–72, with permission of Blackwell Publishing, a subsidiary of John Wiley & Sons Inc.

**Table 13.1** *Regulation of bone cell function*

**1. Hormones**

| | |
|---|---|
| Parathyroid hormone (PTH) | ↑ plasma $Ca^{2+}$ (critical regulator); ↑ OC formation, activity; ↑ OB proliferation, activity → ↑ bone turnover; intermittent PTH ↑ bone formation in vivo; continuous high-dose PTH ↑ bone resorption → bone loss |
| 1,25(OH)$_2$ vitamin D | ↑ gut $Ca^{2+}$ uptake, plasma $Ca^{2+}$; ↑ OC formation, activity; ↓ OB proliferation, ↑ OB (and skin cell) differentiation; required for normal matrix mineralization; deficiency → osteomalacia, rickets |
| Calcitonin | ↓ plasma $Ca^{2+}$ in young/hypercalcaemic animals; ↓ OC formation, activity; 'emergency' hormone, not much effect in normal adults |
| Glucocorticoids | Necessary for normal bone development/function; excess → bone loss/osteoporosis; required for bone formation in vitro |
| Growth hormone | Required for normal bone growth |
| Sex steroids (oestrogens and androgens) | Critical long-term, beneficial effects on bone maintenance; ↓ OC formation, activity; ••↑ OB activity; deficiency → ↑ bone turnover, osteoporosis |

**2. Local (paracrine/autocrine) factors**

| | |
|---|---|
| Growth factors | Mitogens; many produced by OB and other connective tissue cells, e.g. TGFβ, bone morphogenetic proteins, IGF-I, -II, PDGF, FGFs; generally ↑ OC recruitment and activity, ↑ proliferation of OB and other cells |
| Cytokines | Products of immune and other cells; IL-1, -2, -4, -6, -11, -13 and -17, TNFα, RANK ligand, M-CSF ↑ OC formation/activity; IL -4, -10, -12, -13 and -18, interferon-γ and GM-CSF ↓ OC formation; ILs may mediate some actions of PTH, 1,25(OH)$_2$ vitamin D and sex steroids |
| Other molecules | Prostaglandins (normal OB product) ↑ OC recruitment, ↑↓ OC activity; mediate some actions of growth factors, cytokines, responses to mechanical stimuli and hypoxia. Leukotrienes ↑ OC formation/activity. Extracellular ATP ↑ OC formation/activity, ↓ OB activity; possible mediator of inflammatory bone loss. Bradykinin ↑ OC formation/activity; CGRP ↓ OC formation/activity |

**3. Inorganic agents (local/systemic)**

| | |
|---|---|
| Ions | Extracellular $H^+$ (pH< ≈7.2) ↑ OC (required for OC activation), ↓ OB function (mineralization). $PO_4^{3-}$ ↓ OC formation/activity. $Ca^{2+}$ ↓ OC formation/activity (small effect). $Sr^{2+}$ ↑ bone formation; $F^-$ ↑ bone formation |
| Oxygen and free radicals | Hypoxia ($PO_2$ ≤ 5%) ↑ OC formation, ↓ OB function. Nitric oxide ↑↓ OC formation/activity; ↑↓ OB activity; required for normal bone remodelling, mediates responses to loading |

**4. Mechanical effects**

| | |
|---|---|
| | Cyclical loading ↑ OB activity, bone formation; unloading (bed rest, microgravity) ↑ OC formation/activity; large changes in hydrostatic pressure ↑ osteocyte death |

↑ = increases; ↓ = decreases; → = results in; ATP = adenosine triphosphate; CGRP = calcitonin-gene-related peptide; FGF = fibroblast growth factor; GM-CSF = granulocyte–macrophage colony-stimulating factor; IGF = insulin-like growth factor; IL = interleukin; M-CSF = macrophage colony-stimulating factor; OB = osteoblast; OC = osteoclast; PDGF = platelet-derived growth factor; PTH = parathyroid hormone; TGF = transforming growth factor; TNF = tumour necrosis factor. Courtesy of Dr T.R. Arnett.

osteoblast, the concentration of many of the osteogenic markers seen in the osteoprogenitor cells increases and there is still some limited proliferation. The cell is relatively undifferentiated and there is little roughened endoplasmic reticulum. In the postmitotic osteoblast, even more activity of the markers first seen in preosteoblasts is present and there is marked development of roughened endoplasmic reticulum and Golgi material. In addition, new molecules related to mineralization (e.g. osteocalcin) and cell adhesion molecules make their appearance.

The differentiation of osteoblasts and their subsequent lifecycle is regulated by numerous factors, among which will be transcription factors (e.g. TAZ, Msx2, Dlx5 and Osterix), growth factors and cytokines (e.g. BMP, TGFβ, IGF, IL-1) (Fig. 13.21), and hormones (e.g. glucocorticoids, parathyroid hormone). The actions of such molecules may differ according to

the stage of differentiation and concentration (Table 13.1). The final stage of the osteoblast concerns its entrapment in bone matrix, where it becomes the osteocyte.

## FORMATION OF OSTEOCLASTS

Unlike the other cells associated with bone (e.g. osteoblasts, osteocytes, bone-lining cells), osteoclasts are derived not from stromal cells but from blood cells. The pluripotent stem cell is of the monocyte/macrophage lineage. Early important transcription factors indicative of its eventual fate are c-Fos and PU-1. Differentiation from the myeloid progenitor to the mononuclear osteoclast precursor involves the activity of many factors, two of the most important of which are M-CSF and receptor activator of

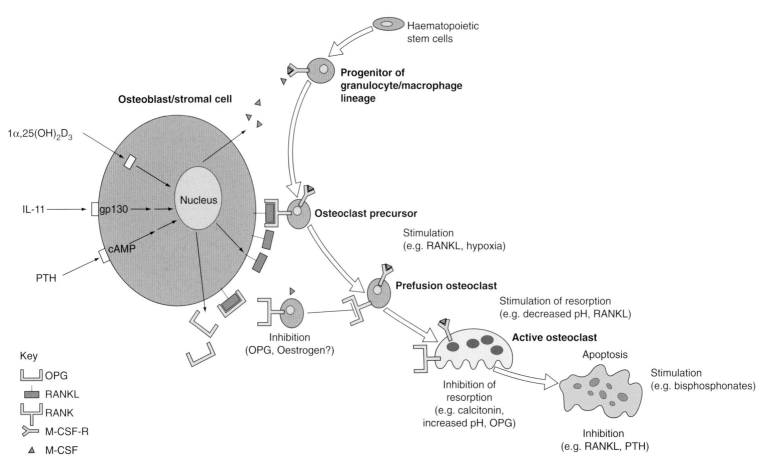

**Fig. 13.22** Factors controlling osteoblast–osteoclast interactions. M-CSF-R = macrophage colony-stimulating factor receptor; OPG = osteoprotegerin; PTH = parathyroid hormone; RANK = receptor activator of nuclear factor κ B; RANKL = receptor activator of nuclear factor κ B ligand. Courtesy of Drs A. Grigoriadis and T. Arnett.

**Fig. 13.23** Effect of pH on osteoclastic resorption, as measured by the number of resorption pits beneath rat osteoclasts cultured on polished cow bone slices.

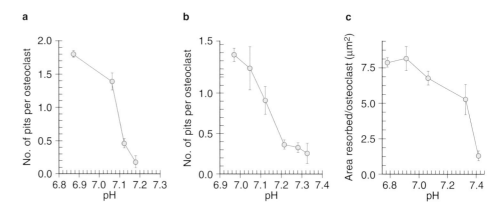

nuclear factor κ B ligand (RANKL), also known as ODF (osteoclast differentiation factor), OPGL (osteoprotegerin ligand) and TRANCE (TNF-related activation-induced cytokine). These two factors are produced by osteoblast/stromal cells. As osteoclast progenitors have a receptor for M-CSF (c-Fms) and a receptor (RANK) for RANKL, close association between the two cell types drives the differentiation of the osteoclast precursors into mononuclear preosteoclasts. As a method of controlling the rate of formation of osteoclast precursors, the osteoblast also secretes osteoprotegerin (OPG), which acts as a soluble decoy molecule by binding with RANKL and thereby inhibiting osteoclast formation. Preosteoclasts also contain receptors for calcitonin. The interrelationships of some of these molecules are shown in Figure 13.22.

Fusion of mononuclear osteoclasts into multinucleated osteoclasts and their subsequent activation is also driven by the RANKL/RANK system. Many complex membrane interactions must occur when cells are undergoing fusion to become multinucleated. Initially, the cell is non-polarized and it is only on attaching to bone by cell–matrix interactions (involving transmembrane receptors such as integrins and matrix components such

as collagen and osteopontin) that the osteoclast becomes polarized and develops the ruffled border, sealing zone and systems to successfully demineralize bone and degrade its organic matrix. Following its resorptive phase, osteoclasts are thought to be removed by apoptosis.

Two additional important factors involved in the activation of osteoclasts are acidification and hypoxia.

Acidification   In appropriate media, osteoclasts cultured on bone at pH 7.4 (physiological or blood pH) are virtually inactive. However, when the pH is lowered to 7.0, there is a large increase in resorption (Fig. 13.23). This reduction in pH also acts synergistically with osteolytic agents such as RANKL. As has been seen above, RANKL is an important agent driving the development and activation of osteoclasts. However, when added to osteoclasts in culture, RANKL by itself has little effect on bone resorption at physiological pH of blood (approximately pH 7.4) but, when combined with low pH, there is a dramatic increase in resorption (Fig. 13.24). In this respect, it is worth noting that the activity of a number of cytokines and growth factors results in the release of hydrogen ions from the affected cells.

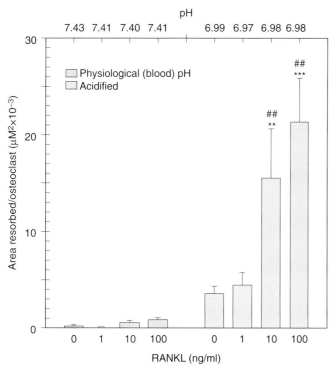

pH

7.43  7.41  7.40  7.41          6.99  6.97  6.98  6.98

**Fig. 13.24** The combined effect of RANKL and pH on osteoclastic resorption. From Arnett TR 2003 Regulation of bone cell function by acid-base balance. *Proceedings of the Nutrition Society* 62: 511–520.

Hypoxia    There is evidence to suggest that a reduction in oxygen levels in the microenvironment of bone tissue provides a stimulus for osteoclasis, although the mechanism is poorly understood. The hypoxia may be associated with acidification, or it may cause the release of factors such as prostaglandins and vascular endothelial growth factor.

The importance of factors listed above in association with the formation and activity of osteoclasts has been deduced from studies designed to produce deficiencies or overexpression of the factor. Thus, mice lacking the ability to produce either M-CSF, RANKL or RANK do not develop osteoclasts. They are therefore unable to resorb bone and thick bone is produced (osteopetrosis). Their teeth may be prevented from erupting (because of the inability to resorb bone overlying the erupting teeth) but this can be corrected by restoring the missing factor. In contrast, mice lacking the ability to produce OPG (the osteoclast inhibitor) have increased numbers of osteoclasts and develop osteoporosis.

## RESORPTION AND FORMATION OF BONE DURING REMODELLING

The processes of bone resorption and formation at sites of remodelling do not occur randomly. Clearly, there must be tight control to ensure a balance between the two processes, as any disruption of this balance can lead to metabolic bone disease. This is referred to as coupling. From a resting state, the sequence of remodelling consists of four main phases:

■ **resorption**: recruitment, migration and activation of osteoclasts causing bone resorption (Fig. 13.25a)

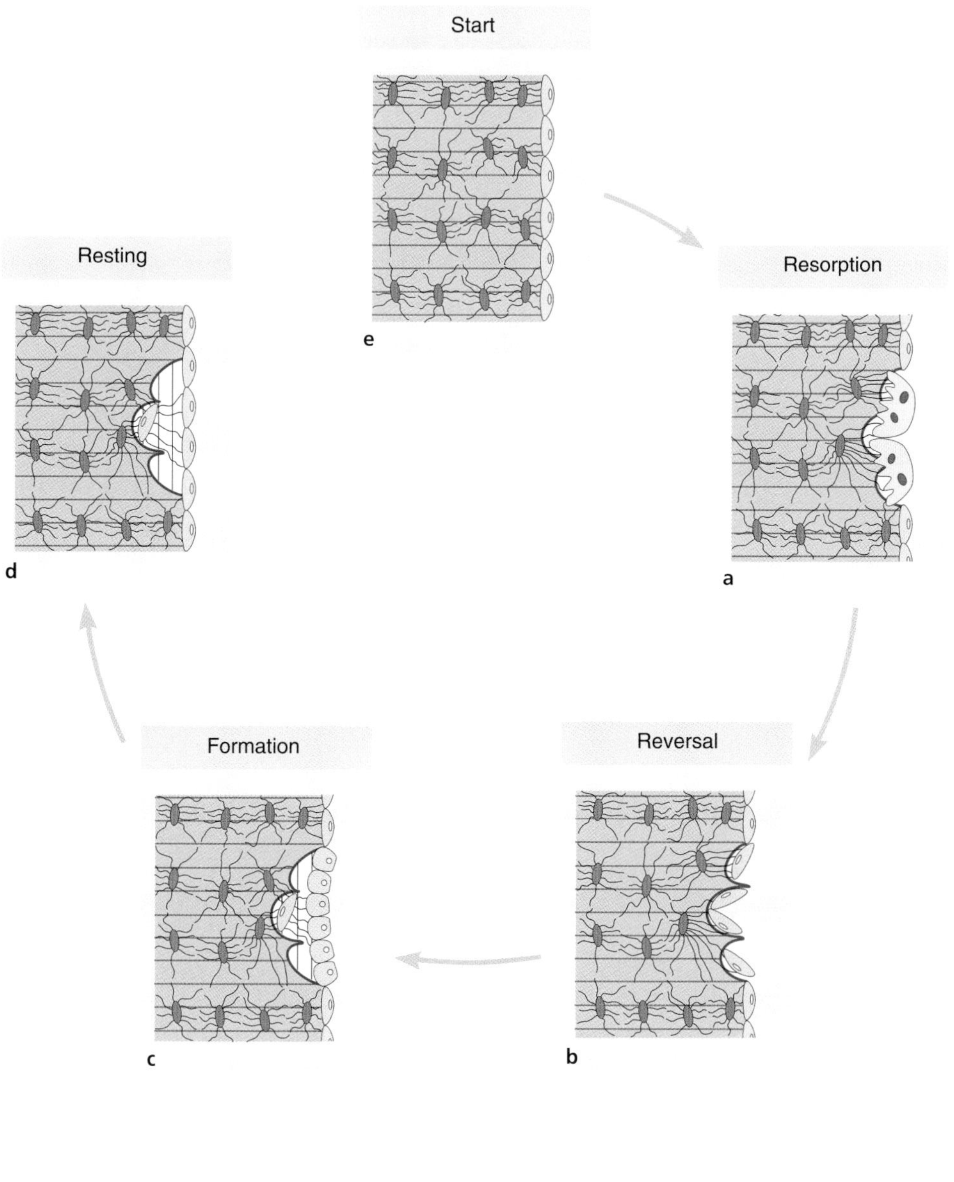

**Fig. 13.25** The sequence of events during bone remodelling. A reversal line is indicated in red. See text for description.

Start

e

Resting

Resorption

d

a

Formation

Reversal

c

b

**Fig. 13.26** A cutting cone. (a) Longitudinal section along a haversian system showing the four main phases of the remodelling cycle. (b) Cross-sections of the haversian system showing the corresponding appearance of each of the four main phases of the remodelling cycle.

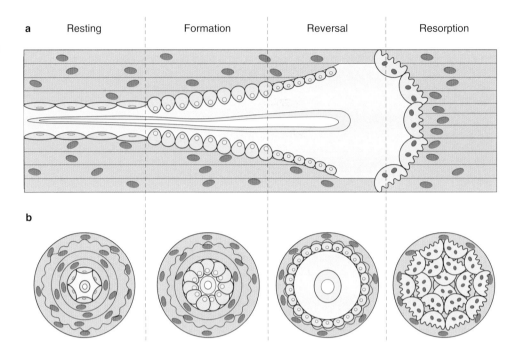

- **reversal**: cessation of resorption and disappearance of osteoclasts by apoptosis or migration; the site becomes occupied by mononuclear cells (Fig. 13.25b)
- **formation**: osteoblast recruitment, migration, differentiation and formation of new bone in the resorption site (Fig. 13.25c)
- **resting**: formation of bone ceases and the surface is lined by a flattened layer of cells (Fig. 13.25d).

In this manner, an initial 'cutting cone' of osteoclastic resorption moves along the central canal of an osteon at about 50 μm/day, followed by a 'closing zone' of osteoblastic activity (Fig. 13.26).The changeover from resorption to deposition is characterized by a reversal (cement) line (Fig. 13.27; see also Fig. 13.43). This reversal line is rich in osteopontin and acid phosphatase (Fig. 13.27).

Many of the biological molecules capable of causing bone resorption, such as parathyroid hormone, interleukins (IL-11), and vitamin $D_3$, have their primary effect on osteoblasts, driving the production of RANKL, OPG and M-CSF: however, each may drive the production via a different route (Fig. 13.22). A close association of these cells with osteoclasts and their precursors is a further requirement necessary for the activation of bone resorption. As previously mentioned (see pages 214–215), ambient pH and levels of oxygen are also important factors affecting resorption.

There is evidence that osteoclasts can be activated, and begin resorption, when they contact the mineralized surface of bone. Initially, therefore, any bone-lining cells or osteoblasts will have to retract or migrate away from the surface in order to expose the bone surface. Following this, any covering of osteoid will need to be removed. Osteoblasts/bone-lining cells have been implicated in this removal, possibly releasing enzymes (e.g. MMP-1) to degrade the osteoid. Molecules in this milieu may then be chemotactic to osteoclasts.

The precise signals responsible for causing the cessation of resorption and a reversal to osteoblast differentiation and activation of bone formation are not known. However, the release of molecules such as growth factors initially bound up in the bone matrix but exposed/activated by the resorption process may be involved. For example, BMPs and IGF released from bone may stimulate osteoblasis, while TGFβ released from bone may inhibit osteoclasis while stimulating osteoblasis.

As a reduction in the mechanical loads impinging on bone is associated with bone loss, it can be assumed that such loading is normally required to stimulate the modelling/remodelling processes of bone necessary to maintain normal bone structure. Strains need to be intermittent (rather than continuous) and the osteogenic response is dependent upon the size of the load and the frequency and rate of application. To maintain bone mass may only require the application of relatively few loading cycles.

The molecular mechanisms whereby forces impinging on the bone are transduced into bone resorption or deposition remain elusive, although many theories have been proposed. Osteocytes, together with the surface layer of osteoblasts/bone lining cells, appear to be the most obvious candidates for detecting strain within bone as 1) they are present throughout bone, 2) they maintain contact with neighbouring osteocytes and with osteoblasts/bone-lining cells via gap junctions, and 3) they are able to modify their volume, which in turn alters their sensitivity to loading. A widely held view envisages that deformation of bone following loading deforms the cell processes/cell membranes either directly or indirectly through movement of tissue fluid residing in the lacunocanalicular system. Signals are then transduced via the cell membrane at the surface (e.g. involving $K^+$ and $Ca^{2+}$ ion channels and integrins) to cytoskeletal elements within the cell, with stimulation of secondary messengers. These changes eventually lead to the production and release of molecules that initiate an osteogenic response. Among the important molecules whose activity is upregulated in osteocytes (and osteoblasts) following the application of mechanical strain are prostaglandins, interleukins, nitric oxide and certain growth factors (e.g. IGFs). Changes in the microenvironment need also to be considered, such as pH, oxygen tension, electric potential and concentration of ions such as calcium and sodium.

Radiographic techniques readily demonstrate that bone is continually remodelling to adapt to the different functional regimens impinging on it. In this context, newly formed bone is less dense (and therefore more radiolucent) than mature bone (Figs 13.28, 13.29). As mentioned previously, spongy bone remodels about 25% of its mass each year, compared with only about 3% for cortical bone.

There are a considerable number of factors that can influence bone remodelling, some of the more common being listed in Table 13.1. Some

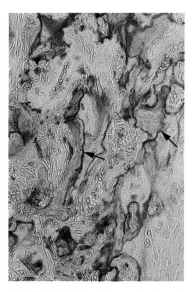

**Fig. 13.27** Portion of bone showing the scalloped outline of a reversal line staining positively (red) for acid phosphatase (arrows) (×100). Courtesy of Dr A. Grigoriadis.

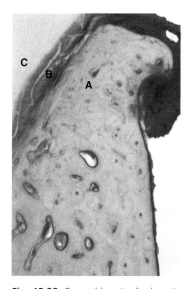

**Fig. 13.28** Ground longitudinal section of alveolar bone at the alveolar crest. A = alveolar bone; B = periodontal space; C = root (×16). Courtesy of R.V. Hawkins.

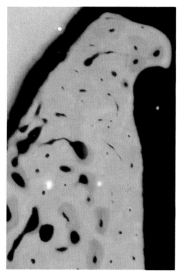

**Fig. 13.29** Microradiograph of section shown in Fig. 13.16. The varying densities of alveolar bone indicate its active remodelling, the darker, radiolucent areas being most recently formed and less mineralized. Courtesy of R.V. Hawkins.

notion of the complexity of the topic is given by the fact that some reagents can affect both formation and resorption of bone, while others can produce opposite effects, depending on concentration. Synergism must also be taken into account.

## MICRODAMAGE IN BONE

Microdamage within bone may result from the cumulative effects of mechanical stress or loading and takes the form of microcracks/microfractures, only visible under the microscope. A major difficulty related to studying this subject concerns the ability of distinguishing real bone microcracks from artefacts created during specimen preparation for microscopy. The development of such features, together with the death (or apoptosis) of osteocytes, may represent the signal that stimulates remodelling of the affected bone, primarily to repair the crack and presumably also to redistribute the functional loads more appropriately throughout the skeleton. Some authorities suggest that any remodelling involves initial resorption of the affected bone, while others claim that cracks are removed by calcified matrix filling alone, without prior resorption. This latter view is supported by the observation that, when osteocytes die, their lacuna and canaliculi may also ossify without resort to prior resorption.

## SCANNING ELECTRON MICROSCOPE APPEARANCES OF THE ALVEOLAR BONE SURFACE

Scanning electron microscopy provides a useful technique for visualizing the appearance of large areas of bone surfaces at high magnification. Cells and the organic material in any covering osteoid layer are removed by substances such as sodium hypochlorite, producing an anorganic preparation and revealing the underlying mineralized or mineralizing surface layer.

An alveolar bone surface on which bone formation is occurring is characterized by the presence of numerous small, calcified nodules within and around collagen fibrils. Sharpey fibres with a central unmineralized core may be encountered as small, dark, circular areas and larger ovoid areas represent lacunae occupied in vivo by osteocytes becoming entombed in bone (Fig. 13.30). If the forming alveolar bone surface is rendered only partially anorganic, the smallest calcified nodules

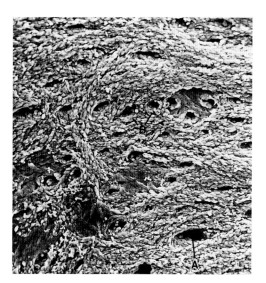

**Fig. 13.30** SEM appearance of alveolar bone surface where bone formation is occurring, characterized by numerous small calcific nodules in partly mineralized intrinsic collagen, masking the underlying collagen fibrils. The larger, dark, elongated areas represent the lacunae of osteoblasts becoming entombed as osteocytes (A), while the smaller circular dark areas (B) represent the unmineralized cores of the Sharpey fibres (Anorganic preparation; ×550). Courtesy of Professor S.J. Jones.

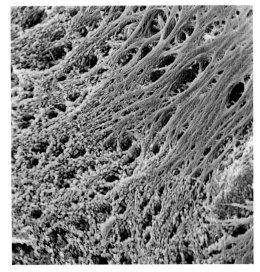

Fig. 13.31

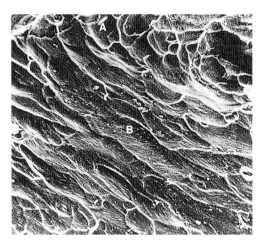

Fig. 13.32

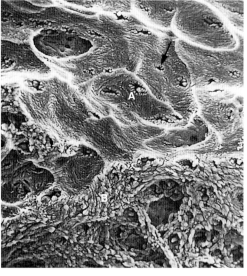

Fig. 13.33

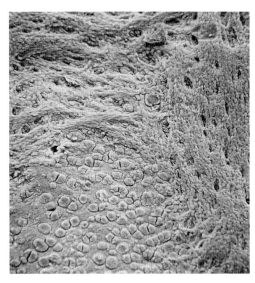

Fig. 13.34

**Fig. 13.31** SEM appearance of alveolar bone surface where bone formation is occurring, as evidenced by the numerous small nodules in the lower and left part of the field. However, the surface has been rendered only partly anorganic to show the collagen fibres of the extracellular matrix (Partial anorganic preparation; ×550). Courtesy of Professor S.J. Jones.

**Fig. 13.32** SEM of periosteal surface of bone (lacking Sharpey fibres) undergoing resorption. In addition to pit-like resorption lacunae (A), elongated 'snail-track' resorption lacunae are evident (B) (Anorganic preparation; ×300). Courtesy of Professor S.J. Jones.

**Fig. 13.33** SEM of alveolar bone surface contrasting the appearance of an area of bone resorption (A) with an adjacent area of bone formation (B). Note the presence of Sharpey fibres with unmineralized cores in the resorbing areas (arrowed) (Anorganic preparation; ×300). Courtesy of Professor S.J. Jones.

**Fig. 13.34** SEM of resting alveolar bone surface (lower left part of field) characterized by projections marking the sites of mineralized extrinsic Sharpey fibres separated by smooth areas. This contrasts with the granular appearance of the forming bone surface in the upper right part of the field, where the Sharpey fibres whose cores have not yet fully mineralized are seen as holes (Anorganic preparation; ×500). Courtesy of Professor S.J. Jones.

**Fig. 13.35** TEM of a Sharpey fibre (A) entering the surface of alveolar bone (B). Note the periodicity evident on the collagen fibrils (Decalcified section; ×10 500).

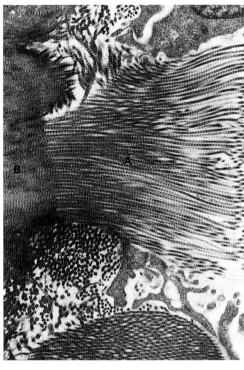

Fig. 13.35

of bone may be seen depositing on the intrinsic collagen fibrils, and the orientation of the collagen parallel to the bone surface is also visualized (Fig. 13.31).

An alveolar bone surface on which bone resorption is occurring is characterized by the presence of Howship's resorption lacunae (Fig. 13.32). If a periosteal surface is examined, there may be no Sharpey fibres present. In addition to localized, pit-like resorption lacunae, bone may also exhibit longer 'snail-track' resorption lacunae. In contrast to a periosteal surface, the appearance of an area of resorption in bundle bone (periodontal surface) shows the presence of Sharpey fibres in the resorbing areas (Fig. 13.33).

When neither bone deposition nor resorption is occurring the surface of the bone is described as a resting surface. The resting surface may be characterized by projections marking the sites of extrinsic mineralized Sharpey fibres, separated by smooth areas containing intrinsic mineralized collagen fibres. This contrasts with the granular appearance of the mineral of the intrinsic fibres of any adjacent forming surface (Fig. 13.34).

## SHARPEY FIBRES

In addition to intrinsic fibres secreted by osteoblasts, which are aligned parallel to the bone surface, alveolar bone contains extrinsic Sharpey fibres that enter bone perpendicular to the surface (Fig. 13.35). Extrinsic fibres, inserting into the cribriform plate as Sharpey fibres, are derived from the principal fibres of the periodontal ligament. Sharpey fibres are particularly prominent in the cervical portion (alveolar crest region) of the cribriform plate. Sharpey fibres entering alveolar bone are less numerous but thicker than those at the cementum surface (Fig. 13.36). There is evidence that traces of type III collagen are found at the periphery of Sharpey fibres (Fig. 13.37). Because of the attachments of numerous bundles of collagen fibres, the cribriform plate has also been called bundle bone. Bundle bone usually comprises thin lamellae running parallel to each other and to the root surface (see Fig. 13.42).

Scanning electron micrographs of anorganic preparations of the periodontal surfaces of alveolar bone show that the Sharpey fibres have two

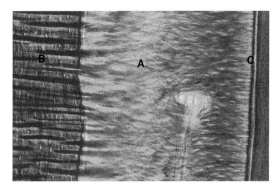

Fig. 13.36

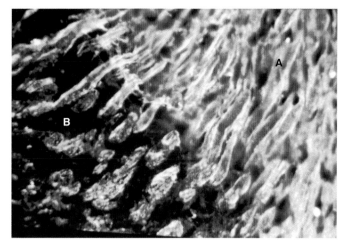

Fig. 13.37

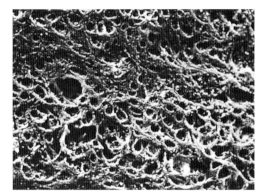

Fig. 13.38

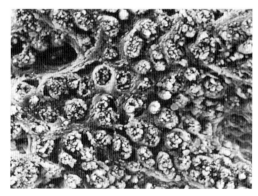

Fig. 13.39

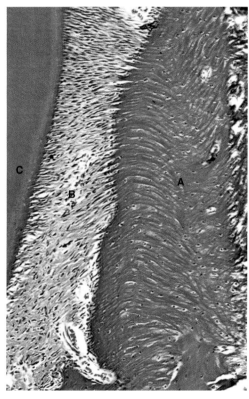

Fig. 13.40

**Fig. 13.36** Section of a root of a tooth showing Sharpey fibres from the periodontal ligament (A) entering alveolar bone (B). The Sharpey fibres in bone are seen to be thicker but less numerous than those entering the cementum on the tooth surface (C) (Decalcified section; aldehyde fuchsin and van Gieson; ×250). Courtesy of Professor S.J. Jones.

**Fig. 13.37** Sharpey fibre insertion from the periodontal ligament (A) into alveolar bone (B), showing peripheral staining of inserting collagen bundles with immunofluorescent stain for collagen type III (×350). From Sloan P, Carter DH 1995 Structural organisation of the fibres of the periodontal ligament. In: Berkovitz BKB, Moxham BJ, Newman H (eds) *The periodontal ligament in health and disease*, 2nd edn. Mosby–Wolfe, London, pp 35–53.

**Fig. 13.38** SEM of Sharpey fibres in alveolar bone with unmineralized centres, which are removed by the hypochlorite used to prepare this anorganic specimen (×300). Courtesy of Professor P. Sloan.

**Fig. 13.39** SEM of Sharpey fibres in alveolar bone, which are mineralized beyond the surface of the bone and remain as small, calcified projections into the periodontal ligament (Anorganic preparation; ×300). Courtesy of Professor P. Sloan.

**Fig. 13.40** Mesiodistal section of interdental bone (A), showing Sharpey fibres from the periodontal ligament (B) appearing to pass more or less completely through the full thickness of bone between two adjacent teeth. C = root. (Decalcified longitudinal section; Masson's trichrome; ×100).

main appearances, depending upon the degree of mineralization. In one, the embedded fibres may remain unmineralized at their centres, and removal of their organic material results in a series of hollow centres (Fig. 13.38). Conversely, the inserting fibres may be fully mineralized and project beyond the surface of the bone as small, calcified prominences into the periodontal ligament (Fig. 13.39).

In the cervical part of the interdental septum, where the bone type is mainly compact, Sharpey fibres entering the bone in the mesiodistal plane may pass straight through to become continuous with similar fibres from the root of the adjacent tooth. These are called transalveolar fibres (Fig. 13.40). A similar pattern exists in the interradicular bone, although in this situation the fibres link roots of the same tooth. Transalveolar fibres also pass through the entire thickness of the alveolar bone in the buccal and lingual planes, intermingling with the overlying periosteum or with the lamina propria of the gingiva (Fig. 13.41). However, where the alveolar bone is cancellous no transalveolar fibres are seen.

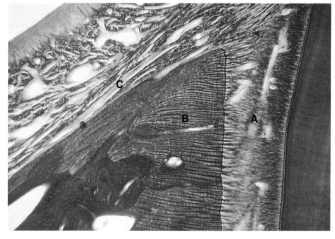

**Fig. 13.41** Buccolingual section of tooth in situ appearing to show Sharpey fibres passing from the periodontal ligament (A) through the compact alveolar bone (B) in the cervical region to reach the lamina propria of the attached gingiva (C) (Decalcified longitudinal section; van Gieson; ×80). Courtesy of Professor S.J. Jones.

## STRUCTURAL LINES IN BONE

Bone is laid down rhythmically, which results in the formation of regular parallel lines that, because they are formed in periods of relative quiescence, are termed resting lines. Such resting lines differ biochemically from adjacent bone. These lines are prominent in bundle bone on the distal surface of the socket wall during physiological mesial drift of the teeth (Fig. 13.42). Bone will also contain reversal lines, representing the site of change from bone resorption to bone deposition (see page 216). Such reversal lines will show evidence of a scalloped outline, reflecting the position of Howship's lacunae (Figs 13.25, 13.27 and 13.43).

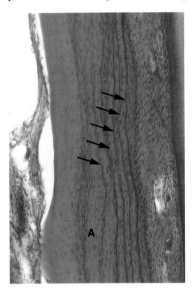

**Fig. 13.42** Alveolar bone (A) on the distal wall of a tooth socket undergoing mesial drift, showing many vertical resting lines (arrows) due to rhythmic deposition of bone with periods of quiescence (H & E; ×40).

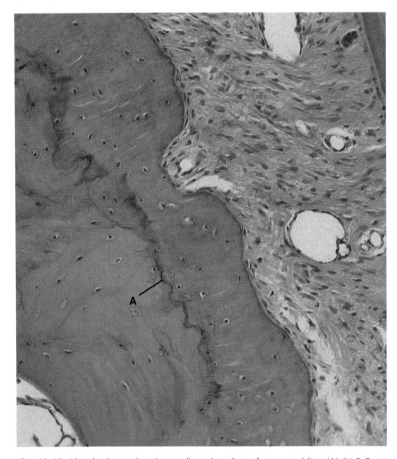

**Fig. 13.43** Alveolar bone showing scalloped outline of a reversal line (A) (H & E; ×250).

## CLINICAL CONSIDERATIONS

As maintenance of bone mass is dependent on suitable functional stimuli, alveolar bone tends to atrophy when tensile functional occlusal loading (transmitted via the periodontal ligament) is decreased. Thus, following tooth extraction, alveolar bone will resorb unless the remaining ridge is loaded. Even the placement of a denture over the remaining alveolar ridge may retard total bone loss. However, if the prosthesis produces excessive compression, the denture-bearing area may show accelerated resorption.

The ability of alveolar bone to remodel throughout life allows teeth to be repositioned during orthodontic treatment, with resorption of bone in front of the moving tooth matched by deposition of bone behind. However, as osteoclasts cannot fully differentiate between dentine, cementum and bone, excessive orthodontic forces can cause root resorption, ranging from blunting the apices in minor cases up to destruction of a considerable portion of the root (Fig. 13.44). As a consequence, many techniques are being examined to enhance orthodontic treatment and limit damage, including electrical pulses (note that this may stimulate the surrounding striated muscles, in turn deforming the bone), magnetic pulses and local injections of mediators of the inflammatory response. As yet no technique has been shown to consistently enhance tooth movement or longevity.

The possible role of oxygen tension on osteoclast activity may help provide an explanation for the loss of bone that is seen to accompany many clinical conditions where the blood supply is compromised and hypoxia is encountered, such as following inflammation, radiation damage, fractures and ageing.

Localized alveolar bone loss is found in periodontal disease (and in periapical abscesses) in response to the inflammatory process associated with the chronic presence of dental plaque and calculus at the cervical margins (see pages 126–128). Among important bioactive molecules implicated in this resorption process are cytokines and prostaglandins, as well as protons (as inflamed tissue is generally acidic). As differences exist between the collagen and the ground substance of bone and periodontal ligament, analysis of their breakdown products in the local serum exudates contributing to gingival crevicular fluid may provide a marker to distinguish those patients who are more at risk of losing alveolar bone. Levels of such molecules will also be found to increase when crevicular fluid is analysed in patients undergoing orthodontic tooth movement.

Apart from localized inflammation, more generalized conditions exist where the normal balance between bone formation and bone resorption is disturbed. A knowledge of the normal histological and radiological appearance of bone helps in diagnosing disease. For example, osteopetrosis is a heterogeneous disorder characterized by impaired osteoclast function. In one type, there is a deficiency of the enzyme carbonic anhydrase type II

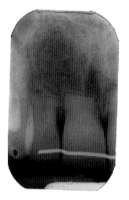
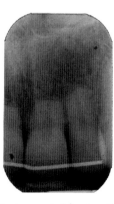

**Fig. 13.44** A 32-year-old patient presented for an orthodontic consultation following 5 years of fixed orthodontic appliances. Two long-cone periapical radiographs of the four anterior segment show significant root resorption in all four incisors. The horizontal white line is a fixed retainer. Courtesy of Professor F. McDonald.

and, although bone formation occurs, the defective osteoclasts lose their ability to resorb normally formed bone, which becomes increasingly thickened. An analogous condition in rodents prevents teeth from erupting because of the inability of osteoclasts to resorb the overlying bone. The cause of one such condition is a lack of production of M-CSF. If the missing factor is replaced, osteoclasts can be switched on to allow alveolar bone resorption and normal eruption.

A number of different strategies can be considered to combat the reverse situation that follows when uncoupling results in more resorption than formation (primarily in cancellous bone), eventually leading to osteoporosis. This is a bone disorder characterized by a low bone mass but of normal constitution. It particularly affects trabecular bone, which has a higher turnover rate than compact bone, and predisposes the patient to spontaneous or low trauma energy level fractures as, once lost, the bone mass is not usually replaced. Vulnerable sites include the neck of the femur and the lumbar vertebrae. Osteoporosis can be age related and particularly affects postmenopausal women, but is of less importance for the jaws, which have comparatively small amounts of cancellous bone and therefore more mineralized tissue per unit volume than many other parts of the skeleton. The precise cause of osteoporosis is not known, although a number of factors, including sex hormone (particularly oestrogen) deficiency, lack of mechanical loading and glucocorticoid excess, have been identified (see Table 13.1). From a knowledge of the different stages in the lifecycle of the osteoclast (Fig. 13.22), a number of therapeutic strategies could be adopted to counteract bone resorption by administering drugs that might:

- enhance the OPG:RANKL ratio and interfere with the formation of osteoclasts (e.g. oestrogens, TGFβ)
- interfere with the attachment mechanisms of osteoclasts (e.g. calcitonin)
- speed up apoptosis in osteoclasts (e.g. oestrogens, bisphosphonates, TGFβ)
- block the activity of degradative enzymes (e.g. doxycycline).

Analyses of various molecules in the blood and/or urine are also of importance in diagnosing conditions affecting the turnover rate of bone. These molecules include calcium, parathormone, acid phosphatase and alkaline phosphatase. In addition, collagen type I cross-linked N-terminals result from the proteolytic cleavage caused by osteoclasts and their levels in serum or urine are indicative of turnover rates, as are the levels of hydroxyproline and hydroxylysine.

Another important clinical area where knowledge of bone biology is important concerns the field of implantology. Whereas a foreign material placed into bone is normally regarded as 'non-self' and becomes surrounded by a capsule of fibrous tissue running parallel to the foreign material surface, some materials allow for a direct structural osseous union. When inserted into the jaw to provide the basis of support for a crown, denture or orthodontic appliance, this union between the dental implant and adjacent living bone is termed osseointegration. The materials most commonly used in the jaws are based on titanium or its aluminium/vanadium alloys, the spontaneously formed metal oxide (ceramic) surfaces being critical to integration. A narrow interface (20–40 nm) between the bone and implant contains non-collagenous bone matrix proteins such as osteopontin and bone sialoprotein. The successful long-term retention of an implant depends on: 1) Correct surgical technique to ensure minimum trauma, heating and infection at the implant site, 2) absence of excessive micromotion following implantation, and 3) factors related to the implant (such as shape, topography, stiffness, composition and surface chemistry. The host responses essential for a successful clinical outcome include blood clot formation in which the necessary factors for successful osteogenesis, such as cytokines, growth factors and osteoprogenitor cells are present. If thermal control has not been optimal during placement, the bone immediately adjacent to the implant may be compromised.

Normally, adjacent to the implant, bone to a depth of 1 mm may necrose and be remodelled and replaced by new bone, a period of about 17 weeks being required for the establishment of a suitable viable bone interface with the implant. Some modern implantation techniques can, however, allow immediate function if the implant is rigidly held in good quality dense cortical bone. From a knowledge of basic bone biology, implants are being used that are coated with materials thought likely to encourage osseointegration, such as cell adhesion molecules and hydroxyapatite crystals, although delamination of material layers in such a hostile environment can cause long-term problems.

As fractures involving the face and jaws are common, an understanding of the principles involved in bone healing is essential in the clinical situation. Similarly, after tooth extraction, the empty socket will initially fill with a blood clot. In this clot, granulation tissue will form and stem cells and osteoprogenitor cells will soon appear. These cells will eventually differentiate into osteoblasts, this process involving cell–matrix interactions. The initial immature (woven) bone will ultimately be remodelled to form mature, fine-fibred bone, having served its purpose by achieving an initial rapid fracture repair.

In some clinical situations, in particular the replacement of bone lost in trauma or malignant disease, the need for larger amounts of bone may require additional techniques. Requirements may be met by either autologous bone grafts (taken from the patient), allografts (taken from another person) or xenografts (taken from a different species, typically BioOssbovine bone chips®, Fig. 13.45).

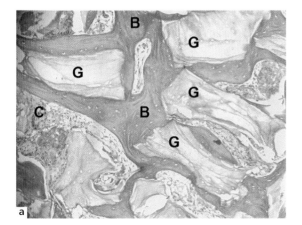

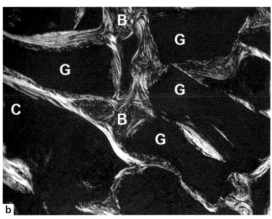

**Fig. 13.45** (a) Demineralized section showing a well healed, granular bovine xenograft (G) placed in an extraction socket to augment the alveolar bone prior to implant placement. New compact lamellar bone (B) and supporting connective tissue (C) have grown through the deproteinated, mineral graft (H & E; ×90). (b) Same section as in (a) but viewed under polarized light. Unlike the ordered collagen fibres of the new lamellar bone, the deproteinated graft does not show the birefringence patterns in polarized light and remains black (H & E; ×90). Courtesy of Dr R.J. Cook.

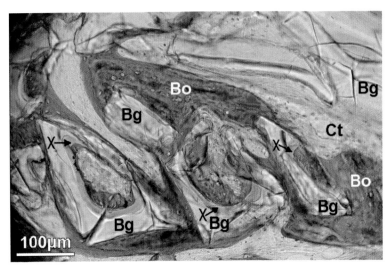

**Fig. 13.46** Plastic embedded ground section showing fully integrated soluble bioactive glass granules (Bg) placed in a human mandible to augment an extraction socket prior to implant placement. New bone (Bo) and connective tissue (Ct) have grown into and bonded directly to the new hydroxyapatite surfaces, formed on the outer silica gel layer (X) of the reacted glass particles (A Sanderson's rapid bone stain; ×150). Courtesy of Dr R.J. Cook.

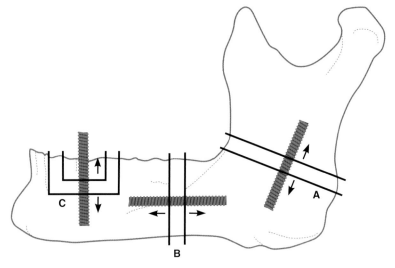

**Fig. 13.47** Schematic diagram of the mandible showing osteotomy sites for distraction osteogenesis allowing for increase in height of ramus (A), increase in length of body of mandible (B) and increase in height of alveolus to allow for implants (C). A cut across the mandibular symphysis would allow for increase in width.

However, major advances are being made to apply tissue engineering techniques to produce laboratory-based materials either to substitute for bone or provide scaffolds and stimuli to promote more rapid bony healing in adverse lesions and those otherwise too large to heal themselves. The three components to be considered in tissue engineering are: 1) the scaffold, 2) the cells and 3) additional molecules to drive osteogenesis.

The scaffold must clearly be biocompatible and must have a special configuration that allows osteogenic cells to migrate, differentiate and mineralize the artificial matrix. It must also allow for angiogenesis and the possibility of being resorbed as new bone is formed within it, ultimately leaving no residual foreign body as an infection hazard. Among the materials under investigation are organic compounds such as collagen matrices and synthetic polymers (polylactic/polyglycolic acid fibres), inorganic osteoconductive ceramic materials (such as deproteinated corals and synthetic hydroxyapatites) and soluble bioactive glasses (Fig. 13.46). The latter materials' ionic dissolution products – including silicon – accelerate mature functioning osteoblast production within a wound site, as well as providing an osteoconductive surface over which new bone may grow.

The most important cells that are required to enter the graft material or scaffold are stem cells of the osteogenic line. These may be derived from the patient's own cells that have been isolated, selected, their numbers boosted by tissue culture and then seeded into the scaffold in vitro, or in vivo by migration to wound sites directly. An alternative approach for the future is to develop lines of stem cells from embryos that may be safely seeded into a scaffold without fear of rejection by the immune system of the patient.

A large number of molecules such as cytokines, growth factors and cell–matrix adhesion factors are required for the successful differentiation of stem cells into functional osteoblasts. It is not surprising, therefore, that much experimental work has been devoted to integration of these molecules into graft matrices in the hope of improving the properties of such artificial bone implants. However, much further work is required to iden-

tify the best method of placement of such molecules. For example, if it was thought that the presence of a bone morphogenetic protein was beneficial to the development of active osteoblasts, is it better to add this protein externally to the scaffold material before implantation, or to try to genetically manipulate the genes of stem cells used to seed the matrix to produce more of this factor themselves?

The rate of fracture repair appears to slow down with age, the precise reason for which remains to be clarified. It may be that there is a reduction in the number of viable stem cells in bone with age. An approach to speed up fracture repair in older patients is to isolate some stem cells from the patient's bone, culture them to increase their numbers and then seed them in a suitable framework that is then placed in the fracture site.

Distraction osteogenesis refers to the technique whereby a bone is sectioned (an osteotomy) and, after an initial interval of 5–7 days, a slow, controlled separation (about 0.5–1 mm/day) of the two bone fragments is undertaken to allow length augmentation by the sustained addition of new woven bone at the fracture site, formed under tension. When adequate length has been achieved, the two bone ends are immobilized for some weeks to allow the woven bone callus to be reinforced and ultimately replaced by mature dense lamellar bone. For success, the original periosteum and blood supply must be retained. Although this technique was initially developed to increase the length of long bones, it has been adapted for use in craniofacial situations where there is marked bony underdevelopment, such as the small mandible of micrognathia. The mandible can be increased in length and height, depending on the orientation of the pre-planned osteotomies. (Fig. 13.47).

When teeth have been extracted, the alveolar bone atrophies. In such cases, distraction osteogenesis may allow for an increase alveolar height to render the site suitable for implants. There is some evidence that, during the early phase of bone remodelling in the distraction site, there is a marked level of osteoclastic activity that may be reflected in root resorption of teeth being orthodontically moved into the distraction site.

Whereas the skin is dry and provides the covering for the external surface of the body, the alimentary tract is lined with a moist mucosa (mucous membrane). The mucosa is specialized in each region of the alimentary tract, but the basic pattern of an epithelium with an underlying connective tissue (the lamina propria) is maintained and is analogous to the epidermis and dermis of the skin respectively. In many regions, a third layer (the submucosa) is found between the lamina propria and the underlying bone (palate) or muscle (cheeks and lips).

The oral mucosa shows specializations that allow it to fulfil several roles:

- It is protective mechanically against both compressive and shearing forces.
- It provides a barrier to microorganisms, toxins and various antigens.
- It has a role in immunological defence, both humoral and cell mediated.
- Minor glands within the oral mucosa provide lubrication and buffering as well as secretion of some antibodies. The viscoelastic mucous film also acts as a barrier, helping to retain water and electrolytes.
- The mucosa is richly innervated, providing input for touch, proprioception, pain and taste.

Two distinct layers are readily recognized in the oral mucosa for all regions of the mouth (Fig. 14.1). The outer layer is a stratified squamous epithelium that in areas subjected to masticatory forces (e.g. gingiva, palate and dorsum of tongue) is keratinized. The epithelium is derived embryologically from either ectoderm or endoderm. Beneath the epithelium is the connective tissue, comprising the lamina propria. The submucosa consists of a looser connective tissue containing fat deposits and glands. Larger nerves and blood vessels run in the submucosa. The boundary between the connective tissues of the lamina propria and the submucosa is often indistinct.

The oral mucosa may be classified into three types: masticatory, lining and specialized mucosa. Masticatory mucosa is found where there is high compression and friction and is characterized by a keratinized epithelium and a thick lamina propria, which is usually bound down directly and tightly to underlying bone (mucoperiosteum).

## EPITHELIUM

Several layers of cells of distinct morphologies may be recognized in the stratified squamous epithelium lining the oral cavity (Fig. 14.2):

- basal layer (stratum germinativum or stratum basale)
- prickle cell layer (stratum spinosum)
- granular layer (stratum granulosum)
- keratinized (cornified) layer (stratum corneum).

All four layers are present in masticatory mucosa and, as the end product is a covering layer of cells filled with cytokeratins, the cells are termed keratinocytes. Other proteins related to the cell membrane, such as loricrin, involucrin and filaggrin, are synthesized as the cells differentiate. In the case of lining mucosa, the outer two layers (granular and keratinized layers) are absent. Epithelial cells exhibit endocytosis and therefore have the capacity to internalize small particles.

Unlike skin, the oral mucosa does not have a clear layer (stratum lucidum) between the granular and keratinized layers.

The different layers of the oral epithelium represent a progressive maturation process. Cells from the most superficial keratinized layer are continuously being shed and replaced from below. Turnover time is fastest (about 5 days) in the region of the junctional and sulcular epithelia, which are located immediately adjacent to the tooth surface. This is probably about twice as fast as the turnover time in lining mucosa such as the cheek. Turnover time in masticatory mucosa appears to be a little slower than that in non-masticatory (lining) mucosa.

## BASAL LAYER

The basal layer is the single cell layer adjacent to the lamina propria and demarcated from it by a basal lamina (see pages 232, 233). It consists of

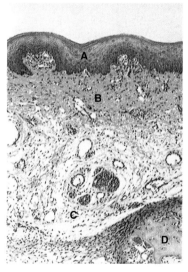

**Fig. 14.1** Section showing regions of oral mucosa. A = stratified squamous epithelium; B = lamina propria; C = submucosa; D = bone (Masson's trichrome; ×35).

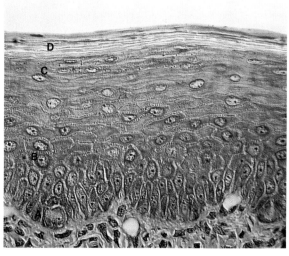

**Fig. 14.2** Section showing layers of keratinized oral epithelium. A = basal layer; B = prickle cell layer; C = granular layer; D = keratinized layer (×180).

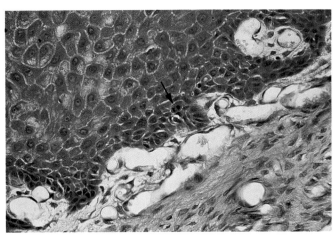

**Fig. 14.3** Section of oral epithelium showing a mitotic figure (arrow) near the basal layer (H & E; ×200). Courtesy of Dr R. O'Sullivan.

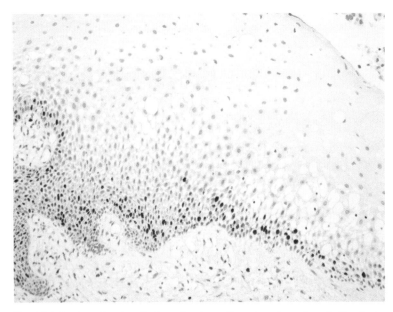

**Fig. 14.4** Section of oral epithelium showing cells undergoing cell replication (red stain) (Stained with MIB1 and counterstained with haematoxylin ×100). Courtesy of Professor P.R. Morgan.

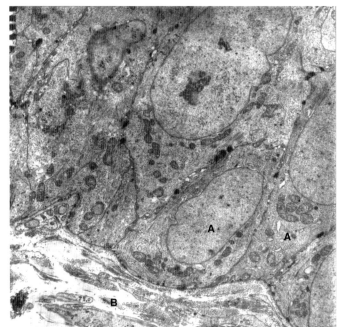

**Fig. 14.5** Electron micrograph of basal layer of keratinized stratified squamous epithelium. The cells (A) are undifferentiated, contain various intracellular organelles such as mitochondria, free ribosomes and microfilaments and rest on a basal lamina. B = lamina propria (×4000). Courtesy of Professor M.M. Smith.

cuboidal cells, among which is a population of stem cells. Stem cells on mitosis give rise to two daughter cells, one of which at least remains a stem cell. Stem cells generate transit-amplifying cells that will undergo a number of further cell divisions, migrate from the basal cell layer and differentiate to give rise to replacement keratinocytes in the epithelial layers above. The stem cells within the basal layer are found mainly at the base of the epithelial ridges (rete) that project into the lamina propria. Not all cells dividing in the basal layer are true stem cells. Stem cells appear to express antiapoptotic proteins (e.g. Bcl2 protein) and it has been claimed that this allows them to remain stem cells. Mitotic figures can occasionally be seen with routine staining (Fig. 14.3). However, they are clearly in evidence when using special stains (Fig. 14.4).

The cells of the basal layer are the least differentiated within the oral epithelium and this is reflected in their ultrastructural appearance. They contain a limited amount of the intracellular organelles associated with the synthesis and secretion of proteins (such as endoplasmic reticulum, Golgi material, mitochondria) in relation to the formation of components of the basal lamina, as well as some tonofilaments of keratin, reflecting their epithelial nature (Fig. 14.5). Cell contacts in the form of desmosomes, hemidesmosomes, intermediate and gap junctions are present, allowing for adhesion, cell signalling and other functions.

It is not known what triggers the start of differentiation in the basal layer but it does not appear to be simply a matter of displacement away from the basal layer, as tissue culture studies indicate that, if cells are prevented from migrating away from the basal lamina, differentiation still occurs. Rather, the onset of differentiation seems to change the adhesive properties of the cell, perhaps involving the nature of its integrins, and leads to its 'expulsion' from the basal layer. Further movement upwards towards the surface and final desquamation will involve much activity relating to the development, quality, turnover and breakdown of cell attachments and adhesion molecules.

## PRICKLE CELL LAYER

Above the basal layer round or ovoid cells form a layer several cells thick called the prickle cell layer (Fig. 14.2). These cells show the first stages of maturation, being larger and rounder than those in the basal layer. The transition from basal to prickle cell layer is characterized by the appearance of new cytokeratin types (see pages 227, 228). They contribute to the formation of the tonofilaments, which become thicker and more conspicuous. Involucrin (the soluble precursor protein of the cornified envelope eventually found in the cornified layer) appears first in the prickle cell layer. There is a progressive decrease in synthetic activity through the layer.

In the upper part of the prickle cell layer small, intracellular membrane-coating granules (approximately 0.25 μm in length) appear. These granules are rich in phospholipids and, in keratinized epithelium, consist of a series of parallel lamellae. They probably originate from the Golgi apparatus. In the more superficial layers of the stratum spinosum the granules come to lie close to the cell membrane.

Within the prickle cell layer, desmosomes increase in number and become more obvious than in the basal layer (Figs 14.6, 14.7). The slight shrinkage that occurs in most histological preparations causes the cells to separate at all points where desmosomes do not anchor them together. This gives the cells their 'spiny' appearance. Desmosomes eventually come to occupy about 50% of the intercellular space.

The term 'parabasal' is used to refer to the deepest layer of cells of the prickle cell layer that lie next to the basal layer. They may show features similar to that of the basal layer in that they may be elongated and undergo cell proliferation.

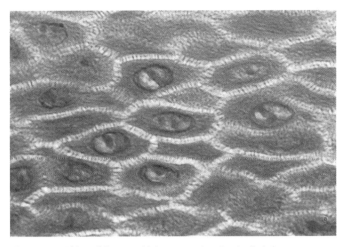

**Fig. 14.6** Prickle cell layer at high power showing 'spiky' desmosomes connecting adjacent cells (H & E; ×1000). Courtesy of Professor M.M. Smith.

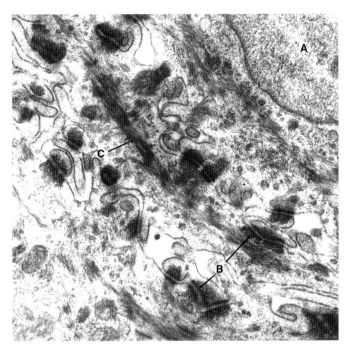

**Fig. 14.7** Electron micrograph of the prickle cell layer. A = nucleus; B = desmosome surrounded by inserting tonofilaments; C = tonofilaments of keratin (×20 000). Courtesy of Professor M.M. Smith.

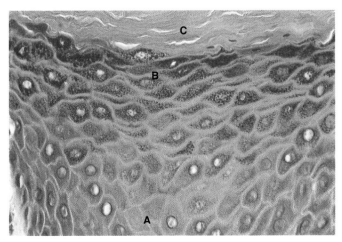

**Fig. 14.8** Section showing upper part of prickle cell layer (A), the granular layer (B) and the keratinized layer (C). Note the granular nature of the cells in the granular layer (H & E; ×350). Courtesy of Professor M.M. Smith.

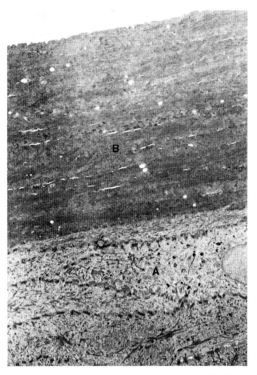

**Fig. 14.9** Electron micrograph showing granular (A) and keratinized (B) layers. Within the cells of the granular layer can be seen the keratohyalin granules, while the cells of the keratin layer lack nuclei and other organelles (×2800). Courtesy of Professor C.A. Squier.

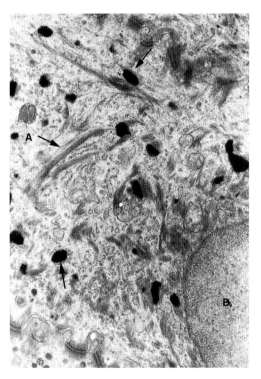

**Fig. 14.10** Higher power electron micrograph of a cell of the granular layer. A = tonofibril; B = nucleus. Keratohyalin granule arrowed (×12 000). Courtesy of Professor C.A. Squier.

## GRANULAR LAYER

The cells of the granular layer (Fig. 14.2) show a further increase in maturation compared with those of the basal and prickle cell layers. Many organelles are reduced or lost, such that the cytoplasm is predominantly occupied by the tonofilaments and tonofibrils. The cells are larger and flatter (Figs 14.8, 14.9) but, most significantly, now contain large numbers of small granules, 0.5–1.0 μm in length, called keratohyaline granules (Fig. 14.10). These contain profilaggrin, the precursor to the protein

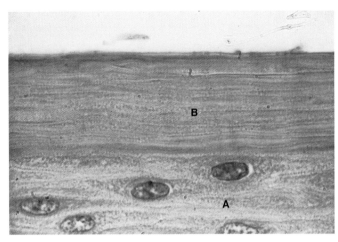

**Fig. 14.11** Section showing the granular (A) and keratinized layers (B) (H & E; ×1000). Courtesy of Dr D. Adams.

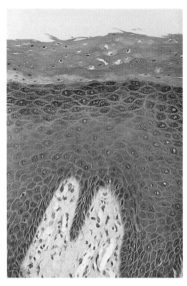

**Fig. 14.12** Section of parakeratinized oral epithelium from the gingiva. The superficial layer stains more heavily for keratin but nuclei are retained (H & E; ×100). Courtesy of Dr A.W. Barrett.

filaggrin that eventually binds the keratin filaments together into a stable network. The membrane-coating granules first seen in the prickle cell layer move towards the superficial surface of the keratinocyte and discharge their lipid-rich contents into the intercellular space. This intercellular 'cement', together with the cell contacts (especially tight junctions in the upper region of the granular layer), helps limit the permeability of the layer and prevents water loss. Synthesis of additional proteins, loricrin and involucrin, that will help form a more resistant cell wall (envelope) is evident in the granular layer.

## KERATINIZED LAYER

In keratinized epithelium the final stage in the maturation of the epithelial cells results in the loss of all organelles (including nuclei and keratohyaline granules) (Figs 14.8, 14.9, 14.11). This autolysis is probably due to the release of proteases within the cell. The cells of the keratinized layer become filled entirely with closely packed tonofilaments surrounded by the matrix protein filaggrin. This mixture of proteins is collectively called keratin. The keratin is also strongly cross-linked by disulphide bonds, contributing to the mechanical and chemical resistance of the layer.

In the cornified layer involucrin becomes cross-linked (by the enzyme transglutaminase) to form a thin (10 nm), highly resistant, electron-dense, cornified envelope just beneath the plasma membrane. The trigger for this is probably cell death and the influx of calcium ions. Approximately 75% of the cornified envelope is loricrin. Although only constituting 5% of the cell envelope, involucrin is an important component on the internal aspect, acting as a binding site for lipids that are extruded to form a water-insoluble barrier.

The cells of the keratinized layer may be termed epithelial squames; it is these cells that are shed (the process of desquamation), necessitating the constant turnover of epithelial cells. Desmosomes weaken and disappear to allow for this desquamation.

The keratinized layer provides the mechanical protective function to the mucosa. It varies in thickness (up to 20 cells) and is thicker for the oral mucosa than for most areas of skin (except for the palms of the hands and the soles of the feet). In some areas such as the gingiva the nuclei may be retained, although small and shrunken. These cells are described as para-keratinized (in contrast to the more usual orthokeratinized cells without nuclei) (Fig. 14.12).

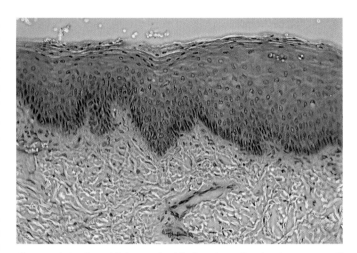

**Fig. 14.13** Section of lining oral epithelium from the alveolar mucosa. There is an absence of keratin in the superficial layer. (H & E; ×80). Courtesy of Professor M.M. Smith.

## LINING EPITHELIUM

In lining epithelium, the cells are non-keratinized at the surface (Fig. 14.13). Like the cells in keratinized epithelia, those in lining epithelium enlarge and flatten as they shift towards the surface. Ultrastructurally, the surface layers differ from the cells of keratinized epithelia in that they lack keratohyaline granules. This absence of filaggrin also accounts for the less developed and dispersed tonofilaments present in lining epithelium. There are also more organelles in the surface layers compared with those in keratinized cells, although there are still considerably fewer than in the basal layer. Above the prickle cell layer, the layers are not as clearly defined as in a keratinized epithelium. The outer layers are usually termed the intermediate (stratum intermedium) and superficial (stratum superficiale) layers. Nuclei persist within the surface layers (Fig. 14.14). The membrane-coating granules are smaller and lack the lipid-rich lamellar structure of those in keratinizing epithelia. This is thought to account for the greater permeability of lining epithelium compared to keratinized epithelium. Lining epithelium generally lacks filaggrin (Fig. 14.15a) and loricrin, but contains involucrin (Fig. 14.15b).

## CELL KINETICS

Although the processes involved in controlling the proliferation and maturation of keratinocytes are not fully known, many growth factors (e.g. epidermal growth factor, platelet derived growth factor, transforming growth factor (TGF), keratinocyte growth factor and cytokines (e.g. interleukins (ILs), produced by either the keratinocyte or adjacent fibroblasts, can affect the rate of proliferation and differentiation. The nature of adjacent adhesion molecules and their interaction with integrins are also of importance. Epithelial cells themselves will have numerous cell-surface receptors and molecules important in regulating cell behaviour. Maturing cells are believed to produce growth inhibitors that restrict further cell division by negative feedback. The precise mechanism of inhibitor release is not known but, as the mitotic rate shows diurnal variation, systemic factors may be implicated.

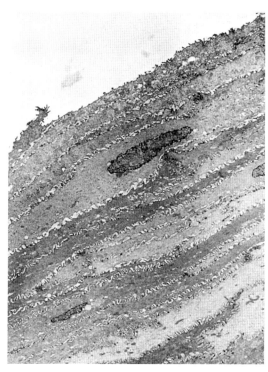

**Fig. 14.14** Electron micrograph of surface layers in non-keratinized lining epithelium. Note the retention of nuclei (×2000). Courtesy of Professor C.A. Squier.

## CYTOKERATINS

In epithelial cells the cytoskeleton is composed of microfilaments, microtubules and intermediate filaments. Microfilaments are approximately 4–6 nm in diameter and have a molecular weight of the order of 43 kDa. By contrast, microtubules are 25 nm in diameter with a molecular weight of 55 kDa. Although intermediate in terms of diameter (7–11 nm), the intermediate filaments have a molecular weight ranging from 40 kDa to as high as 200 kDa. In contrast with microfilaments and microtubules, which are ubiquitous proteins, intermediate filaments have a high degree of tissue specificity. Six major classes of intermediate filament have been identified, including the cytokeratins (CK), which have a high specificity for epithelial cells. 'Moll' numbers were assigned to the CK proteins, which are the products of two gene families and translate into at least 22 main CK polypeptides. The products of each CK gene family are divided into the neutral or basic type II CK (numbered 1–8) and the acidic type I CK (numbered 9–20). They occur in pairs. The type I CK is the smaller of each pair, ranging between 40 and 56.5 kDa and always about 8 kDa smaller than its type II counterpart, which has a molecular weight of 53–67 kDa (Table 14.1).

CK expression conforms to several 'rules', each epithelial cell expressing at least one CK pair comprising one type I and one type II. The ultimate CK phenotype reflects the differentiation pathway the cell has followed. Because they are only expressed in simple epithelia, such as ductal luminal cells, CKs 7, 8 and 18 are designated 'simple'. The best-characterized CKs associated with epithelial stratification are pairs 5 and 14, 4 and 13, and 1 and 10.

Within epithelial cells CK filaments function as components of the cytoskeleton and cell contacts (desmosomes and hemidesmosomes). However, the physiological reason for the large number of CKs remains obscure. Some insight into their functional significance can be obtained from analysis of congenital or experimental CK abnormalities. For example, in some forms of epidermolysis bullosa (a group of mucocutaneous lesions, all of which produce subepithelial blistering) there is a mutant form of CK14. Some CKs may be important in maintaining the metabolic homeostasis of the cell.

Apart from their structural role in the cytoskeleton, there is evidence for other roles for CKs, possibly related to their location. For example, CK14 is most strongly positive in the basal layer. The fact that CK14-positive basal cells in palatal and lingual epithelium synthesize neurogenic peptides may be related to the innervation of the superficial oral mucosa. This view is supported by work that showed that denervation of rodent taste buds causes loss of CK expression and is consistent with a possible role for CK in signal transduction.

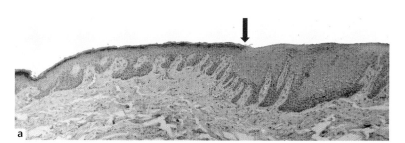

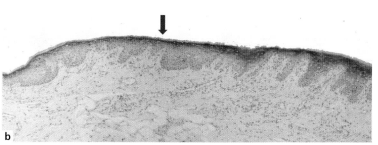

**Fig. 14.15** (a) Section across lip stained immunohistochemically for filaggrin, showing its positive (brown) staining at the surface of the keratinized vermilion layer (left of arrow) and its absence over the non-keratinized labial mucosa (right of arrow). (b) Section across lip stained immunohistologically for involucrin, showing positive staining (brown) at the surface of the keratinized vermilion (left of arrow) and the labial mucosa (right of arrow) (Streptavidin-biotinylated immunoperoxidase stain; ×20). With permission from Barrett AW, Morgan M, Nwaeze G et al 2005 The differentiation profile of epithelium of the human lip. *Archives of Oral Biology* 50: 431–438.

**Table 14.1** *Distribution of cytokeratins in human stratified squamous epithelium (SSE)*

| | CK pair | |
|---|---|---|
| | Type II, basic, higher MW. | Type I, acidic, lower MW. |
| Suprabasal, keratinized SSE | 1, 2 and 3 | 10 and 11 |
| Cornea | 3 | 12 |
| Suprabasal, non-keratinized SSE | 4 | 13 |
| Basal keratinocytes (all SSE) | 5 | 14 |
| Hyperproliferative epithelia | 6 | 16 |
| Simple epithelia | 8 | 18 |
| Some simple epithelia, pilosebaceous tracts, basal cell carcinomas | ? | 17 |
| Basal keratinocytes in non-keratinized SSE, some simple or 'plastic' epithelia (e.g. odontogenic) | ? | 19 |

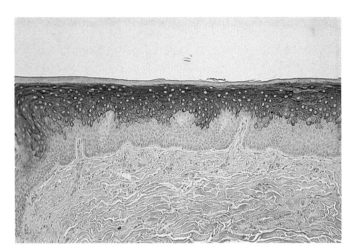

**Fig. 14.17** Section of orthokeratinized epithelium from the hard palate stained for cytokeratin 10, showing positive suprabasal staining (brown) (Streptavidin-biotinylated immunoperoxidase stain; ×50). Courtesy of Dr A.W. Barrett.

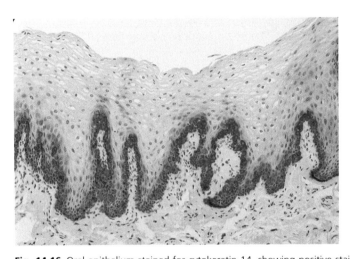

**Fig. 14.16** Oral epithelium stained for cytokeratin 14, showing positive staining (purple) restricted to the basal cell layer (Streptavidin-biotinylated immunoperoxidase alkaline phosphatase stain; ×100). Courtesy of Dr A.W. Barrett.

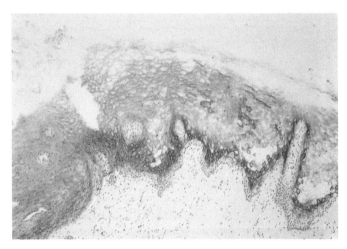

**Fig. 14.18** Section of non-keratinized epithelium from the cheek stained for cytokeratin 4, showing positive staining (brown) throughout except for the basal layer (Streptavidin-biotinylated immunoperoxidase stain; ×60). Courtesy of Dr A.W. Barrett.

## MAJOR DISTRIBUTION PATTERNS OF CYTOKERATINS IN ORAL EPITHELIUM (Table 14.1)

CK5 and 14 are usually restricted to the basal and parabasal layers (Fig. 14.16), although CK14 may also be expressed by suprabasal keratinocytes. CK1 and 10 (or CK2 and 11) are characteristically found in the suprabasal layers of masticatory mucosa and are associated with terminal differentiation and keratinization (Fig. 14.17). The keratin layer itself is negative. In lining mucosa, the suprabasal keratinocytes stain primarily for CK4 (Fig. 14.18) and 13 rather than the CK1 and 10 found in masticatory mucosa. There is variable expression of other cytokeratins. CK6 and 16 are associated with rapid turnover epithelia. CK19 may also be a marker for basal keratinocytes in lining mucosa but reports concerning its presence are inconsistent. Variations in the CK distribution of non-keratinized oral epithelium at different anatomical sites have been reported. The epithelium lining the ventral surface of the tongue may be distinguished from other lining oral epithelium by its increased expression of CK5, 6 and 14. However, most unusual is the epithelium covering the soft palate, which apparently expresses the simple cytokeratins (CK7, 8 and 18) as well as high levels of CK19.

## OTHER SECRETORY PRODUCTS OF KERATINOCYTES

In addition to synthesizing cytokeratins that remain inside the cell, keratinocytes can produce bioactive molecules such as interleukins, tumour necrosis factor-α and colony stimulating factors. Such molecules can influence the biology of both the epithelium and the underlying connective tissue of the lamina propria.

### FACTORS CONTROLLING ORAL EPITHELIAL PHENOTYPE

In reviewing the nature of the oral epithelium, it has been shown that regional specificity exists throughout life, even though there is a continuous and rapid replacement of the components. This poses questions as to the nature of the factor(s) determining such specificity. The specificity may be considered as being the result of extrinsic inductive stimuli from the underlying lamina propria or an intrinsic property of the basal layer of the epithelium. Knowledge of the underlying mechanisms has clinical relevance as, following surgical removal of the dentogingival tissues, the three distinctive epithelia of the oral gingiva, sulcular epithelium and junctional

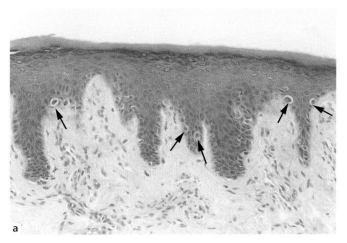
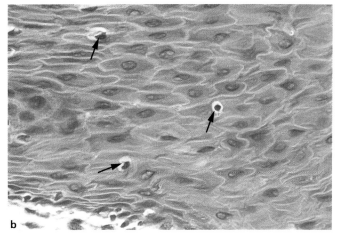

**Fig. 14.19** (a) Section of red zone of lip showing clear cells (arrows) in the basal layer, representing mainly melanocytes (×80). (b) Clear cells in the upper layers of the epithelium (arrowed), mainly representing Langerhans cells (H & E; ×350; Courtesy of Professor M.M. Smith).

epithelium do regenerate, presumably from the remaining oral gingival epithelium. Furthermore, conditions exist where non-keratinized zones of epithelia are encountered in regions of masticatory epithelia and treatment may be geared towards attempting to replace these zones with the appropriate keratinized epithelium.

As regards the view that specificity is the result of epithelial–mesenchymal interactions, this has been well established during tooth development (see pages 305–310). The role of mesenchyme in determining the phenotype of the overlying epithelium, and its ability to maintain this property and therefore redirect patterns of epithelial morphogenesis in the adult, has been investigated by a number of researchers using classical methods in which portions of oral mucosa were transplanted to different regions or were separated into their epithelial and connective tissue components and then homo- and heterotypically recombined and transplanted. Such studies support the view that the underlying lamina propria is primarily responsible for the specificity of the overlying epithelia, in terms of both morphology and CK content. Thus, lining oral epithelium combined with lamina propria from masticatory mucosa took on the features of a masticatory mucosa, while masticatory epithelium combined with lamina propria from lining mucosa modulated to lining epithelium. Such modulation does not appear to require a vital lamina propria as a similar effect was seen even after the connective tissue was frozen. These fundamental changes are not only seen in subcutaneous sites in animal experiments but have also been reported in clinical situations. Deep connective tissue, however, was not able to facilitate such changes. In this context, gingival fibroblasts also produce substances, such as keratinocyte growth factor and scatter factor, that are important in the growth and maintenance of the overlying epithelium, and these factors themselves are influenced by other growth factors and cytokines (such as TGFβ and IL-1β). This relationship may be of clinical significance when considering the junctional epithelium in health and disease.

Other evidence confirming the existence of epithelial/mesenchymal interactions is shown from experiments in which normal epithelium is combined with carcinogen-treated (and transformed) mesenchyme, when the epithelium is seen to show an increased mitotic activity and irregular nuclei. However, although there is considerable evidence for the importance of the underlying mesenchyme in specifying the form and phenotype of the overlying epithelium, both during development and in the adult, there is also evidence for some regionally related variations in the competence of epithelia to respond to these influences.

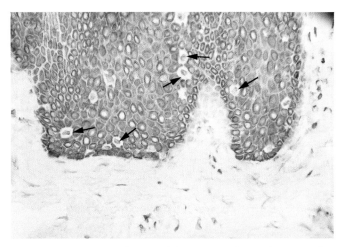

**Fig. 14.20** Basal region of oral epithelium stained for cytokeratin 14 (brown) and illustrating clear cells (arrows) lacking cytokeratin and representing mainly melanocytes (×200). Courtesy of Professor P.R. Morgan.

## NON-KERATINOCYTES

As many as 10% of the cells in the oral epithelium are non-keratinocytes, and include melanocytes, Langerhans cells and Merkel cells. All lack the tonofilaments and desmosomes characteristic of keratinocytes (except for the Merkel cells). Non-keratinocytes may appear as clear cells in sections stained routinely with haematoxylin and eosin (Fig. 14.19). Lacking the typical cytokeratins associated with normal keratinocytes, they remain unstained in sections of epithelium stained for cytokeratins (Fig. 14.20) except for Merkel cells. Some non-keratinocytes are inflammatory cells that have migrated through the epithelium. Lymphocytes are the most common type of inflammatory cell, though polymorphonuclear leukocytes and plasma cells are also encountered. Lymphocytes are retained within the epithelial layer by binding to integrins that may increase in disease. The greater degree of permeability of non-keratinized epithelium may account for the larger number of inflammatory cells said to occur there compared with the masticatory epithelium.

## MELANOCYTES

Melanocytes are pigment-producing cells located in the basal layer. They are derived from the neural crest and are present in the skin at about 8 weeks of intrauterine life. Once located in the epithelium, they are assumed to be long-lived but with some powers of self-replication and are seen to divide in vitro. Melanocytes have long processes that extend in several

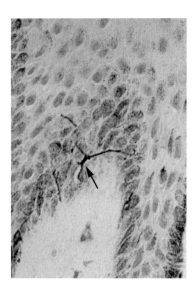

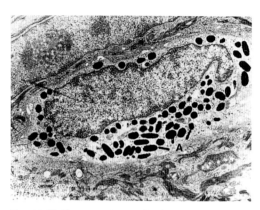

**Fig. 14.22** Electron micrograph of a melanocyte packed with melanosomes (A) (×60 000). Courtesy of Professor C.A. Squier.

**Fig. 14.21** Section of oral epithelium illustrating a melanocyte (arrowed) (Masson's Fontana stain; ×280). Courtesy of Professor I. Mackenzie.

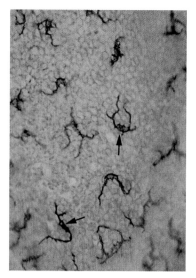

**Fig. 14.23** Section of superficial layers of oral epithelium showing Langerhans cells (arrowed) (Lead capture staining for ATPase; ×200). Courtesy of Professor I. Mackenzie.

directions and across several epithelial layers. As suggested by their name, melanocytes produce the pigment melanin, using the enzyme tyrosinase (which is lacking in albinos). They can be identified by special staining (Fig. 14.21).

Ultrastructurally, in addition to mitochondria, endoplasmic reticulum and Golgi material, the cytoplasm of melanocytes characteristically contains pigment that is packaged in small granules termed melanosomes (Fig. 14.22). The long processes of the melanocyte extend between adjacent keratinocytes and each melanocyte establishes contact with about 30–40 keratinocytes. Indeed, keratinocytes release numerous mediators that are essential for normal melanocyte function. As the melanosomes mature under the activity of tyrosinase, their content of melanin increases. The pigment is passed to adjacent keratinocytes (and hair cortex cells) as the tips of the dendrites are actively phagocytosed by the keratinocytes. Melanin pigmentation is usually not pronounced in the buccal mucosa, tongue, hard palate or gingiva.

The number of melanocytes varies in different regions but the difference in the degree of pigmentation between ethnic groups is the result of a combination of the size and degree of branching of the cells (rather than the absolute number), the size of the melanosomes, the number and degree of dispersion of the melanosomes, the degree of melanization of the melanosomes and the rate of degradation of the pigment.

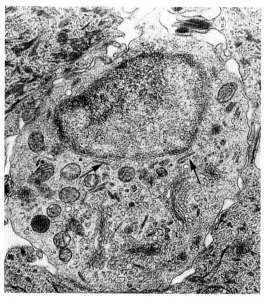

**Fig. 14.24** Electron micrograph of Langerhans cell showing the characteristic Birbeck granules (arrows) (×15 000). Courtesy of Dr N.G. El-Labban.

## LANGERHANS CELLS

Langerhans cells are dendritic cells situated in the layers above the basal layer. They are derived from bone marrow precursors that are probably related to the monocyte lineage and leave the bloodstream to enter the lamina propria before penetrating the basal lamina to reach the epithelium. Such migration may relate to certain chemokines released by keratinocytes with surface receptors on the Langerhans cells. Langerhans cells act as part of the immune system as antigen-presenting cells. They express class II molecules of the major histocompatibility complex and Fc receptors and move back and forth from the epithelium via dermal lymphatics to local lymph nodes, presenting antigenic material to T lymphocytes. Indeed, lymphocytes present within the oral epithelium are commonly associated with Langerhans cells. Langerhans cells play an important role in skin in producing contact hypersensitivity reactions, in antitumour immunity and in graft rejection; they also react as propagators of human immunodeficiency virus (HIV)-1 transmission to T cells. The cells may be localized because of the presence of ATPase on the cell membrane (Fig. 14.23).

Ultrastructurally, the Langerhans cell contains characteristic, trilaminar, rod-shaped granules called Birbeck granules (Fig. 14.24). These may be up to 50 nm long and 4 nm wide with a vesicular swelling at one end, resembling a tennis racquet. Foreign antigens penetrate the superficial layers and bind to dendritic antigen-presenting cells such as Langerhans cells, which stimulate helper T lymphocytes, and Granstein cells, which stimulate specific suppressor T lymphocytes. T cells also receive a signal in the form of a cytokine (IL-1) from both keratinocytes and dendritic cells, then secrete a lymphokine (IL-2) that causes the proliferation of T cells.

## MERKEL CELLS

The Merkel cell is found in the basal layer, often closely apposed to nerve fibres. It is thought to act as a receptor and is derived from the neural crest. As they contain CK filaments, Merkel cells can be identified by immuno-

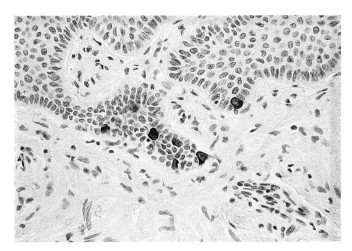

**Fig. 14.25** Section showing Merkel cells in basal layer of epithelium staining positively (brown) for cytokeratin18 (Streptavidin-biotinylated immunoperoxidase stain; ×200). Courtesy of Dr W.A. Barrett.

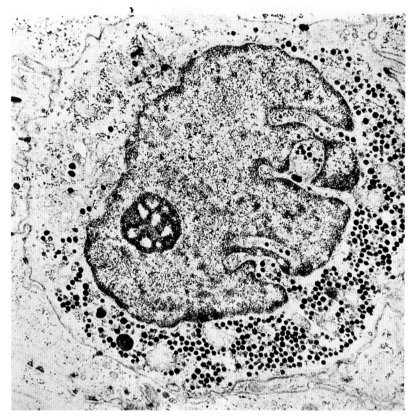

**Fig. 14.26** Electron micrograph of Merkel cell. Note the indented nucleus and nuclear rodlet. The cytoplasm contains numerous characteristic dense granules 80–180 nm in diameter (×16000). Courtesy of Dr S.-Y. Chen.

histochemical techniques using antibodies for CK 8/18 and 20 (Fig. 14.25). Merkel cells are common in masticatory epithelia such as the gingiva but less frequent in lining mucosa such as the buccal mucosa.

Ultrastructurally, the nucleus of the Merkel cell is often deeply invaginated and may contain a characteristic rodlet (Fig. 14.26). The cytoplasm contains numerous mitochondria, abundant free ribosomes and a collection of electron-dense granules (80–180 nm in diameter), the function of which is unknown. In addition, there are many small vesicles in the region adjacent to the nerve terminal. The granules may liberate a transmitter towards the terminal, giving the cell a sensory function. Desmosomes are associated with the cell membrane. Free nerve endings not associated with a Merkel cell are also found within the epithelium. These are nociceptors.

## LAMINA PROPRIA

The connective tissue underlying the oral epithelium can be described as having two layers: a superficial, papillary layer between the epithelial ridges, in which the collagen fibres are thin and loosely arranged; and, beneath this, a deep, reticular layer dominated by thick, parallel bundles of collagen fibres. The lamina propria provides mechanical support for the epithelium as well as nutrition. Its nerves have an important sensory function, while its blood cells and salivary glands have important defensive roles. Vascular concentration shows regional variation and this, associated with the rate of blood flow, may account for the vary small differences in temperature that are found (e.g. the temperature of the more vascularized alveolar mucosa is on average 0.67°C higher than that of the attached gingival mucosa). Furthermore, a similar slight temperature increase can be achieved following stimulation using an electric toothbrush.

As with other soft connective tissues, the principal cell of the lamina propria is the fibroblast. In outline their shape varies, a number appearing spindle-shaped. They contain the full complement of synthetic organelles

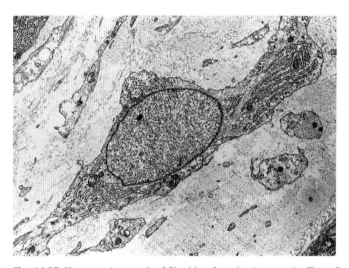

**Fig. 14.27** Electron micrograph of fibroblast from lamina propria. The cell contains a full complement of all the intracellular organelles associated with collagen synthesis. Note the conspicuous rough endoplasmic reticulum (×11000). Courtesy of Professor C.A. Squier.

consistent with their role in the continuous production and secretion of extracellular fibres and ground substance for the lamina propria (Fig. 14.27). There is evidence of heterogeneity among the fibroblast-like cells. In addition to a stem cell population, tissue-culture experiments have isolated clones of fibroblast-like cells that have different responses to the same bioactive molecule and that synthesize different ratios of extracellular matrix molecules. Gingival fibroblasts also produce substances such as keratinocyte growth factor and scatter factor that are important in the growth and maintenance of the overlying epithelium. This relationship may be of considerable clinical significance when considering the junctional epithelium.

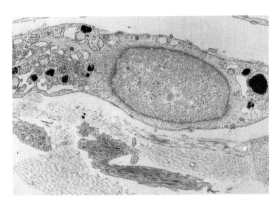

**Fig. 14.28** Electron micrograph of macrophage in lamina propria. It contains many lysosomes but little endoplasmic reticulum (×10000). Courtesy of Professor C.A. Squier.

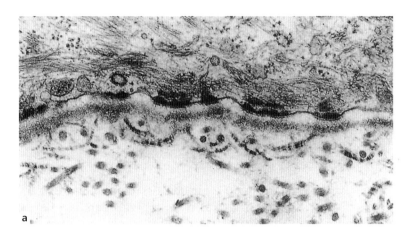

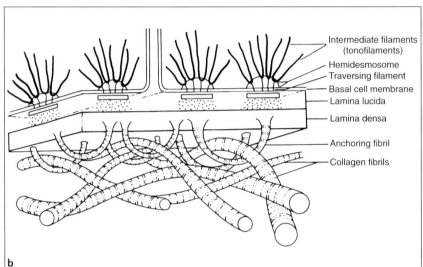

**Fig. 14.29** Electron micrograph showing appearance of basal lamina (×34000). Courtesy of Professor C.A. Squier.

The extracellular matrix of the lamina propria contains numerous collagen fibres. The majority are type I (about 90%) with about 8% type III. In addition there are small amounts of other types of collagen, including types IV and VII (associated with the presence of basement membranes) and types V and VI. Elastin fibres are also present, their number depending on site, while some oxytalan fibres have also been described in regions of the oral mucosa. The ground substance of the lamina propria consists of a hydrated gel of proteoglycans and glycoproteins. As with all general connective tissues, the usual defence cells are present. Macrophages are seen in the lamina propria. In their fixed, inactive stage, they are known as histiocytes and are difficult to distinguish from fibroblasts. They have a smaller, darker nucleus than fibroblasts and contain lysosomes but little endoplasmic reticulum (Fig. 14.28). As well as having a phagocytic role, macrophages act as antigen-presenting cells. Mast cells are mononuclear, spherical or elliptical in shape, and contain histamine and heparin intracellular granules (see page 195). They play a role in vascular homeostasis, in inflammation and in cell-mediated immunity, and are responsible for anaphylactic (type 1) hypersensitivity. Lymphocytes are also found in small numbers in healthy mucosa, but increase dramatically in inflammation.

## EPITHELIAL–CONNECTIVE TISSUE INTERFACE

### BASEMENT MEMBRANE/BASAL LAMINA

A complex arrangement links the surface epithelium to the underlying lamina propria in the oral mucosa. In the light microscope, a layer 1–2 μm thick is seen on the lamina propria side of the junction. This is termed the **basement membrane**. Under the electron microscope, the layer appears

much thinner and is then termed the **basal lamina**. The thicker appearance under the light microscope is probably due to the inclusion of some of the subepithelial collagen fibres, which in this region have staining properties similar to those of the basal lamina. All the major products of the basal lamina appear to be synthesized by the epithelial cells.

Ultrastructurally, the cell membrane possesses specialized attachment plaques, the hemidesmosomes, along its length, where there is an increased density in structure. Cytoplasmic keratin filaments insert into the hemidesmosome. Immediately adjacent to the cell membrane is the basal lamina. In routine electron microscopy, the basal lamina is seen to consist of two layers (Fig. 14.29):

- an electron-lucent lamina lucida (20–40 nm thick) that lies immediately under the epithelium.
- a thicker (20–120 nm) lamina densa.

However, there is evidence that the lamina lucida is a preparation artefact.

The basal lamina is composed of a network of type IV (non-fibrillar) collagen in which is found a number of important proteoglycan and glycoprotein molecules. Among these are fibronectin, laminin and perlecan (heparin sulphate proteoglycan). Transmembrane molecules such as integrins and bullous pemphigoid antigens (BPAG-1 and BPA-2) strengthen the link between the cell and the basal lamina. The bond is further strengthened by looping fibrils of type VII collagen that bind to the type IV collagen of the basal lamina and interdigitate with type I and type II collagen of the extracellular matrix.

Apart from providing a mechanism of attachment, the hemidesmosome/basal lamina complex allows for control of biological behaviour of the epithelial cells. The basal lamina acts as a molecular barrier and plays a

**Table 14.2** *Principal features and regional variations of the oral mucosa*

| Region | Epithelium | | Lamina propria | | Submucosa | | Type of mucosa |
|---|---|---|---|---|---|---|---|
| | Thickness | Keratinization | Papillae | Fibre types | Density | Attachment | |
| Labial and buccal mucosa | Thick | Non-keratinized | Short and irregular | Collagen and some elastic fibres | Dense | Firmly to underlying muscle | Lining |
| Vermilion (red) zone of lip | Thin | Keratinized | Long and narrow | Collagen and some elastic fibres | Dense | Firmly to underlying muscle | Specialized |
| Alveolar mucosa | Thin | Non-keratinized | Short or absent | Many elastic fibres | Loose | Loose attachment to periosteum | Lining |
| Attached gingiva | Thick | Keratinized and parakeratinized | Long and narrow | Dense collagen firmly attached to underlying periosteum | No distinct submucosa | | Masticatory |
| Floor of mouth | Thin | Non-keratinized | Short and broad | Collagen and some elastic fibres | Loose | Loose attachment to underlying muscle | Lining |
| Ventral surface of tongue | Thin | Non-keratinized | Short and numerous | Collagen and some elastic fibres | Not very distinct layer; attached to underlying muscle | | Lining |
| Dorsum of tongue (anterior two-thirds) | Thick | Primarily keratinized | Long | Collagen and some elastic fibres | Not very distinct layer; attached to underlying muscle | | Specialized gustatory |
| Dorsum of tongue (posterior one-third) | Variable | Generally non-keratinized | Short or absent | Collagen and some elastic fibres | Not very distinct layer; attached to underlying muscle | | Lining gustatory |
| Hard palate | Thick | Keratinized | Long | Dense collagen in submucosa laterally, but lamina propria firmly bound to periosteum without submucosa in midline | | | Masticatory |
| Soft palate | Thick | Non-keratinized | Short | Many elastic fibres | Loose | Loose attachment to underlying tissues | Lining |

role in the response to tissue injury. As will be seen when considering the development of certain dental tissues, the basal lamina is important when considering epithelial/mesenchymal interactions. It is not surprising therefore, to find that abnormalities resulting in defects in the composition of the hemidesmosomal/basal lamina complex is associated with pathologies (see pages 250, 251).

## REGIONAL VARIATIONS IN THE STRUCTURE OF THE ORAL MUCOSA

In different parts of the mouth, the mucosa has different roles and experiences different degrees and types of stress during mastication, speech and facial expression. As a consequence, the structure of the oral mucosa varies in terms of the thickness of the epithelium, the degree of keratinization, the complexity of the connective tissue–epithelium interface, the composition of the lamina propria and the presence or absence of the submucosa.

There are three types of oral mucosa: masticatory, lining and specialized mucosa. Masticatory mucosa is found where there is high compression and friction, and is characterized by a keratinized epithelium and a thick lamina propria. The mucosa of the gingiva and palate is masticatory, the bulk of which is firmly bound down directly and tightly to underlying bone (mucoperiosteum), except for the region at the side of the palate, where a submucosa is present. Lining mucosa is not subject to high levels of friction but must be mobile and distensible. It is thus non-keratinized and has a loose lamina propria. Within the lamina propria, the collagen fibres are arranged as a network to allow free movement, and the elastic fibres allow recoil to prevent the mucosa being chewed. Commonly, lining mucosa also has a submucosa. The lips, cheeks, alveolus, floor of the mouth, ventral surface of the tongue and soft palate have a lining mucosa. Two areas of specialized mucosa occur: the specialized gustatory mucosa of the dorsum of the tongue and where the vermilion zone forms a transition between the skin and the oral mucosa.

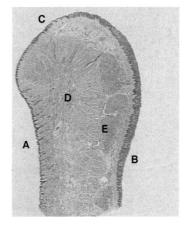

**Fig. 14.30** Transverse section of the lip. A = skin on external surface; B = labial mucosa on inner surface; C = vermilion (red) zone; D = striated muscles of orbicularis oris; E = minor salivary glands (H & E; ×2). Courtesy of S. Kariyawasam.

Within the oral cavity about 60% of the mucosa is lining mucosa, about 25% of the mucosa is masticatory mucosa and the remaining 15% specialized mucosa.

Regional variations of the oral mucosa are summarized in Table 14.2.

## LIP

The lip has skin on its outer surface and labial mucosa on its inner surface. Between these two tissues lies the vermilion zone (also known as the red or transitional zone of the lip) (Fig. 14.30). The lips have striated muscles in their core that are part of the muscles of facial expression. Substantial amounts of minor mucous salivary glands are present in the submucosa beneath the oral mucosa. The epithelial thickness gradually increases from the skin to the mucosal aspect.

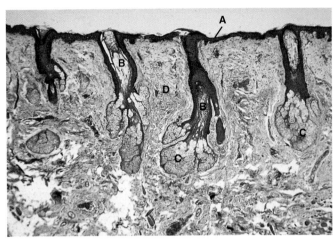

**Fig. 14.31** Section of skin of lip. A = keratinized epidermis; B = shaft of hair; C = sebaceous gland; D = dermis (Masson's trichrome; ×30).

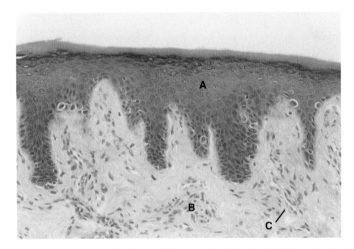

**Fig. 14.32** Section of red zone of lip. A = keratinized epithelium; B = lamina propria. Note the folded interface between epithelium and lamina propria bringing blood vessels (C) close to the surface (×80).

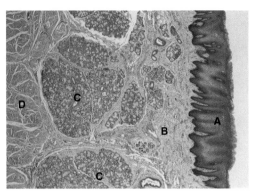

**Fig. 14.33** Section of labial mucosa. A = non-keratinized oral epithelium; B = lamina propria; C = minor salivary gland in submucosa; D = fibres of orbicularis oris (H & E; ×15). Courtesy of S. Kariyawasam.

**Table 14.3** *Staining patterns of principal cytokeratins in the stratified squamous epithelium of the lip (From Barrett AW, Morgan M, Nwaeze et al 2005 The differentiation profile of epithelium of the human lip. Archives of Oral Biology 50: 431–438 and courtesy of the editors of Archives of Oral Biology)*

| | Layer | CK1 | CK10 | CK4 | CK13 | CK5 | CK14 | CK19 |
|---|---|---|---|---|---|---|---|---|
| Labial skin | Basal layer | – | – | – | – | + | + | – |
| | Prickle cell layer | + | + | – | – | +/– | – | – |
| | Granular layer | + | + | – | – | – | – | – |
| | Keratinized layer | – | – | – | – | – | – | – |
| Vermilion | Basal layer | – | – | – | – | + | + | – |
| | Prickle cell layer | + | + | – | – | +/– | +/– | – |
| | Granular layer | + | + | – | – | +/– | +/– | – |
| | Keratinized layer | – | – | – | – | – | – | – |
| Intermediate zone | Basal layer | – | – | – | – | + | + | +/– |
| | Prickle cell layer | +/– | +/– | +/– | +/– | +/– | +/– | +/– |
| | Keratinized layer | – | – | – | – | – | – | – |
| Labial mucosa | Basal layer | – | – | – | – | + | + | + |
| | Prickle cell layer | +/– | – | + | + | +/– | +/– | +/– |

– = Negative staining; + = positive; +/– = positive (with variable intensity of staining) or negative. Positive controls were: cytokeratins (CK)1 and 10 – suprabasal keratinocytes in abdominal epidermis and palatal mucosa; CK4 and 13 – suprabasal keratinocytes in non-keratinized cheek mucosal stratified squamous epithelium; CK5 and 14 – basal keratinocytes; CK9 – basal keratinocytes of gingival and cheek mucosal stratified squamous epithelium, outer root sheath of hair follicles, luminal cells lining the ducts of sweat and minor salivary glands.

The skin on the outer surface of the lip shows all the features of skin elsewhere (Fig. 14.31). A keratinized layer of epidermis lies on a bed of connective tissue, the dermis. The border between epidermis and dermis in this area is relatively flattened. The connective tissue contains sweat glands; sebaceous glands and the bases of hair follicles pass through the epithelium. The epidermis is, in fact, continuous around the bases of the follicles and is responsible for producing the keratin of which the hair is formed. Sebaceous glands drain either into the hair follicles or occasionally directly on to the skin surface.

## Vermilion

The vermilion zone lacks the appendages of skin. However, very occasional sebaceous glands may be found, especially at the angles of the mouth. As the vermilion zone also lacks mucous glands, it requires constant moistening with saliva by the tongue to prevent drying. The epithelium of the vermilion zone is keratinized, but thin and translucent. The connective tissue papillae of the lamina propria are relatively long and narrow, and contain capillary loops (Fig. 14.32). The proximity of these vessels to the surface, combined with the translucency of the epithelium, gives the surface a red appearance – hence its name. This red appearance is a human characteristic. The junctional region between the vermilion zone and the labial mucosa is known as the intermediate zone. It lacks a granular layer and tends to have a thick parakeratinized layer. In infants this becomes thickened and forms the suckling pad.

## Labial mucosa

The inner surface of the lip, the labial mucosa, is covered by a relatively thick, non-keratinized epithelium. The lamina propria is also wide but the papillae are short and irregular. A submucosa containing many minor salivary glands is present (Fig. 14.33). Strands of dense connective tissue bind the mucosa down to the underlying orbicularis oris muscle.

As the vermilion and intermediate zone (when identifiable) separate the keratinized skin from the lining mucosa, the question arises as to their particular phenotype. From a study of the distribution of cytokeratins and other epithelial proteins, it has been concluded that a unique transitional phenotype with features of both epidermis and labial epithelium occurs across the vermilion and particularly the intermediate zone of the upper lip (Tables 14.3, 14.4).

**Table 14.4** *Staining patterns of filaggrin, loricrin and involucrin in the stratified squamous epithelium of the lip (From Barrett AW, Morgan M, Nwaeze et al 2005 The differentiation profile of epithelium of the human lip. Archives of Oral Biology 50: 431–438 and courtesy of the editors of Archives of Oral Biology)*

|  | Layer | Profilaggrin/ filaggrin | Loricrin | Involucrin |
|---|---|---|---|---|
| Labial skin | Basal layer | – | – | – |
|  | Prickle cell layer | – | – | – |
|  | Granular layer | + | + | + |
|  | Keratinized layer | – | – | – |
| Vermilion | Basal layer | – | – | – |
|  | Prickle cell layer | – | +/– | +/– |
|  | Granular layer | + | + | + |
|  | Keratinized layer | – | – | + |
| Intermediate zone | Basal layer | – | – | – |
|  | Prickle cell layer | – | +/– | +/– |
|  | Keratinized layer | – | – | – |
| Labial mucosa | Basal layer | – | – | – |
|  | Prickle cell layer | + |  | + |

– = Negative staining; + = positive; +/– = positive or negative. Positive control was granular layer of epidermis.

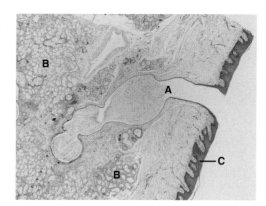

**Fig. 14.35** Section of the buccal mucosa showing collecting duct (A) from a minor salivary gland (B) penetrating the overlying lining epithelium (C) (H & E; ×40).

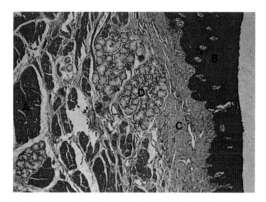

**Fig. 14.34** Section of buccal mucosa. B = non-keratinized oral epithelium; C = lamina propria; D = minor salivary gland in submucosa; A = fibres of buccinator muscle (H & E; ×15).

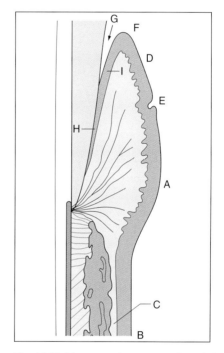

**Fig. 14.36** Diagrammatic representation of gingiva. A = attached gingiva; B = alveolar mucosa; C = submucosa associated with alveolar mucosa; D = free gingiva; E = free gingival groove; F = gingival margin; G = gingival sulcus; H = junctional epithelium; I = crevicular epithelium.

## CHEEK

The buccal mucosa lining the cheeks is, like the labial mucosa, a lining mucosa. The epithelium is non-keratinized and the lamina propria is dense with short, irregular papillae. A submucosa is present with many minor mucous salivary glands, beneath which lie fibres of the buccinator muscle (Fig. 14.34). The main collecting ducts of the minor salivary glands penetrate the overlying oral epithelium to drain into the vestibule of the mouth (Fig. 14.35). Sometimes, along a line coincident with the occlusal plane, the epithelium becomes keratinized, forming a white line, the linea alba (see Fig. 1.25). Sebaceous glands are sometimes present and seem to become more obvious after puberty in the male and after menopause in the female, when they appear as small yellow patches. These patches are termed Fordyce spots (see page 5). The role, if any, of sebaceous glands in this location is unknown, although it is important to differentiate them from pathological changes.

## GINGIVA AND ALVEOLAR MUCOSA

The gingiva is that portion of the oral mucosa that surrounds, and is attached to, the teeth and the alveolar bone. It has two recognized regions (Fig. 14.36). The main component is the attached gingiva, which is directly bound down to the underlying alveolar bone and tooth. Coronal to the attached gingiva is the free gingiva, which is the narrow rim of mucosa that is not bound down to underlying hard tissue. Its junction with the attached gingiva is sometimes demarcated by a shallow groove, the free gingival groove. Its coronal limit is the gingival margin. The unattached region between the free gingiva and the tooth is the gingival sulcus. The region apical to this, where the gingiva is bound to the underlying tooth, is the junctional epithelium.

Apically, the attached gingiva is demarcated from the alveolar mucosa (which is loosely attached to the lower part of the alveolar bone) by the mucogingival junction, which normally lies 3–5 mm below the level of the alveolar crest. The height of the gingiva above this junction is about 4–6 mm. The alveolar mucosa has a submucosa.

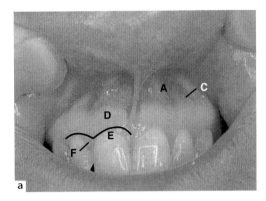

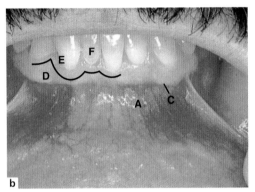

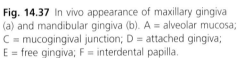

**Fig. 14.37** In vivo appearance of maxillary gingiva (a) and mandibular gingiva (b). A = alveolar mucosa; C = mucogingival junction; D = attached gingiva; E = free gingiva; F = interdental papilla.

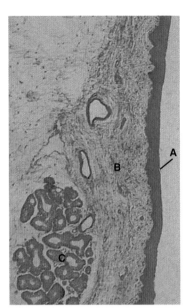

**Fig. 14.38** Section of alveolar mucosa. A = non-keratinized oral epithelium; B = lamina propria; C = minor salivary gland in submucosa (H & E; ×15).

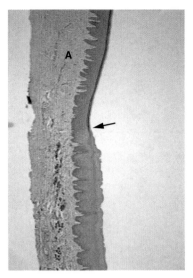

**Fig. 14.39** Section of the attached gingiva (A) and alveolar mucosa stripped off from underlying bone. The arrow points to the sharp demarcation site of the mucogingival junction. Note the keratinized epithelium covering the attached gingiva, the non-keratinized epithelium covering the alveolar mucosa and the numerous blood vessels in the alveolar mucosa (Papanicolaou stain; ×20). Courtesy of Professor C.A. Squier.

The appearance of the gingiva and alveolar mucosa in the maxilla and mandible in vivo is seen in Figure 14.37. The alveolar mucosa lines the lower part of the alveolus and is reflected over the buccal and labial sulcus to meet the buccal and labial mucosa respectively. It has a loose submucosa that allows for wide degrees of movement. The submucosa on its deep aspect is firmly attached to the underlying periosteum. The mucogingival junction (or health line) demarcates the boundary between attached gingiva and alveolar mucosa. The difference in appearance between the alveolar mucosa and the attached gingiva is due to differences in keratinization and translucency. The alveolar mucosa epithelium is translucent and the blood vessels lie superficially. Small blood vessels are clearly seen. The junction may be scalloped, paralleling the contours of the gingival margin. The free gingival groove that separates the attached gingiva from the free gingiva is apparent in only about 40% of teeth. It follows the contours of the cement–enamel junction. The groove may be produced by the bundles of principal collagen fibres that run from the cervical cementum to the gingiva, or may correspond to a heavy epithelial ridge. When present, the free gingival groove lies approximately at the level of the cement–enamel junction. Healthy attached gingiva often shows surface stippling, which corresponds to sites of intersecting epithelial ridges. In some cases, when the free gingival groove is absent, an irregularly aligned line of stipples marks the junction between attached and free gingiva. The free gingiva is smooth. The widths of both the free and attached gingivae vary regionally. The interdental papilla is that part of the gingiva that fills the space between the teeth. Its shape in three dimensions, and its histological appearance, depend on the shape and nature of contact between the adjacent teeth.

On the palatal surface of the maxillary teeth, there is no alveolar mucosa. Here, the attached gingiva merges with the palatal mucosa, with no clearly demarcated boundary (see Fig. 1.10).

## Alveolar mucosa

The alveolar mucosa comprises a thin, non-keratinized epithelium overlying a lamina propria that shows poorly developed dermal papillae. Underlying blood vessels lie near the surface (Fig. 14.38). The extensive

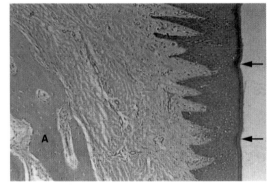

**Fig. 14.40** Section of the attached gingiva. The epithelium is a keratinized stratified squamous epithelium. The lamina propria is dense and relatively avascular and the interface with the epithelium is highly folded. The lamina propria is directly attached to the underlying alveolar bone (A), forming a mucoperiosteum. Arrows indicate surface stippling (H & E; ×75).

submucosa houses many minor mucous salivary glands and, near the vestibular sulcus, is loosely attached with numerous elastin fibres, allowing for free movement. Where it adjoins the attached gingiva the alveolar mucosa is thicker than elsewhere (and commonly thicker than the adjacent keratinized epithelium). The demarcation between keratinized and non-keratinized epithelium (the mucogingival junction) is well defined and submucosal vessels and glands are limited to the alveolar mucosa (Fig. 14.39).

## Gingiva

### Attached gingiva

The mucosa of the attached gingiva on its external surface (oral gingival epithelium) is a masticatory mucosa (Figs 14.39, 14.40). It is keratinized, but the degree and extent vary considerably between and within individuals. Orthokeratinization is the norm in mucosa unimpeded by inflammation; however, as much as 75% of the surface may be parakeratinized (i.e. the surface shows a strong pink stain with haematoxylin and eosin, as for keratin, but nuclei are retained in the surface layer – Fig. 14.41) and as much as 10% non-keratinized. Papillation is variable, the papillae

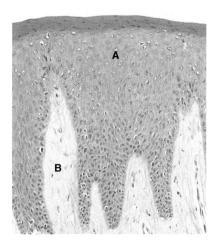

Fig. 14.41

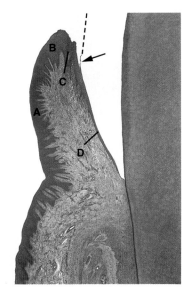

Fig. 14.42

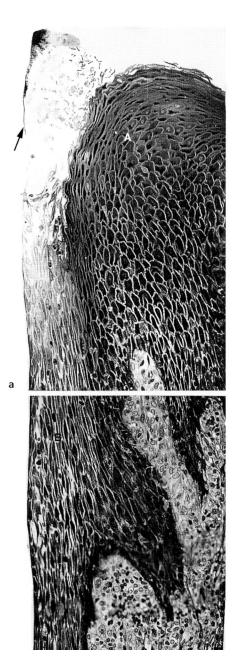

a

b

Fig. 14.43

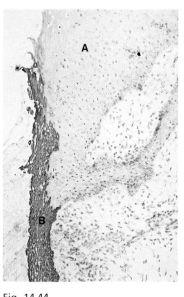

Fig. 14.44

**Fig. 14.41** Section of the gingival mucosa. The epithelium (A) is parakeratinized with nuclei being retained in the superficial keratinized layer. B = lamina propria (H & E; ×100). Courtesy of Dr A.E. Barrett.

**Fig. 14.42** Demineralized section showing the dentogingival junction. The outline of the original enamel surface is indicated by the broken black line. A = region of attached gingiva covered by masticatory epithelium; B = region of free gingiva covered externally by masticatory epithelium; C = non-keratinized crevicular epithelium; D = non-keratinized junctional epithelium. Note the tag of enamel cuticle (arrow) that helps to delineate the oral sulcular epithelium from the junctional epithelium (H & E; ×30). Courtesy of Professor H.E. Schroeder.

**Fig. 14.43** Section of gingiva showing the crevicular epithelium (a) and the upper portion of the junctional epithelium (b). At this site the junctional epithelium may be 15–30 cells thick. Note the tag of enamel cuticle (arrow) helping to delineate the two types of epithelia (×200). Courtesy of Professor H.E. Schroeder.

**Fig. 14.44** Demineralized section of gingiva showing sulcular (A) and junctional epithelium (B) staining for cytokeratin 19. The junctional epithelium stains positively (brown) (×150). Courtesy of Professor P.R. Morgan.

often being aligned in rows (especially at the margin). As little as 0.08 mm may separate the tips of some papillae from the surface. The surface is stippled, the stipples arising from intersecting epithelial ridges. There is no submucosa, the lamina propria being bound directly to bone, forming a mucoperiosteum (Figs 14.39, 14.40).

### Free gingiva

The mucosa of the free gingiva is indistinguishable from that of the attached gingiva (Fig. 14.42), but may be demarcated from it by the free gingival groove (or a line of stipples). The gingival margin marks the boundary with the **gingival crevice** or **sulcus**. In germ-free animals, and in strictly healthy, plaque-free gingivae, the crevice is absent and the gingival margin corresponds to the coronal extent of the junctional epithelium. In clinically healthy mouths, the clinical crevice is 0.5–2.0 mm deep. Crevices deeper than 3 mm (measured clinically) are generally accepted as diseased and are described as 'periodontal pockets'. In routine decalcified sections, the enamel will be lost, but its position must be envisaged in order to appreciate the approximate position of the gingival crevice and thus distinguish between the crevicular (sulcular) epithelium, which faces

the gingival crevice, and the junctional epithelium, which is in direct contact with the enamel surface at the base of the crevice (Fig. 14.42).

### Crevicular (sulcular) epithelium

The epithelium on the inner surface of the gingiva constitutes the crevicular epithelium and the junctional epithelium, both of which are non-keratinized and therefore lack a granular layer. These form the so-called gingival cuff at the site where the oral mucosa meets the tooth. Histologically, the crevicular epithelium may be distinguished from the junctional epithelium by having a more folded interface with the underlying connective tissue. In addition, tags of an enamel cuticle may be seen at the interface between the two epithelia (Figs 14.42, 14.43). The two epithelia can also be distinguished by their different cytokeratin profiles. As is to be expected, the superficial layers of the crevicular epithelium stain positive for CK4, typical of lining epithelium. However, unusually, junctional epithelium not only lacks CK4 (even though it can be considered a lining mucosa) but characteristically expresses the basal keratinocyte markers CK5, 14 and 19 throughout all its layers (Fig. 14.44), indicating that it is a non-differentiating tissue. This CK profile is similar to that of

**Fig. 14.45** Demineralized section of gingiva showing non-keratinized stratified squamous epithelium forming junctional epithelium (B). Note the smooth interface with the underlying lamina propria (C). A = enamel space (H & E; ×150).

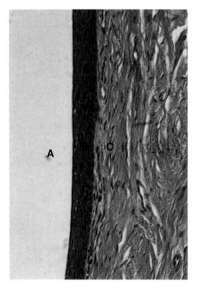

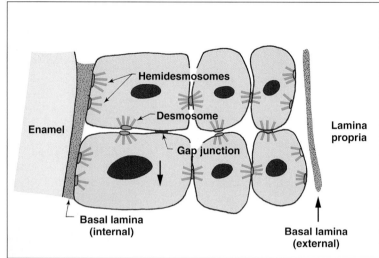

**Fig. 14.46** Diagrammatic representation of junctional epithelium.

the reduced enamel epithelium from which it is derived. Unlike the oral sulcular epithelium, the junctional epithelium also has receptors for, and expresses, epidermal growth factor.

The gingival crevice (Figs 14.36, 14.42) is bounded by the gingival margin above and the junctional epithelium below. The epithelium is non-keratinized and thinner. The crevicular epithelium merges with the junctional epithelium and a distinct boundary is not usually seen. Externally, the base of the gingival crevice corresponds approximately with the free gingival groove, when present.

### Junctional epithelium

The junctional epithelium is an epithelial collar that surrounds the tooth and extends from the region of the cementum–enamel junction to the bottom of the gingival crevice (Figs 14.42–14.45). It may extend for up to 2 mm. Coronally the junctional epithelium may be 15–30 cells thick (up to 100 μm – Fig. 14.43), while apically it narrows to only 1–3 cells thick. It consists of two zones: a single cell layer of cuboidal cells (the stratum germinativum) overlying several layers of flattened cells equivalent to a stratum spinosum. There is no stratum granulosum or corneum. The junctional epithelium has a high rate of turnover (in the order of 5–6 days) and its cells are exfoliated coronally into the gingival crevice. It is derived from the rapidly replaced reduced enamel epithelium (probably from the stratum intermedium component of that tissue) and this may explain why its cytokeratin profile resembles odontogenic epithelium rather than the lining stratified squamous epithelium typical of oral mucosa (Fig. 14.44). The cells of the stratum germinativum rest on a typical lamina propria, which shows many capillaries and appears to be more cellular than other parts of the gingiva. The connective tissue interface is smooth (Fig. 14.45).

The principal features of the junctional epithelium are shown diagrammatically in Figure 14.46. The cells of the junctional epithelium immediately adjacent to the tooth attach themselves to the tooth by hemidesmosomes and a basal lamina. The combination of the hemidesmosomes and basal lamina is known as the attachment apparatus or epithelial attachment. The basal lamina in contact with the tooth is termed the internal basal lamina. On the other surface of the junctional epithelium in contact with the lamina propria is the normal basal lamina (the external basal lamina). The junctional epithelium is therefore unique in having two basal laminae. However, differences exist between the two basal laminae (see below). Like epithelial cells elsewhere, the cells of the junctional epithelium are joined by desmosomes and gap junctions; tight junctions are rare. However, the desmosomes are fewer in number, and this is correlated with larger inter-

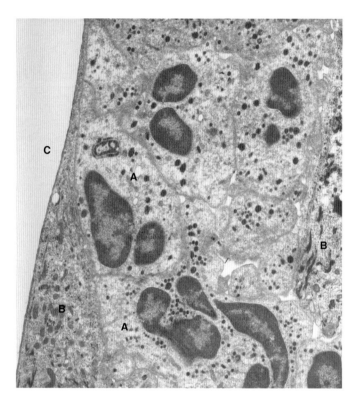

**Fig. 14.47** Electron micrograph of demineralized section of junctional epithelium showing defence cells (leukocytes, A) migrating through junctional epithelial cells (B). C = enamel space (×10 000). Courtesy of Professor M.M. Smith.

cellular spaces that may comprise up to 5% of the volume of the tissue. This has profound clinical significance because not only crevicular fluid but also defence cells can pass across the junctional epithelium (Fig. 14.47). Indeed, even healthy gingival tissue may exhibit neutrophils in the intercellular spaces, indicative of its protective role. The lack of membrane-coating granules (see page 224) may also assist the permeability of the cell layer. In this context, cells of the junctional epithelium, together with underlying fibroblasts and endothelial cells, express intercellular adhesion molecule (ICAM)-1, which helps in the transmigration of neutrophils from the adjacent capillaries and through the junctional epithelium. The turnover rate for cells of the junctional epithelium is the highest of any oral mucosa. There is also evidence for a high turnover rate for the internal basal lamina.

Ultrastructural examination of junctional epithelial cells interfacing with enamel will show that the attachment of the cell to the enamel is

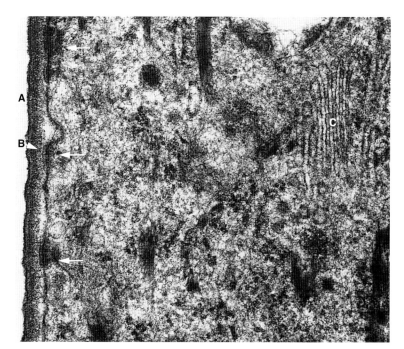

**Fig. 14.48** Electron micrograph of demineralized section of part of junctional epithelial cell adjacent to enamel space (A). B = lamina lucida and lamina densa of basal lamina; C = Golgi complex; arrows indicate hemidesmosomes (×70 000). Courtesy of Professor J.V. Soames.

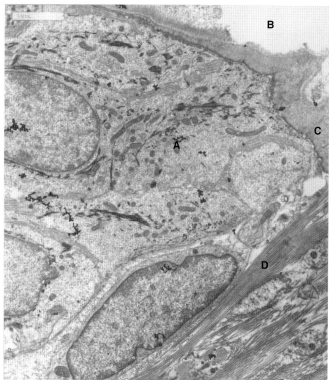

**Fig. 14.49** Electron micrograph of demineralized section showing the apical limit of the junctional epithelial cells (A) at the cement-enamel junction. B = enamel space; C = cementum; D = collagen fibre of gingiva (×2500). Courtesy of Professor M.M. Smith.

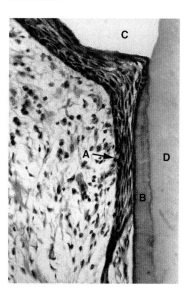

**Fig. 14.50** Demineralized section showing junctional epithelium (A) having proliferated rootwards to lie on cemental surface of root (B). C = enamel space; D = dentine. (H & E; ×120). Courtesy of Dr D. Adams.

mediated by hemidesmosomes and a basal lamina (Fig. 14.48). The internal basal lamina, as elsewhere, is seen to contain two zones: an electron-lucent zone adjacent to the cell (which may represent a preparation artefact) and an electron-dense layer against the tooth surface. The pattern of a lamina densa and lamina lucida is apparently not as clear as in other basal laminae, the lamina densa not always being clearly delineated, but the combined thickness is similar (100–140 nm). The internal basal lamina also differs from the external basal lamina in lacking type IV collagen and anchoring fibrils. It is therefore not surprising that the composition of the internal basal lamina differs from the external basal lamina in lacking laminin. The basement membrane seen in light microscopy adjacent to the connective tissue would appear much thicker than in electron micrographs because of a reticular component derived from the connective tissue. The hemidesmosomes consist of thickenings of the inner leaflet of the plasma membrane (called the attachment plaque). Opposite the attachment plaque at the enamel surface there is a peripheral dense line comparable to that seen in the lamina lucida of the basal lamina between epithelium and connective tissue.

The nature of the adhesive mechanisms associated with the cells of the gingiva has been studied by observing the distribution of the integrin α6β4. As this transmembrane receptor glycoprotein is a component of hemidesmosomes, it is present in both basal laminae of the junctional epithelium (compared with the crevicular epithelium where it is only found in the single basal lamina). However, the α6 component is also associated with all the remaining cells of the junctional epithelium, allowing these cells to be distinguished from those of the crevicular epithelium, which lack the α6 component. This, together with the distribution of CK19, implies a difference in adhesive mechanisms within the junctional and crevicular epithelia.

In addition, as the components of the basal lamina must also be synthesized, transported and secreted by junctional epithelial cells, the cytoplasm of the cells contains numerous free ribosomes, cisternae of rough endoplasmic reticulum and a prominent Golgi complex (Fig. 14.48). There is an absence of both membrane-coating granules and keratohyaline granules, and few cytokeratin filaments are present.

An element not visible in decalcified preparations is the enamel cuticle (see pages 124, 125). This cuticle is a non-mineralized structure interposed between the junctional epithelium and the underlying hard tissue. It varies in extent and is not always present. When present, it is patchy and most prominent when filling depressions in the calcified surface. The cuticle is ultrastucturally amorphous and biochemically distinct from the basal lamina. It is probably proteinaceous and may be derived from serum.

The length of the junctional epithelium attached to the enamel surface varies according to the stage of eruption (see Fig. 26.9). When the tooth first erupts into the oral cavity, most of the enamel will be covered by junctional epithelium. By the time the tooth reaches the occlusal plane, about one-quarter of the enamel surface is still covered by junctional epithelium. Eventually it will come to lie close to the cementum–enamel junction (Figs 14.42, 14.49). In patients with exposure of the roots, the junctional epithelium proliferates apically and, as a consequence, may establish a firm union with the surface of the cementum (Fig. 14.50), also

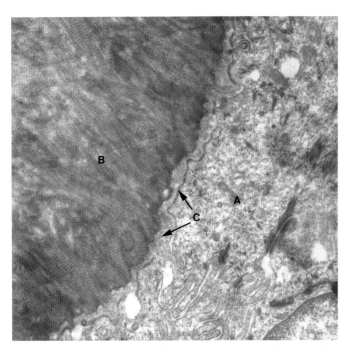

**Fig. 14.51** Electron micrograph of demineralized section of junctional epithelium (A), which has proliferated rootwards to lie on cementum (B), the collagen fibrils of which are evident. The epithelial cells are attached to the cementum by a basal lamina/cuticle (C) (×20000). Courtesy of Professor M.M. Smith.

via a basal lamina (Fig. 14.51). When this occurs, and in the absence of obvious periodontal inflammatory disease, the question arises as to whether it is a physiological age change (passive eruption) or whether, as there must have been some associated loss of collagen fibres at the cervix of the tooth to allow for epithelial proliferation apically, it is the result of a disease process.

The lamina propria associated with the junctional epithelium has a rich blood supply arranged as a complex anastomosing network, the major vessels representing postcapillary venules. This crevicular plexus is separated from the surrounding looping vessels that lie within the dermal papillae of the attached gingiva (see Fig. 12.58). The crevicular plexus is the obvious source of gingival crevicular fluid. The vessels of the plexus are very sensitive to stimulation and are likely to vasodilate under the slightest of insults. In response to plaque, they may become more permeable, increasing the production of crevicular fluid. The junctional epithelium has a rich plexus of nerves close to its basal layer, with many endings penetrating into the epithelium itself.

The dentogingival junction seals the underlying connective tissue of the periodontium from the oral environment. The strength of the seal is thought to be dependent not only upon the attachment of the junctional epithelium to the tooth but also upon the pressure exerted by the fibres and tissue fluid of the underlying connective tissue. The weakness of the dentogingival junction derives from its situation, the enamel being a non-shedding surface, allowing persistent bacterial colonization. The epithelium is therefore exposed to toxic products emanating from the consequent bacterial accumulation.

The turnover of the junctional epithelium is rapid. The epithelial cells migrate in a coronal direction, to be shed into the oral cavity via the gingival crevice. The continual breakdown and reformation of lamina densa, hemidesmosomes and desmosomes allows cells to alter their relationship as they migrate through the junctional epithelium. The rate of turnover is dependent on the demands placed upon the tissue and appears to be directly related to the degree of inflammation. Following the surgical removal of the gingiva, a new junctional epithelium rapidly forms that has all the original characteristics. As the newly reformed dentogingival junction can have been derived only from the gingival epithelium (which is

keratinized), it can be assumed that proliferating epithelial cells from this surface are modified by underlying connective tissue cells closer to the tooth surface to express a different phenotype (see pages 228, 229).

### Gingival crevicular fluid

The junctional epithelium is permeable. Indeed, tissue fluid and cells (as well as experimental substances such as dyes, carbon particles and horse-radish peroxidase) pass readily through the epithelium from the connective tissue into the gingival crevice. This is known as gingival crevicular fluid (GCF) and it can be collected using capillary tubing, gingival washing or absorbent paper strips. It is thought by some, however, that fluid only passes into the crevice as a response to pathological stimuli and is absent from perfectly healthy gingiva.

The permeability of the junctional epithelium may be related to the presence of particularly wide intercellular spaces. GCF contains material of low molecular weight that is said to pass continuously from the sub-epithelial tissue into the gingival crevice. Other oral epithelial surfaces do not show such exudation of tissue fluid. GCF contains immunoglobulins, complement, polymorphonucleocytes and epithelial squames. In addition, plaque bacteria and their products will also be present. Once the immunological and phagocytic properties of the fluid undertake their defensive activity against the plaque, other inflammatory products will be present in the plaque, such as cytokines and metalloproteinases. The products of the protective inflammatory reaction, however, can lead to damage of the host tissue.

The composition of the GCF provides an indicator of the state of health of the underlying periodontium. For example, following the application of orthodontic loads, there are significant increases in the levels of molecules associated with remodelling of alveolar bone and the periodontal ligament, such as cathepsin B, prostaglandins, ILs, tumour necrosis factor and epidermal growth factor. Breakdown products of the extracellular matrix of bone and periodontal ligament may be distinguishable in GCF because of known differences in composition between their extracellular matrices. Breakdown products of basal lamina components in GCF may indicate the status of the junctional epithelium. Analysis of the GCF may eventually help indicate the severity of inflammatory periodontal disease and may allow for the development of markers to assist in identifying those in the general population who are most vulnerable to the spread of infection from a simple gingivitis into a periodontitis.

### Interdental gingiva

The interdental gingiva is the part of the gingiva between adjacent teeth. The shape and arrangement of the gingival tissues between the teeth depend on the shape of the contact between the teeth (although free and attached gingivae are always present). The interdental gingiva occupies the space between the teeth and conforms to its shape. From the buccal or lingual aspects, the interdental gingiva has a wedge-shaped appearance (Fig. 14.37). Between the anterior teeth (which contact only at a small point), it would appear similarly 'pointed' when viewed in a buccolingual plane. In the posterior cheek teeth, which have a broader area of contact, the appearance from the buccal or lingual side would show the typical wedge shape (Fig. 14.52) but across its buccolingual plane there are two peaks on the buccal and lingual aspects with a curved depression between them (the **interdental col**), which follows the contour around the contact point (Fig. 14.53).

The epithelium of the col is continuous with the junctional epithelium on each side. It is similarly non-keratinized and initially derived from the reduced enamel epithelium. Its epithelium is thin and, as the region is not easy to keep plaque-free, inflammatory cells may be seen infiltrating the underlying lamina propria (Fig. 14.54). When teeth are spaced, the col

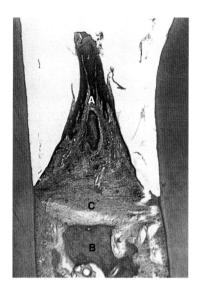

**Fig. 14.52** Demineralized section showing the interdental gingiva (A) between two cheek teeth in the anteroposterior plane. B = alveolar crest; C = transseptal group of gingival fibres (H & E; ×20).

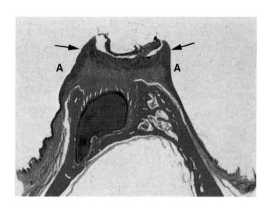

**Fig. 14.53** Demineralized section of the interdental papilla cut in the buccolingual plane between two cheek teeth showing the 'interdental col'. The buccal and lingual margins (arrows) of the attached gingiva externally (A) are raised above the central concavity of the col, whose margin passes below the contact points of the teeth (H & E; ×4).

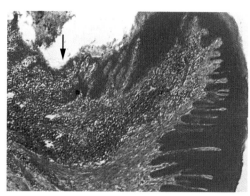

**Fig. 14.54** Higher-power view of the thin, non-keratinized epithelium of the interdental col (arrow). There is a substantial infiltrate of inflammatory cells in the area (H & E; ×40).

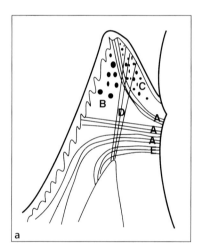

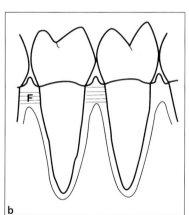

**Fig. 14.55** Diagram showing arrangement of principal collagen fibre groups in the lamina propria of the gingiva. (a) buccolingual section; (b) mesiodistal section; (c) horizontal section; (d) buccolingual section along interdental col. A = dentogingival fibres; B = longitudinal fibres; C = circular fibres; D = alveolo-gingival fibres; E = dentoperiosteal fibres; F = transseptal fibres; G = semicircular fibres; H = transgingival fibres; I = interdental fibres; J = vertical fibres.

**Fig. 14.56** Demineralized section showing direction of dentogingival fibres (arrowed) passing over the alveolar crest (A) and inserting into the lamina propria of the attached gingiva (B). C = root of tooth; D = periodontal ligament (Masson's trichrome; ×80).

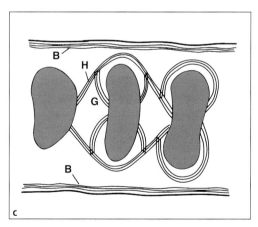

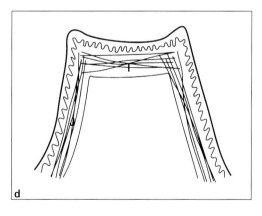

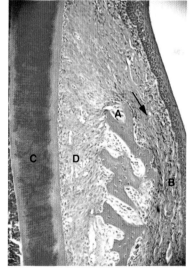

Fig. 14.55                                                      Fig. 14.56

does not exist and an often very flat gingiva is seen, which is covered by a keratinized epithelium.

The vast majority of collagen fibres of the gingiva are composed of type I collagen. These are in the form of dense principal bundles the functions of which include support of the free gingiva, binding of the attached gingiva to the alveolar bone and tooth, thereby resisting masticatory loads, and linkage of teeth one to another. These principal fibre groups have been given names based upon their orientation and attachments, although whether they always exist as such discrete and definable groups is debat-

able (Fig. 14.55). The turnover rate of gingival collagen appears to be faster than in other parts of the oral cavity.

*Dentogingival fibres* arise from the root surface above the alveolar crest and radiate to insert into the lamina propria of the gingiva. The most superficial fibres lie beneath the crevicular epithelium, a middle group lies almost horizontally and the deepest group courses between the gingiva and the alveolar bone (Fig. 14.56).

*Longitudinal fibres* extend for long distances within the free gingiva, some possibly for the whole length of the arch.

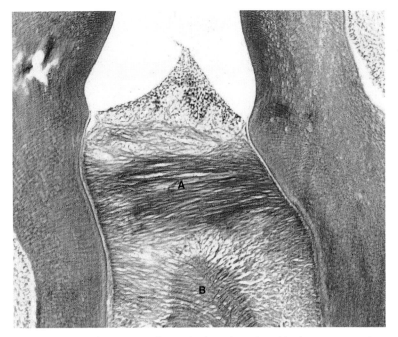

**Fig. 14.57** Decalcified section of two cheek teeth sectioned in the anteroposterior plane showing transseptal fibres (A) passing from the cementum of one tooth over the alveolar crest (B) to attach into the cementum of the adjacent tooth (von Gieson; ×140). Courtesy of Dr M.E. Atkinson.

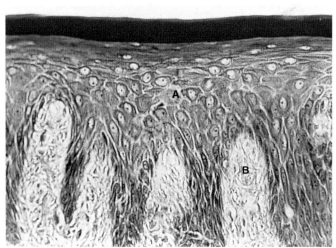

**Fig. 14.58** Section of the masticatory keratinized epithelium (A) of the hard palate. Note the highly folded interface with the lamina propria (B) (H & E; ×250). Courtesy of Dr D. Adams.

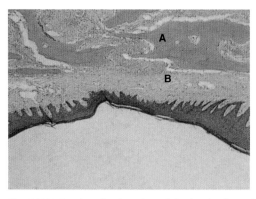

**Fig. 14.59** Demineralized section of the hard palate. The keratinized epithelium exhibits deep epithelial rete. The dense lamina propria (B) is attached to the bone of the hard palate (A) in the absence of a submucosa, forming a mucoperiosteum (H & E; ×20).

*Circular fibres* encircle each tooth within the marginal and interdental gingiva. Some attach to cementum, some to alveolar bone. Some cross interdentally to join the fibre group of the adjacent tooth.

*Alveologingival fibres* run from the crest of the alveolar bone and interdental septum, radiating coronally into the overlying lamina propria of the gingiva.

*Dentoperiosteal fibres* occur only in labial/buccal and lingual gingiva. They arise from cementum and pass over the alveolar crest to insert into the periosteum.

*Transseptal fibres* pass horizontally from the root of one tooth, above the alveolar crest, to be inserted into the root of the adjacent tooth (Figs 14.52, 14.57). Such fibres provide an anatomical basis for linking all the teeth in the dentition. They have been implicated in the mechanism of mesial drift (pages 373, 374).

*Semicircular fibres* emanate from cementum near the cementum–enamel junction, cross the free marginal gingiva and insert into a similar position on the opposite side of the tooth.

*Transgingival fibres* reinforce the circular and semicircular fibres. The fibres arise from the cervical cementum and extend into the marginal gingiva of the adjacent tooth, merging with the circular fibres.

*Interdental fibres* pass through the coronal portion of the interdental gingiva in the buccolingual direction, connecting buccal and lingual papillae.

*Vertical fibres* arise in alveolar mucosa or attached gingiva and pass coronally towards the marginal gingiva and interdental papilla.

The lamina propria of the gingiva has properties that distinguish it from the connective tissue of the periodontal ligament (see Ch. 12). For example, the fibroblasts lack alkaline phosphatase, have less contractile proteins and can release more prostaglandin in response to histamine. The extracellular matrix has less ground substance and less type III collagen, is hyaluronan-rich and has a lower turnover rate. Such differences in properties may be relevant when considering periodontal regeneration (see pages 355–357).

The vasculature of the lamina propria of the gingiva is very rich and forms two plexuses, one beneath the oral gingival epithelium, the other beneath the oral sulcular epithelium. These plexuses allow the tissues to respond very quickly to stimuli. Each dermal papilla of the lamina propria beneath the oral gingival epithelium possesses an ascending arterial loop and a descending venous loop, between which lies a terminal capillary loop. Beneath the junctional epithelium lies a complex vascular plexus comprising postcapillary venules. From this region is derived the gingival crevicular fluid. Specializations also allow for the rapid passage of cells and molecules across the junctional epithelium.

## PALATE

### Hard palate

The mucosa of the hard palate is a typical masticatory mucosa with a keratinized (or parakeratinized) epithelium (Fig. 14.58). In much of the central region there is no submucosa and the dense lamina propria binds down directly to bone (mucoperiosteum; Fig. 14.59). The same arrangement is seen in much of the attached gingiva (Fig. 14.40). Where the palate joins the alveolus, a submucosa is present and contains the main neurovascular bundles. There are also minor mucous glands (predominantly posteriorly) that open on to the surface by ducts (Fig. 14.60) and adipose tissue (predominantly anteriorly).

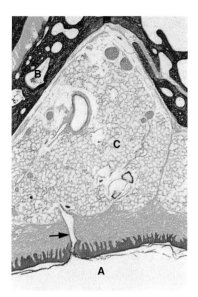

**Fig. 14.60** Demineralized section of posterior part of the hard palate at its junction with the alveolar process showing the presence of a submucosa (C) containing minor mucous salivary glands with a duct (arrow) opening on to the surface. A = oral cavity; B = bone. Note the masticatory mucosa lining the surface (Masson's trichrome; ×15).

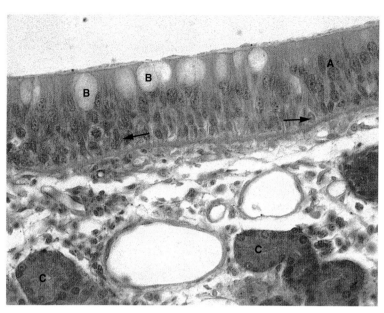

**Fig. 14.62** Section of nasal surface of hard palate from Fig. 14.61. A = ciliated columnar epithelium; B = goblet cell; C = minor gland; arrows indicate basal cells in epithelium (H & E; ×500). Courtesy of Dr M.E. Atkinson.

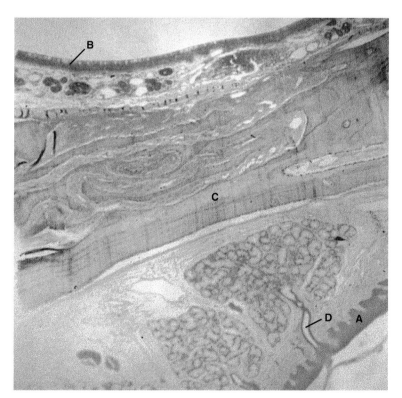

**Fig. 14.61** Demineralized section of the hard palate showing the oral surface (A) lined by masticatory epithelium and the nasal surface (B) lined by a respiratory epithelium. C = bone of hard palate; D = duct from mucous gland opening on to surface (H & E; ×110). Courtesy of Dr M.E. Atkinson.

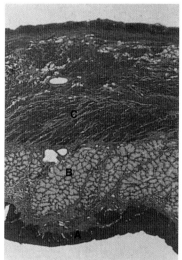

**Fig. 14.63** Section of soft palate showing the oral surface being covered by a non-keratinized lining mucosa (A). Numerous minor salivary glands lie in the submucosa (B), beneath which is seen the palatal musculature (C). The nasal surface is lined by a pseudostratified ciliated columnar epithelium (H & E; ×20).

While the oral surface of the hard palate is lined by masticatory epithelium, the nasal surface of the hard palate is lined by a respiratory mucosa (Fig. 14.61). The respiratory mucosa consists of ciliated columnar epithelial cells with many goblet cells (Fig. 14.62). The ciliated cells contain 'simple' cytokeratin types (i.e. 7, 8 and 18). In addition, there are proliferative basal cells characterized by cytokeratin types 5 and 14.

Beneath the respiratory epithelium there is a vascular submucosa containing minor glands of both mucous and serous types.

## Soft palate

The mucosa covering the oral surface of the soft palate is a non-keratinized lining mucosa (Fig. 14.63). Thus, the connective tissue papillae are short and broad. The lamina propria contains many elastic fibres and its collagen bundles are relatively thin. There is a broad submucosa containing many small mucous glands. The submucosa attaches into the palatal muscles. The nasal surface of the soft palate is lined by a respiratory mucosa of ciliated columnar epithelium.

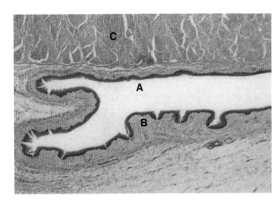

**Fig. 14.64** Section showing the ventral surface of the tongue (A) and floor of mouth (B) being lined by non-keratinized lining epithelium. The submucosa in the floor of the mouth is indistinct, the thin lamina propria being bound to the underlying tongue musculature (C) (H & E; ×20).

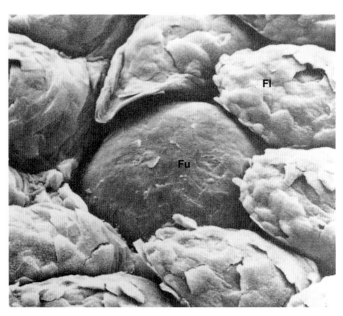

**Fig. 14.65** Scanning electron micrograph showing filiform papillae (Fl) surrounding a fungiform papilla (Fu) (×90). Courtesy of S. Franey.

## TONGUE AND FLOOR OF THE MOUTH

The ventral surface of the tongue and the floor of the mouth are covered by typical lining mucosa (Fig. 14.64). There is little wear and tear but a need for considerable mobility. The epithelium is thin, non-keratinized and shows short papillae. The submucosa is extensive on the floor of the mouth but indistinct (if not absent) on the ventral surface of the tongue where the mucosa binds down to the tongue muscles. The thinness of the epithelium and the vascularity of the connective tissue make this a route by which some drugs can rapidly reach the blood stream.

An indistinct groove, the sulcus terminalis (see Fig. 1.15) divides the tongue into an anterior two-thirds (palatal surface) and a posterior one-third (pharyngeal surface). The anterior two-thirds of the tongue is covered with numerous papillae, which can be classified into four types: filiform, fungiform, foliate and circumvallate papillae (see Figs 1.16–1.18). The posterior one-third of the tongue is studded with small lymphatic nodules (or follicles). In addition to its mechanical functions, the tongue has important sensory functions (particularly taste) and is regarded as a specialized mucosa.

The mucosa on the dorsum of the anterior two-thirds of the tongue is classified as a masticatory mucosa as a large part of it is covered by the numerous keratinized (or parakeratinized) filiform papillae (Fig. 14.65). The overlying stratified squamous epithelium is keratinized and forms hair-like tufts, although the regions between the papillae are non-keratinized (Fig. 14.66). Each **filiform papilla** consists of a central core of lamina propria with smaller, secondary papillae branching from it. The filiform papillae are highly abrasive during mastication when the bolus is compressed against the palate.

The simplest model of homeostasis in stratified epithelia is that all basal epithelial cells divide in a fairly homogeneous manner, and that increased basal cell 'pressure' generated by dividing cells results in an upward random migration of keratinocytes destined for desquamation. However, it is now clear that many renewing tissues (including oral epithelium) are organized in a much more complicated way, as reference to the mouse filiform papilla shows (Fig. 14.67a). Each mouse filiform papilla comprises several columns of cells around a central connective tissue core. The anterior column is two cells wide and has well defined boundaries that result from the difference in cell size and differentiation on either side of each boundary. The posterior column of 16–20 cells piled one on top of another gradually inclines as cells move upwards so that the top cell desquamates backwards (towards the pharynx). The buttress column appears to fill in the rear of the papilla structure to 'buttress' the posterior column.

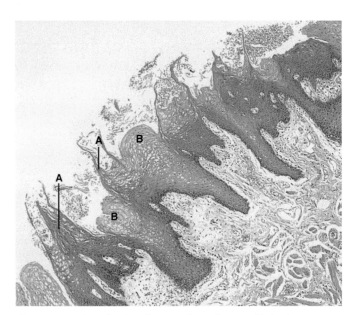

**Fig. 14.66** Section showing dorsum of anterior two-thirds of tongue covered by keratinized filiform papillae (A) with non-keratinized regions between (B) (H & E; ×35). Courtesy of Professor P.R. Morgan.

Note the maturity of basal cells over the apex of the connective tissue core and the method used to number individual cell positions within each column. The posterior column shows keratinization (its cytokeratin profile containing CK1 and 10), while the anterior column is non-keratinized (its cytokeratin profile containing CK4 and 13).

A schematic representation of column boundaries and cell migration patterns in the mouse filiform papilla is shown in Figure 14.67b. The stem cell population is at position 1, next to column boundaries. As cells move bodily along the basement membrane their capacity for proliferation decreases so that, by the time they reach the highest cell position number,

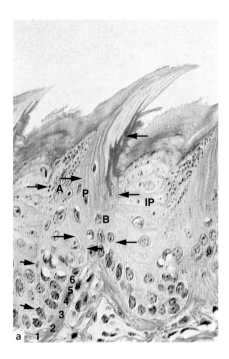
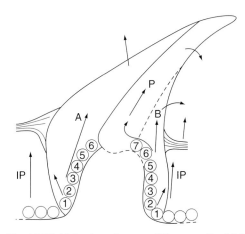

**Fig. 14.67** (a) Section of mouse filiform papilla. (b) Schematic representation of column boundaries and cell migration patterns. A = anterior column; B = buttress column; IP = interpapillary epithelium; P = posterior column (Masson's trichrome ×120). Courtesy of Professor W.J. Hume.

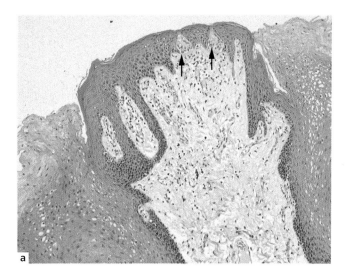
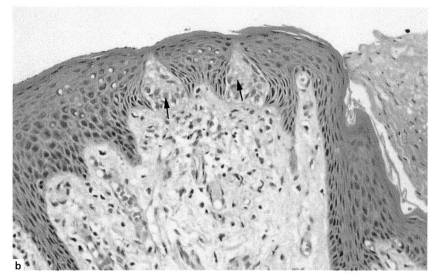

**Fig. 14.68** (a) Section of fungiform papilla on dorsal surface of anterior part of tongue showing taste buds (arrowed). The papilla is keratinized (H & E; ×120). (b) High-power view of surface of fungiform papilla seen in (a), showing taste buds (arrows) (×240). Courtesy of Professor P.R. Morgan.

they are postmitotic, differentiating cells. This model implies that, because of rapid desquamation of cells, four or five cells per day in the posterior column are the stem cells. There is some suprabasal migration in the anterior column in addition to migration along the basement membrane. The posterior column is derived from lateral cell migration and the buttress column from suprabasal migration from the stem cell population at the rear of the papilla. Thus, each of these columns is one cell wide whereas the anterior column is two cells wide.

**Fungiform papillae** are found as isolated, elevated mushroom-shaped papillae scattered between the filiform papillae and are approximately 150–400 µm in diameter (Fig. 14.65). They are covered by a relatively thin epithelium that may or may not be keratinized and have a vascular core of lamina propria. Taste buds may be found on the surface (Figs 14.68, 14.69).

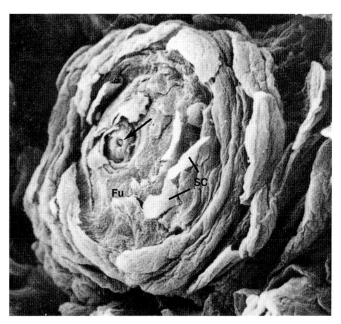

**Fig. 14.69** Scanning electron micrograph of fungiform papilla (Fu) showing opening (pore) of taste bud on surface (arrow). SC = surface keratinocytes (×175). Courtesy of S. Franey.

**Foliate papillae** may be present as one or two longitudinal clefts at the side of the posterior part of the tongue (see Fig. 1.18). Taste buds may be found within the non-keratinized epithelium of these papillae (Fig. 14.70).

**Circumvallate papillae** are large and rounded. They are surrounded by a trench-like feature and do not project beyond the normal surface level of the tongue (Figs 14.71, 14.72; see also Fig. 1.15). The circumvallate papilla is generally covered by a non-keratinized epithelium. Taste buds predominate on the internal wall of the trench in the epithelium. Small serous glands (of von Ebner) empty into the base of the trench (Fig. 14.73). Groups of mucous glands are also seen within the muscle of the tongue, particularly in the posterior part, and these are unencapsulated.

The **taste buds**, the special chemoreceptive organs responsible for taste, are located within the epithelium, particularly around the walls of the circumvallate papillae (Figs 14.72, 14.74) and also in small numbers on the upper surface of fungiform papillae, in the lateral walls of foliate papillae, in the mucosa of the soft palate and in the epiglottis. Two types of cell are present in the taste bud: the supporting cell and the taste cell. A small pore opens from the surface into the taste bud (Fig. 14.75).

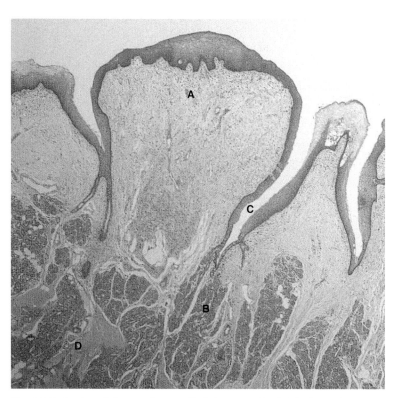

**Fig. 14.72** Section of circumvallate papilla (A). Serous glands (B) of von Ebner empty via ducts into the base of the trench (C) surrounding the papilla, which is not raised above the surface of the tongue. D = muscle of tongue (H & E; ×35). Courtesy of Professor P.R. Morgan.

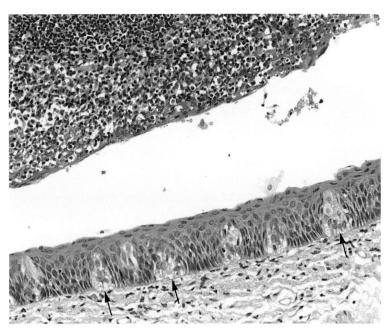

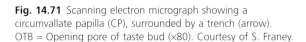

**Fig. 14.70** Section of foliate papilla showing taste buds (arrowed). Note the adjacent lymphoid material characteristic of the posterior part of the tongue (×200).

**Fig. 14.71** Scanning electron micrograph showing a circumvallate papilla (CP), surrounded by a trench (arrow). OTB = Opening pore of taste bud (×80). Courtesy of S. Franey.

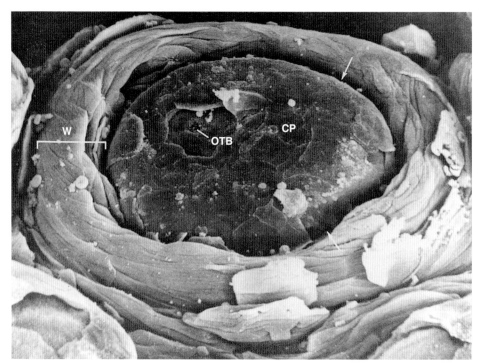

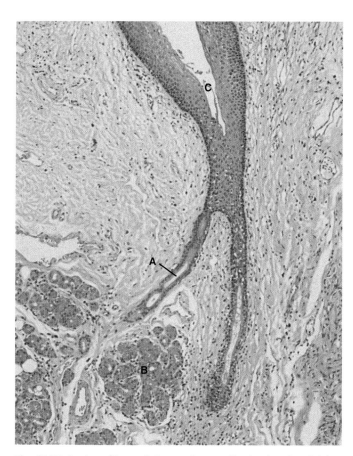

**Fig. 14.73** Section of base of circumvallate papilla showing duct (A) from serous gland (B) emptying into the base of the trench (C) (H & E; ×130). Courtesy of Professor P.R. Morgan.

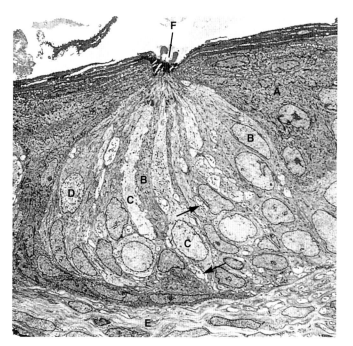

**Fig. 14.75** Electron micrograph of a taste bud. A = epithelial cells adjacent to taste bud; B = darker type I cells; C = lighter type II cells; D = lighter type III cell; E = underlying connective tissue; F = taste pore; arrows indicate where type I and type III cells form synapses with intragemmal nerves (×11 000). Courtesy of Drs S.M. Royer and J.C. Kinnamon.

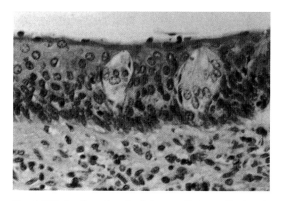

**Fig. 14.74** Section of wall of circumvallate papilla showing two pale barrel-shaped areas representing two taste buds (Masson's trichrome; ×300).

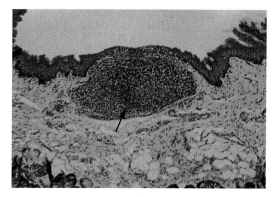

**Fig. 14.76** Section of dorsal surface of posterior one-third of tongue containing a lymphoid follicle (arrow). This part of the tongue is covered by a non-keratinized lining epithelium (H & E; ×40).

At the ultrastructural level the cells of the taste bud are clearly demarcated from the adjacent epithelial cells (Fig. 14.75). The morphology of a taste bud may vary according to species and site. Four distinct cell types have been described: the relatively undifferentiated type IV cells are distinguished by their basal position and the presence of intermediate filaments; type I cells have a dark appearance, while types II and III cells are lighter. Types I and III cells may form synapses with intragemmal nerves. The taste bud is separated from the underlying connective tissue by a basal lamina.

The collection of lymphoid follicles on the posterior one-third of the tongue is collectively known as the **lingual tonsil** and forms a component of Waldeyer's ring, which protects the opening into the pharynx (with the palatine tonsil, and the tubal and pharyngeal tonsils within the nasopharynx). The follicles are deep crypts lined with epithelium and containing a mass of lymphoid material (Fig. 14.76). The follicles usually open onto the surface of the tongue. The mucosa in this region also contains many mucous glands. Some small mucous glands also occasionally occur at the margin and tip of the anterior two-thirds of the tongue.

Simple cytokeratins are expressed by taste buds: most are positive for CK7, 8 and 19, with fewer expressing CK18.

## CLINICAL CONSIDERATIONS

In dealing with the oral mucosa, the student needs to be able to distinguish between conditions reflecting normal variation, benign conditions and those that may be premalignant.

As an example of variation in normal anatomy, lymphoid tissue exhibits considerable size variation, especially in the young. Lingual tonsils may show localized symmetrical swelling, being symptomless and without the

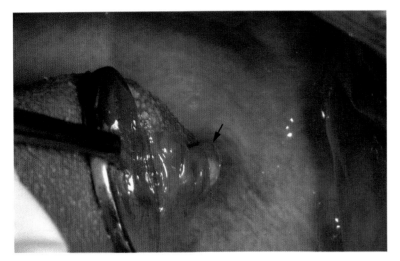

**Fig. 14.77** Side view of tongue showing localized enlargement of a lingual follicle and foliate papillae (arrow). Courtesy of Professor P.R. Morgan.

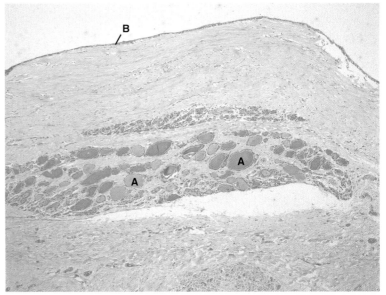

**Fig. 14.79** Section taken from thyroglossal duct cyst removed from the back of the tongue showing the presence of thyroid tissue (A). B = epithelial lining of cyst cavity (H & E; ×50). Courtesy of Professor P.R. Morgan.

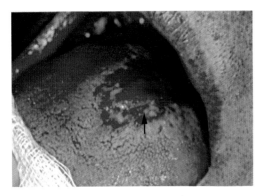

**Fig. 14.78** View of back of tongue showing a lingual thyroid (arrow). Courtesy of Professor J.D. Langdon.

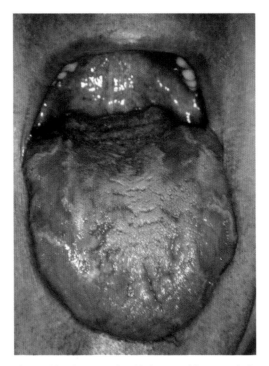

**Fig. 14.80** Migratory glossitis (geographic tongue). Courtesy of Professor P.R. Morgan.

presence of any observable underlying pathology (Fig. 14.77). An example of a benign developmental condition is the lingual thyroid. The dorsum of the posterior one-third of the tongue may show a midline swelling that represents active thyroid gland tissue that has failed to migrate from its developmental situation at the site of the foramen caecum (Fig. 14.78, see also page 297). Remnants of the migrating thyroid gland may also form thyroglossal duct cysts in the neck. The diagnosis can be confirmed using a radioactive iodine test and by means of a biopsy that reveals the presence of thyroid tissue (Fig. 14.79).

Another example of a common benign condition is migratory glossitis. This is an inflammatory condition of unknown cause characterized by the presence of smooth, red regions on the tongue related to atrophy of the filiform papillae that are surrounded by a grey-white, irregular boundary (Fig. 14.80). The appearance has been likened to the outline of continents on a map, hence the more familiar name of 'geographical tongue'. A characteristic of the condition is that the outlines of the 'map' change, even from day to day, and the area covered may wax and wane. It may be symptomless, although some patients may complain of a burning sensation. Migratory glossitis occurs in about 3% of the population and affects adults more often than children. The red coloration of affected areas coincides histologically with thickening of the epithelium and the presence of inflammatory cells in the region. In the grey-white borders, the epithelium contains the highest concentration of neutrophils (Fig. 14.81).

White lesions are common in the oral cavity, being associated with areas of keratinization in normally non-keratinized lining mucosa. Of major significance is the need to differentiate those that are benign from those that may give rise to malignancies. At its mildest, in buccal mucosa and

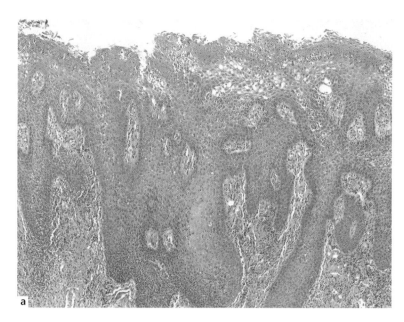

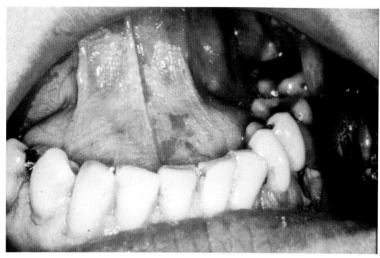

**Fig. 14.82** White patch in the floor of the mouth (sometimes referred to as sublingual keratosis) associated with smoking. Note the smooth surface lesion with a characteristic rippling outline caused by alternation of parakeratinized and normal lining epithelium. Courtesy of Professor P.R. Morgan.

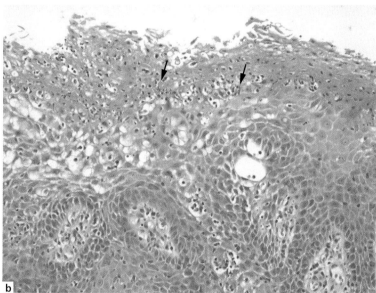

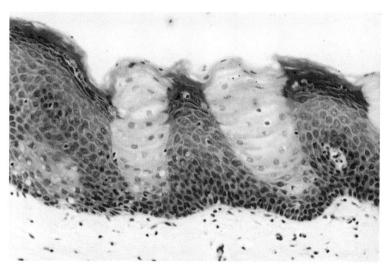

**Fig. 14.81** Micrograph in grey-white area at the border of a lesion of migratory glossitis. (a) Low power, showing loss of filiform papillae (H & E; ×50). (b) Higher power, showing neutrophil infiltration of epithelium (arrows) (×125). Courtesy of Professor P.R. Morgan.

**Fig. 14.83** Section of biopsy from sublingual keratosis from lesion similar to that seen in Fig. 14.82. The epithelium shows alternation of normal non-keratinized and parakeratinized epithelium (H & E; ×150). Courtesy of Professor P.R. Morgan.

level with the occlusal plane, a linear, slightly raised whitish ridge may be seen, the linea alba, commonly the result of low-grade, intermittent trauma due to folds of cheek mucosa being trapped between the teeth. The constant irritation converts the surface epithelium from its normal non-keratinized state into a parakeratinized layer (see page 226). One site in which a white patch is most conspicuous is the floor of the mouth, here associated with friction or smoking. In one form a smooth surfaced, white patch shows a characteristic rippling pattern, with the normal non-keratinized lining epithelium alternating with areas of keratinized epithelium (Figs 14.82, 14.83).

Occasionally white patch lesions do progress to malignancy (rather less than 1% by general consensus) and therefore they must be kept under observation. A change in form to a speckled appearance associated with a firmness on palpation (induration) may signify a malignant change (Fig. 14.84).

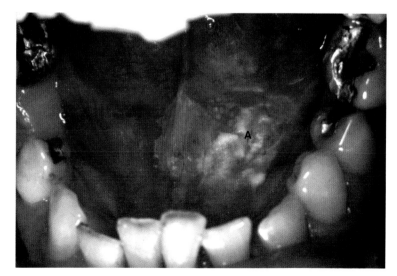

**Fig. 14.84** White patch lesion in the floor of the mouth (A) showing the speckled appearance that, together with firmness on palpation (induration) is indicative of a malignancy. Courtesy of Professor P.R. Morgan.

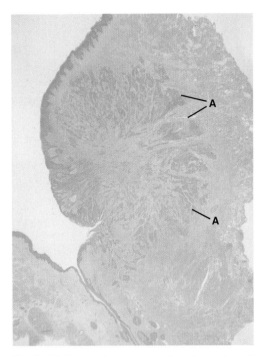

**Fig. 14.85** Biopsy of squamous cell carcinoma from the lateral border of the tongue revealing invasion of darker epithelial tissue (A) into deeper, muscular tissues (H & E; ×4). Courtesy of Professor P.R. Morgan.

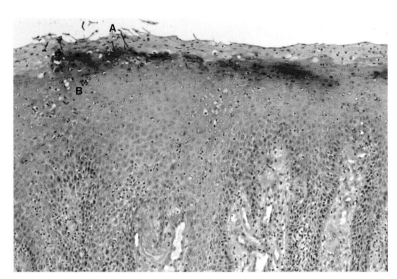

**Fig. 14.87** Biopsy of lesion shown in Fig. 14.86 showing presence within the epithelial layer of red-staining fungal hyphae of *Candida albicans* filaments (A), while clusters of neutrophils (B) are present nearby (Periodic-acid–Schiff stain; ×100). Courtesy of Professor P.R. Morgan.

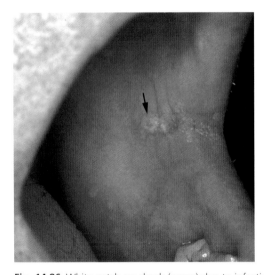

**Fig. 14.86** White patch on cheek (arrow) due to infection with *Candida albicans*. Courtesy of Professor P.R. Morgan.

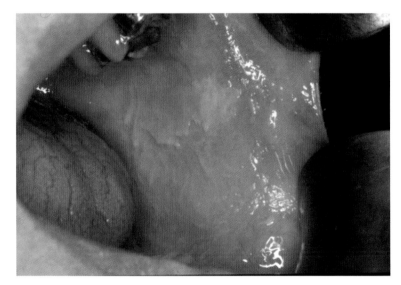

**Fig. 14.88** White sponge naevus on the buccal mucosa. Courtesy of Professor P.R. Morgan.

Such a change can be confirmed by a biopsy showing invasion of the epithelium into the deeper tissues (Fig. 14.85).

White patches associated with infections caused by the fungus *Candida albicans* may also appear in lining mucosa (Fig. 14.86) and can be diagnosed with the aid of stains to reveal the causal organism within the epithelium (Fig. 14.87).

White patches are also a feature of white sponge naevus (a rare, benign, autosomal dominant condition). Here, areas of thick, white, soft plaques cover both sides of the non-keratinized regions of the oral mucosa, par-

ticularly the tongue and cheek (Fig. 14.88). Histological features reveal a thickened epithelium showing parakeratinization with widespread vacuolation of the suprabasal epithelium (Fig. 14.89). The underlying cause of this condition appears to be a mutation affecting the structure of CK13 and/or CK4.

The importance of the basement membrane complex in uniting the epithelium and lamina propria is apparent when disorders in this region occur. The commonest example of such a disorder in the mouth is mucous membrane pemphigoid in which autoantibodies are produced by the patient

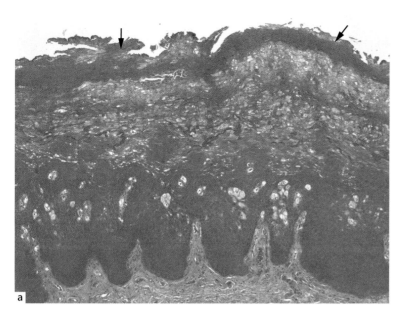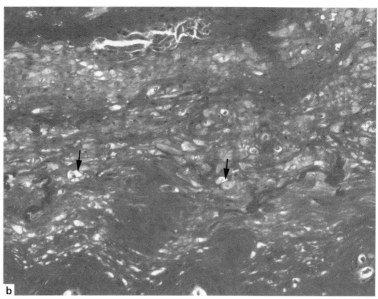

**Fig. 14.89** (a) Low-power section of biopsy from a white sponge nevus showing the superficial layers of the epithelium parakeratinized (arrows) (H & E; ×50). (b) Higher-power view of middle epithelial layers showing extensive vacuolization of cells (arrows) and irregular keratinization (darker red) (×125). Courtesy of Professor P.R. Morgan.

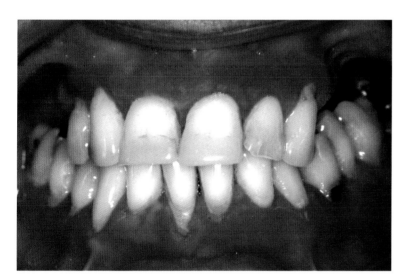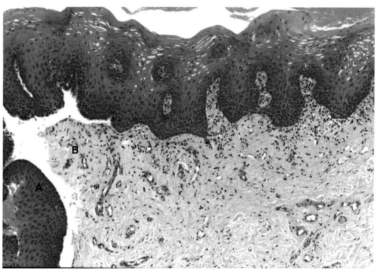

**Fig. 14.90** Red, inflamed appearance of gingiva in mouth of patient suffering with mucous membrane pemphigoid. Courtesy of Professor P.R. Morgan.

**Fig. 14.91** Micrograph of biopsy from patient with mucous membrane pemphigoid, showing splitting between epithelium (A) and lamina propria (B). Note the presence of inflammatory cells beneath the epithelium (H & E; ×50). Courtesy of Professor P.R. Morgan.

and directed against the transmembrane molecules bullous pemphigoid antigens (BP180 and BP230), important components in the hemidesmosomes of the basement membrane complex (see pages 232, 233). This weakens the bond between the epithelium and lamina propria, resulting in splitting between them with associated inflammation, further producing blisters and ulcers within the mouth (Figs 14.90, 14.91).

In pathological situations, the usual cytokeratin profiles of masticatory (e.g. CK1 and 10) and lining epithelium (e.g. CK4 and 13) may be altered. For example, some masticatory epithelium may show a reduction in, or

even disappearance of, CK1 and 10 and an increased expression of CK4 and 13. This feature has been related to the presence of an underlying gingival inflammation (which may also produce CK19 expression in basal and parabasal layers).

It was quickly recognized that there was potential to exploit the epithelial specificity of cytokeratins in diagnostic histopathology, principally in the determination of the tissue of origin of poorly differentiated neoplasms. A further possibility was that dysplastic lesions would 'declare' themselves by an alteration in cytokeratin profiles, thus enabling those

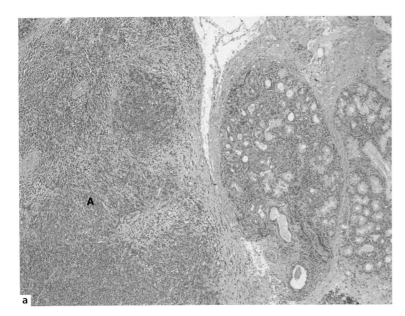
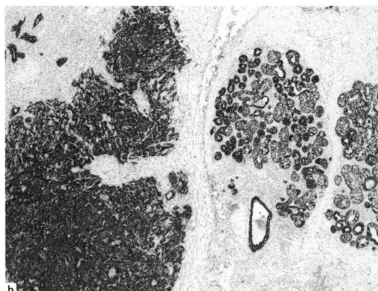

**Fig. 14.92** (a) Section of a mass of poorly differentiated cells in the left part of the micrograph (A) representing an oral squamous cell carcinoma. The right part of the section represents an adjacent minor salivary gland (H & E; ×50). (b) Immunohistological staining of a section similar to (a) using a pankeratin antibody (AE1/3) that confirms the diagnosis of a squamous cell carcinoma by giving a positive response (brown stain) to the majority of the undifferentiated epithelial cells on the left side. Many of the unstained cells on the left represent lymphocytes. The normal salivary gland tissue on the right also stains positive (brown), acting as an internal control for the pancytokeratin antibody (Streptavidin-biotinylated immunoperoxidase staining; haematoxylin counterstain; ×50). Courtesy of Professor P.R. Morgan.

with invasive potential to be identified early. In terms of the latter, these hopes have not yet reached fruition, but pancytokeratin antibodies helping to determine whether an anaplastic neoplasm is, for example, a poorly differentiated carcinoma or a lymphoma, are now in widespread use (Fig. 14.92). It is to be remembered, however, that some malignancies are too poorly differentiated to synthesize appropriate intermediate filaments. Furthermore, other normal cell types (e.g. endothelial and mesenchymal cells) may express cytokeratins (usually at low levels) as may other malignant cell lineages which are expressing other abnormal phenotypes.

# Temporomandibular joint | 15

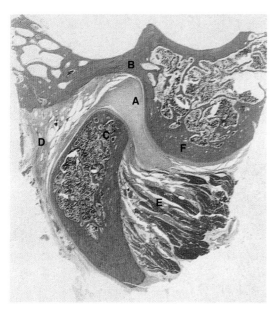

**Fig. 15.1** Low-power sagittal section showing general distribution of tissues of the temporomandibular joint. A = intra-articular disc; B = mandibular (glenoid) fossa; C = condyle of mandible; D = capsule of joint; E = lateral pterygoid muscle; F = articular eminence (H & E; ×3). Courtesy of S. Kariyawasam.

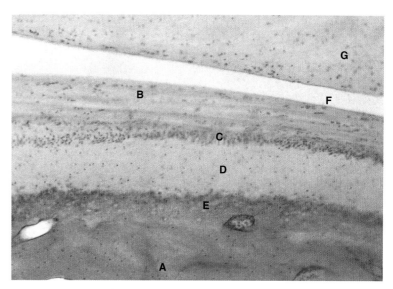

**Fig. 15.2** Articular surface of adult condyle showing the four main layers covering the bone. A = bone of condylar head; B – fibrous articular surface layer; C = cell rich layer; D = fibrocartilaginous layer; E = layer of calcified cartilage; F = lower joint space; G = intra-articular disc (H & E; ×100).

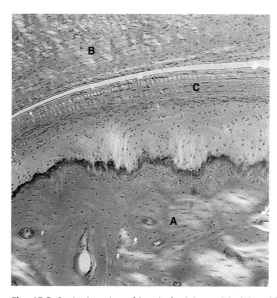

**Fig. 15.3** Sagittal section of head of adult condyle (A) and lower part of intra-articular disc (B), viewed in partial polarized light. The alternating dark and light bands seen in the fibrous articular layer of the condyle (C) are indicative of the collagen being crimped. Crimping is also evident in the disc. Note that the bony surface is composed of compact bone (×77). Courtesy of Professor M.M. Smith.

The temporomandibular joint is the synovial articulation between the condyle of the mandible and the mandibular fossa of the temporal bone. It is also known as the craniomandibular joint. Being a synovial joint, it allows considerable movement and has a joint cavity filled with synovial fluid. The synovial membrane that secretes the synovial fluid lines the internal surface of the joint capsule. The gross anatomy of the temporomandibular joint is described on pages 62–65.

The temporomandibular joint has a number of unusual features:

- The joint space is divided into two joint cavities (upper and lower) by an intra-articular disc (Fig. 15.1): the upper joint cavity allows for gliding movements, the lower joint cavity for hinge movements.
- The articular surfaces are not composed of hyaline cartilage but of fibrous tissue (reflecting the joint's intramembranous development – see pages 293, 294).
- A secondary condylar cartilage is present in the head of the condyle until adolescence.
- Movements of the joint are influenced by the teeth.

## ARTICULAR SURFACES OF THE TEMPOROMANDIBULAR JOINT

Four distinct layers have been described covering the bony head of the adult condyle (Fig. 15.2).

- The most superficial layer forms the articular surface and is composed of fibrous tissue. Although most of the fibres are collagenous, some elastin fibres are also present. The collagen fibres in the superficial layers are arranged parallel to the surface and, when viewed between crossed polars in a polarizing microscope, show alternating light and dark bands that indicate the fibres are wavy or crimped

(Figs 15.3, 15.4). The collagen fibres in the deeper layers run more vertically. Fibroblasts/fibrocytes within the surface layer are sparsely distributed.
- Beneath the articular surface layer is a more cellular zone (cell-rich zone) in which proliferation occurs, providing a source of cells to replenish adjacent layers.
- Beneath the cell-rich zone is another fibrous layer that can have a variable appearance. However, as a number of the cells are rounded and have an appearance reminiscent of cartilage-like cells, the layer is generally referred to as the fibrocartilaginous layer.

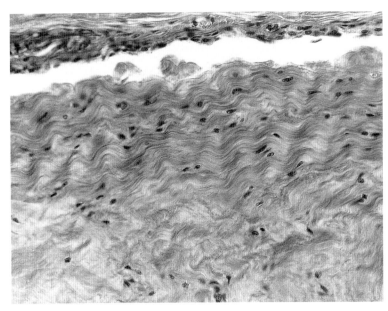

**Fig. 15.4** Sagittal section of part of articular fibrous layer of condyle viewed with interference microscopy to directly demonstrate the crimped nature of the collagen fibres (×300). From Berkovitz BKB 2000 Collagen crimping in the intra-articular disc and articular surfaces of the human temporomandibular joint. *Archives of Oral Biology* 45: 749–756.

- Immediately covering the bone is a thin zone of calcified cartilage, distinguished from the bone by its different staining properties. This calcified cartilage is a remnant of the secondary condylar cartilage (see page 294).

The articular surface covering the mandibular fossa of the temporal bone is similar to that of the condyle. Although generally thinner, it thickens as it passes over the articular eminence. It also shows crimping of the superficial collagen fibres.

## INTRA-ARTICULAR DISC

The gross anatomy of the intra-articular disc has been described on pages 64, 65. Like other soft, dense connective tissues, the intra-articular disc contains cells embedded in a matrix composed of fibres and ground substance. The majority of fibres consist of type I collagen, although traces of other types of collagen have been recorded. There is also a small quantity of elastin fibres present in the disc whose amount varies according to species. Up to 80% of the disc is composed of water.

## COLLAGEN FIBRES

In addition to the presence of type I collagen, which comprises about 80% (dry weight) of the disc, traces of other types of collagen (e.g. types III, VI, IX and XII) have also been reported within the intra-articular disc. The apparent presence of localized areas of fibrocartilage (see below) might also account for the presence of small amounts of type II collagen in some species.

Collagen fibres in the thinner, central region of the intra-articular disc (also known as the intermediate zone) run mainly in an anteroposterior direction. In the thicker anterior and posterior portions (also known as the anterior and posterior bands respectively), prominent fibre bundles also run transversely (mediolateral orientation) and superoinferiorly, giving the fibres a much more convoluted appearance (Fig. 15.5). Around the periphery of the disc, the collagen fibre bundles are arranged circumferentially. When viewed in polarized light, the collagen fibres show alternating dark and light bands, indicating that they are wavy or crimped. Using specialized interference microscopy, the crimped nature of the collagen can be

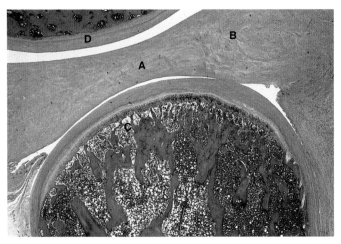

**Fig. 15.5** Sagittal section of the temporomandibular joint of a child showing the collagen fibres of the central portion of the intra-articular disc (A) being more regularly aligned than at the periphery (B). Compare with Fig. 15.3, and note the larger marrow spaces and the lack of a layer of compact bone at the surface of the condyle (C). D = articular surface of mandibular fossa (×5). Courtesy of Professor M.M. Smith.

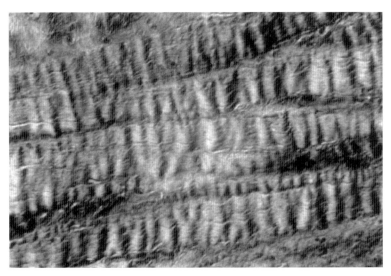

**Fig. 15.6** Sagittal section of intra-articular disc viewed with interference microscopy to directly demonstrate the crimped nature of the collagen fibres (×150).

visualized directly (Fig. 15.6). Such crimping is seen in a wide variety of animal discs. It is unlikely to be the result of a fixation artefact as it is evident even in fresh, unfixed material. As collagen crimping is a characteristic feature of the ligamentous attachment of muscles, it may be inferred that the intra-articular disc is similarly subjected to tensional loads. This does not preclude the presence of compressive loading falling on the intra-articular disc as well. In an intervertebral disc, for example, although the central portion is adapted to resist compressive loading, circumferential bundles of collagen at the periphery are crimped, presumably as an adaptation to tensional loads being generated at that site.

Ultrastructural studies show that collagen fibril diameters generally tend to be small (about 45 nm) with a unimodal distribution. This pattern is often associated with connective tissues subjected to compression. However, regional variation also exists, as collagen fibrils with larger diameters (mean of 70 nm, but with some fibrils reaching a diameter of 150 nm) and a non-unimodal distribution have also been reported. These dimensions are typically associated with a connective tissue subjected to tension (such as a ligament) (see page 182).

## ELASTIN FIBRES

Elastin fibres are also present in the intra-articular disc and are said to decrease with age. They are conspicuous within the upper part of the

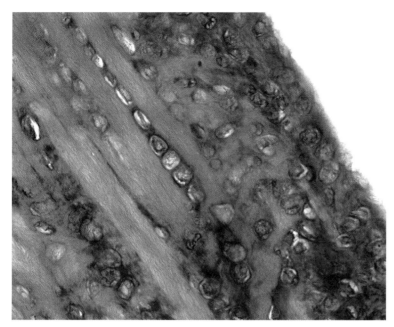

**Fig. 15.7** Section of intra-articular disc. The blue staining (arrows) surrounding the more rounded cells indicates the presence of chondroitin-sulphate-containing proteoglycans (Alcian blue/PAS stain ×300). Courtesy of Professor P.R. Morgan.

bilaminar zone and may function in recovery processes following disc loading or displacement.

## GROUND SUBSTANCE

The ground substance of the disc comprises about 5% of its dry weight. There is species as well as regional variation. In addition, compositional changes may occur with age. The major glycosaminoglycans are chondroitin sulphate and dermatan sulphate, with additional traces of hyaluronan and heparin sulphate. Because of their anionic charge, these dominant glycosaminoglycans absorb water and adapt the intra-articular disc to resist compressive loading. Presumably, the compressive loading in one part of the disc will generate tensional loads elsewhere that can be resisted by the crimped collagen. Chondroitin sulphate is associated with proteins to form large-molecular-weight proteoglycans. These resemble aggrecan, an important component of the ground substance of cartilage. These proteoglycans are particularly localized at the periphery of the more rounded cartilage-like cells of the intra-articular disc (Fig. 15.7). Fibronectin and tenascin have also been located in the intra-articular disc.

## CELLS

Cells in the intra-articular disc seem to be more numerous at the time of birth (Fig. 15.8), and become more sparsely distributed in the adult (Fig. 15.9). The cells show an outline varying between flattened (fibroblast-like) and rounded (chondrocyte-like). The more rounded cells possess considerable amounts of cytoplasm. Cell kinetics are poorly understood. However, as the cells contain anti-apoptotic proteins (e.g. Bcl-2), this has suggested to some authors that the cells have a considerable life span. When the cells are isolated and placed in tissue culture medium, however, they show a rapid degree of cell proliferation.

At the ultrastructural level, the cells show moderate amounts of the intracellular organelles normally associated in fibroblasts with the synthesis and secretion of components of the extracellular matrix (such as endoplasmic reticulum, mitochondria, Golgi material and vesicles (Fig. 15.10)). This might indicate that there is reasonable turnover of the extracellular matrix (but see later). Some cells also exhibit considerable quantities of intermediate filaments (Fig. 15.11) whose diameter (approximately 9 nm) suggests the presence of vimentin. The cell membrane is closely

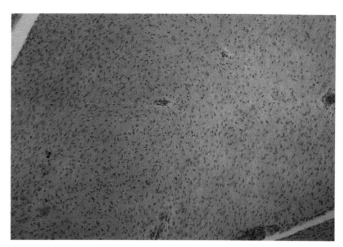

**Fig. 15.8** Sagittal section of the intra-articular disc of a neonate showing the presence of numerous fibroblasts (H & E; ×100). Courtesy of Professor M.M. Smith.

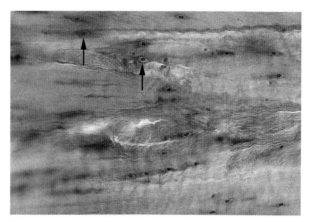

**Fig. 15.9** Sagittal section of an adult intra-articular disc showing the sparse distribution of cells compared with Fig. 15.8. Note the rounded cartilage-like appearance of some cells (arrow) (H & E; ×150).

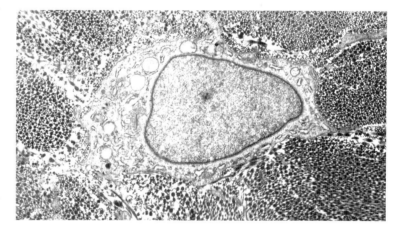

**Fig. 15.10** Electron micrograph of fibroblast from the intra-articular disc showing moderate amounts of rough endoplasmic reticulum, and mitochondria. The extracellular matrix shows collagen fibrils lying close to the cell membrane (×8000). From Berkovitz BKB, Pacy J 2002 Ultrastructure of the human intra-articular disc of the temporomandibular joint. *European Journal of Orthodontics* 24: 151–158.

opposed to the collagen fibrils of the extracellular matrix (Figs 15.10, 15.11).

The fluorescent marker phalloidin binds to the intracellular cytoskeletal filament F-actin within a cell and is small enough to penetrate the cell membrane in a thin block of tissue, thus highlighting the outline of the cell body and any processes. Studies using this technique have revealed new information about the cells in the intra-articular disc. When viewed in a confocal microscope that can optically section a cell and show its three-dimensional appearance, the cells are seen to possess numerous long,

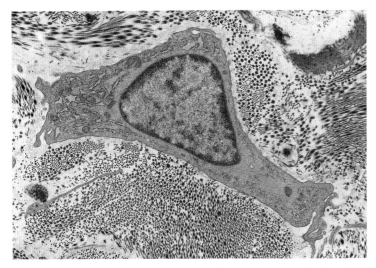

**Fig. 15.11** Electron micrograph of fibroblast from the intra-articular disc. The left part of the cell contains rough endoplasmic reticulum, while surrounding the nucleus and projecting into the right side of the cell is a clear zone containing microfilamentous material. The extracellular matrix shows transversely sectioned collagen fibrils (×8000). From Berkovitz BKB, Pacy J 2002 Ultrastructure of the human intra-articular disc of the temporomandibular joint. *European Journal of Orthodontics* 24: 151–158.

fine processes. These processes are present throughout the tissue (Figs 15.12, 15.13), with some extending for distances of up to 100 μm or more. As the processes might be expected to contact those of other cells, the tissue has also been double-stained with both phalloidin and antibodies for the gap junction protein, connexin 43. The results reveal the presence of dense punctate staining for this gap junction protein throughout the numerous and extensive cell processes (Fig. 15.14).

The significance of the presence of a complex system of cell processes containing considerable quantities of gap junction protein is unclear. The precise route whereby the cells of the disc obtain their nutrition is not known, but the two sources are the local blood vessels and/or the synovial fluid. In the case of the blood vessels, these are situated at the periphery of the disc, the bulk of the central part of the disc being avascular (Figs 15.5, 15.9). As one of the functions of the connexin family of transmembrane proteins is to permit the passage of small molecules between contacting cell processes, it could be suggested that the role of the cell processes in the intra-articular disc is to allow for the passage of nutrients and fluid from the peripheral blood vessels to the central avascular regions of the disc. That some diffusion of nutrients can occur at the surface of the disc seems evident from the observation that it is possible to maintain vital cells in thin intra-articular discs (e.g. rat) in tissue culture.

A characteristic feature of true cartilage cells is the presence at the ultrastructural level of a pericellular matrix intervening between the cell membrane and the adjacent type II collagen fibrils of the extracellular matrix. This pericellular matrix contains microfilamentous material and is delineated by a pericellular capsule. As the rounded cells in the intra-

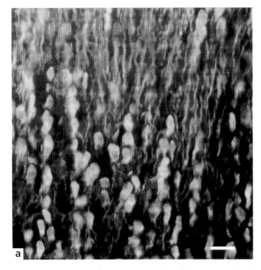
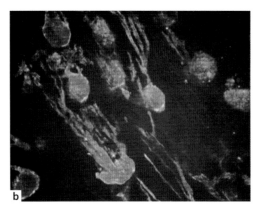
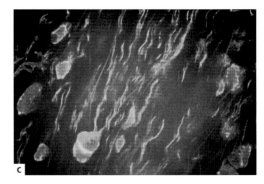

**Fig. 15.12** (a) Confocal micrograph of intra-articular disc cells labelled with phalloidin. Note the numerous cell processes (×300). (b, c) Higher-power micrographs (×500). From Berkovitz BKB, Becker D 2002 The detailed morphology and distribution of gap junction protein associated with cells from the intra-articular disc of the rat temporomandibular joint. *Connective Tissue Research* 203: 12–18.

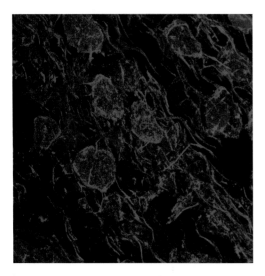

**Fig. 15.13** Confocal micrograph representing a stacked series of 211 sections, each 0.2 μm thick, showing cells of the intra-articular disc stained with phalloidin and showing profusion of cell processes (×900). From Berkovitz BKB, Becker D 2002 The detailed morphology and distribution of gap junction protein associated with cells from the intra-articular disc of the rat temporomandibular joint. *Connective Tissue Research* 203: 12–18.

**Fig. 15.14** Confocal image representing a stacked series of 14 sections, each 3 μm thick, showing cells of the intra-articular disc double-stained with phalloidin (green) and an antibody to the gap junction protein connexin 43 (red). Note the rich concentrations of red stain in the cell processes (×250). From Berkovitz BKB, Becker D 2002 The detailed morphology and distribution of gap junction protein associated with cells from the intra-articular disc of the rat temporomandibular joint. *Connective Tissue Research* 203: 12–18.

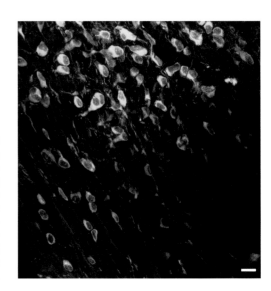

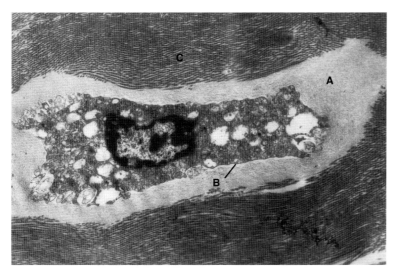

**Fig. 15.15** Electron micrograph of a cell from an adult marmoset intra-articular disc. Note the presence of a pericellular matrix (A) between the cell membrane (B) and the collagen fibrils of the extracellular matrix (C) (×7000).

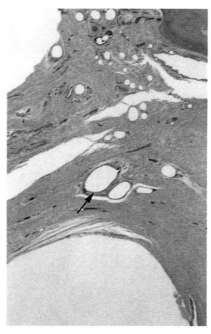

**Fig. 15.16** Section of the superior lamella of the intra-articular disc showing considerable vascularity (arrowed) compared with the rest of the disc, which is relatively avascular (H & E; ×14).

articular disc have been considered to be cartilage-like, ultramicroscopic studies have been undertaken to see whether these cells also possess a pericellular matrix. The results indicate that most cells do not (Figs 15.10, 15.11). However, a pericellular matrix can be seen surrounding the cells of some older specimens (of the rat and marmoset) (Fig. 15.15), suggesting that their presence is related to age. Unlike the cells in hyaline cartilage, but like cells in fibrocartilage from other sites (e.g. at the insertion of tendons), cartilage-like cells in these older intra-articular discs lack a pericellular capsule at the periphery of the pericellular matrix. The presence of a pericellular matrix has yet to be confirmed in the cells of healthy intra-articular discs of humans.

A general question arises as to the terminology to be used for the cells of the intra-articular disc. If the intracellular organelles present in the cells of the disc are mainly associated with the secretion and turnover of extracellular matrix (collagen and ground substance), then the moderate amounts of such organelles would indicate that the cells are reasonably active and could be referred to as fibroblasts. However, if these organelles are more concerned with the synthesis of gap junction protein and collagen turnover is slow, then the cells could be termed fibrocytes. This is partly supported by the absence of intracellular collagen profiles, usually indicative of a rapid turnover rate of collagen (see pages 188, 189). Future studies designed to determine the turnover rate of collagen in the disc should help clarify the situation.

The term fibrocartilage has been widely used to describe the tissue comprising the intra-articular disc. The features associated with cartilage include:

- the presence of type II collagen
- the presence of high-molecular-weight chondroitin-sulphate-containing proteoglycans
- the presence of a pericellular matrix surrounding the cells
- chondrocyte-like cells that exhibit a rounded morphology with short, microvillus-like processes
- the absence of cell contacts
- the absence of blood vessels within the tissue.

With regard to the above features, the intra-articular disc lacks blood vessels (especially in its central portion) and exhibits high-molecular-weight chondroitin-sulphate-containing proteoglycans. However, it may lack, or only have traces of, type II collagen and its some-

what rounded cells are not surrounded by a pericellular matrix (except in relation to age) and possess numerous processes that form connections with adjacent cells. The term fibrochondrocyte has therefore been used by some authors to describe the rounded cells of the intra-articular disc.

## BLOOD VESSELS

Although blood vessels are present in the intra-articular disc at the time of birth, the majority are soon lost and the bulk of the intra-articular disc, especially the central region, becomes avascular (Figs 15.5, 15.9), blood vessels being localized to the periphery of the disc. Similarly, there is a lack of lymphatics. However, posteriorly in the bilaminar zone where the disc divides into superior and inferior lamellae (see pages 64, 65), the region of the superior lamella possesses numerous blood vascular spaces (Fig. 15.16). As the tendon of the lateral pterygoid muscle pulls the disc forwards during jaw opening, blood flows into the back part of the disc to fill the space behind the migrating mandibular condyle. The volume of this retrodiscal tissue appears to increase four to five times as a result of venous engorgement as the jaw is opened. This venous engorgement is not the result of the tissue having erectile properties but more the result of continuity with the pterygoid venous plexus lying medial to the condyle. As the mandibular condyle moves backwards during jaw closure, blood leaves the retrodiscal tissues. Elastic tissue in the superior lamella has been regarded by some authors as providing elastic recoil, aiding the backward movement of the disc during jaw closure. Others believe that the return of the disc is entirely passive. The inferior lamella is relatively avascular and inelastic. The posterior discal attachment tissues also appear to contain some type III collagen. Some have interpreted this feature as providing increased distensibility and being an aetiological factor in eventual joint dysfunction.

## SYNOVIAL MEMBRANE

The synovial membrane lines the inner surface of the fibrous capsule of the temporomandibular joint and the margins of the intra-articular disc

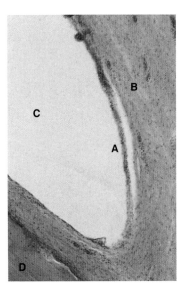

**Fig. 15.17** Section showing the synovial membrane (A) lining the margins of the inferior joint cavity (C). B = articular disc; D = condyle (H & E; ×60).

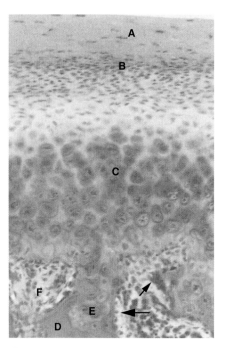

**Fig. 15.18** Section through the condyle of a child. A = fibrous articular layer; B = cell-rich proliferative layer; C = hypertrophic chondrocytes of the secondary condylar cartilage; D = woven bone being deposited around a template of calcified cartilage (E); F = marrow space; small arrow = multinucleated osteoclast; large arrow = osteoblast layer depositing bone on calcified cartilage (×130). Courtesy of Dr D.A. Luke.

(Fig. 15.17). It obviously does not cover the articular surfaces, where it would be rapidly worn away. The synovial membrane consists of a layer of flattened endothelial-like cells resting on a vascular layer. The cells comprising the superficial layer are of two types: a macrophage-like cell type, which is phagocytic, and a fibroblast-like cell type. The synovial membrane shows high metabolic activity and has considerable powers of regeneration. The synovial membrane may be folded at rest, these folds flattening out during movements of the joint. With age, the number and size of the projections increase.

The synovial membrane secretes the synovial fluid that occupies the joint cavities. The inferior joint cavity holds about 1 ml of synovial fluid, while the slightly larger superior joint cavity contains a little more. Synovial fluid lubricates the joint. Important components of the synovial fluid that aid lubrication are the proteoglycans. Hyaluronan can also bind to fibronectin to maintain surface non-adherence. Normal synovial fluid contains various proinflammatory cytokines such as interleukins and tumour necrosis factors the level of which is elevated in certain temporomandibular joint disorders. At rest, the hydrostatic pressure of the synovial fluid has been reported as being subatmospheric, but is greatly elevated during mastication. Raised fluid pressures may also be clinically relevant in patients who continually clench their teeth (bruxists).

## CONDYLE OF THE CHILD

The histological appearance of the mandibular condyle varies according to age. This is due to the presence of the secondary condylar cartilage during childhood. This cartilage appears initially at about the 10th week of intrauterine life (see page 294) and remains as a zone of proliferating cartilage until adolescence.

Like that of the adult, the mandibular condyle of a child is lined by a layer of fibrous tissue, beneath which is a proliferative layer of undifferentiated cells that shows more activity. Cells from this proliferative layer divide to give rise to fibroblast-like cells that subsequently differentiate into chondrocytes, which form the secondary condylar cartilage (Fig. 15.18). Like cartilage elsewhere, the collagen is chiefly type II. Chondrocytes in the deep part of the condylar cartilage hypertrophy and synthesize type X collagen, following which the matrix undergoes endochondral ossification. In brief, this process involves mineralization of the cartilage matrix and subsequent apoptosis of the hypertrophic chondrocytes. Part of

the calcified cartilage is resorbed by large, multinucleated osteoclasts. Subsequently, bone-forming cells, the osteoblasts, deposit woven bone around the template of calcified cartilage. Eventually, this area will be remodelled to produce mature bone. Unlike the chondrocytes in a typical growth plate, the chondrocytes of the condylar cartilage are not aligned into columns and do not secrete as much intercellular matrix. The possible role of the condylar cartilage in growth of the mandible is controversial and is discussed on page 294. The condyle of the young child is not lined by a distinct layer of compact bone as is that of the adult (compare Figs 15.3 and 15.5).

## SPHENO-OCCIPITAL SYNCHONDROSIS

The spheno-occipital synchondrosis, an example of a primary cartilage, is described here to provide a comparison between a primary cartilage and a secondary cartilage, as exemplified by the condylar cartilage. Developmentally, the primary cartilage appears first and maps out the shape of the future bone. In the case of the condylar cartilage, the ramus has already formed in membrane before this secondary cartilage appears. Primary cartilages have inherent growth potential, as is evidenced when they are transferred to tissue culture. The condylar cartilage has little intrinsic growth potential when placed in tissue culture. In the spheno-occipital synchondrosis, proliferative zones lie on either side of the central region of the cartilage, and proliferation involves cartilage cells. This contrasts with the condylar cartilage, where it is undifferentiated fibroblast-like cells that undergo proliferation. In the synchondrosis, the chondrocytes are aligned in columns in the direction of growth on both sides of the cartilage (Figs 15.19, 15.20) and there is considerable production of extracellular matrix which, together with the original cell proliferation and the absorption of water by the proteoglycans, is responsible for providing the growth force. In the secondary condylar cartilage, however, there is far less production of extracellular matrix and there is no alignment of the hypertrophic chondrocytes into columns. This might relate to the

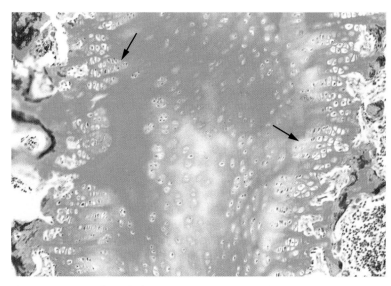

**Fig. 15.19** Section through the spheno-occipital synchondrosis. Chondrocytes aligned in columns on each side of the cartilage (arrows). The reddish zones at both sides indicate the sites of endochondral ossification. Note the large amounts of extracellular matrix compared with that seen in Fig. 15.18.

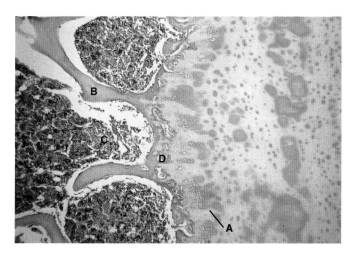

**Fig. 15.20** Section at one surface of the spheno-occipital synchondrosis showing the alignment of chondrocytes into columns (A). B = bone; C = marrow space; D = endochondral ossification front (×80). Courtesy of Dr M.E. Atkinson.

ability of the secondary cartilage to produce some growth in more than one direction. In the case of an epiphyseal growth plate (as opposed to a synchondrosis), columns of cartilage cells are produced only on one side of the cartilage.

## CLINICAL CONSIDERATIONS

Temporomandibular joint disorders are multifactorial in origin, although they may present with common symptoms, such as pain in the jaw joint or face, clicking sounds in the joint and limited mouth opening.

During movement at the temporomandibular joint, there is little friction generated at the surface of the intra-articular disc because of the lubricating properties of the synovial fluid and the smoothness of the articular surfaces. Frictional forces on the disc are increased when synovial fluid is replaced with a less viscous substitute (e.g. phosphate-buffered saline). Like other synovial joints, the temporomandibular joint is prone to inflammatory and degenerative conditions, such as rheumatoid and osteoarthritis. In these situations, damage to the articular surfaces will subject the articular disc to increased friction that may lead to degenerative changes within the disc. Experimental removal of the intra-articular disc results in degenerative changes being produced in the mandibular condyle.

The intra-articular disc may gradually become displaced from its normal position between the articular surfaces. With the more usual anteromedial displacement (see Fig. 3.11), the posterior part of the disc may end up between the bony articular surfaces and be subjected to abnormal loading. This may result in a loss of proteoglycans that, together with an increased water content, may affect the biomechanical properties of the tissues. Degenerative changes are seen in the disc with subsequent changes in its shape. The associated loss of structure may be accompanied by an invasion of blood vessels, with the disc eventually becoming perforated. The accompanying degenerative changes may also result in exposure of bone at the articular surfaces. Inflammatory changes and increased permeability of the vessels of the synovial membrane may raise the intra-articular fluid pressure and change the composition of the synovial fluid. The synovial fluid in temporomandibular joint disorders may show an increased content in molecules such as proinflammatory cytokines (e.g. interleukin, tumour necrosis factor), matrix metalloproteinases and vascular endothelial growth factor. Irrigating and aspirating the joint (arthrocentesis) may reduce symptoms and improve mobility.

Estimates indicate that a considerable proportion of the population suffer in varying degrees from temporomandibular joint disorders. These disorders are not easily treated. For those most severely affected, joint implants have been designed. As far as a damaged disc is concerned, part of the difficulty in treating the condition is due to its lack of healing properties, perhaps related to the lack of blood vessels. For this reason, work is under way to attempt to construct replaceable substitute intra-articular discs using tissue engineering techniques, although attaching such a disc to the capsule is likely to provide a surgical challenge.

During examination of children in their early teens, it may be evident that the mandible is developing at a greater or lesser rate than the maxilla and that this imbalance is likely to lead to a malocclusion and/or facial disharmony. Unlike some aspects of sutural growth in the upper jaw, which are amenable to intervention and improvement, growth is less easy to modulate in the mandible. Nevertheless, orthodontic appliances have been designed to try to modify any growth contributed by the condylar cartilage (although there is little evidence that the cartilage plays any significant role in the growth process). Thus, appliances that push the mandible back and compress the condylar cartilage against the mandibular fossa are used to try to retard mandibular growth. Conversely, in situations where the mandible is underdeveloped, appliances that reposition the condyle in a forward position have been used to enhance development of the condyle in an attempt to produce a more forward positioned lower dental arch. However, the success of such procedures is not always predictable.

# 16 Salivary glands

Salivary glands are compound, tubuloacinar, merocrine, exocrine glands the ducts of which open into the oral cavity. The term compound refers to the fact that a salivary gland has more than one tubule entering the main duct; tubuloacinar describes the morphology of the secreting cells; merocrine indicates that only the secretion of the cell is released; exocrine describes a gland that secretes fluid on to a free surface.

Secretion of saliva is a reflex function emanating from salivary centres that is dependent on afferent stimulation (e.g. taste and mastication) and involves complex integration from salivary centres. Species differences exist, which accounts for some of the controversy surrounding this topic.

Saliva is over 99% water, yet the very small amount of additional inorganic and organic compounds (such as proteins, glycoproteins and enzymes) allows it to perform many important functions. A major role is related to the production of mucin, which acts as a lubricant during mastication, swallowing and speech. The mucous film protects the mucosa and keeps it moist. Saliva brings substances into solution so that they can be tasted. It also limits the activity of bacteria by causing their aggregation. Saliva contains minerals and acts as a buffer; both features help to maintain the integrity of the dental enamel. Peptide growth factors (e.g. epidermal growth factor, nerve growth factor) are produced by the submandibular gland. Their precise functions are not known but epidermal growth factor may be involved in wound healing and (together with mucin) maintaining gastro-oesophageal epithelial integrity. Saliva contains small quantities of numerous other proteins, to which many different functions have been ascribed. Among these are cystatin (inhibitors of harmful cysteine-proteinases produced by bacteria and dying neutrophils), lysozyme histatin and lactoferrin (antibacterial agents), statherin (inhibitor of mineralization) and gustin (detection of taste). Immunoglobulins (mainly IgA) are produced by plasma cells within the stroma of the salivary glands and secreted into saliva to function as part of a widespread mucosal immune system that also includes lymphoid tissue in the gut and bronchi. A polysaccharide-hydrolysing enzyme (amylase) is present in saliva to aid digestion. Also present in saliva are kallikrein (a serine protease) and blood group substances.

The varied functions of saliva can be taken for granted and it is only when salivary production and flow are disrupted that its true importance to the general well-being of the individual is realized: with an ageing population this is of potential clinical importance (see page 274).

Salivary glands consist of two main elements: the glandular secretory tissue (the parenchyma) and the supporting connective tissue (the stroma). From the stroma of the capsule surrounding and protecting the gland pass septa that subdivide the gland into major lobes; lobes are further subdivided into lobules. Each lobe contains numerous secretory units consisting of clusters of grape-like structures (the acini) positioned around a lumen (Fig. 16.1). A secretory acinus may be serous, mucous or mixed. Serous acini can be distinguished from mucous acini according to the nature of the secretion produced and, in structural terms, the morphology of their secretory granules. Serous cells secrete more protein and less carbohydrate than mucous cells. The acinus, via its lumen, empties into an intercalated duct lined with cuboidal epithelium, which in turn joins a larger striated duct formed of columnar cells. Both the intercalated and striated ducts are intralobular and affect the composition of the secretion passing through them. The striated ducts empty into the collecting ducts, which are mainly interlobular. Basal cells are present and are sparsely distributed in the striated ducts and more densely distributed in the collecting ducts. The collecting ducts join until the main duct is formed at the hilum. The main duct carries the saliva to the mucosal surface and may be lined near its termination by a layer of stratified squamous epithelial cells.

The connective tissue septa carry the blood and nerve supply into the parenchyma. Apart from fibroblasts and collagen, the connective tissue also contains fat cells, which show much variability in the case of the parotid gland. Plasma cells (which secrete the immunoglobulins) are found in the stroma of the gland around the intralobular ducts. With age, there is a decrease in the number of secretory cells. Unlike endocrine glands, the secretion of which is controlled by the activity of hormones, the secretion of saliva by the salivary glands is under the control of the autonomic nervous system.

The acini of the parenchyma are responsible for the production of the primary secretion. Saliva is the product of an active secretory process and is not an ultrafiltrate of blood. The serous cells produce a watery proteinaceous fluid and are the source of amylase. The secretory product of mucous cells contains proteins linked to a greater amount of carbohydrate, forming a more viscous, mucin-rich product. Both serous and mucous cells are arranged as acini, although groups of mucous cells may have a more tubular form. Acini may contain either serous or mucous cells, or may be mixed. When mixed, the serous cells have been traditionally described as forming a cap or demilune outside the mucous cells (Fig. 16.2), although the results of recent studies have challenged this view (see pages 268, 269). Around the acini and intercalated ductal cells, contractile cells with several processes are present and represent the myoepithelial (basket) cells.

Salivary glands may be classified according to size (major and minor) and/or the types of secretion (mucous, serous or mixed). The three, paired, major salivary glands are the parotid, submandibular and sublingual glands. The numerous minor salivary glands are scattered throughout the oral mucosa and include the labial, buccal, palatoglossal, palatal and lingual glands. Salivary glands are not present in the gingiva or the dorsum of the anterior two-thirds of the tongue.

There is a low level of secretion of saliva throughout the day, with periodic large additions from the major glands (e.g. at meal times). With

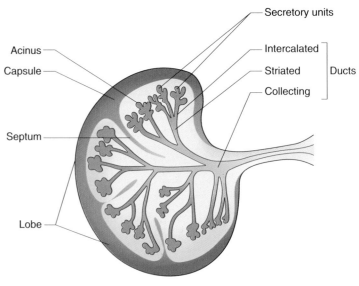

**Fig. 16.1** The general organization of a salivary gland.

**Fig. 16.2** The secretory and ductal elements in a mixed salivary gland. However, as discussed later, the serous demilunes are artefacts of preparation.

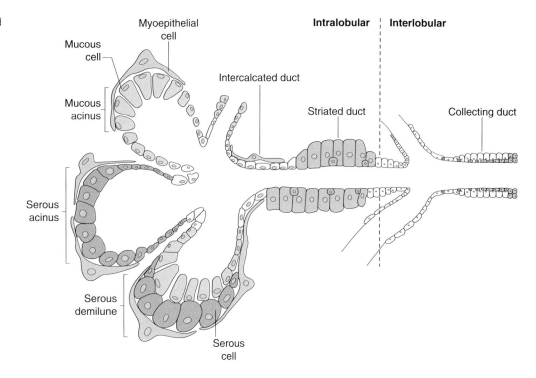

an average salivary flow rate of 0.3ml/min, it has been calculated that 500–750 ml of saliva is secreted each day (with about 90% derived from the major salivary glands). A very small contribution to the pooled saliva is derived from gingival fluid and from sebaceous glands. The sublingual gland and the minor salivary glands spontaneously secrete saliva, but the bulk of this secretion is nerve-mediated. The parotid and submandibular glands do not secrete saliva spontaneously and their secretion is entirely nerve-mediated. Thus, during anaesthesia, secretion ceases almost entirely.

## METHODS OF SALIVARY SECRETION

There are two methods of protein secretion involved in salivary acini. In the first and *main regulated* pathway, the cells store, and then secrete, protein by a process of stored granule exocytosis upon receipt of a neuronal signal (Fig. 16.3); the time taken from synthesis to exocytosis is at least 3.5 hours. As it has been found that some proteins (e.g. kallikrein) can be secreted within about half an hour of synthesis, irrespective of whether the cells are being stimulated, a second pathway must also be involved. For this pathway, cells do not store the protein but secrete it continuously by a vesicular mechanism, vesicles travelling directly from the Golgi complex to the plasma membrane (Fig. 16.4). Whereas some proteins pass in this way into the lumina, others may pass in the opposite direction to reach the interstitial tissue where they can gain access to the blood. In the latter context, the salivary glands should not be considered endocrine glands in the conventional sense, but any movement of molecules into the blood may contribute to widespread effects if they are not inactivated. This second pathway has been termed a *constitutive pathway* to indicate that some proteins may be secreted as they are synthesized. In addition, there is also transcytosis, whereby substances such as IgA that are present in the interstitial tissue pass across the cell from the basolateral to the apical membrane (Fig. 16.4). How such transcytosis interacts with the other vesicular pathways described and whether it is responsible for the delivery of other non-salivary cell proteins into saliva is unclear.

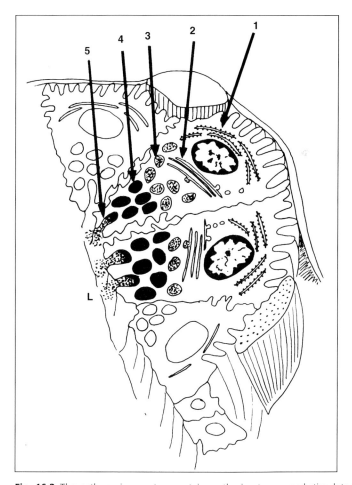

**Fig. 16.3** The pathway in secretory protein synthesis, storage and stimulated exocytosis. 1 = protein synthesis in the rough endoplasmic reticulum; 2 = transport via the Golgi complex to the *trans*-face; 3 = initial storage within immature granules; 4 = concentration of secretory proteins in mature storage granules; 5 = exocytosis of stored proteins into the lumen of the acinus. L = lumen surface. Courtesy of Professor G. Proctor and Karger Press.

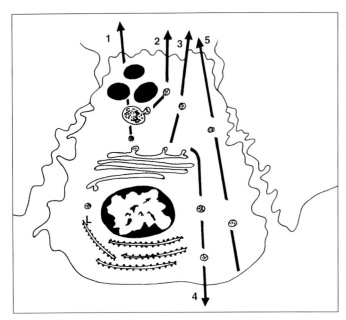

**Fig. 16.4** The vesicular protein secretory pathways likely to be operating in parotid acinar cells. 1 = storage granule pathway; 2 = constitutive-like pathway; 3 = constitutive pathway to the apical membrane; 4 = constitutive pathway to the basolateral membrane; 5 = transcytosis from the basolateral to the apical membrane. Courtesy of Professor G. Proctor and the Karger Press.

## PAROTID GLAND

### SEROUS CELLS

The parotid gland is the largest of the salivary glands. It is enclosed within a well defined capsule, the parotid capsule. The acini of the gland are serous, although mucous cells are occasionally present. The cells have a characteristic granular appearance with routine haematoxylin and eosin staining (Fig. 16.5). Connective tissue septa can be seen subdividing the secretory parenchyma into lobes and then further into lobules. The connective tissue contains blood vessels, nerves and collecting ducts. The lumina of the acini are very narrow (Fig. 16.6). The prominent nuclei are round and located in the basal third of the cell, which is basophilic (because of the presence of rough endoplasmic reticulum). The granular appearance of the serous acinar cell results from the numerous refractile granules in

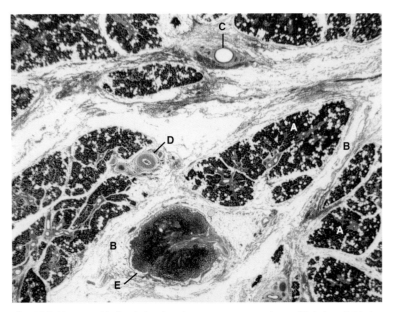

**Fig. 16.5** The parotid gland showing the secretory parenchyma (A) being divided into lobules by septa of the stromal connective tissue (B). C = interlobular collecting duct; D = interlobular artery. E = lymph node (H & E; ×13). Courtesy of Dr J.D. Harrison.

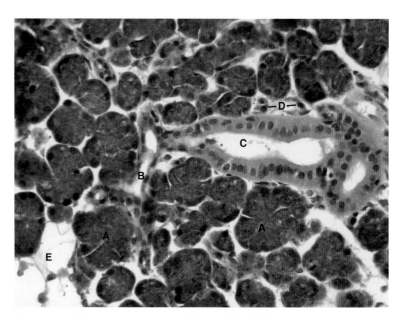

**Fig. 16.6** Darkly staining serous acini of parotid gland (A). B = intercalated duct; C = striated duct; D = plasma cell; E = fat cell (H & E; ×360). Courtesy of Dr J.D. Harrison.

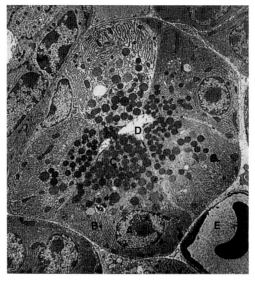

**Fig. 16.7** TEM of serous acinus. A = nucleus in basal part of cell; B = rough endoplasmic reticulum; C = secretory granules in luminal part of cell; D = central lumen; E = capillary (×2000). Courtesy of Mr P.F. Heap.

the luminal portion of the cell (adjacent to the lumen). Intercalated ducts pass from the acini and open into striated ducts, which are well represented in the parotid gland.

The ultrastructural appearance of a serous acinus is illustrated in Figure 16.7. The cells have a wedge-shaped outline, the basal surface being broader, and surround the central lumen. The cell membrane shows numerous microvilli and infoldings. The basal part of each serous cell is delineated from the surrounding connective tissue by a basal lamina. This region of the cell contains the nucleus and rough endoplasmic reticulum and capillaries are seen in close approximation to this surface. The luminal part of the cell contains dense, round secretory granules. Many narrow canaliculi run between the cells and join the lumen. Both the canaliculi and the lumen are lined by short microvilli. Adjacent cell membranes contact at desmosomes, gap junctions and tight junctions.

Over 99% of saliva is water, which passes both across the cell membrane (transcellularly) and between adjacent cells (paracellularly) as a result of chloride secretion into the lumen. The proteinaceous components are packaged in granules for release into the luminal system by exocytosis at the luminal surface of the cells. For this reason, the cells are highly

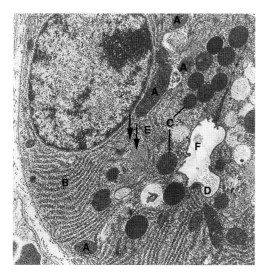

**Fig. 16.8** TEM of part of a serous cell showing secretory pathway. A = mitochondria; B = rough endoplasmic reticulum; C = secretory granules; D = site of discharge of granule by exocytosis into lumen; E = Golgi material; F = lumen of acinus. Note that the granules are initially pale (arrows) but become more electron dense as they mature (×6700). Courtesy of Mr P.F. Heap.

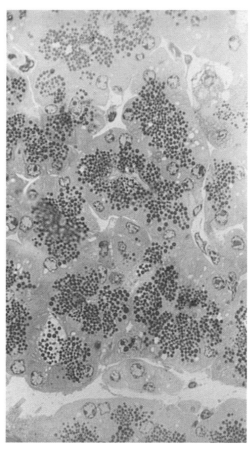

**Fig. 16.9** Following synthesis of secretory products, resting (unstimulated) serous cells contain numerous secretory granules in the distal parts of their cytoplasm (Toluidine blue; ×600). Courtesy of Mr P.F. Heap.

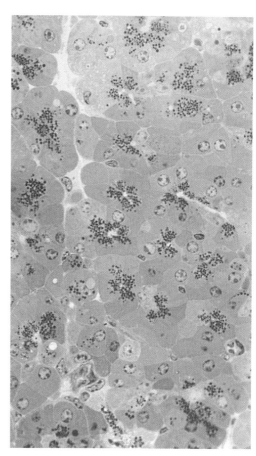

**Fig. 16.10** Soon after stimulation, the secretory granules are depleted after being discharged into the lumen of the acini by exocytosis (compare with Fig. 16.9) (Toluidine blue; ×600). Courtesy of Mr P.F. Heap.

polarized. Like proteins in other cells, those in the serous cells of the parotid gland are assembled by the ribosomes of the rough endoplasmic reticulum and move into the cisternae of the endoplasmic reticulum and from there to the Golgi material. Here the proteins are glycosylated and released in vacuoles that become secretory granules. Initially, the immature granules are of pale electron density but, as they move to the luminal plasma membrane, they become more electron-dense as the protein content is concentrated (Fig. 16.8). Following this maturation period, the granules are discharged by exocytosis when required. Mitochondria within the cell supply the energy for the synthetic and secretory process.

The appearance of serous cells will clearly vary with the levels of secretory activity. Following the synthesis of secretory products, resting (unstimulated) serous cells will contain numerous secretory granules in the luminal parts of their cytoplasm (Fig. 16.9). With reflex stimulation of salivary flow during mastication at mealtimes, the number of granules will be severely depleted after being discharged into the lumen by exocytosis (Fig. 16.10).

Both parasympathetic and sympathetic fibres innervate the acini and act collaboratively in the production of saliva during feeding. The main neurotransmitter for parasympathetic nerves is acetylcholine and that for sympathetic nerves is noradrenaline (norepinephrine). In addition to these substances, each axon contains arrays of neuropeptides (such as vasoactive intestinal polypeptide, substance P and calcitonin-gene-related peptide). These neuropeptides are not necessarily uniform for each type of nerve, nor are all present within every nerve of the same type. Embryologically, the transmitters are likely to influence the genetic expression of the glandular cells and, conversely, the cell types are likely to influence the neuropeptides in the axons innervating them. Some neuroeffector sites occur beneath the basal lamina in direct contact with the plasma membrane

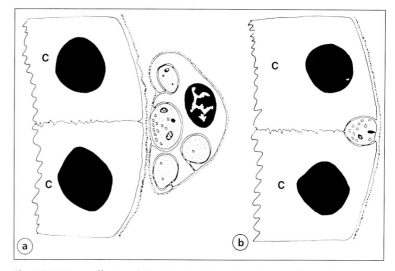

**Fig. 16.11** Neuroeffector relationships in salivary glands. a = epilemmal; b = hypolemmal; C = parenchymal cells. Courtesy of Professor J.R. Garrett and Karger Press.

(hypolemmal), while others remain outside the basal lamina (epilemmal) (Figs 16.11–16.13). Neuroeffector sites of either type probably affect the cell if transmitter vesicles are present. In electron micrographs, the conventional neurotransmitters are contained in small vesicles while the neuropeptides are contained in larger, dense-cored vesicles (Fig. 16.14). Parasympathetic drive causes formation and secretion of secretory granules and fluid by the secretory units; sympathetic drive usually increases the output of preformed components from the cells. Both pathways cause contraction of the myoepithelial cells, which helps direct fluid from the acinar lumen out along the duct system.

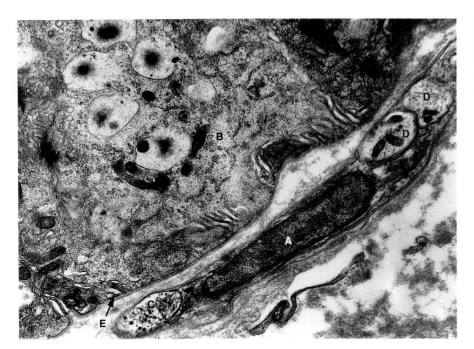

**Fig. 16.12** TEM showing the Schwann cell nucleus (A) of an epilemmal nerve fibre in association with a parotid acinus cell (B). C = adrenergic axon; D = two cholinergic axons; E = basal lamina of acinus. Note the small translucent vesicles and the dense-cored vesicles (with neuropeptides) in the axons (×14 000). Courtesy of Professor J.R. Garrett and the editor of the *Archives of Oral Biology*.

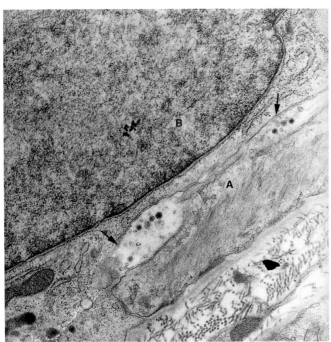

**Fig. 16.13** TEM of submandibular gland showing hypolemmal axons (arrowed) containing many large dense-cored vesicles, and lying between a myoepithelial cell (A) and a central acinar cell (B) (×15 000). Courtesy of Professor J.R. Garrett and the editor of *Microscopy Research and Technique*.

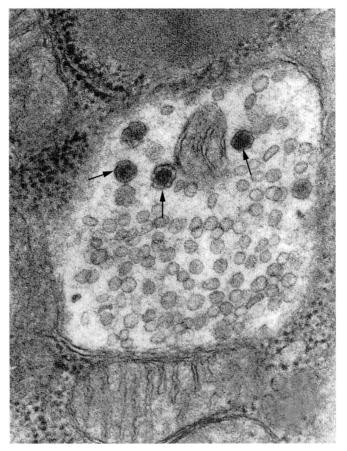

**Fig. 16.14** TEM of neuroeffector part of a hypolemmal parasympathetic axon showing small agranular vesicles that contained acetylcholine and larger dense-cored granular vesicles (arrow) that contained neuropeptides (×60 000). Courtesy of Professor J.R. Garrett and the editor of *Microscopy Research and Technique*.

Salivary gland acinar cells make up a salt-secreting epithelium, that is, sodium and chloride, bicarbonate and other less abundant anions are transported into acinar lumina. This process forms the basis of salivary secretion as the generation of an environment in lumina that is hypertonic with respect to the adjacent blood capillaries and interstitial fluid enables the movement of water into lumina. Figure 16.15 summarizes the key events in this process. Anion channels in the apical acinar cell membrane, which are permeable to chloride and bicarbonate, are opened when acinar cells receive signals from autonomic nerves (principally acetylcholine from parasympathetic nerves). The electrochemical gradient created by chloride leads to sodium movement into the acinar lumen and the osmotic gradient thus created leads to the movement of water into the lumen. The latter may occur by a transcellular route through aquaporin water channels. The isotonic saliva generated in the acinar lumen is rendered hypotonic by the removal of sodium, chloride and bicarbonate as it passes through striated ducts, which are impermeable to water.

## DUCT SYSTEM

The smallest (and most distal) of the ducts is the intercalated duct. This leads from the serous acini into the striated duct and is usually compressed between the acini (Figs 16.2, 16.6 and 16.16). It is lined by cuboidal epithelial cells. The nuclei in the duct cells appear prominent, owing to the relatively scanty cytoplasm. At the ultrastructural level, intercalated ducts are seen to consist of a simple cuboidal epithelial tube. Both luminal and basal surfaces of the duct cells are smooth and desmosomes unite adjacent cells (Fig. 16.17). The cells sometimes contain apical secretory granules

**Fig. 16.15** Salivary fluid secretion by acinar cells and the resorption of salt in striated duct cells. See text for description. Courtesy of Professor G. Proctor.

**Fig. 16.16** Parotid gland showing intercalated ducts (A) leading from serous acini and into the striated duct (B). C = fat cell. Note the cuboidal epithelial cells lining the intercalated ducts have prominent nuclei due to their scanty cytoplasm. The nuclei in the striated ducts are more centrally positioned within the cells (H & E; ×360). Courtesy of Dr E.H. Batten.

**Fig. 16.17** TEM of an intercalated duct. The cuboidal lining cells of the duct (A) possess only small amounts of the intracellular organelles associated with protein synthesis. Some secretory granules are evident (arrow). The cells are united by desmosomes and both the luminal and abluminal surfaces are smooth. Myoepithelial cells are present (B) (×2520). Courtesy of Dr J.D. Harrison.

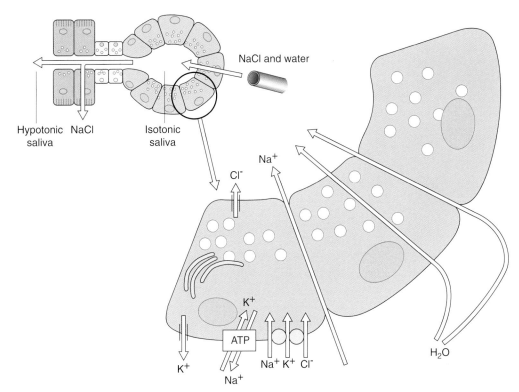

Fiq. 16.15

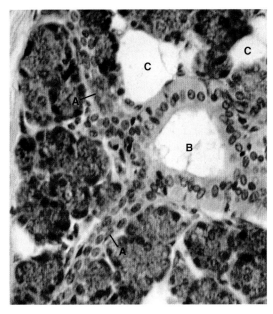

Fig. 16.16

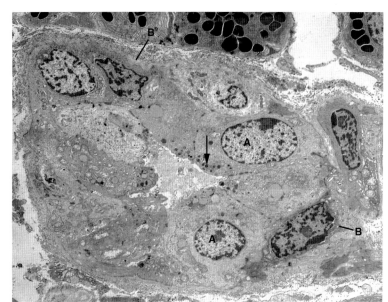

Fig. 16.17

and there are only small amounts of the organelles normally associated with protein synthesis. However, the intercalated ducts appear to contribute to the primary secretion. Several acini drain into each intercalated duct. In the parotid gland, intercalated ducts are characteristically long, narrow and branching.

The striated ducts are intralobular and form a much longer and more active component of the duct system than the intercalated ducts. The cells of the striated ducts have a large amount of cytoplasm and a large, spherical, centrally positioned nucleus that makes them easy to identify (Fig. 16.16). The cells of the striated duct are highly polarized. Their luminal surfaces have short microvilli. The duct's basal (abluminal) surface, adjacent to the basal lamina separating it from the adjacent connective tissue, shows numerous striations in the light microscope. Ultrastructurally, the striations correspond to multiple infoldings of the plasma membrane at

the base of the cell (Fig. 16.18). Vertically aligned mitochondria are packed between the infoldings. Adjacent cells are intertwined in a complex pattern and anchored together by desmosomes. This large surface area, supplied with high levels of energy from the mitochondria, is clearly involved in active transport. The striated ducts are the site of electrolyte resorption (especially of sodium and chloride) and secretion (potassium and bicarbonate) without loss of water. As this resorption is against a concentration gradient, it requires substantial amounts of energy. The effect on the material in the lumen is to convert an isotonic or slightly hypertonic fluid (with concentrations similar to those in the plasma) into a hypotonic fluid. The cells of the striated duct exhibit small secretory granules on the luminal side that may contain epidermal growth factor, lysozyme, kallikrein and secretory IgA. The granules are less abundant in humans than in many other species and less abundant in the parotid than in the submandibular gland.

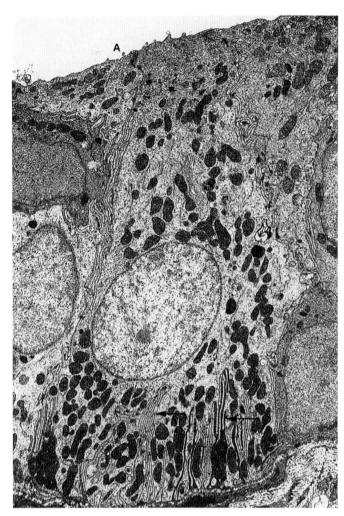

**Fig. 16.18** TEM of striated duct cells. The nucleus is centrally positioned within the cell because of the large amount of cytoplasmic material. Adjacent cell membranes are intertwined in a complex pattern and united by numerous desmosomes. Note the multiple infoldings of the plasma membrane at the base of the cell (arrowed), between which are packed numerous mitochondria. A = lumen surface of duct (×12 000). Courtesy of Mr P.F. Heap.

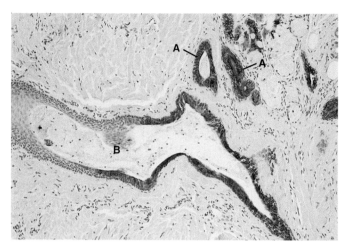

**Fig. 16.19** Striated ducts staining positive (brown) for cytokeratin 8 and 18 using immunohistochemical techniques (A), typical of the type of cytokeratin intermediate filaments associated with simple ducts. The early part of a collecting duct also stains positively, but this is lost as the duct becomes stratified near the surface (B) (×80). Courtesy of Dr A.W. Barrett.

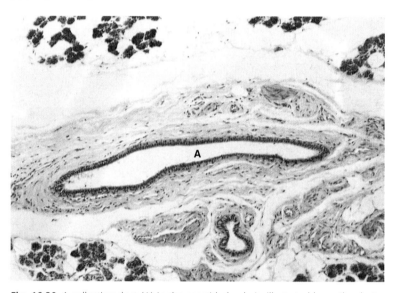

**Fig. 16.20** A collecting duct (A) in the parotid gland. As illustrated here, the duct may have two layers of cells (H & E; ×60).

The luminal cells of the intercalated, striated and collecting ducts contain the low-molecular-weight cytokeratin intermediate filaments 7, 8, 18 and 19 (Fig. 16.19).

The striated duct leads into the collecting duct (Fig. 16.20). Whereas the intercalated and striated ducts modify the composition of the saliva (as well as transport it) and may be termed secretory ducts, the main function of the collecting ducts is to transport it. In addition to the columnar layer (which now lacks striations), the collecting duct situated in the interlobular region may have a layer of basal cells. As it enlarges, the main parotid duct appears like many excretory passages and contains two layers: the mucosa and the outer connective tissue adventitia. Near its termination the lining of the main duct becomes stratified as it merges with the stratified squamous epithelium of the surface oral epithelium. When stratified, the duct epithelium contains keratin intermediate filament types typical of stratified epithelium in the oral mucosa (Table 14.1).

## MYOEPITHELIAL CELLS

Myoepithelial cells lie between the basal lamina and the basal membranes of the acinar secretory cells and the intercalated duct cells. Myoepithelial cells around acini are dendritic cells, consisting of a stellate-shaped body containing the nucleus and a number of tapering processes radiating from it. A different arrangement exists around the intercalated ducts, where the myoepithelial cells are elongated, run longitudinally along the duct and

have few, short, processes. Around the acini, the processes lie in gutters on the surface of the secretory cells so the outline of the acinus remains smooth; around the intercalated ducts, the cells lie more superficially and produce a bulge in the outline of the duct. Although salivary myoepithelial cells in some species stain positively for alkaline phosphatase, those in humans do not. Myoepithelial cells contract as a result of activity of both parasympathetic and sympathetic stimulation, supporting the view that the two autonomic divisions act in concert, not in conflict.

Ultrastructurally, the nucleus tends to be flattened and intracellular organelles associated with protein synthesis are not particularly abundant. However, the cell contains numerous contractile actin microfilaments about 7 nm in diameter (Figs 16.13, 16.21). Myoepithelial cells have desmosomal attachments with underlying parenchymal cells, gap junctions with adjacent myoepithelial cells, and hemidesmosomal attachments with the basal lamina, the last suggesting that some of their activity is transmitted via the basal lamina. Myoepithelial cells (and the basal cells of double-layered ducts) also contain cytokeratin intermediate filament (Figs 16.22 and 16.23) and contractile actin filaments (Figs 16.22 and 16.24), which can be used to help identify them using immunocytochemistry. The presence of cytokeratin confirms the epithelial origin of the myoepithelial cell. Pinocytotic vesicles and dense attachment areas are associated with that part of the plasma membrane of the myoepithelial cell covered by the basal

**Fig. 16.21** TEM showing a myoepithelial cell (A) with a dendritic process (B) surrounding some serous cells (C). Bundles of contractile myofilaments (arrowed) are evident in the process. Note also the variable appearance and density of the secretory granules in the serous cells (×6500). Courtesy of Dr J.D. Harrison.

**Fig. 16.22** Immunohistochemical double staining of parenchymal cells showing evidence of proliferation in normal parotid gland. Positive reaction of nuclei (red staining, indicated by arrows) for the cell proliferation marker Ki67 is seen: (a) in acinar cells, the cytoplasm of which has been stained brown using an antibody to cytokeratin 18; (b) in an intercalated duct cell, the cytoplasm of which has been stained brown using an antibody to cytokeratin 7; (c) in a myoepithelial cell, the cytoplasm of which has been stained brown using an antibody to a-actin; (d) in basal cells of a collecting duct, the cytoplasm of which has been stained brown using an antibody to cytokeratin 14 (All ×300). Courtesy of Dr S. Ihrler.

**Fig. 16.23** Myoepithelial cells staining positively (brown) for the antibody to cytokeratin 14 using immunohistochemical techniques (arrows) (×240). Courtesy of Dr A.W. Barrett.

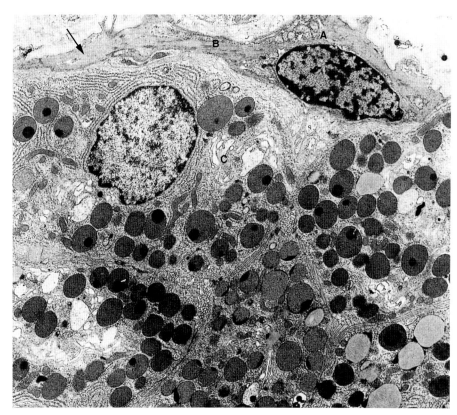

Fig. 16.21

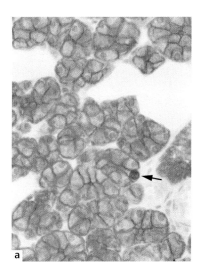

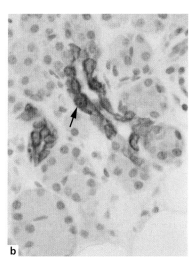

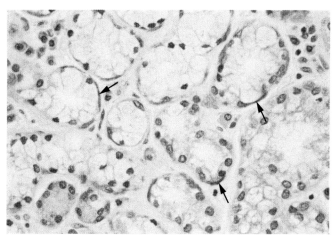

Fig. 16.23

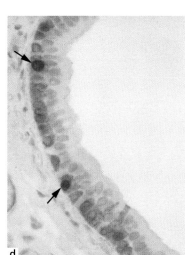

Fig. 16.22

lamina. At the cell membranes where myoepithelial cells contact serous acinar cells, CD44 is expressed in both cell types. As CD44 in other tissues is involved in many basic processes associated with cell proliferation and differentiation, it may play a similar role in salivary glands in both the normal and neoplastic state.

Functional studies clearly indicate that myoepithelial activity can:

- support the underlying parenchyma and reduce back-permeation of fluid
- accelerate the initial outflow of saliva
- reduce luminal volume
- contribute to the secretory pressure
- help salivary flow to overcome increases in peripheral resistance – but if this is excessive it may lead to sialectatic damage of striated ducts, thereby increasing overall permeability.

Other possible functions include assistance for some parenchymal cells to expel their contents and a milking effect on any underlying extracellular fluid, assisting passage via parenchymal tight junctions.

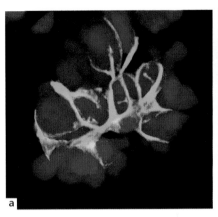
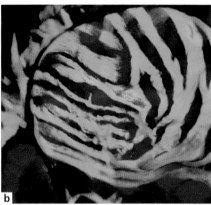

**Fig. 16.24** Myoepithelial cells and their numerous dendritic processes staining positively (green) for antibody to F-actin (bodipy-phallacidin) around secretory acini (stained red with ethidium homodimer 1). (a) Submandibular gland. (b) Sublingual gland (×1000). Courtesy of Dr Y. Satoh.

## BASAL CELLS

A population of basal cells is present in the striated and collecting ducts. They are sparsely distributed in the striated ducts and more densely distributed in the collecting ducts, in which they form a continuous layer as the ducts pass further towards the hilum (Fig. 16.22d). On the abluminal surface of ductal cells associated with both striated and collecting ducts is found a small population of basal cells. These cells can be distinguished from other parenchymal cells by a combination of their morphology, their coexpression of cytokeratin 14 and the antiapoptotic factor bcl-2, and a proliferative index of about 3% that is the highest of any cell in the region. Basal cells have been implicated as potential stem cells during turnover and/or cell regeneration in salivary glands and during metaplasia when oncocytes and sebaceous cells may appear. However, some cell division is seen in all parenchymal cell types, including myoepithelial cells (Fig. 16.22), and all these cells may be involved in salivary gland regeneration.

## LYMPH NODES

Lymph nodes are situated both on the surface and within the parotid gland (Fig. 16.5) but are not found within the other salivary glands.

## SUBMANDIBULAR GLAND

The second largest of the salivary glands, the submandibular gland, produces a mixed mucous/serous secretion. The overall mean of the proportional volume of mucous cells is 8% of the total acinar volume, although it varies between 1% and 33%. The gland has a well formed connective tissue capsule. The serous cells, duct system, myoepithelial cells and basal cells as described for the parotid gland also apply to the submandibular gland. The intercalated ducts are shorter and the striated ducts are longer and more conspicuous.

## MUCOUS CELLS

In routine microscopy, the collections of mucous acini within the submandibular gland are readily distinguished in the resting gland from the darker-staining and granular serous acini because the mucous acini are paler since their mucin content does not readily take up routine stains. In addition, their nuclei tend to be compressed into the basal part of the cell. Small, crescent-shaped collections of serous cells may be found in routine sections at the most distal ends of the mucous acini; these are referred to as serous demilunes (Figs 16.25, 16.26).

The traditional, and widely held, view relating to the disposition of serous demilunes and the ultrastructural morphology of the mucous cell has recently been challenged: it has been shown to be the result of an

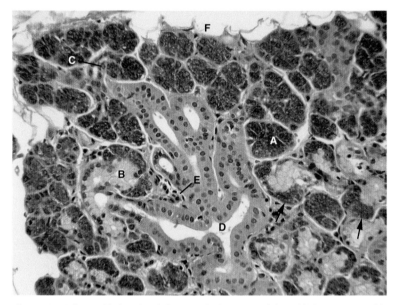

**Fig. 16.25** Submandibular gland showing darker serous (A) and lighter mucous (B) acini. Crescent-shaped collections of serous cells form serous demilunes (arrows) (but see text). C = intercalated duct; D = striated duct; E = plasma cells; F = fat cell (H & E; ×245). Courtesy of Dr J.D. Harrison.

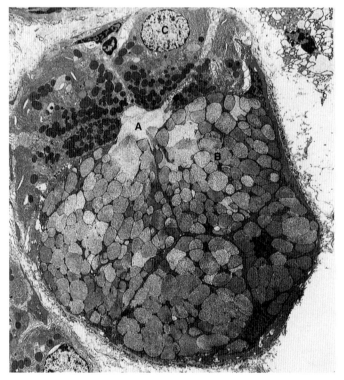

**Fig. 16.26** TEM of the submandibular gland showing serous cells (C) forming a serous demilune capping a mucous acinus (B). A = lumen (×1600). Courtesy of Dr J.D. Harrison.

**Fig. 16.27** TEM of the terminal portion of a mixed gland prepared by rapid freezing and freeze-substitution method. In the mucous cell (A) all secretory granules are round and discrete. The serous cell (B) is aligned to surround the common lumen (C) and no serous demilune could be detected. The nucleus (not shown) is centrally located (×10 000). Courtesy of Dr S. Yamashida and the editor of the *Archives of Histology and Cytology*.

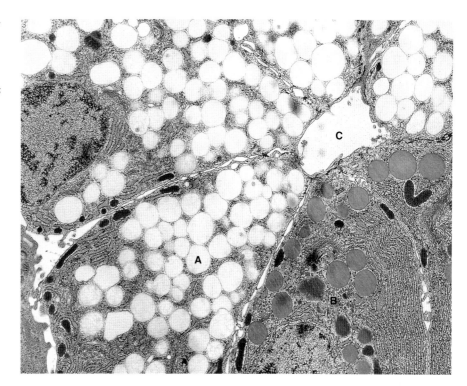

**Fig. 16.28** TEM of the terminal portion of a mixed gland prepared by conventional immersion fixation in glutaraldehyde. Secretory granules of mucous cells (A) are enlarged and some have coalesced because of the disruption of limiting membranes. Serous cells (B) are compressed by the distended mucous cells towards the peripheral portion of the acinus, forming the demilune structure (×5500). Courtesy of Dr S. Yamashida and the editor of the *Archives of Histology and Cytology*.

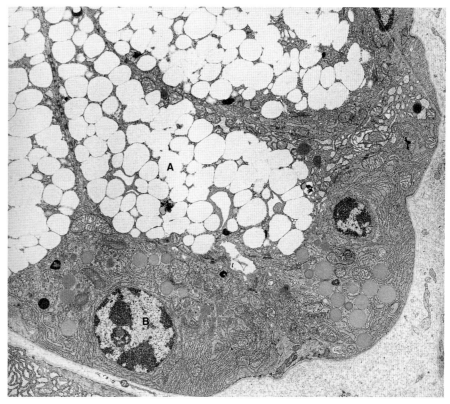

artefact of preparation. Using methods of rapid freezing and freeze-substitution to obtain minimal distortion and dimensional changes during fixation, it has now been demonstrated that all the serous cells align with mucous cells to surround a common lumen, leaving no demilune structure (Fig. 16.27), whereas samples fixed by conventional methods resulted in distended mucous cells that displaced the serous cells towards the basal portion of the acinus to form the demilune structure (Fig. 16.28). This has been confirmed using three-dimensional reconstruction techniques (Fig. 16.29). In addition, the distension caused by mucous granules within each cell results in a flattening and displacement of the nucleus into the basal cytoplasm. (This feature is further illustrated in Fig. 16.30.)

The mucous cell can be readily distinguished from the serous cell at the ultrastructural level. In the early stages of synthesis of its secretory products, large amounts of rough endoplasmic reticulum are present in mucous cells together with a few secretory granules. Compared with serous cells, mucous cells have a more conspicuous Golgi apparatus (because of the greater amount of carbohydrate that is added to the secretory protein). At a later phase of its secretory cycle, the mucous cell exhibits numerous round and isolated secretory granules that are readily distinguished from those of serous cells by their pale appearance (Fig. 16.27). The cell membrane shows fewer microvilli and infoldings than that of a serous cell.

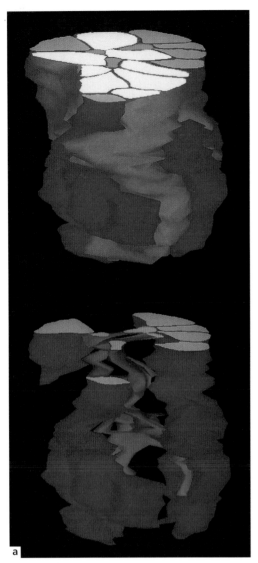
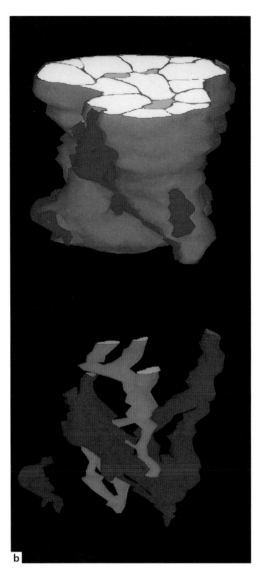

Fig. 16.29

**Fig. 16.29** Computer reconstruction of a terminal portion of the submandibular gland showing mucous (purple) and serous (red) cells and luminal space (green). (a) In the upper diagram, following rapid freezing, a surface view indicates that the terminal portion consists of mucous and serous cells distributed not only at the most fundal portion of the acinus but also in the portion nearest the duct. In the lower diagram, the mucous cells have been deleted from the reconstruction to show more clearly the relation of the serous cells to the luminal space. All serous cells prepared by the rapid freezing method are found to have a direct connection with the luminal space. (b) In the upper diagram, following conventional immersion fixation, the acinus illustrated is found to be branched and serous cells appear attached to the outer wall of the acinus formed by mucous cells. In the lower diagram, the mucous cells have been deleted from the reconstruction to show more clearly the relation of the serous cells to the luminal space. The serous cells are found to be disconnected from the luminal space, giving a floating appearance. Courtesy of Dr S. Yamashida and the editor of the *Archives of Histology and Cytology*.

**Fig. 16.30** TEM of mucous cell using conventional immersion fixation leading to swelling of the secretory granules. The cell illustrated is in a late secretory phase with numerous granules (B) of irregular size (due to coalescence by the disruption of limiting membranes) occupying most of the cell and compressing the organelles and nucleus (C) to the periphery. The granules will discharge into the lumen (A) by exocytosis (×5000). Courtesy of Mr P.F. Heap.

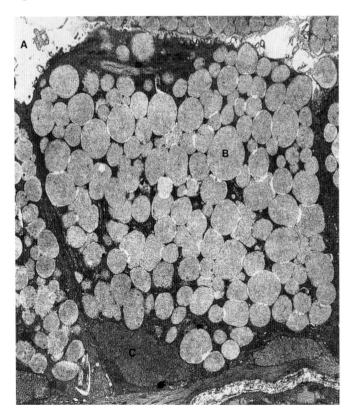

Fig. 16.30

The nuclei of mucous cells are round and centrally located. This account of the ultrastructure of the mucous cell contains two features that distinguish it from accounts derived using conventional immersion fixation. In conventional fixation there is distension of the mucous secretory granules, which show discontinuous limiting membranes and coalescence to form irregularly shaped secretory granules, and the nucleus is flattened and displaced into the basal part of the cell (Figs 16.26 and 16.30).

As in the serous cell, the granules discharge into the lumen by exocytosis. The depletion in granule content of mucous cells in the recently stimulated and unstimulated cells is illustrated ultrastucturally in Figures 16.31 and 16.32. Clearly, the nucleus will be less compressed against the basal surface of the cell following discharge of the mucous granules.

## SALIVARY GLYCOPROTEINS AND CALCIUM

The salivary glands contain a mixture of salivary glycoproteins that range from neutral to acidic. This is easily demonstrated by staining with Alcian blue at pH 2.5, which stains any acidic groups present in the glycoproteins, such as carboxyl or sulphate and then with periodic-acid–Schiff, which stains the glycol groups present in all glycoproteins. This technique has shown that 1) serous cells in the parotid gland contains neutral glycoproteins, 2) mucous cells in the submandibular, sublingual and minor salivary glands contain mainly acidic glycoproteins, 3) serous cells in the

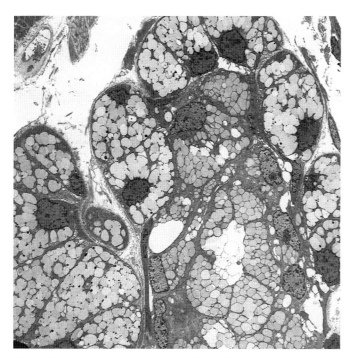

**Fig. 16.31** Unstimulated mucous cells filled with secretory granules; consequently their nuclei are compressed into the basal parts of the cells (Conventional immersion fixation; TEM; ×1000).

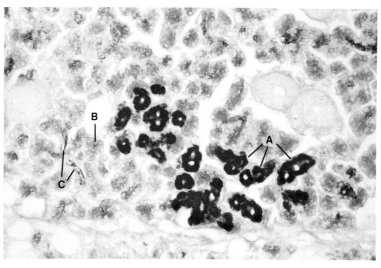

**Fig. 16.33** Submandibular gland showing diffuse royal blue staining of acid glycoprotein in mucous cells (A) and discretely stained secretory granules in serous cells (B) and intercalated duct cells (C) that variously contain neutral glycoprotein stained red and acidic glycoprotein stained royal blue (Alcian blue at pH2.5 followed by periodic-acid–Schiff; ×190). Courtesy of Dr J.D. Harrison.

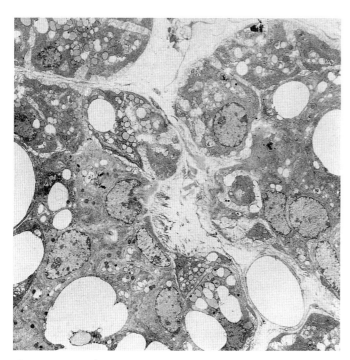

**Fig. 16.32** TEM of mucous cells in a recently stimulated submandibular gland. The mucous cells have lost their secretory granules and consequently their nuclei are more prominent (×1000).

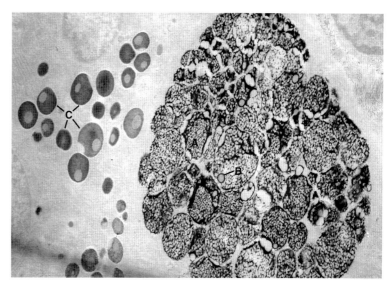

**Fig. 16.34** TEM of mucous cell packed with secretory granules (A) that contain stained glycoprotein and small unstained spherules that contain protein (B). An adjacent serous cell shows scattered secretory granules (C) composed of stained glycoprotein and unstained spherules of protein (Phosphotungstic acid stain; ×6130). Courtesy of Dr J.D. Harrison.

submandibular gland contain a mixture of neutral and acidic glycoproteins, 4) intercalated duct cells often contain glycoproteins that are a mixture of both neutral and acidic forms and 5) striated duct cells often contain neutral glycoproteins (Fig. 16.33).

Thus, although the division of salivary acinar cells into serous and mucous types in routine sections stained with haematoxylin and eosin is clear cut, histochemical methods do not contribute further to the ease of identification as serous cells can synthesize carbohydrates that are histochemically similar to those of mucous cells. This is reflected in the considerable variation seen among the secretory granules in serous acini (Figs 16.21, 16.34).

Calcium is incorporated into the secretory granule during its formation in order that the negatively charged parts of the glycoprotein (which would normally repel each other) can be neutralized by the positive charge on the calcium. This allows the molecule to condense in the secretory granule. The more acidic the glycoprotein, the more calcium is needed. Thus, the secretory granules of the mucous acini and the serous acini of the submandibular gland contain more calcium (Fig. 16.35) than those of the serous acini in the parotid gland, while the secretory granules of the striated ducts contain no demonstrable calcium. The calcium in the secretory granules, when released, may precipitate on exposed phospholipids of damaged membranes to form sialomicroliths (see page 273).

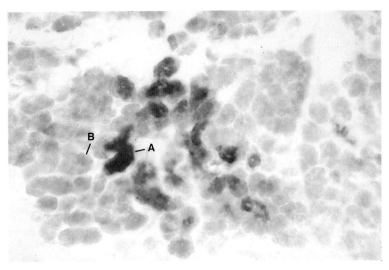

**Fig. 16.35** Submandibular gland showing strong staining for calcium (orange) in mucous cells (A) and moderate to weak staining in serous cells (B) (Schafer's modified GBHA; ×190). Courtesy of Dr J.D. Harrison.

## SUBLINGUAL GLAND

The human sublingual gland is not a single unit like the parotid and submandibular glands, but is made up of a posterior part (the greater sublingual gland) and an anterior part (the lesser sublingual gland) of 8–30 small salivary glands, each having its own duct system emptying into the sublingual fold (see Fig. 1.13).

The sublingual gland has been conventionally considered to be a mixed gland but with a preponderance of mucous elements. Although with routine staining at the light microscope level, it is seen to consist of many groups of pale staining mucous cells with darker staining so-called serous acini and demilunes (Fig. 16.36), there is evidence that the so-called serous cells in this gland are immature mucous cells. The histological structure of the greater and lesser sublingual glands is identical to that of the mucous minor salivary glands.

## DUCT SYSTEM

The duct system is much less well developed than in the other major salivary glands and striated ducts are usually absent. The acini sometimes lead to intercalated ducts but these may be absent and the acini lead to collecting ducts, which lack the basal striations that characterize striated ducts. The sublingual saliva is therefore rich in sodium. The greater sublingual gland usually drains into a main duct, and the lesser sublingual glands drain independently through many smaller ducts that open directly into the overlying oral mucosa.

## MINOR SALIVARY GLANDS

The minor salivary glands are classified by their anatomical location: buccal, labial, palatal, palatoglossal and lingual. It has been estimated that they may number between 450 and 750. They are primarily mucous except for the serous glands of von Ebner, which drain into the trench of the circumvallate papillae (see Figs 14.72, 14.73). Labial and buccal glands are illustrated in Figs 14.33, 14.34. The palatoglossal glands are located in the region of the pharyngeal isthmus. The palatal glands lie in both the soft and the hard palate (Fig. 16.37 and page 242). The anterior lingual glands are embedded within muscle near the ventral surface of the tongue and have short ducts opening near the lingual frenulum. The posterior glands are located in the root of the tongue. Minor salivary glands have collecting ducts, but intercalated and striated ducts are generally absent. This duct system does not remove as much salt, so that the final saliva released from them is isotonic and rich in sodium. Whereas the sympathetic innervation appears to be important in evoking reflex protein secretion from major glands, such nerves sparsely innervate the secretory tissue of minor salivary glands, and so mucous secretion here is entirely mediated by parasympathetic nerve impulses. However, the minor salivary glands secrete spontaneously and continuously, as do the sublingual glands.

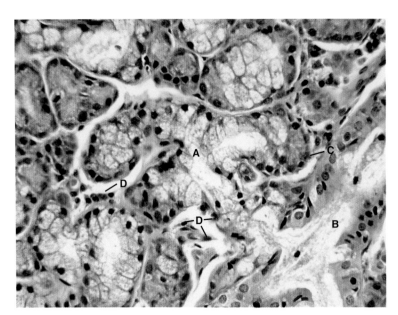

**Fig. 16.36** Pale-staining mucous acini of the sublingual gland (A) draining into collecting duct (B). Note the appearance of serous demilunes (C). Plasma cells are present interstitially (D) (H & E; ×360). Courtesy of Dr J.D. Harrison.

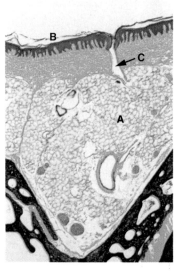

**Fig. 16.37** Minor mucous gland (A) in hard palate. B = keratinized masticatory mucosa; C = collecting duct of gland opening on to surface (Masson's trichrome; demineralized section; ×15).

## SIALOMICROLITHS

Sialomicroliths are small, hard masses (concrements) that are only evident microscopically in the salivary glands and may occur in the parenchymal cells, in the lumina or in the stroma. They contain variable amounts of both mineral (in the form of calcium phosphates, including hydroxyapatite) as well as non-mineralized components in the form of condensed organic secretory material (Fig. 16.38). Sialomicroliths are often associated with atrophic foci (Fig. 16.39), and both increase in number with age. They remain small as they are formed in small spaces.

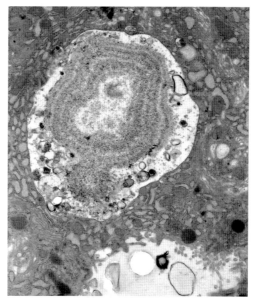

**Fig. 16.40** TEM of an autophagosome in an acinar cell of the sublingual gland in which crystals of hydroxyapatite are being deposited in secretory material associated with membranous debris to form a sialomicrolith. The sialomicrolith will pass from the acinar cell into the lumen (×920). Courtesy of Dr J.D. Harrison.

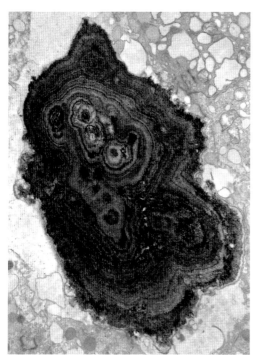

**Fig. 16.38** TEM of a sialomicrolith in the acinar lumen of the sublingual gland. The presence of numerous cores and lamellae indicates that smaller sialomicroliths had accreted (fused together) to form this microlith (×15 100). Courtesy of Dr J.D. Harrison.

Sialomicroliths in parenchymal cells arise as a result of the degradation of superfluous secretory granules and other organelles during periods of secretory inactivity. These materials, rich in calcium, are engulfed by autophagosomes and the calcium released may precipitate on remnants of membranes to form sialomicroliths (Fig. 16.40),which may pass from the parenchymal cells into the lumina. They may also form within the lumina in the presence of stagnant secretory material. They remain small following their formation in small spaces and may be flushed away in saliva or scavenged by macrophages. Sialomicroliths, therefore, do not enlarge to become the larger, macroscopic salivary stones (sialoliths) seen in the large collecting ducts (see Figs 16.47, 16.48 and page 275).

Sialomicroliths are present in all normal submandibular glands and 20% of normal parotid glands. This frequency appears to relate to the higher concentration of calcium in the submandibular gland. Sialomicroliths are rare in sublingual glands and minor salivary glands where secretion is continuous and stagnation is less likely.

## ONCOCYTES

Oncocytes are epithelial cells occurring singly or in small groups in the acini and ducts of normal salivary glands (as well as in other tissues such as the thyroid and parathyroid glands, the kidneys and regions of the vocal tracts). They are acidophilic with haematoxylin and eosin staining (Fig. 16.41) and appear granular due to a large increase in the number of mitochondria that, although initially having a normal morphology, subsequently display an abnormal morphology (Fig. 16.42) and are probably biochemically deficient. This increase in numbers of mitochondria is accompanied by a great reduction in other types of organelle. Oncocytes increase with age and are thought to arise as the result of degeneration of normal cells.

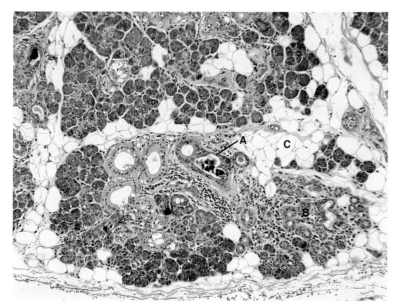

**Fig. 16.39** Submandibular gland showing sialomicroliths (A) occluding the lumen of a striated duct that has led to the formation of an inflamed, atrophic focus (B). C = fat cells. Secretory inactivity leads to an increase in sialomicroliths and allows microbes to ascend the ducts and settle in the atrophic foci out of reach of microbicidal saliva (H & E; ×95). Courtesy of Dr J.D. Harrison.

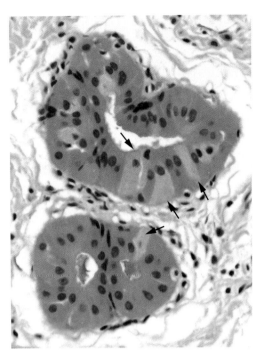

**Fig. 16.41** Oncocytes (arrowed) in striated duct of parotid gland (H & E; ×375). Courtesy of Dr A.W. Barrett.

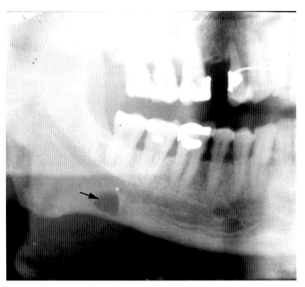

**Fig. 16.43** Radiograph of a Staphne's cavity near the angle of the ramus of the mandible (arrowed). Courtesy of Professor D. Smith.

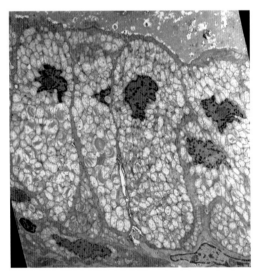

**Fig. 16.42** TEM of oncocytes. Note that the cytoplasm is filled with mitochondria, many having an abnormal morphology (×2250). Courtesy of Dr J.D. Harrison.

## AGE CHANGES

A wide range of age changes has been documented in salivary glands. These include a decrease in the amount of glandular tissue (over 50 years) and an increase in the amount of fibrous tissue, fat cells, inflammatory cells and oncocytes. An increase in duct volume has also been described, although some of this increase may be due to shrinkage of acini, giving the appearance of duct-like forms.

With such a significant loss of parenchyma (in both major and minor glands), it might be assumed that there would be a reduction in the amount of saliva produced in the aged population, giving rise to the clinical condition of xerostomia (dry mouth). However, in healthy, unmedicated individuals, this is not the case and this could be interpreted as being the result of salivary glands being able to produce more saliva than is needed.

## CLINICAL CONSIDERATIONS

### XEROSTOMIA

Older patients frequently complain of a dry mouth (xerostomia), with all the unpleasant symptoms one might expect from a consideration of the important functions of saliva. This was once thought to be a reflection of decreased salivary production associated with the ageing process. However, this does not usually appear to be the case and it is likely that many drugs depress salivary production, sometimes centrally as well as peripherally, with unstimulated salivary flow rates falling from approximately 0.3 ml/min to less than half this value, and many are anticholinergic, such as some antidepressants and antihistamines.

Loss of salivary tissue is also a consequence of radiotherapy treatment for certain tumours in the region of the jaws, or of Sjögren's syndrome, where there is invasion and destruction of the parenchyma by lymphoid tissue. As saliva is important in the maintenance of oral health, decreased secretion from the salivary glands results in an increased incidence of oral conditions such as periodontal disease, dental caries and candidal infections ('thrush'). Partial relief may be obtained by the frequent administration of artificial salivas.

### STAPHNE'S CAVITY (CYST)

A portion of the submandibular gland may invaginate into the lingual surface of the mandible, typically in the region of the ramus below the mandibular canal, near the angle of the ramus. On a radiograph, this will give the appearance of a circumscribed, unilateral radiolucent lesion with a radiopaque border (Fig. 16.43). It can be distinguished from other lesions

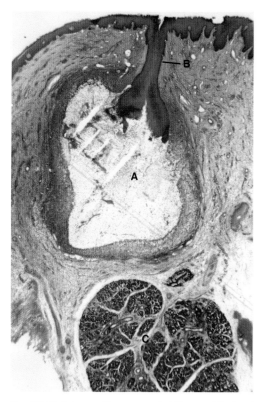

**Fig. 16.44** Extravasation mucocele (A) caused by tearing the main duct (B). The affected minor salivary gland (C) may have to be surgically removed to prevent the continued extravasation of mucus (H & E; ×15). Courtesy of Dr J.D. Harrison.

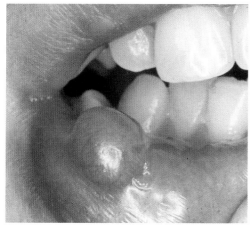

**Fig. 16.45** Extravasation mucocele on the lower lip. Courtesy of Dr J.D. Harrison.

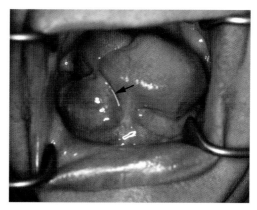

**Fig. 16.46** Ranula (arrowed) in floor of mouth caused by trauma that damaged the floor of the mouth and also the tongue. Courtesy of Dr J.D. Harrison.

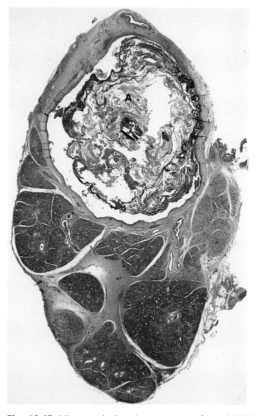

**Fig. 16.47** Micrograph showing presence of a sialolith (A) in a large, dilated duct of the submandibular gland following chronic submandibular sialadenitis with associated inflammation, fibrosis and atrophy of normal parenchyma (H & E; ×5). Courtesy of Dr J.D. Harrison.

by careful computed tomography imaging and by sialography, when a radiolucent dye injected in the submandibular duct will spread into the radiolucency (see Fig. 2.133). A similar but rarer radiolucency can occur in the anterior region of the mandible where it is due to an invagination related to the sublingual gland.

## MUCOCELES AND RANULAS

Damage to the ducts of minor and sublingual salivary glands may result in the extravasation of mucus into the surrounding soft tissues (Fig. 16.44). When the extravasation persists an extravasation mucocele is formed (Fig. 16.45). In the case of the sublingual gland, it is also termed a ranula because the swelling it causes to the floor of the mouth somewhat resembles the belly of a frog. When a ranula is situated above the mylohyoid muscle (oral ranula), it produces a painless swelling that may displace the

tongue (Fig. 16.46). If it penetrates the mylohyoid (cervical ranula), it produces a swelling in the neck. Treatment of these conditions may necessitate the surgical removal of the affected sublingual gland.

## SIALOLITHS

Blockage may occur of the main collecting duct of a major salivary gland (usually the submandibular, but occasionally the parotid). The cause is usually the sialolith (stone or calculus) (Figs 16.47, 16.48) but sometimes is a stricture or an inflammatory exudate. A sphincter has been variously described near the opening of the submandibular duct but this is not supported by one recent study. The lack of access to the mouth caused by the blockage results in swelling of the gland at mealtimes, together with pain and subsequent discharge as saliva gradually flows past the obstruction.

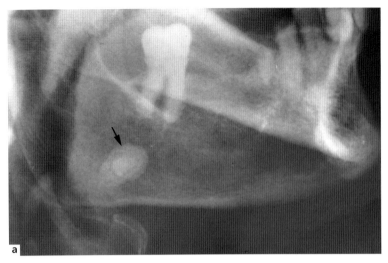

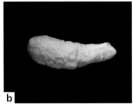

**Fig. 16.48** (a) Radiograph showing presence of a sialolith (arrow) at the proximal end of the submandibular duct at the hilum of the submandibular gland. Courtesy of Dr J.D. Harrison. (b) Sialolith removed from a submandibular duct. The length of this sialolith is 2.2 cm. Courtesy of Professor J. Freher.

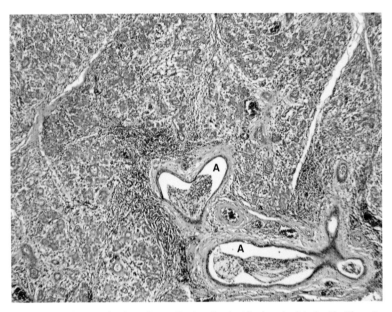

**Fig. 16.49** Micrograph of a submandibular gland with chronic sialadenitis. There is widespread inflammation and atrophy of normal parenchymal tissue. The collecting ducts (A) are dilated and contain mucus and inflammatory cells resulting in the release of mucopus into the mouth. The stroma around these ducts is fibrotic (H & E; ×160). Courtesy of Dr J.D. Harrison.

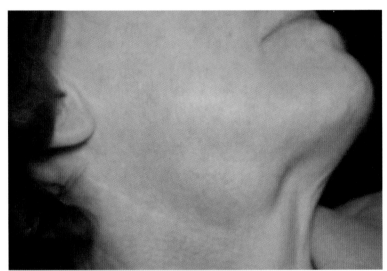

**Fig. 16.50** Swelling in the neck produced by enlargement of the submandibular gland as a result of chronic submandibular sialadenitis. Courtesy of Dr J.D. Harrison.

## SIALOMICROLITHS AND CHRONIC SUBMANDIBULAR SIALADENITIS

Though present in normal submandibular glands (and less frequently, in normal parotid glands), sialomicroliths (Fig. 16.39) may be associated with chronic submandibular sialadenitis (inflammation of the submandibular gland – Fig. 16.49), which may produce symptoms of pain, swelling (Fig. 16.50) and discharge from the gland and sialolithiasis (sialolith or stone formation) The sequence of events is shown in Table 16.1.

## TISSUE ENGINEERING AND SALIVARY GLAND REGENERATION

Salivary glands have some capacity for regeneration. There is considerable proliferation in the presence of noxious stimuli, as in chronic sialadenitis, which is the biological basis for the excellent results of the conservative

**Table 16.1** *Natural history of chronic sialadenitis and sialolithiasis*

| | |
|---|---|
| 1 | Secretory inactivity in normal gland |
| 2 | Accumulation of sialomicroliths causes foci of obstructive atrophy |
| 3 | Microbes ascend main duct and proliferate in foci of obstructive atrophy, aided by the lack of flushing and bactericidal activity of saliva |
| 4 | Inflammation with fluid exudate |
| 5 | Compression of surrounding parenchyma with further atrophy |
| 6 | Further ascent by and proliferation of microbes |
| 7 | Further inflammation with fluid exudate |
| 8 | Compression of large duct with partial obstruction |
| 9 | Stagnation of secretory material and released calcium |
| 10 | Formation of sialolith as calcium precipitates on phospholipids of degenerate membranes |
| 11 | Further obstructive atrophy, ascent by microbes and inflammation |

With permission from Harrison JD 2005 Histology and pathology of sialolithiasis. In: Witt RL (ed) *Salivary gland diseases: surgical and medical management.* Georg Thieme, Stuttgart, pp 71–78.

treatment of this disease (rather than surgical removal of the gland). It has been assumed that this regeneration was essentially the property of the basal cell population associated with the striated and collecting ducts, as these showed the highest proliferative index (approximately 3%). However, recent research has shown the presence of a low baseline proliferation of mature acinar, intercalated ductal and myoepithelial cells (Fig. 16.22), indicating that these cells also have the capacity to contribute to parenchymal regeneration. As with other dental tissues, investigations are being undertaken in the hope of increasing salivary gland regeneration following the loss of parenchymal tissue associated with tumours and other disorders by injecting or grafting stem cell populations into the glandular remains.

## AGE CHANGES

Age changes need to be taken into account when examining the salivary glands histologically in clinical diagnosis. This is particularly so when biopsies of lower labial salivary glands are examined in an attempt to diagnose Sjögren's syndrome, in which there are characteristic changes in the parotid and, to a lesser extent, other salivary glands that involve an infiltration by lymphocytes. However, there is an infiltration by lymphocytes to form lymphocytic foci in salivary glands that increases with age and may be as great as what has been considered to be diagnostic of Sjögren's syndrome in the lower labial glands.

# Development of the face

The face develops in the human between the 4th and 10th weeks of intra-uterine life. During the 4th week in utero, the primitive oral cavity (stomodeum) is bounded by five facial swellings, produced by proliferating zones of mesenchyme lying beneath the surface ectoderm (Fig. 17.1). These are the unpaired frontonasal process and the paired mandibular and maxillary processes. The frontonasal process lies above, the two mandibular processes lie below and the two maxillary processes are located to the sides of the stomodeum. The frontonasal process is formed from the mesenchyme in front of the developing forebrain. The maxillary and mandibular processes are derived from the first pharyngeal (branchial) arches. The facial processes are demarcated by grooves that, in the course of normal development, become flattened out by the proliferative and migratory activity of the underlying mesenchyme. Although it was once believed that epithelial sheets partitioned the facial processes, and that these sheets had to break down for facial development to proceed, such sheets do not exist and facial clefts cannot therefore be related to such epithelial sheets and to their failure to break down. However, in this regard, some attention has been paid to an epithelial sheet termed the nasal fin that lies in the developing upper lip region (see below)

At an early stage of development (week 4), a membrane (the oropharyngeal membrane) separates the primitive oral cavity from the developing pharynx. This membrane is bilaminar, being composed of an outer ectodermal layer and an inner endodermal layer. The oropharyngeal membrane soon breaks down to establish continuity between the ectoderm-lined oral cavity and the endoderm-lined pharynx. Although not detectable in the adult, the demarcation zone between mucosa derived from ectoderm and endoderm is said to correspond to a region lying just behind the permanent third molar tooth.

In a 5-week-old embryo (Fig. 17.2), localized thickenings of ectoderm give rise to the nasal and optic placodes. These placodes will form the olfactory epithelium and the lenses of the eyes, respectively (see page 280). The nasal placodes sink into the underlying mesenchyme, forming two blind-ended nasal pits (the primitive nasal cavities). Proliferation of

mesenchyme from the frontonasal process around the openings of the nasal pits produces the medial and lateral nasal processes. In addition, the maxillary processes enlarge and grow forwards and medially.

In the 6-week-old embryo (Fig. 17.3), the two mandibular processes fuse in the midline to form the tissues of the lower jaw. The mandibular processes and maxillary processes are continuous at the angle of the mouth, thus defining its outline. From the upper corners of the mouth, the maxillary processes grow below the lateral nasal processes and towards the medial nasal processes (Fig. 17.3b). Between the merging maxillary and the lateral nasal processes lie the naso-optic furrows (alternatively termed the nasolacrimal grooves). From each furrow, a solid ectodermal rod of cells sinks below the surface and canalizes to form the nasolacrimal duct.

Two differing accounts have been given for the continued development of the upper lip beyond the 6th week of intra-uterine life. One view suggests that the maxillary processes overgrow the medial nasal processes to meet in the midline and thus contribute all the tissue for the upper lip. A different slant on this view suggests that the mesenchyme of the maxillary processes entirely displaces the mesenchyme of the medial nasal processes. This idea of the development of the upper lip is based upon an appreciation of the innervation of the fully formed upper lip (i.e. the infraorbital branch of the maxillary division of the trigeminal nerve), the maxillary processes being supplied by the maxillary nerve and the frontonasal process by the ophthalmic nerve. Alternatively, it has been suggested that the maxillary processes meet the medial nasal processes without such overgrowth or mesenchyme invasion, the middle third of the upper lip (the intermaxillary segment) being therefore derived from the merged medial nasal processes of the frontonasal process. While histological evidence favours the latter explanation, at present too little is known about the behaviour of the mesenchyme of the facial processes after the initial fusion, thereby not excluding the possibility of subsequent migration of tissue derived from the maxillary processes towards the midline. The possible contributions to the adult face from the embryonic facial processes

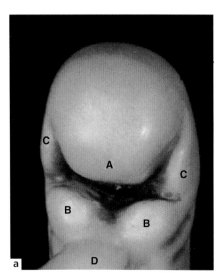

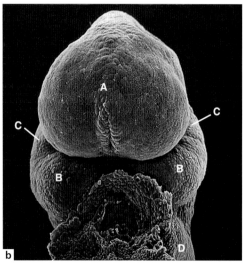

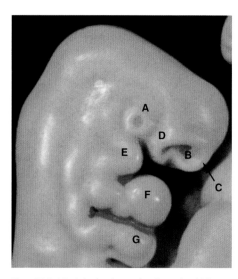

**Fig. 17.2** Model of a face of a 5-week-old human embryo (lateral aspect). A = optic placode; B = nasal pit; C = medial nasal process; D = lateral nasal process; E = maxillary process; F = mandibular process; G = second pharyngeal arch.

**Fig. 17.1** (a) Model of a face of a 4-week-old human embryo (frontal aspect). (b) SEM of the face at an equivalent stage to 4 weeks in the rat (frontal aspect). A = frontonasal process; B = mandibular processes; C = maxillary processes; D = pericardial swelling. Courtesy of Professor A.G.S. Lumsden.

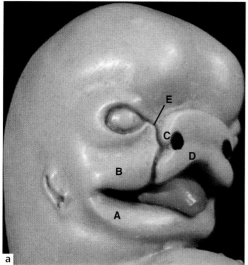
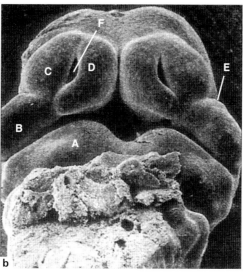
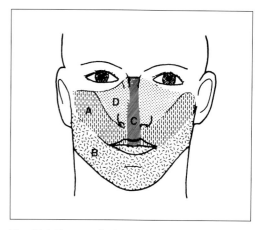

**Fig. 17.4** The contributions to the adult face from the embryonic facial processes. A = maxillary processes; B = mandibular processes; C = medial nasal processes; D = lateral nasal processes.

**Fig. 17.3** (a) Model of a face of a 6-week-old human embryo (lateral aspect). A = mandibular process; B = maxillary process; C = lateral nasal process; D = medial nasal process; E = naso-optic furrow. (b) SEM of developing rat upper jaw and lip at an equivalent stage to 6 weeks showing the merging maxillary and medial nasal processes; F = nasal pit. Courtesy of Professor A.G.S. Lumsden.

(based upon the suggestion that the middle third of the upper lip is derived from the frontonasal process) are described in Figure 17.4. The facial derivatives shown are therefore at odds with the sensory distribution of the adult face, because (as previously mentioned) the fully developed lip is supplied only by the maxillary division of the trigeminal nerve and has no contribution from the ophthalmic division. The facial muscles are derived from mesenchyme of the second pharyngeal arches that migrates into the primitive lips and cheeks, and these muscles are therefore innervated by the facial nerve.

Some controversy persists concerning the so-called intermaxillary segment that is formed initially by the merged medial nasal processes. First, as mentioned above, there are different views concerning the contribution of the intermaxillary segment to the developing upper lip. Second, some embryologists persist with the notion of a 'premaxilla' at the site of development of the maxillary incisor teeth. While a premaxilla is seen in apes, where there are sutures between this region and the rest of the maxilla and where there is a separate centre of ossification, this does not apply to the human situation. As mentioned in Chapter 18, the primary palate is initially formed from the caudal aspect of the merged medial nasal processes of the frontonasal process.

The cells that make up the mesenchyme of the facial primordia are derived from two main sources: connective tissue cells migrating from the neural crest and muscle cells from the paraxial mesenchyme. It has been reported that the mesenchyme of the frontonasal process is derived entirely from cranial neural crest, whereas the mesenchyme of the maxillary and mandibular processes originates from both cranial neural crest and mesoderm. However, fate mapping of the cells suggests that this notion is oversimplified. Although the two types of mesenchyme have distinct developmental histories, there are considerable and significant interactions between them. The signalling mechanisms are however as yet relatively poorly understood. The development of the craniofacial region involves the four fundamental mechanisms that underlie all embryonic development: growth, morphogenesis, cell differentiation and pattern formation. The last mechanism leads to the spatial ordering of cell differentiation. Present research into the development of the face is geared towards understanding the basis of all these mechanisms.

The size of the cell populations is of key importance and is controlled, at least in part, by growth factors. These may also be of significance in the epithelial–mesenchymal interactions known to induce cartilage, bone and tooth differentiation within facial primordia. Pattern formation in developing limbs is, in part, controlled by vitamin A derivatives (retinoids), which form morphogenetic gradients within the limb bud. While such gradients have not yet been demonstrated in the face, a similar mechanism seems likely as the facial primordia are sensitive to exogenous retinoic acid and the mesenchymal cells contain specific retinoic acid receptors.

Quantitative electron microscopic studies (Fig. 17.5) show that, at the time of fusion of the facial processes, there is a marked increase in the number of small projections/processes from the mesenchymal cells. This increase is consistent with reports that changes within the epithelial cells occur and may be related to intercellular signalling between the mesenchymal cells at the time of fusion of the upper lip (i.e. just before the onset of major histiogenic events).

It is worth noting that the brain and facial mesenchyme have been shown to express particular genes at key times in their development. These 'homeobox' (Hox) genes were discovered in embryos of the fruit fly *Drosophila* and are responsible for the spatial organization of the developing *Drosophila* embryo. Similar genes are expected to be of major importance in mammalian development and are the subject of intensive research. It has been shown that neural crest cells that form the frontonasal process and the maxillary and mandibular primordium do not express *Hox* genes but express closely related factors such as the *Dlx* and *Msx* family. It has also been reported that *Hoxa2* is expressed in the second, but not the first, pharyngeal arch. Loss of *Hoxa2* function in the first arch results in the formation of second arch structures. There is much evidence that the neural crest cells of the facial processes acquire significant patterning information from the surrounding epithelia and that the surface ectoderm plays an important role in initiating outgrowth of the frontonasal process. Patterning in the region requires integration of signals between neural crest, ectoderm and endoderm and it is noteworthy that neural crest transplantation experiments show that the neural crest can pattern the face. Recent studies have also highlighted the importance of *Dlx* genes in the development of the pharyngeal arches, including the mandibular and maxillary processes.

Sonic hedgehog (Shh) is a protein switched on by retinoic acid, which, along with fibroblast growth factor (FGF), has been located in the ectoderm of the frontonasal and maxillary processes in chick embryos. Their function is unclear, but it is possible that Shh may act as an organizer of morphogenesis, whereas FGF may be involved in the stimulation of the mesenchyme of the facial processes to produce growth. Indeed, Shh is

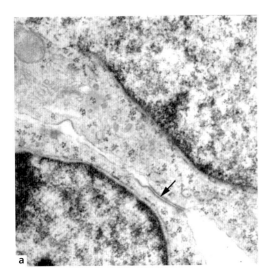
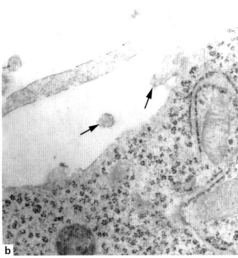

**Fig. 17.5** Electron micrographs of the mesenchyme within the maxillary facial processes (TEM; ×15000). (a) Shows cell junction (arrow). (b) Shows small cell processes (arrows). Courtesy of D. Symons.

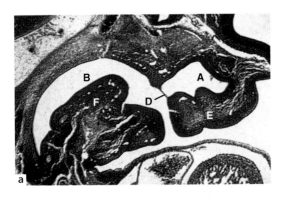
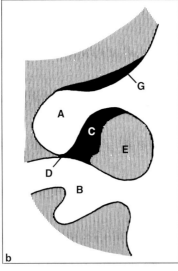

**Fig. 17.6** Sagittal sections of the head illustrating aspects of the development of the nasal cavity. A = nasal pit; B = oral cavity; C = nasal fin; D = oronasal membrane; E = maxillary isthmus; F = developing tongue; G = nasal placode in root of nasal pit. (a) (Toluidine blue; ×30). Courtesy of Dr D.A. Luke. (b) Courtesy of Professor A.G.S. Lumsden.

a critical factor in regulating craniofacial development. Shh is expressed by the facial ectoderm, the pharyngeal endoderm and mesoderm of the prechordal plate (underlying the forebrain). In this respect, there is a 'frontonasal–ectodermal zone' that is the junction between regions expressing FGF8 and Shh. This zone is the initial site of the outgrowth of the frontonasal process and, in avians, sets up the dorsoventral axis for development of the upper beak. When facial ectoderm not expressing Shh is removed there is no effect, whereas removal of ectoderm expressing Shh results in the arrest of the outgrowth of the maxillary processes. Transgenic experiments have also shown that there are severe effects in craniofacial development in mice with mutations in *Shh*-expressing genes. Thus, there is ample evidence showing that there is 'cross-talk' between ectodermal, neural crest and endodermal tissues in the craniofacial region that relies upon Shh signalling pathways. Furthermore, there is evidence for signalling pathways involving FGF, Wnt and BMP.

Three sets of facial placodes are seen on the developing face: nasal placodes, lens placodes and otic placodes. These placodes are thickenings of the surface ectoderm. The nasal placodes are situated towards the front of the developing head and give rise to the olfactory epithelia. The lens placodes invaginate and eventually become internalized to form the lens vesicles, which, as indicated by the name, become the lenses of the eyes. The otic placodes are the first part of the ears to develop. They appear over the regions of the developing hindbrain and, like the lens placodes, invaginate and become internalized to form the otic vesicles, which ultimately will develop into the internal ears (the primordium of the membranous labyrinths).

The nasal placodes invaginate from the surface but do not become completely internalized and help form two blind-ended pits, the nasal pits (see page 278). They are separated in the midline by the primary nasal septum. The nasal pits continue to deepen (at least in part because of the growth of the surrounding medial and lateral nasal processes) and the nasal placodes come to lie in the roof of the nasal pits (Fig. 17.6b), where they will form the olfactory epithelium. Eventually, the roof of the primitive oral cavity is partitioned from the floor of each nasal pit by a sheet of epithelium termed the nasal fin. The nasal fin thins to form an oronasal membrane separating the nasal pit from the developing oral cavity. By the end of the 5th week, the oronasal membrane ruptures to produce communication between oral and nasal cavities.

The nasal fin (the sheet of epithelium seen below each nasal pit) does not, as was once thought, form a complete epithelial partition between the maxillary and medial nasal processes. A bridge of mesenchyme, the maxillary isthmus, joins the two processes in front of the nasal fin. Figure 17.6b shows a sagittal section through the developing nasal and oral cavities and the positions of the nasal fin, the oronasal membrane between the nasal pit and the developing oral cavity, and the maxillary isthmus at the end of the 5th week of development. The nasal fin eventually becomes incorporated into the walls of the nasal pit and, at the roof of the developing oral cavity, thins to form the oronasal membrane. However, should the fin become enlarged, it may constitute a line of weakness between the mesenchyme of the maxillary and medial nasal processes and eventually lead to a cleft in this region.

**Fig. 17.7** Example of extreme holoprosencephaly in a human embryo exhibiting cyclopia. (a) External features. Note the appearance and position of the nose (A) and ears (B). (b) Skull exposed to reveal the central orbit. Courtesy of the Royal College of Surgeons of England.

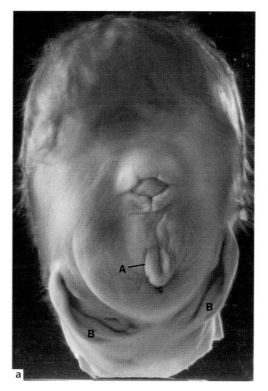
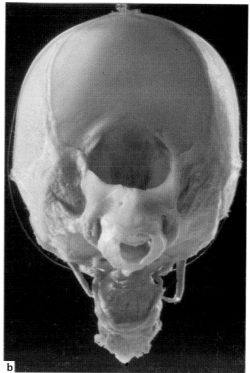

## CLINICAL CONSIDERATIONS

Holoprosencephaly is a congenital abnormality in which the developing forebrain fails to divide into two separate hemispheres and ventricles. It occurs at a rate of 1:5–10000 live births. The cause is unknown, although between 25% and 50% of affected individuals have either a numerical chromosomal abnormality (syndromic hydroprosencephaly) or a gene mutation (non-syndromic hydroprosencephaly). Among environmental factors that may be relevant are maternal diabetes, infections during pregnancy (e.g. syphilis, rubella) and drugs during pregnancy (e.g. retinoic acid, alcohol, anticonvulsants). From the preceding account of facial development, it is not surprising that one of the important mutated genes is *Shh* (as well as its receptor, *PATCHED*). Other mutated genes include *Tgif*, *Six3* and *Zic2*.

Patients with holoprosencephaly display a spectrum of facial anomalies, especially of midline structures. In its severest form, there may be cyclopia (with a single or partially divided eye within a single midline orbit, Fig. 17.7), absence or severe reduction of nasal structures, microcephaly, cleft palate and cleft lip. Among dental abnormalities there may be a single first maxillary incisor.

Disturbances in the relationship between the mandibular and maxillary processes may give rise to macrostomia (enlarged oral orifice), microstomia (small oral orifice) or, rarely, astomia (lack of an oral orifice). Persistence of the naso-optic furrow (nasolacrimal groove) may produce an oblique facial cleft (Fig. 17.8c). Rarely, persistence of a midline groove between the two merging mandibular processes produces a mandibular cleft (Fig. 17.8e).

Failure of fusion of the maxillary and medial nasal processes produces the common congenital malformation of cleft lip, which may be unilateral (Fig. 17.9) or bilateral (Figs 17.8b, 17.10). Failure of the medial nasal processes to merge may be responsible for the formation of median cleft lip (Fig. 17.8a). Most clefts of the lip have a multifactorial aetiology, being associated with both genetic and environmental disturbances. The critical period for such disturbances is during the 6th and 7th weeks of intrauterine life. Candidate genes for clefts of the lip are now being recognized. For example, *Dlx1/2/5/6* (associated with FGF8 growth factor and *Arnt2*

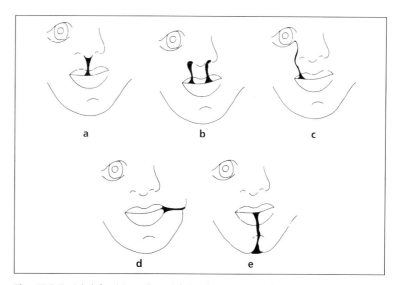

**Fig. 17.8** Facial clefts. (a) Median cleft lip. (b) Bilateral cleft lip. (c) Oblique facial cleft. (d) Lateral facial cleft. (e) Median mandibular cleft.

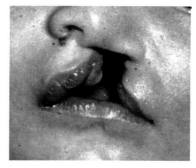
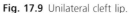
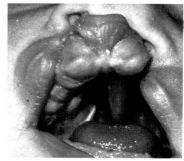

**Fig. 17.9** Unilateral cleft lip.   **Fig. 17.10** Bilateral cleft lip.

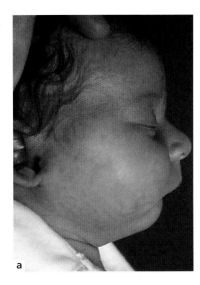
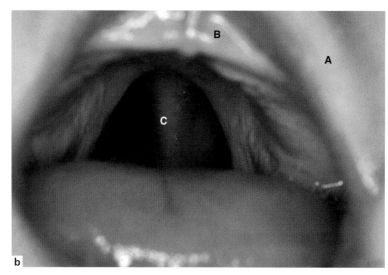

**Fig. 17.11** Pierre Robin's sequence. (a) Neonate with a poorly developed mandible (micrognathia). (b) U-shaped palatal cleft viewed from the mouth. A = upper lip; B = maxillary alveolus; C = nasal septum. Courtesy of Professor R.G. Oliver; copyright Cardiff & Vale NHS Trust.

cell signalling), *Irf6* (associated with FGFR1 growth factor and BMP4 cell signalling) and *Lhx8* (associated with SK11 growth factor and GABRB3 cell signalling) are candidate genes for non-syndromic cleft lip (with or without cleft palate). A comparison between clefts of the lip and clefts of the palate is provided in Table 18.1.

Most congenital abnormalities of the craniofacial region involve transformation of the pharyngeal arch apparatus. The so-called 'first arch syndromes/sequences', including Pierre Robin's sequence and Treacher Collins' syndrome, affect all or most of the structures derived from the first pharyngeal arch (i.e. the mandibular and maxillary processes). First arch syndromes/sequences are caused either by insufficient migration of neural crest cells into the region of the first pharyngeal arch during week 4 of intra-uterine life, by decreased cell proliferation or by increased cell death.

Pierre Robin's sequence (Fig. 17.11) is a heterogeneous birth defect found in about 1 : 8500 live births. In its usual manifestation, it is found equally in males and females. However, there is an X-linked form. Pierre Robin's sequence is characterized by micrognathia (underdeveloped mandible), glossoptosis (abnormal downward or backward placement of the tongue, which may produce respiratory distress and difficulty in feeding), ear defects, speech defects due to velopharyngeal insufficiency, and clefts of the lips and palate. In its normal form, Pierre Robin's sequence is an autosomal recessive hereditary condition.

Treacher Collins' syndrome is found in 1 : 10 000 live births. Typically, the syndrome is characterized by downward-slanting eyes, coloboma of the eye (a notch-like defect (keyhole appearance) in the inferior part of the iris resulting from failure of closure of the retinal fissure of the developing eye), micrognathia, absent or malformed ears, and clefts of the lips and palate. Mutations in the *Tcof1* gene (at chromosome 5q32–q33.1) can cause this syndrome; the mutation results in disturbance in the synthesis of a protein called treacle, which is particularly important in craniofacial development for the survival of the neural crest progenitors and for neural crest proliferation. The disorder is an autosomal dominant condition.

# Development of the palate 18

The definitive palate (or secondary palate) appears in the human fetus between the 6th and 8th weeks of intra-uterine life (1 week later for females). Palatogenesis is a complex event and is often disturbed, producing the congenital defect known as cleft palate (see pages 290–292). Consequently, the events and mechanisms responsible for the development of the palate have been much studied, although some controversy remains.

By the 6th week of development (Fig. 18.1), the primitive nasal cavities are separated by a primary nasal septum and are partitioned from the primitive oral cavity by a primary palate. Both the primary nasal septum and the primary palate are derived from the frontonasal process. The stomodeal chamber is divided at this stage into the small primitive oral cavity beneath the primary palate and the relatively large oronasal cavity behind the primary palate. As shown in Figure 18.2, during the 6th week of development, two lateral palatal shelves develop behind the primary palate from the maxillary processes. A secondary nasal septum grows down from the roof of the stomodeum behind the primary nasal septum, thus dividing the nasal part of the oronasal cavity into two. Evidence suggests that the mesenchyme within the palatal shelves originates from the neural crest.

During the 7th week of development, the oral part of the oronasal cavity becomes completely filled by the developing tongue (Fig. 18.3). Growth

of the palatal shelves continues such that they come to lie vertically. This orientation is characteristic of mammalians but the reason for this is unknown. It has been suggested that the potential space in the oronasal cavity is insufficient because of the evolution of a large tongue in mammals. Two peaks of DNA synthesis occur as the palatal shelves are formed: during initial shelf outgrowth and during vertical shelf elongation.

During the 8th week of development (Fig. 18.4), the stomodeum enlarges, the tongue 'drops' and the vertically inclined palatal shelves become horizontal. It has been suggested that the descent of the tongue is related to mandibular growth and/or a change in the shape of the tongue. On becoming horizontal, the palatal shelves contact each other (and the secondary nasal septum) in the midline to form the definitive (or secondary) palate. The shelves contact the primary palate anteriorly so that the oronasal cavity becomes subdivided into its constituent oral and nasal cavities (Fig. 18.5). After contact, the medial edge epithelia of the two shelves fuse to form a midline epithelial seam. Subsequently, this seam degenerates so that mesenchymal continuity is established across the now

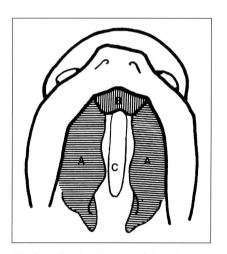

**Fig. 18.2** The development of the palate during the 6th week of intra-uterine life. A = lateral palatal shelves; B = primary palate; C = secondary nasal septum.

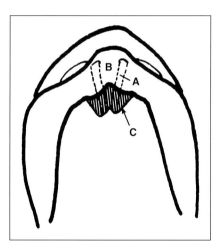

**Fig. 18.1** The state of development of the palate by the 6th week of intra-uterine life. A = primitive nasal cavities; B = primary nasal septum; C = primary palate.

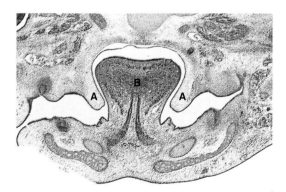

**Fig. 18.3** Coronal section through the developing head during the 7th week of development showing the palatal shelves (A). B = developing tongue (Masson's trichrome; ×30).

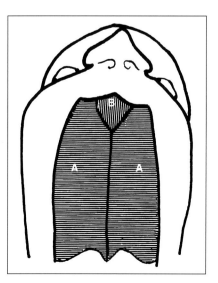

**Fig. 18.4** The state of development of the palate during the 8th week of intra-uterine life. A = palatal shelves; B = primary palate.

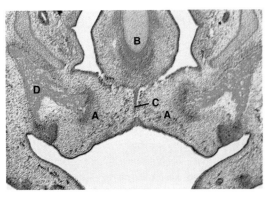

**Fig. 18.5** Coronal section through developing oronasal regions following contact of the palatal shelves (A) and secondary nasal septum (B). C = midline epithelial seam; D = developing bone of maxilla (Masson's trichrome; ×30).

intact and horizontal secondary palate. Fusion of the palatal processes is complete by the 12th week of development. Behind the secondary nasal septum, the palatal shelves fuse to form the soft palate and uvula.

Recent research on palatogenesis has concentrated on two main events: palatal shelf elevation and the initial stages of fusion of the shelves.

## PALATAL SHELF ELEVATION

Elevation of the palatal shelves from the vertical to the horizontal position takes place very rapidly. Several mechanisms have been proposed to account for the rapid movement of the palatal shelves. Although it was once thought that extrinsic forces might be responsible (e.g. from forces derived from the tongue or jaw movements or as a result of differential

pressures above and below the palatal shelves), research has primarily focused on the search for a force intrinsic to the palatal shelf and within its mesenchyme. It has been proposed that the intrinsic shelf elevation force might develop as a result of hydration of extracellular matrix components (principally hyaluronan) in the shelf mesenchyme, or as a result of mesenchymal cell activity. The intrinsic shelf elevating force might be multifactorial, although there is as yet no experimental evidence to support what otherwise might be considered this commonsense view.

The changing amounts of glycosaminoglycans (GAGs) during development of the anterior (presumptive hard) and posterior (presumptive soft) palates are illustrated in Figure 18.6. Stage A occurs immediately before shelf elevation, stage B immediately after shelf elevation, stage C during shelf fusion and early histogenesis and stage D when there is marked histogenesis after fusion. The most significant changes occur after elevation: during the time of elevation there are no differences between the anterior and posterior regions of the shelves even though, in the species studied in Figure 18.6 (the rat), the posterior region of the shelf does not elevate but grows initially with a horizontal disposition. Three GAG types are found in vivo: hyaluronan, heparan sulphate and chondroitin 4-sulphate (Fig. 18.7). If palatal shelves are cultured in vitro, dermatan sulphate is also present, highlighting the difficulties of extrapolating from the findings of tissue culture to the in vivo situation.

A section through a vertical (pre-elevation) palatal shelf, stained using the hyaluronectin/antihyaluronectin technique, is shown in Figure 18.8. Note the intense staining for hyaluronan within the palatal shelf mesenchyme. It has been proposed that hyaluronan is a GAG involved in shelf elevation because it is a highly electrostatically charged, open-coil molecule capable of binding up to 10 times its own weight in water. The changing concentrations of hyaluronan within the anterior and posterior regions of palatal shelves are illustrated in Figure 18.9. The stages of palatogenesis (A–D) are the same as those described in Figure 18.6. Note

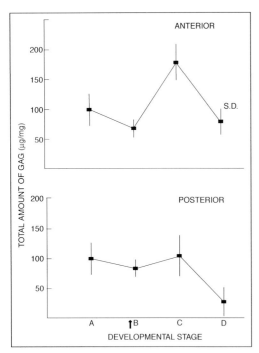

**Fig. 18.6** Graphs illustrating the changing amounts of glycosaminoglycans (GAGs) during development of the anterior (presumptive hard) and posterior (presumptive soft) palates. Stage A = before shelf elevation; stage B = after shelf elevation; stage C = during shelf fusion and early histogenesis; stage D = a stage of marked histogenesis after fusion. Arrow indicates time of shelf elevation. Courtesy of Dr G.D. Singh and the editor of the *Archives of Oral Biology*.

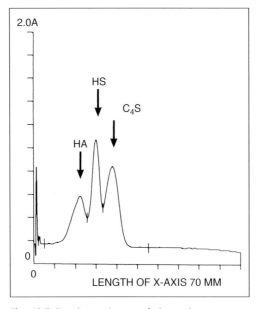

**Fig. 18.7** Densitometric scan of electrophoretograms showing the GAGs within the palatal shelves in vivo. HA = hyaluronan; HS = heparan sulphate; C$_4$S = chondroitin 4-sulphate. Courtesy of Dr G.D. Singh and the editor of the *Archives of Oral Biology*.

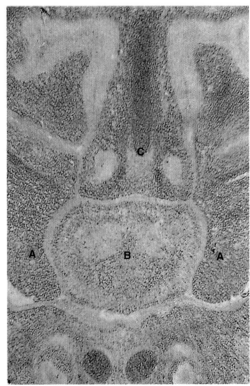

**Fig. 18.8** Coronal section through a vertical (pre-elevation) palatal shelf (A) stained using the hyaluronectin/antihyaluronectin technique. Positive brown staining shows presence of hyaluronan in shelf mesenchyme. B = tongue; C = nasal septum (×30). Courtesy of Professor M.W.J. Fergusson.

that, statistically, there is significantly more hyaluronan in the shelves immediately before elevation than immediately after; however, the data do not agree with some reports that there is less hyaluronan posteriorly than anteriorly, and again the pattern of change in hyaluronan is similar both anteriorly and posteriorly even though the posterior region does not undergo elevation to become horizontal.

Studies have revealed the presence during palatogenesis of enzymes associated with hyaluronan synthesis, of a cell-surface receptor associated with hyaluronan, of the hyaluronan binding extracellular matrix components versican and hyaluronectin, and of hyaluronan binding sites (Fig. 18.10). Furthermore, using an organ-culture system (Figs 18.11–18.14), agents that alter hyaluronan content or size, disrupt GAG substitution on proteoglycans, or alter the balance of matrix molecules secreted via the Golgi complex and hyaluronan produced at the cell surface all affect palatogenesis. However, while all agents prevent palatal fusion, there are variable effects on shelf elevation. For example, hyaluronidase digestion results in failure of elevation (Fig. 18.11), and treatment with a drug that blocks secretion from the Golgi material, while still allowing hyaluronan production, also prevents elevation (Fig. 18.14). On the other hand, displacement of nascent hyaluronan with oligosaccharides allowed elevation (although the shelves were incorrectly oriented) (Fig. 18.12) and treatment

with an agent that disrupts GAG assembly on proteoglycans resulted in abnormal elevation (Fig. 18.13). Overall, therefore, recent research indicates that hyaluronan is crucial to shelf elevation. To add to such findings, a reduced-molecular-weight hyaluronan leads to palate dysmorphogenesis (Fig. 18.13), suggesting that a minimum hyaluronan size is required to achieve normal palatogenesis.

Other matrix components, including proteoglycans, are of importance to shelf elevation. Versican and decorin have been identified at a range of molecular weights corresponding to various processed forms (Fig. 18.15). Link protein is absent within the mesenchyme of the palatal shelves (although present in other parts of the developing mouth) (Fig. 18.16). This could be important, since link protein 'stabilizes' proteoglycans in the extracellular matrix and its absence could mean that there is greater

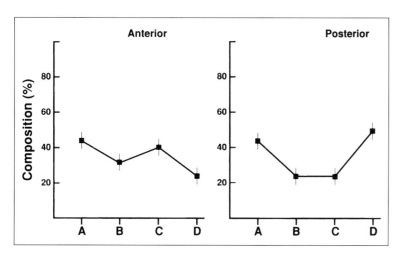

**Fig. 18.9** Graphs showing the changing concentrations of hyaluronan within the anterior and posterior regions of palatal shelves. A–D = stages of palatogenesis described in Fig. 18.6. From Singh GD, Moxham BJ, Langley MS, Embery G 1994 Changes in the composition of glycosaminoglycans during normal palatogenesis in the rat. *Archives of Oral Biology* 39: 401–407.

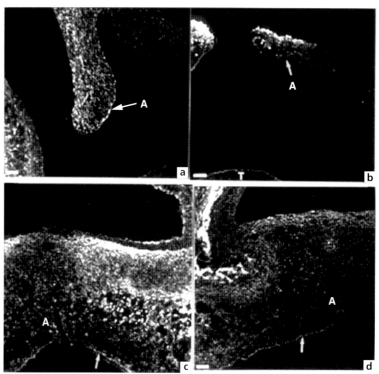

**Fig. 18.10** The palatal shelves before (a) and after (b–d) elevation showing the presence of binding for the glycosaminoglycan hyaluronan (white label) using CD44 antibody immunohistochemistry. A = palatal shelves (Fluorescent immuno-histochemistry; ×80). Courtesy of S. Thomas, R. Hall and B.J. Moxham.

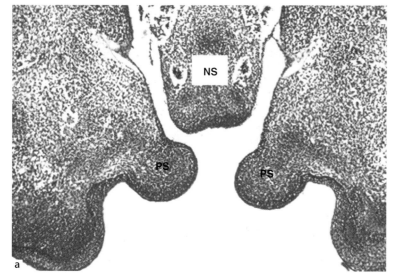

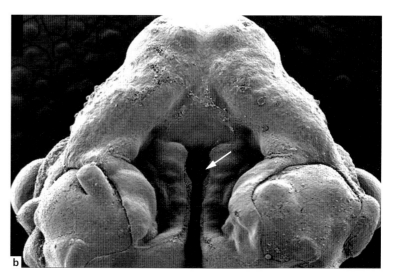

**Fig. 18.11** The effects of *Streptomyces* hyaluronidase on the developing palate in organ culture. Clefts are produced, suggesting that palate development is disrupted in the absence of the glycosaminoglycan hyaluronan. (a) Section through a cleft palate resulting from hyaluronidase treatment. NS = nasal septum; PS = unfused palatal shelves (×60). (b) SEM showing the cleft (arrowed) (×30). Courtesy of S. Thomas, R. Hall and B.J. Moxham.

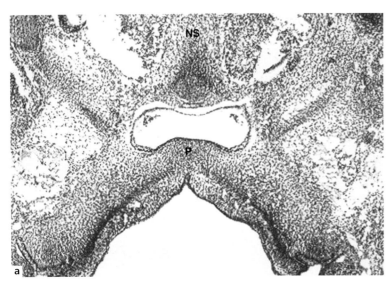

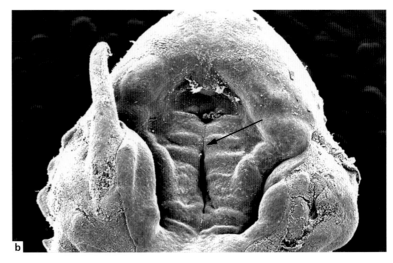

**Fig. 18.12** The effects of UDP-xylose on the developing palate in organ culture. UDP-xylose is a natural inhibitor of UDPGD, the enzyme responsible for the conversion of UDP-glucose to UDP-glucuronic acid. Normal palatogenesis with UDP-xylose suggests that inhibition of UDPGD has no effect on palate development or that it may not be entering the tissue. (a) Section through a normally developing palate following UDP-xylose treatment. NS = nasal septum; P = fused palatal shelves (×50). (b) SEM showing normal palatogenesis (arrowed) (×25). Courtesy of S. Thomas, R. Hall and B.J. Moxham.

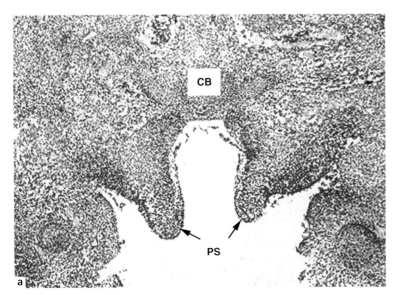

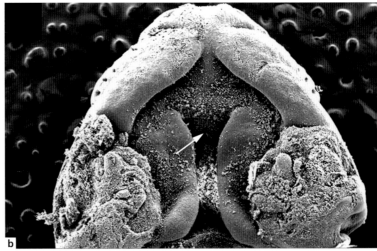

**Fig. 18.13** The effects of chlorcyclizine (CHLR) on the developing palate in organ culture. CHLR enhances degradation of hyaluronan and chondroitin sulphate to lower-molecular-weight products, with little effect on their synthesis and on DNA synthesis. Clefts are produced, suggesting that the size of the glycosaminoglycan chain may influence palatogenesis. (a) Section through a cleft palate resulting from CHLR treatment. CB = cranial base; PS = unfused palatal shelves (×50). (b) SEM showing the cleft (arrowed) (×25). Courtesy of S. Thomas, R. Hall and B.J. Moxham.

aggregation and disaggregation of the proteoglycans as palatogenesis proceeds. The role of collagen within the palatal shelves is disputed, although immunocytochemically type I collagen can easily be identified (Fig. 18.17). Stout bundles of collagen can be seen running down the centre of the palatal shelf, oriented from the base towards the tip of the shelf. It has been suggested that the shelf elevation force is directed by these collagen fibres.

The role of the mesenchymal cells within the palatal shelves has also attracted some controversy. There is evidence that a critical number of cells are required for palatal shelf elevation to occur but there is no reliable evidence that these cells, by their rapid division and proliferation, and by migration or by contraction, can effect a palatal shelf elevation force (particularly in view of the rapidity of shelf elevation). Using a special silver staining technique, the degree of activity of the mesenchymal cells in the palatal shelf mesenchyme can be assessed. To determine whether cell activity changes at different stages of palatogenesis, the Ag–NOR staining technique has been employed; this produces grains in the nucleolar region (Fig. 18.18). The number and configuration of these 'grains' reflect the

overall degree of protein synthesis by the cells. This staining procedure confirmed that the rate of protein synthesis during palatogenesis is high, is higher pre-elevation than post-elevation and is higher still during later stages of histogenesis. These results accord with the changes occurring in GAG synthesis at various stages of palatogenesis. The staining technique is, however, unable to demonstrate major differences between anterior and posterior regions within the rat fetus where differences might have been expected. Quantitative electron microscopy of the cells within the palatal shelves has also not produced evidence that such cells can generate a shelf elevation force. Research has been undertaken to study the cell surface receptors for hyaluronan (CD44 receptors) and there is evidence that there is a transient and dynamic expression of CD44 splice variants during palatogenesis, particularly after shelf elevation. This suggests that, although hyaluronan in the palatal shelves is most often associated with the development of a turgor pressure for shelf elevation via attraction of water molecules, this GAG might also influence cellular activity. For example, hyaluronan produces large intercellular spaces during early palatogenesis to prevent cell–cell and cell–matrix interactions, allowing assembly of

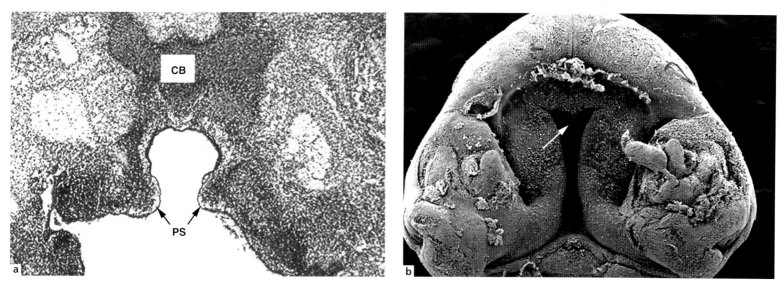

**Fig. 18.14** The effects of brefeldin A (BFA) on the developing palate in organ culture. BFA inhibits vesicular transport through the Golgi complex. Hyaluronan synthesis is not affected as this GAG, unlike other GAGs, undergoes a different synthetic pathway at, or near, the plasma membrane. Clefts are produced, suggesting that a set of macromolecules other than hyaluronan and synthesized in the Golgi play an important role in normal palatogenesis. (a) Coronal section through a cleft palate resulting from BFA treatment. CB = cranial base; PS = unfused palatal shelves (×50). (b) SEM showing the cleft (arrowed) (×25). Courtesy of S. Thomas, R. Hall and B.J. Moxham.

**Fig. 18.15** The presence of some proteoglycans during normal palatogenesis. (a) Decorin (green labelling) beneath the lining epithelial cells of the palatal shelf pre-elevation (biglycan is not found). Note that decorin relocates to the centre of the shelf mesenchyme post-elevation (Fluorescence immuno-histochemistry; ×240). (b) Versican (white labelling) in the palatal shelves (P); T = tongue (Fluorescence immunohistochemistry; ×140). (c) Link protein (white labelling) found in the developing nasal septum (N) but absent in the palatal shelf (P), indicating that the proteoglycans within the shelf are 'labile' (Fluorescence immunohistochemistry; ×60). Courtesy of S. Thomas, R. Hall and B.J. Moxham.

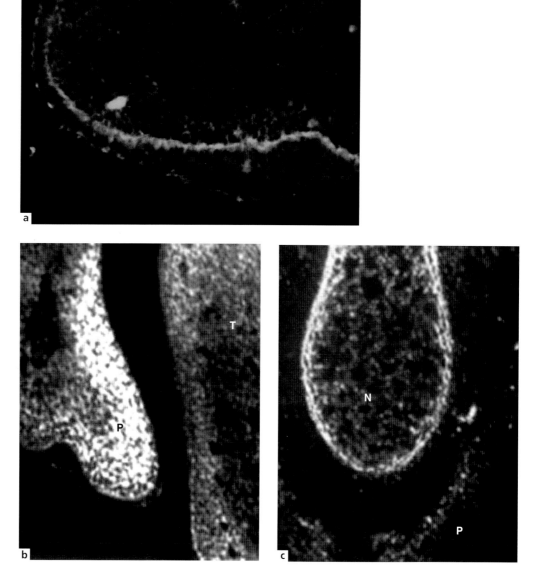

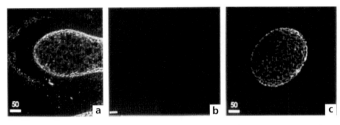

**Fig. 18.16** Use of 8-A-4 antibodies to recognize link protein immunohistochemically. Immunopositivity is observed in the cartilages of the nasal septum (a) and Meckel's cartilage (c) but is absent from the developing palate, both before and after shelf elevation (b) (Bar = 50 μm). Courtesy of S. Thomas, R. Hall and B.J. Moxham.

extracellular constituents and presentation of growth factors that in turn influence cell growth and differentiation by altering the local concentration of intercellular signals. Following shelf elevation, there is a decline in hyaluronan shelf content, probably via CD44-receptor-mediated endocytosis of hyaluronan and via hyaluronidases that produce shorter hyaluronan chains. This enables the onset of palatal tissue differentiation. Hyaluronan that is taken up into cells can bind to intracellular hyaluronan binding proteins (e.g. RHAMM). Such binding induces cell signalling pathways that can, in turn, induce changes in the cytoskeleton. During differentiation, the intercellular matrix becomes more dense where hyaluronan is replaced by proteoglycans, but the remaining hyaluronan binds to such proteoglycans (including hyaluronan-binding proteins such as versican, cell surface RHAMM and CD44) to form a stable extracellular matrix.

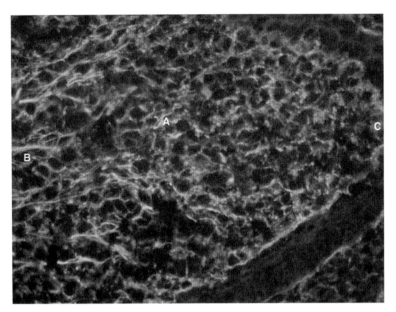

**Fig. 18.17** Coronal section of a palatal shelf labelled immunocytochemically with antibodies against type I collagen showing positive green labelling throughout. A = collagen bundles; B = base of palatal shelf; C = tip of palatal shelf (×240). Courtesy of Professor M.W.J. Fergusson.

## FUSION OF THE PALATAL SHELVES

Once the palatal shelves have elevated, they contact each other (initially in the middle third of the palate) and adhere by means of a 'sticky' glycoprotein, which coats the surface of the medial edge epithelia of the shelves. The epithelial cells develop desmosomes and consequently an epithelial seam is formed (Fig. 18.19). The adherence of the medial edge epithelia is specific as palatal epithelia will not fuse with epithelia from other sites (e.g. the tongue). This may be related to the fact that the protein associated with the formation of desmosomes (desmoplakin) appears specifically on the cell membranes of the medial edge epithelia just before shelf contact.

Disruption of the epithelial seam, with penetration by mesenchymal cells, is shown in Figure 18.20, although the signals that are responsible for such breakdown are not yet fully understood. Nevertheless, the breakdown of the basal lamina is likely to be a significant event. At this early stage of fusion (Fig. 18.21), the basal lamina remains intact. At a later stage of fusion (Fig. 18.22), with migration of the epithelial cells into the mesenchyme, the midline epithelial seam is disrupted and the migrating cells initially carry with them fragments of the disrupted basal lamina.

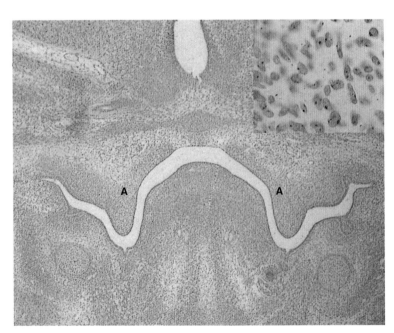

**Fig. 18.18** Ag–NOR staining of the palatal shelves (A) to assess the degree of activity of the mesenchymal cells (Silver stain; ×45). Inset shows black silver grains at higher power (×400).

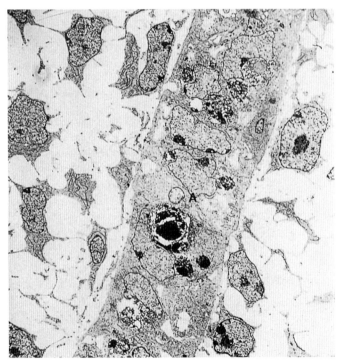

**Fig. 18.19** TEM showing the midline epithelial seam for early fusing palatal shelves. An intact basal lamina lies on either side of the epithelial seam. A = epithelial cells (×3900). Courtesy of Professor M.W.J. Fergusson.

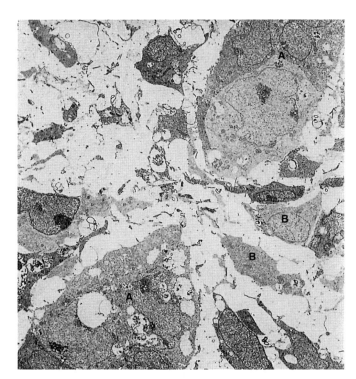

**Fig. 18.20** TEM showing disruption of the epithelial seam (A) with penetration by mesenchymal cells (B) (×3900). Courtesy of Professor M.W.J. Fergusson.

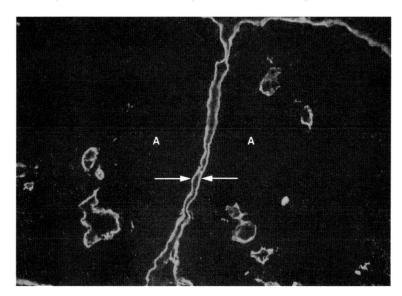

**Fig. 18.21** Fusing palatal shelves (A) immunocytochemically labelled with antibodies against type IV collagen showing positive green labelling in basal lamina (arrowed) (×90). Courtesy of Professor M.W.J. Fergusson.

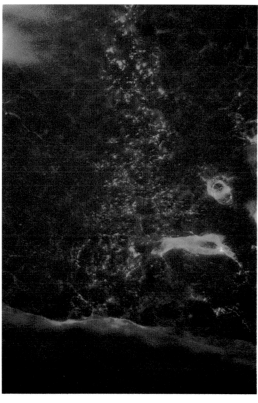

**Fig. 18.22** Late stage of fusion of the palatal shelves immunocytochemically labelled for type IV collagen and showing disruption of the positively green-labelling midline epithelial seam; compare with Fig. 18.19 (×180). Courtesy of Professor M.W.J. Fergusson.

Fibrils comprising tenascin and type III collagen have been shown to run at right angles to the basal lamina and may provide guiding pathways for the migrating epithelial cells. Evidence indicates that the events leading to the breakdown of the epithelial seam occur in single isolated palatal shelves and therefore do not depend upon shelf contact.

Almost as soon as the epithelial seam is formed, it thins to a layer two or three cells thick. This thinning may be the result of three processes. First, the seam is thinned by growth of the palate (in terms of oronasal height) and by epithelial cell migration from the region of the seam onto the oral and nasal aspects of the palate. Second, there is programmed cell death (apoptosis) in the seam. This is shown by the finding that DNA synthesis ceases in the medial edge epithelial cells 1 day before shelf contact. Furthermore, cyclic AMP (cAMP) levels increase just before shelf fusion: exogenous cAMP is associated with precocious cell death in the medial edge epithelia. It has also been shown that epidermal growth factor

(EGF) inhibits medial edge cell death and that this inhibition is blocked by exogenous cAMP. Care must be taken, however, when interpreting the effects of cAMP because physiologically it is an intracellular messenger and may therefore be mediating differential gene expression triggered by other events occurring at the cell surface. Third, there is good evidence that some of the epithelial cells migrate from the seam into the palatal shelf mesenchyme and differentiate into cells indistinguishable from the mesenchymal cells. Indeed, it is well known that epithelial cells can migrate and differentiate into mesenchymal-like cells in other situations during development.

There have been many experiments to help clarify the nature of the epithelial–mesenchymal interactions during fusion of the palatal shelves. In the main, these experiments have involved the separation and then the recombination in culture of the epithelial and mesenchymal components of the shelves. Overall, these experiments have shown that, as with epithelial–mesenchymal interactions for later tooth development (see pages 305–310), it is the mesenchyme that signals epithelial differentiation and behaviour. The nature of this signal is controversial. Although it was once proposed that the palatal mesenchyme could signal epithelial differentiation directly by cell-to-cell contact, mesenchymal–epithelial cell contacts are very rare during palatogenesis. Recent evidence indicates that extracellular matrix molecules may provide the signal and work has been undertaken to assess the role of type IX collagen (Figs 18.23, 18.24). At the earliest stages before shelf elevation, the medial edges of the palatal shelves label poorly for type IX collagen compared with floor of the mouth epithelia (Fig. 18.23). Note that, at the stage of fusion, type IX collagen appears around the surfaces of the medial edge epithelial cells (Fig. 18.24). Present day thinking suggests that the control of the synthesis of type IX collagen is influenced by growth factors.

Immunocytochemical labelling with antibodies against EGF receptors of the mesenchymal cells adjacent to the midline epithelial seam of fusing palatal shelves is shown in Figure 18.25. EGF, or its embryonic

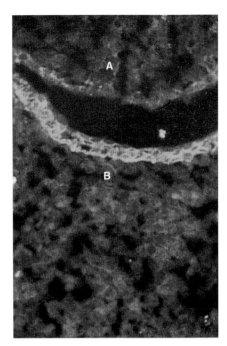

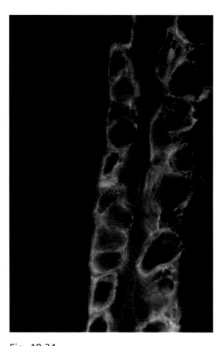

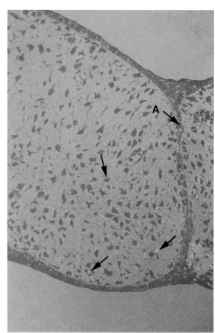

Fig. 18.23

Fig. 18.24

Fig. 18.25

**Fig. 18.23** The medial edge epithelia of palatal shelves (A) labelled immunocyto-chemically for type IX collagen before shelf elevation. Little positive green labelling is evident compared with the epithelium covering the floor of the mouth (B) (×280). Courtesy of Professor M.W.J. Fergusson.

**Fig. 18.24** The medial edge epithelia of palatal shelves labelled immunocytochemi-cally for type IX collagen at a time when medial edge epithelial differentiation

occurs. Compared with Fig. 18.23, positive green labelling is evident (×280). Courtesy of Professor M.W.J. Fergusson.

**Fig. 18.25** Immunocytochemical labelling with antibodies against epidermal growth factor receptors of the mesenchymal cells adjacent to the midline epithelial seam of fusing palatal shelves. White dots indicate positive labelling (arrows). A = epithelial seam (×85). Courtesy of Professor M.W.J. Fergusson and the editor of *Development*.

homologue known as transforming growth factor (TGF)α, is known to inhibit palatal medial edge epithelial cell death in the presence of mesen-chyme. Furthermore, it has been shown that the synthesis of extracellular matrix molecules (including type IX collagen) is stimulated by factors such as TGFα and TGFβ and is inhibited by fibroblast growth factors (FGF). When palatal shelves are organ-cultured with EGF, the medial edge of the palatal shelf shows a nipple-like bulge, medial edge epithelial cell death is absent, and the mesenchyme possesses increased quantities of extracellular matrix molecules. It has been proposed, therefore, that the palatal shelf mesenchyme produces growth factors that either directly signal epithelial differentiation or, by stimulating extracellular matrix pro-duction, indirectly influence differentiation through this matrix. The pho-tomicrograph shown in Figure 18.25 suggests that EGF receptors show regional heterogeneity and that the receptors appear beneath the medial edge of the shelves only when the epithelial seam is degenerating.

Once fusion is complete, the hard palate ossifies intramembranously from four centres of ossification, one in each developing maxilla and one in each developing palatine bone. The maxillary ossification centre lies above the developing deciduous canine tooth germ and appears in the 8th week of development (Fig. 18.5). The palatine centres of ossification are situated in the region forming the future perpendicular plate and appear in the 8th week of development. Incomplete ossification of the palate from these centres defines the median and transverse palatine sutures. There does not appear to be a separate centre of ossification for the primary palate in humans (in other species there being a separate 'premaxilla'). Figure 18.26 provides a coronal section through the developing hard palate to show early ossification.

Areas that remain unossified in the hard palate provide bony canals for the passage of nerves and vessels, namely the incisive canals combining to form an incisive fossa between the primary and secondary palate in the anterior midline, and the greater and lesser palatine canals in the postero-lateral region. During development, transient paired strands of epithelium

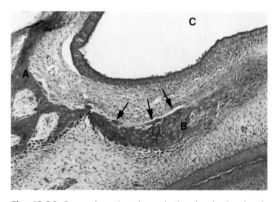

**Fig. 18.26** Coronal section through the developing hard palate showing early ossification. A = developing body of maxilla; B = bone extending from body of maxilla into palate; C = nasal cavity. Note the osteoclasts on the nasal surface (arrowed) and osteoblasts on oral surface (Masson's trichrome; ×80).

are found in the region of the incisive canals termed nasopalatine ducts.

## CLINICAL CONSIDERATIONS

Remnants of the nasopalatine ducts may proliferate to give non-neoplastic cysts that are considered to be the most common of the non-odontogenic cysts in the jaw region. Such cysts are found in the anterior midline region of the maxillae (Figs 18.27, 18.28).

Malformations of palatogenesis may result in the appearance of clefts. Palatal clefts are one of the most common congenital abnormalities (approximately 1:2500 live births) and are more frequent in females (67%). Clefts may result from disturbances of any of the processes involved during palatogenesis (i.e. from defective palatal shelf growth; delayed shelf elevation or failure of elevation; defective shelf fusion or lack of

**Fig. 18.27** Nasopalatine cyst evident as a bluish swelling in the anterior midline region of the palate. Courtesy of Dr J. Potts.

**Fig. 18.28** Radiograph showing a heart-shaped radiolucent nasopalatine cyst in the anterior region of the maxillae. Courtesy of Dr J. Potts.

**Fig. 18.29** Gross clefting of the palate. Courtesy of Dr B.A.W. Brown.

**Fig. 18.30** A cleft uvula (arrows). Courtesy of Dr R.W. Pigott.

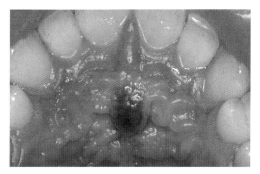

Fig. 18.27

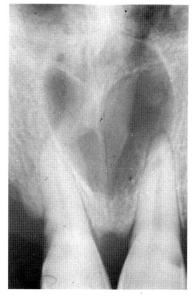

Fig. 18.28

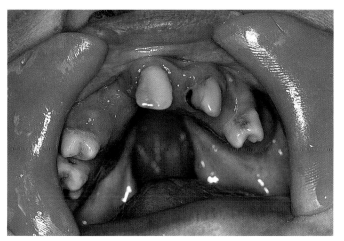

Fig. 18.29

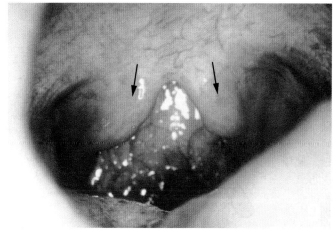

Fig. 18.30

degeneration of the midline epithelial seam; or failure of mesenchymal consolidation and/or differentiation). The mildest form of cleft is that affecting only the uvula, such a disturbance occurring relatively late in the process of palatal malfusion. Disturbances during the early phases of palatogenesis (e.g. during shelf elevation and early fusion) can result in a more extensive cleft involving most of the secondary palate. Should the cleft involve the primary palate, it may extend to the right and/or left of the incisive fossa to include the alveolus, passing between the lateral incisor and canine teeth. Cleft palate may be associated with cleft lip, although the two conditions are independently determined. Dental malformations are commonly associated with a cleft involving the alveolus. A submucous cleft describes a condition where the palatal mucosa is intact but the bone/musculature of the palate is deficient beneath the mucosa. Figure 18.29 shows an extensive cleft of the palate and Figure 18.30 a cleft uvula. Less problematic than clefts (but more common) is the retention of epithelial remnants in the midline that may eventually become cystic (Fig. 18.31).

The most common problem experienced by persons who have clefts of the palate is 'hypernasality' (a speech/resonance disorder caused by velopharyngeal (soft palate–pharyngeal) incompetence and characterized by air escaping through the nasal airway). Hypernasality can make speech incomprehensible and can severely affect quality of life and a person's self-esteem. Children with hypernasality can be 'judged' as unintelligent, unpleasant and unattractive and consequently as social outcasts.

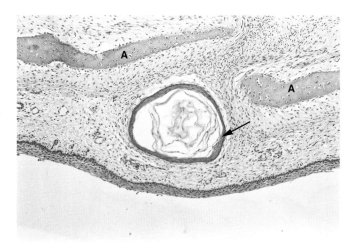

**Fig. 18.31** Section through a developing midline palatine cyst (arrowed). A = bone of hard palate (H & E; ×40).

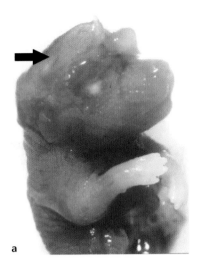

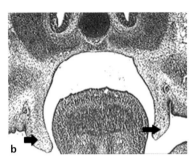

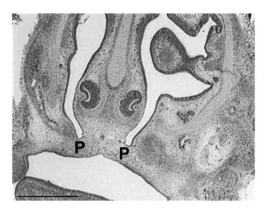

**Fig. 18.33** Normally elevated and fused palatal shelves (P) resulting from supplementation of all-*trans* retinoic acid with calcium folinate. Note that, as shown in Fig. 18.32, all-*trans* retinoic acid alone would produce serious craniofacial abnormalities, including cleft palate. Courtesy of L.J. Richardson, E.-N. Emmanouil-Nikoloussi and B.J. Moxham.

**Fig. 18.32** The effects of high doses of all-*trans* retinoic acid on craniofacial development. (a) Fetal head showing exencephaly – the appearance of the brain close to the surface of the head (arrow). (b) Cleft of the palate produced by failure of elevation of the palatal shelves (arrows). Courtesy of E. Gunston, M. Wise, E.-N. Emmanouil-Nikoloussi and B.J. Moxham 2005 *European Journal of Anatomy* 9(1): 1–16.

Experiments have shown that clefts produced in experimental animals are associated with the synthesis of much less GAGs than normally developing palates, although qualitatively the same types of GAG are still secreted and the percentages of each of these GAGs are unaltered. The Ag–NOR staining technique referred to on page 286 further shows that protein synthesis is severely depressed during cleft formation.

Clefts of the palate, like those of the lip, are multifactorial malformations, involving both genetic (often polygenic) and environmental factors. The aetiology is not related to maternal age and, within a family with a child with a cleft, the probability of another child being affected is estimated as being 2%. Recent data show that clefts that are multifactorial are most common for clefts of the lip (67% of cases). 41% of cleft palates can be ascribed a multifactorial aetiology and 34% of submucous clefts are multifactorial in origin. 20% of cleft palates are monogenic, 5% are caused by teratogens, 1% are associated with chromosomal abnormalities and over 20% are of unknown aetiology. Concerning risk factors, smoking and alcohol abuse by the mother can increase the likelihood of clefting. Furthermore, drugs (both medical and recreational), some viruses and

**Table 18.1** *Clefts of the upper lip and of the palate*

| Cleft lip | Cleft palate |
| --- | --- |
| Unilateral or bilateral<br>With or without cleft palate | Classification with reference to incisive fossa – anterior anomalies (primary palate) and posterior anomalies (secondary palate) |
| 1:1000 births | 1:2500 births |
| Mostly male infants | More common in females |
| 67% with multifactorial aetiology | 41% with multifactorial aetiology |
| Due to failure of fusion of mesenchymes in facial processes | Due to failure of elevation of palatal shelves (major clefts) or failure of fusion of shelves (minor clefts) |

rubella infection can be associated with the development of a cleft. Some clefts may be caused by nutritional factors. For example, excessive vitamin A intake (retinoids) and deficiencies in folic acid can be related to clefting. Figure 18.32 shows the effects on rat fetuses of large doses of all-*trans* retinoic acid and Figure 18.33 indicates that supplements of folinates can 'rescue' these disorders.

Table 18.1 compares clefts of the upper lip and the palate.

## THE MANDIBLE

The mandible initially develops intramembranously but its subsequent growth is related to the appearance of secondary cartilages (the condylar cartilage being the most important). The developing mandible is preceded by the appearance of a rod of cartilage belonging to the first pharyngeal arch. This is known as Meckel's cartilage (Figs 19.1, 19.2) and it first appears at about the 6th week of intra-uterine life. Meckel's cartilage extends from the cartilaginous otic capsule in the region of the developing ear to a midline symphysis. However, it makes little contribution to the adult mandible, merely providing a framework around which the bone of the mandible forms.

The mandible first appears as a band of dense fibrous tissue on the anterolateral aspect of Meckel's cartilage. During the 7th week of intra-uterine life, a centre of ossification appears in this fibrous tissue at a site close to the future mental foramen. From this centre, bone formation spreads rapidly backwards, forwards and upwards, around the inferior alveolar nerve and its terminal branches (the incisive and mental nerves). Further spread of the developing bone in a forwards and backwards direction produces a plate of bone on the lateral side of Meckel's cartilage that corresponds to the future body of the mandible and extends towards the midline, where it comes to lie in close relationship with the bone forming on the opposite side. However, the two plates of bone remain separated by fibrous tissue to form the mandibular symphysis (Fig. 19.1).

At a later stage in the development of the body of the mandible, continued bone formation markedly increases the size of the mandible, with development of the alveolar process occurring to surround the developing tooth germs (Fig. 19.3). At an even later stage, Meckel's cartilage resorbs (Fig. 19.4). The neurovascular bundle that initially was located with the developing tooth germs now becomes contained within its own bony canal and there is considerable development of the alveolar process.

Although Meckel's cartilage contributes no significant tissue to the developing mandible, nodular remnants of cartilage may be seen in the region of the mandibular symphysis until birth and, in its most dorsal part, Meckel's cartilage ossifies to form ear ossicles (the malleus and incus). Behind the body of the mandible the perichondrium of Meckel's cartilage persists as the sphenomandibular and sphenomalleolar ligaments. The sphenomandibular ligament ossifies at its sites of attachment to form the lingula of the mandible and the spine of the sphenoid bone.

As the developing tooth germs reach the bell stage (see page 301), developing bone becomes closely related to it to form the alveolus (Fig. 19.5). The size of the alveolus is dependent upon the size of the growing tooth germ. Resorption occurs on the inner wall of the alveolus (indicated by Howship's lacunae) while, on the outer wall of the alveolus, bone is deposited (indicated by osteoblasts lining an osteoid seam). The developing teeth therefore come to lie in a trough of bone. Later, the teeth become separated from each other by the development of interdental septa. With the onset of root formation, interradicular bone develops in multirooted teeth.

The ramus of the mandible is first mapped out as a condensation of fibrocellular tissue that, although continuous with the developing body of

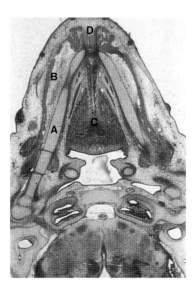
Fig. 19.1

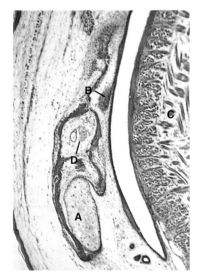
Fig. 19.2

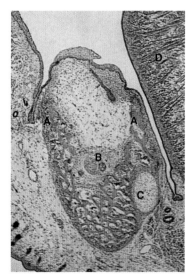
Fig. 19.3

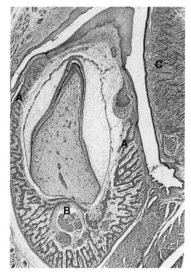
Fig. 19.4

**Fig. 19.1** Meckel's cartilage (A), around which the bone of the mandible (B) is forming in membrane. This is a horizontal section through the developing mandible during the 8th week of intra-uterine life. Note that Meckel's cartilage extends from the cartilaginous otic capsule to the midline symphysis (D), where initially it is separated from its fellow of the opposite side by mesenchyme. C = tongue (Masson's trichrome; ×12).

**Fig. 19.2** Transverse section through the early developing mandible (8th week of development). At this stage, only a small amount of mandibular bone has formed intramembranously on the lateral aspect of Meckel's cartilage (A). Note the beginnings of tooth development in this region as indicated by the dental lamina (B). C = tongue; D = neurovascular bundle (Masson's trichrome; ×60).

**Fig. 19.3** A later stage in the development of the body of the mandible. Continued bone formation has increased the size of the mandible. The alveolar process (A) grows to surround the developing tooth germ. The developing teeth share the same common crypt as the neurovascular bundle (B). Note that Meckel's cartilage (C) is now comparatively small, although it still lies medial to the developing mandibular bone. D = developing tongue (Masson's trichrome; ×25).

**Fig. 19.4** Even later stage in the development of the body of the mandible. Meckel's cartilage has been resorbed. The neurovascular bundle (B) is now contained within its own bony canal and there has been considerable development of the alveolar process (A). C = developing tongue (Masson's trichrome; ×25).

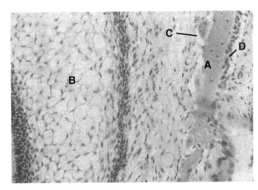

**Fig. 19.5** Development of the mandibular alveolus (A) in the region of a developing tooth (B). Note that resorption is occurring on the inner wall of the alveolus (indicated by Howship's lacunae; C) while, on the outer wall of the alveolus, bone is being deposited (indicated by osteoblasts (D) lining an osteoid seam) (Decalcified section; Masson's trichrome; ×110).

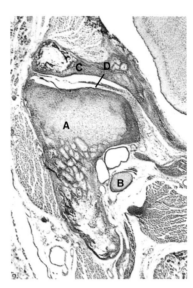

**Fig. 19.7** The early developing condylar cartilage (A) and temporomandibular joint. B = Meckel's cartilage; C = developing bone of mandibular fossa; D = part of developing articular disc of temporomandibular joint (Decalcified section; Masson's trichrome: ×20).

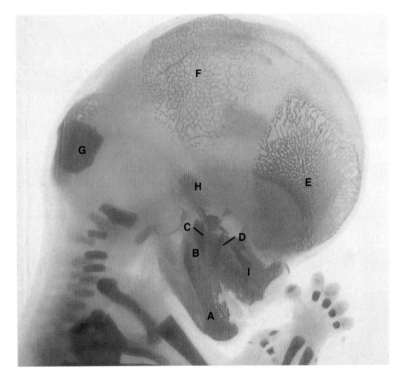

**Fig. 19.6** The appearance of the developing jaws of a human fetus (14 weeks). A = body of mandible; B = ramus of mandible; C = secondary condylar cartilage; D = secondary coronoid cartilage; E = frontal bone; F = parietal bone; G = occipital bone; H = squamous portion of temporal bone; I = maxilla (Cleared alizarin red preparation; ×5).

the mandible, is positioned some way laterally from Meckel's cartilage. Further development of the ramus is associated with a backward spread of ossification from the body and by the appearance of secondary cartilages. Between the 10th and 14th weeks in utero, three secondary cartilages develop within the growing mandible. The largest and most important of these is the condylar cartilage, which, as its name suggests, appears beneath the fibrous articular layer of the future condyle (see Figs 15.18 and 19.7). By proliferation and subsequent ossification, the cartilage is thought by some to serve as an important centre of growth for the mandible, functioning up to about the 16th year of life. Less important, transitory, secondary cartilages are seen associated with the coronoid process and in the region of the mandibular symphysis. The appearance of the developing jaws of a human fetus at 14 weeks is shown in Figure 19.6.

The temporomandibular joint develops from mesenchyme lying between the developing mandibular condyle below and the temporal bone above, which develop intramembranously. During the 12th week of intra-uterine life, two clefts appear in the mesenchyme, producing the upper and lower

joint cavities. The remaining intervening mesenchyme becomes the intra-articular disc. The joint capsule develops from a condensation of mesenchyme surrounding the developing joint. At birth, the mandibular fossa is flat and there is no articular eminence; this eminence becomes prominent only following the eruption of the deciduous dentition. The early developing condylar cartilage and temporomandibular joint are shown in Figure 19.7.

Figure 19.8 illustrates the postnatal development of the mandible by lateral and occlusal views of the mandible at birth, at 6 years and in an adult. The ratio of body to ramus is greater at birth than in the adult, indicating a proportional increase with time in the development of the ramus. At birth, there is no distinct chin and the two halves of the mandible are separated by the mandibular symphysis. Ossification of the symphysis is complete during the second year, the two halves of the mandible uniting to form a single bone. The chin becomes most prominent after puberty (especially in the male). There is some evidence that the angle of the mandible decreases from birth to adulthood.

Some indication of the directions of growth of the mandible can be obtained by superimposing traces of neonatal and adult mandibles (Fig. 19.9). Indeed, there is some evidence that the region around the mental foramen is a 'fixed' point for such an endeavour.

Growth of the mandible occurs by the remodelling of bone. In general terms, increase in the height of the body occurs primarily by formation of alveolar bone, although some bone is also deposited along the lower border of the mandible. Increase in the length of the mandible is accomplished by bone deposition on the posterior surface of the ramus with compensatory resorption on its anterior surface, accompanied by deposition of bone on the posterior surface of the coronoid process and resorption on the anterior surface of the condyle. Increase in the width of the mandible is produced by deposition of bone on the outer surface of the mandible and resorption on the inner surface.

There is some controversy concerning the role of the condylar cartilages in mandibular growth. One view states that continued proliferation of this cartilage is primarily responsible for the increase in both the mandibular length and the height of the ramus. Alternatively, it has been suggested that proliferation of the condylar cartilage is a response to growth and not its cause. The latter view has been supported by experiments showing that mandibular growth is relatively unaffected following condylectomy, provided that normal mandibular function is maintained.

Although the mandible is a single bone, it may be thought of as a number of skeletal units, each associated with one or more soft tissue 'functional matrices'. The behaviour of these matrices primarily determines the growth of each skeletal unit. For example, the coronoid process forms a skeletal unit acted upon by the temporalis muscle. Sectioning of

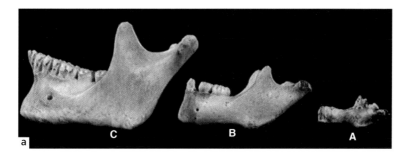

**Fig. 19.8** The postnatal development of the mandible illustrated by lateral (a) and occlusal (b) views of the mandible at birth (A), at 6 years (B) and in an adult (C).

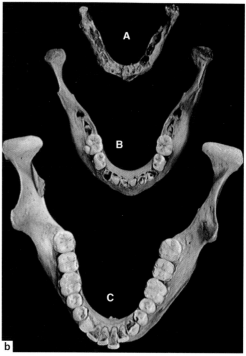

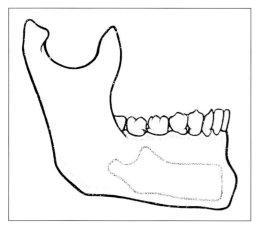

**Fig. 19.9** Superimposed neonatal and adult mandibles. Note that growth of the mandible results in posterior relocation of the ramus of the mandible.

the temporalis muscle during early mandibular development may result in atrophy or complete absence of a coronoid process in the adult mandible. Similarly, the alveolar process is influenced by the teeth, the condyle by the lateral pterygoid muscle, the ramus by the medial pterygoid and masseter muscles and the body by the neurovascular bundle.

## THE MAXILLA

As with the mandible, the maxilla develops intramembranously. The centre of ossification appears during the 8th week of intra-uterine life, close to the site of the developing deciduous canine tooth. Unlike the mandible, maxillary growth and development are not related to the appearance of secondary cartilages. Because of the maxilla's position in the developing skull, its growth is influenced by the development of the orbital, nasal and oral cavities.

From the region of the developing deciduous canine (Fig. 19.10), ossification spreads throughout the developing maxilla into its growing processes (palatine, zygomatic, frontal and alveolar). The appearance of the developing maxilla in a cleared alizarin red preparation may be seen in Figure 19.6. The ossification of the palatine processes is described on page 290.

At one time it was thought that the incisor-bearing part of the maxilla, which develops from the frontonasal process (see page 279), had a separate centre of ossification. It was consequently called the premaxilla. However, it is now clear that ossification spreads from the body of the maxilla into its incisor-bearing component.

Growth of the maxilla occurs by bone remodelling (i.e. surface deposition of bone with associated resorption) and by sutural growth. Among the agents that provide the forces separating the maxilla from the adjacent bones (thus permitting growth at the sutures) are the growing eyeballs,

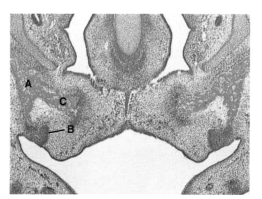

**Fig. 19.10** The early developing maxilla (A) in the region of the developing deciduous canine (B). From this site, ossification spreads throughout the developing maxilla into its growing processes (e.g. palatine process; C) (Decalcified section; Masson's trichrome; ×35).

cartilaginous nasal septum and orbital pad of fat. Thus, growth of the maxilla is not an isolated phenomenon but occurs in association with the development of the orbital, nasal and oral cavities. It has been suggested that the growing nasal septum pulls the maxilla forward by means of a septopremaxillary ligament that runs from the anterior border of the nasal septum posteroinferiorly towards the anterior nasal spine and interpremaxillary suture. As in the lower jaw (page 293), growth in height of the maxilla is related to the development of the alveolar process. It is difficult to determine how much of the adult alveolus is the result of bone deposition and how much is due to bodily displacement of the maxilla. Studies using metal implants suggest that each method of growth contributes equal amounts. Increase in height of the nasal cavity is associated with resorption of bone on the upper surface of the palatine process of the maxilla and deposition of bone on the lower surface (see Fig. 18.26).

The maxillary sinus appears as an outpocketing of the mucosa of the middle meatus of the nose at the beginning of the 4th month of intra-uterine life. Although small at birth, the maxillary sinus is identifiable radiologically. After birth, the maxillary sinus enlarges with the growing maxilla, although it is only fully developed following the eruption of the permanent dentition. Forward growth of the whole face (including the maxillae) is dependent upon growth of the spheno-occipital synchondrosis (see Figs 15.19 and 15.20).

## CLINICAL CONSIDERATIONS

Congenital abnormalities of the jaws are most often associated with 'first pharyngeal (branchial) arch syndromes'. Treacher Collins' syndrome and Pierre Robin's sequence are the two most common types of 'first arch syndrome' and have been described already in relation to the development of the face (see page 282).

Trauma and infection in the region of the temporomandibular joint may lead to an ankylosis of the condyle with the base of the skull. The most obvious sign of this condition would be limitation of jaw opening. The associated lack of function of the mandible may lead to a decreased growth on the affected side, with resultant facial asymmetry.

# Development of the tongue and salivary glands  20

## DEVELOPMENT OF THE TONGUE

The anterior two-thirds of the tongue, the 'oral tongue', develops from three swellings: two distal tongue buds (lateral lingual swellings) and a median tongue bud (tuberculum impar) (Fig. 20.1). Each is formed by proliferation of mesenchyme beneath the endodermal lining of the first pharyngeal (branchial) arch. The caudal border of this part of the developing tongue is marked by the foramen caecum (the site of origin embryologically of the thyroid gland). The distal tongue buds (lateral lingual swellings) expand rapidly to overgrow the median tongue bud (tuberculum impar) and consequently this median swelling contributes little to the adult tongue.

The posterior third of the tongue, the 'pharyngeal tongue', develops from a single midline swelling, the hypopharyngeal eminence, which is derived mainly from the third pharyngeal (branchial) arch (with a small contribution from the fourth arch). The hypopharyngeal eminence rapidly overgrows the second arch (the copula) to merge with the first arch swellings.

The muscles of the tongue develop primarily from paraxial mesoderm from occipital somites that migrate into the developing tongue.

The diverse embryological origin of the tongue explains its diverse sensory supply (see Fig. 4.12). General sensation to the anterior two-thirds of the tongue is supplied by the lingual nerve, a nerve of the first pharyngeal (branchial) arch. General sensation and taste to the posterior third of the tongue is supplied by the glossopharyngeal and superior laryngeal nerves, the nerves of the third and fourth arches. The perception of taste in the anterior two-thirds of the tongue is associated with the chorda tympani nerve, a branch of the facial nerve, the nerve of the second pharyngeal (branchial) arch. As this arch does not contribute tissue to the anterior part of the tongue, in this situation it is termed a 'pretrematic' nerve. Because the muscles of the tongue arise from occipital somites, as they migrate into the developing tongue they carry their nerve supply, the hypoglossal nerve, with them.

As previously mentioned, the thyroid gland develops between the median tongue bud (tuberculum impar) and the copula (on day 24 of intra-uterine life). It is the first endocrine gland to develop. On the fully formed tongue, the site of origin of the thyroid gland is demarcated by a small pit, the foramen caecum (see Fig. 1.15). The thyroid diverticulum remains connected to the embryonic tongue by a thyroglossal duct. This descends into the developing neck anterior to the hyoid bone and trachea. The definitive shape and position of the thyroid gland is complete by the 7th week of intra-uterine life.

## DEVELOPMENT OF THE SALIVARY GLANDS

Salivary glands initial form during the 6th and 7th weeks of intra-uterine life as solid epithelial buds extending from the developing mouth into the underlying mesenchyme. It is this oral epithelial-derived tissue that forms the secretory elements of a salivary gland; the surrounding connective tissue is derived from neural crest. The parotid gland is the first to be formed and appears near the angles of the developing mouth (stomodeum). The epithelial bud for the parotid gland extends towards the developing ears and initially branches to form solid cords. By week 10, the cords canalize to form the salivary ducts and the rounded ends of the cords form the secretory acini. It is 8 weeks later that the acini become functional. The submandibular gland is the second major salivary gland to develop (late in the 6th week of intra-uterine life). The epithelial bud grows posteriorly and laterally to the tongue and, during the 12th week, canalizes to form the ducts and acini. The submandibular gland becomes functional in week 16 of intra-uterine life. The sublingual glands appear late in the 8th week. Part of the gland develops from multiple epithelial buds that appear in the paralingual sulcus of the forming mouth. They canalize to form up to 12 ducts that open independently into the floor of the mouth.

## CLINICAL CONSIDERATIONS

The tongue is prone to many abnormalities, a considerable number of which are congenital. For example, should the lingual frenum on the

**Fig. 20.1** The schema of tongue primordia.
(a) The ventral wall of the pharynx in the 4th week of intra-uterine life. (b) The developing tongue at the 5th month. Numbers 1–4 indicate the positions of the pharyngeal (branchial) arches. Four swellings are seen: two distal tongue buds (lateral lingual swellings; A), the median tongue bud (tuberculum impar; B) and the hypopharyngeal eminence (C).

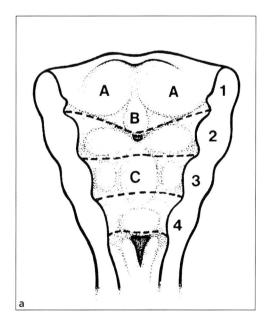
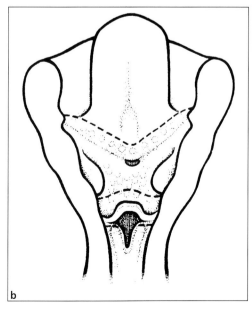

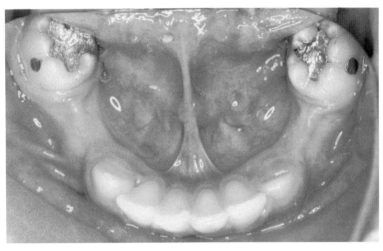

**Fig. 20.2** In this patient, the lingual frenum extends across the floor of the mouth to become attached to the lingual alveolus behind the mandibular incisors, giving an ankyloglossia.

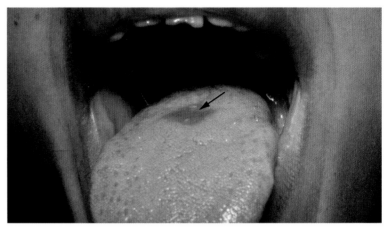

**Fig. 20.4** A median rhomboid glossitis (arrow). Courtesy of Dr J.D. Harrison.

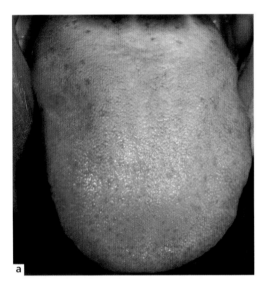

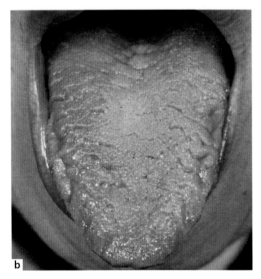

**Fig. 20.3** (a) Normal tongue. The red spots represent fungiform papillae. (b) A fissured tongue where the dorsal surface is grooved. Courtesy of Professor P.R. Morgan.

ventral surface of the tongue extend from the sublingual papilla and across the floor of the mouth, there may be a 'tongue-tie' (ankyloglossia) (Fig. 20.2). This condition is associated with restricted movement of the tongue, which, if untreated, may cause problems with breast-feeding in the newborn and later with speech.

Neonates with an excessively large tongue (macroglossia) can have major problems with breathing and feeding. Bifid tongue occurs when the right and left portions of the tongue do not merge during development. This is usually seen close to the tip of the tongue in the anterior two-thirds (oral tongue). Fissured tongue describes a situation where the surface of the tongue is deeply grooved (Fig. 20.3). As a result, the person with this condition may have to regularly clean his/her tongue in order to remove food debris within the fissures.

Median rhomboid glossitis is a condition characterized by a non-papillated, reddish region in the anterior two-thirds of the tongue in front of the sulcus terminalis and in the midline (Fig. 20.4). As the name suggests, it has a diamond-shaped outline and is usually asymptomatic. Although once thought to represent a congenital malformation, it is now thought to be associated with candidal infection, although the underlying reason for its specific location is not understood.

Although the only remains of the developing thyroid gland on the normal adult tongue is the foramen caecum, in some instances thyroid tissue can be retained at this site. When this occurs, it is referred to as a 'lingual thyroid' (see Fig. 14.78). It possible to have a lingual thyroid secrete sufficient thyroxine hormone to satisfy the metabolic requirements of the individual. Indeed, technetium-99m pertechnetate scans can be employed to detect sites of secretion of the hormone. In this context, accessory thyroid tissue may be found along the midline of the neck in locations related to the track of the migrating thyroid gland during its development. Furthermore, thyroglossal duct cysts may be located along this pathway.

# Early tooth development 21

Tooth development can be divided into three overlapping phases: initiation, morphogenesis and histogenesis. During initiation, the sites of the future teeth are established, with the appearance of tooth germs along an invagination of the oral epithelium called the dental lamina. During morphogenesis, the shape of the tooth is determined by a combination of cell proliferation and cell movement. During histogenesis, differentiation of cells (begun during morphogenesis) proceeds to give rise to the fully formed dental tissues, both mineralized (i.e. enamel, dentine and cementum) and unmineralized (i.e. dental pulp and periodontium). Tooth development is characterized by complex interactions between epithelial and mesenchymal tissues.

The first histological sign of tooth development is the appearance of a condensation of mesenchymal tissue and capillary networks beneath the presumptive dental epithelium of the primitive oral cavity. The mesenchymal cells are ectomesenchymal (neural crest) in origin, having migrated into the jaws from the margins of the neural tube. Recent research on amphibians and mammals suggests that, in addition to oral ectoderm and neural crest mesenchyme, foregut endoderm plays a role in tooth initiation.

Indeed, there is evidence that the specification of dental epithelium takes place in the oral epithelium adjacent to foregut endoderm and above midbrain neural crest cells.

By the 6th week of development, the oral epithelium thickens and invaginates into the mesenchyme to form a primary epithelial band (Fig. 21.1). By the 7th week, the primary epithelial band divides into two processes: a buccally located vestibular lamina and a lingually situated dental lamina (Fig. 21.2). The vestibular lamina contributes to the development of the vestibule of the mouth, delineating the lips and cheeks from the tooth-bearing regions. The dental lamina contributes to the development of the teeth. To form the vestibule of the oral cavity, the cells of the vestibular lamina proliferate, with subsequent degeneration of the central epithelial cells to produce the sulcus of the vestibule (Fig. 21.3). Further development of the dental lamina (Fig. 21.4) is characterized by an increase in length, although it is not known whether this results from active invagination of the lamina or upward proliferation of the mesenchyme. By the 8th week, a series of swellings develops on the deep surface of the dental lamina (Fig. 21.5). The complete dental lamina of the lower

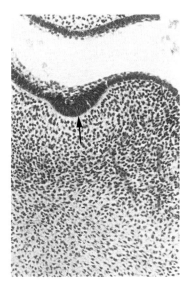

Fig. 21.1

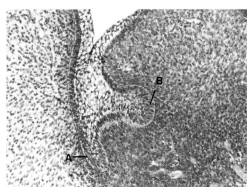

Fig. 21.2

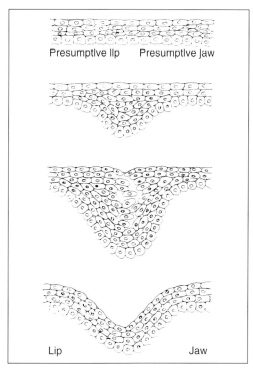

Fig. 21.3

**Fig. 21.1** Primary epithelial band (arrowed) at the 6th week of intra-uterine life (H & E; ×115).

**Fig. 21.2** The vestibular lamina (A) and dental lamina (B) seen at the 7th week of intra-uterine life (H & E; ×120). Courtesy of Dr D. Adams.

**Fig. 21.3** Diagram illustrating the formation of the vestibule of the oral cavity.

**Fig. 21.4** The developing dental lamina (A) (Masson's trichrome; ×55).

**Fig. 21.5** Model showing the stage of tooth development by the 8th week of intra-uterine life when a series of swellings representing developing tooth germs (arrows) develops on the deep surface of the dental lamina. A = vestibular fold.

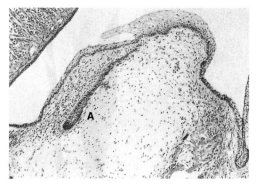

Fig. 21.4

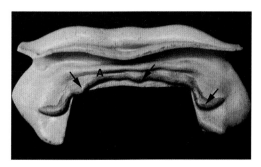

Fig. 21.5

jaw is shown in green on the model and the epithelial swellings indicating early developing tooth germs are arrowed. It is important to appreciate that the dental lamina appears as an arch-shaped band of tissue, which follows the line of the vestibular fold. Although not shown on the model, each epithelial swelling is almost completely surrounded by a mesenchymal condensation.

For descriptive purposes, tooth germs are classified into bud, cap and bell stages according to the degree of morphodifferentiation and histodifferentiation of their epithelial components (enamel organs). Leading up to the late bell stage, the tooth germ changes rapidly both in its size and shape; the cells are dividing and morphogenetic processes are taking place. At the late bell stage, hard tissues are forming and further growth of the crown is related mainly to the deposition of enamel, the rate of cell division being reduced.

## BUD STAGE

The enamel organ in the bud stage (Fig. 21.6) appears as a simple, spherical to ovoid, epithelial condensation that is poorly morphodifferentiated and histodifferentiated. It is surrounded by mesenchyme. The cells of the tooth bud have a higher RNA content than those of the overlying oral epithelium, a lower glycogen content and increased oxidative enzyme activity. It would appear that the epithelium is instructive in tooth initiation (see page 205). Nevertheless, the successful development of the tooth germ relies upon a complex interaction of the mesenchymal and epithelial components since, should these components be separated and cultured individually, neither will differentiate further. The epithelial component is separated from the adjacent mesenchyme by a basement membrane.

## CAP STAGE

By the 11th week, morphogenesis has progressed, the deeper surface of the enamel organ invaginating to form a cap-shaped structure. In the section shown in Figure 21.7, both maxillary and mandibular early cap stages are shown, each enamel organ appearing relatively poorly histodifferentiated. However, a greater distinction develops between the more

rounded cells in the central portion of the enamel organ and the peripheral cells, which are becoming arranged to form the external and internal enamel epithelia.

In the late cap stage of tooth development (Fig. 21.8), by about the 12th week, the central cells of the enlarging enamel organ have become separated (although maintaining contact by desmosomes), the intercellular spaces containing significant quantities of glycosaminoglycans. The resulting tissue is termed the stellate reticulum, although it is not fully developed until the later bell stage. The cells of the external enamel epithelium remain cuboidal, whereas those of the internal enamel epithelium become more columnar. The latter show an increase in RNA content and hydrolytic and oxidative enzyme activity, while the adjacent mesenchymal cells continue to proliferate and surround the enamel organ. The part of the mesenchyme lying beneath the internal enamel epithelium is termed the dental papilla, while that surrounding the tooth germ forms the dental follicle. A model describing the arrangement of deciduous tooth germs at 13 weeks on the dental lamina of the lower jaw is shown in Figure 21.9.

## EARLY BELL STAGE

By the 14th week, further morphodifferentiation and histodifferentiation of the tooth germ lead to the early bell stage (Fig. 21.10). The configura-

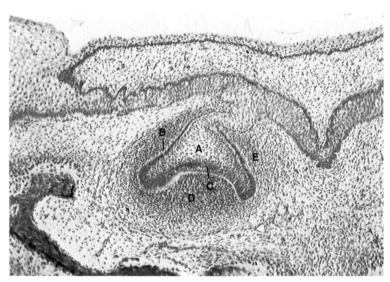

**Fig. 21.8** Late cap stage of tooth development. A = stellate reticulum; B = external enamel epithelium; C = internal enamel epithelium; D = dental papilla; E = dental follicle (H & E; ×75).

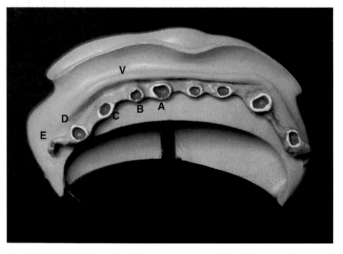

**Fig. 21.9** Model illustrating the arrangement of deciduous tooth germs (identified by the Zsigmondy system) at 13 weeks on the dental lamina of the lower jaw. V = vestibular fold.

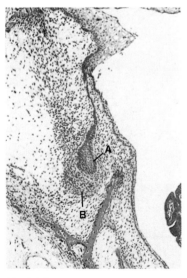
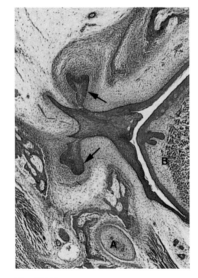

Fig. 21.6                    Fig. 21.7

**Fig. 21.6** Bud stage of tooth development. A = enamel organ; B = mesenchymal condensation (Masson's trichrome; ×60).

**Fig. 21.7** Early cap stage of tooth development (arrows). A = Meckel's cartilage; B = developing tongue (Masson's trichrome; ×32).

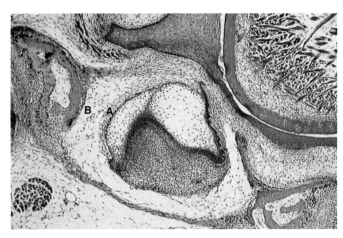

**Fig. 21.10** Early bell stage of tooth development. A = inner investing layer of dental follicle; B = outer layer of dental follicle (Masson's trichrome; ×45).

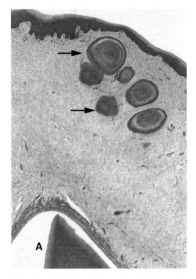

**Fig. 21.11** Epithelial pearls (of Serres) (arrows). A = enamel space (H & E; ×8). Courtesy of Dr D.A. Luke.

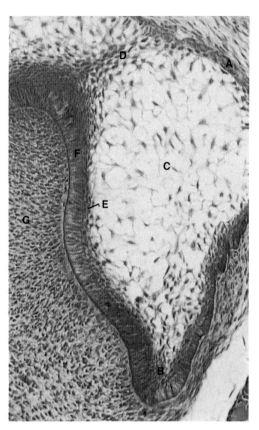

**Fig. 21.12** A high-power view of the early bell. A = external enamel epithelium; B = cervical loop; C = stellate reticulum; D = enamel cord; E = stratum intermedium; F = internal enamel epithelium; G = dental papilla (Masson's trichrome; ×120).

tion of the internal enamel epithelium broadly maps out the occlusal pattern of the crown of the tooth. This folding is related to differential mitosis along the internal enamel epithelium. The future cusps and incisal margins are sites of precocious cell maturation associated with cessation of mitosis, while areas corresponding to the fissures and margins of the tooth remain mitotically active. Thus, cusp height is related more to continued downward growth at the margin and fissures than to upward extension of the cusps. During the bell stage, any bone resorption defects that restrict the space for development of the tooth germ may be associated with the increased folding pattern of the internal enamel epithelium, leading to changes in tooth shape. Consequently, spatial impediment, and the changing mechanical forces that ensue, may be a co-factor in dental morphogenesis.

It is during the bell stage of development that the dental lamina breaks down and the enamel organ loses connection with the oral epithelium. At the same time, the dental lamina between tooth germs also degenerates. Remnants of the dental lamina may remain in the adult mucosa (Fig. 21.11) as clumps of resting cells (epithelial pearls (of Serres)) that may contain keratin and can be involved in the aetiology of cysts.

Interposed between the enamel organ and the wall of the developing bony crypt is the mesenchymal tissue of the dental follicle, which is generally considered to have three layers (Fig. 21.10). The inner investing layer is a vascular, fibrocellular condensation, three to four cells thick, immediately surrounding the tooth germ; the nuclei of the cells tend to be elongated circumferentially. The outer layer of the dental follicle is represented by a vascular mesenchymal layer that lines the developing alveolus.

Between the two layers is loose connective tissue with no marked concentration of blood vessels. There is evidence that the cells of the inner layer of the dental follicle may be derived from the neural crest.

A high degree of histodifferentiation is achieved in the early bell stage (Fig. 21.12). The enamel organ shows four distinct layers: external enamel epithelium, stellate reticulum, stratum intermedium and internal enamel epithelium.

The cervical loop at the margins of the enlarging bell-shaped enamel organ is a site of mitotic activity. Here, the central cells of the stellate reticulum/stratum intermedium may be the site of a stem cell niche providing cells that pass to the internal enamel epithelium and later form ameloblasts. This may be under the control of Notch protein in the epithelium and growth factors, such as BMP4 and FGF10, in the adjacent dental mesenchyme (see pages 342–343).

## EXTERNAL ENAMEL EPITHELIUM

As its name suggests, this forms the outer layer of cuboidal cells that limits the enamel organ. It is separated from the surrounding mesenchymal tissue by a basement membrane 1–2 μm thick, which, at the ultrastructural level, corresponds to the much narrower basal lamina with associated hemidesmosomes (see Fig. 14.29). The external enamel epithelial cells contain large, centrally placed nuclei. Ultrastructurally, they contain relatively small amounts of the intracellular organelles associated with protein synthesis (e.g. endoplasmic reticulum, Golgi material, mitochondria) and they contact each other via desmosomes and gap junctions. The external enamel epithelium is thought to be involved in the maintenance of the shape of the enamel organ and in the exchange of substances between the enamel organ and the environment. The cervical loop, at which there is considerable mitotic activity, lies at the growing margin of the enamel organ where the external enamel epithelium is continuous with the internal enamel epithelium.

## STELLATE RETICULUM

This tissue is most fully developed at the bell stage. The intercellular spaces become filled with fluid, presumably related to osmotic effects arising from the high concentration of glycosaminoglycans. The cells are star-shaped with bodies containing conspicuous nuclei and many branching processes. In addition to glycosaminoglycans, the cells also contain alkaline phosphatase but have only small amounts of RNA and glycogen. The mesenchyme-like features of the stellate reticulum include the synthesis of collagens in the tissue. Collagens types I, II and III are expressed in the cells of the stellate reticulum, although their functional significance is unclear (Fig. 21.13).

The cells of this layer (Fig. 21.14) possess little endoplasmic reticulum and few mitochondria. However, there is a relatively well developed Golgi complex, which, together with the presence of microvilli on the cell

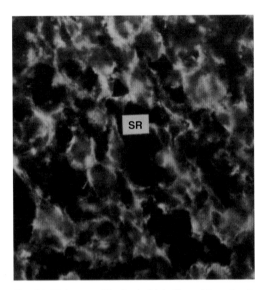

**Fig. 21.13** Immunohistological labelling of type II collagen showing positive (white) labelling in the stellate reticulum (SR) (×350).

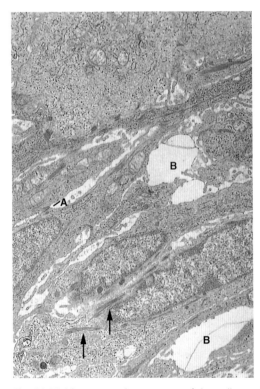

**Fig. 21.14** Ultrastructural appearance of the stellate reticulum. A = desmosomes; B = intercellular space; arrows show tonofilaments (TEM; ×6380). Courtesy of Drs H. Azawa and H. Nakamura.

surface, has been interpreted as indicating that the cells contribute to the secretion of the extracellular material. Numerous tonofilaments are present within the cytoplasm, and desmosomes and gap junctions are present between the cells.

The main function ascribed to the stellate reticulum is a mechanical one. This relates to the protection of the underlying dental tissues against physical disturbance and to the maintenance of tooth shape. It has been suggested that the hydrostatic pressure generated within the stellate reticulum is in equilibrium with that of the dental papilla, allowing the proliferative pattern of the intervening internal enamel epithelium to determine crown morphogenesis. However, a change in either of these pressures might lead to a change in the outline of the internal enamel epithelium, and this could be important for crown morphogenesis.

The stellate reticulum also produces macrophage colony-stimulating factor (MCSF), transforming growth factor (TGF)$\beta_1$ and parathyroid hormone-related protein (PTHrP). These molecules may be released into the dental follicle and help recruit, and activate, the osteoclasts necessary to resorb the adjacent alveolar bone as the developing tooth enlarges and erupts (see page 359).

## STRATUM INTERMEDIUM

This first appears at the bell stage and consists of two or three layers of flattened cells lying over the internal enamel epithelium (and its derivatives). The cells of the stratum intermedium resemble the cells of the stellate reticulum, although their intercellular spaces are smaller and the cells contain much alkaline phosphatase. It has been suggested that the stratum intermedium is concerned with the synthesis of proteins, the transport of materials to and from the enamel-forming cells (the ameloblasts) derived from the internal enamel epithelium and/or the concentration of materials.

## INTERNAL ENAMEL EPITHELIUM

The cells of this layer are columnar at the bell stage but, beginning at the regions associated with the future cusp tips (i.e. the sites of initial enamel formation), the cells become elongated. The internal enamel epithelial cells are rich in RNA but, unlike the stratum intermedium and stellate reticulum, do not contain alkaline phosphatase. Desmosomes connect the internal enamel epithelial cells and link this layer to the stratum intermedium. The internal enamel epithelium is separated from the peripheral cells of the dental papilla by a basement membrane and a cell-free zone 1–2 µm wide.

The differentiation of the dental papilla is less striking than that of the enamel organ. Until the late bell stage, the dental papilla consists of closely packed mesenchymal cells with only a few delicate extracellular fibrils. Histochemically, the dental papilla becomes rich in glycosaminoglycans.

Figure 21.15 provides a model demonstrating the arrangement of deciduous tooth germs at 17 weeks on the dental lamina of a lower jaw quadrant. The dental lamina (green) is beginning to degenerate. Downgrowths on the lingual aspect of the enamel organs indicate the early development of the successional (permanent) teeth.

## LATE BELL STAGE

The late bell stage (appositional stage) of tooth development (Fig. 21.16) is associated with the formation of the dental hard tissues, commencing at about the 18th week. Dentine formation always precedes enamel formation. Detailed accounts of amelogenesis and dentinogenesis are given in Chapters 22 and 23. In the section shown in Figure 21.16, downgrowths of the external enamel epithelium appear from the lingual sides of the

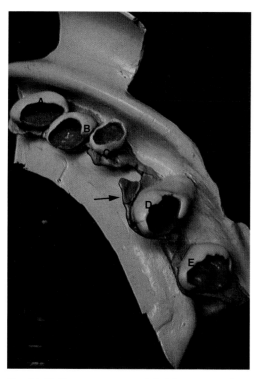

**Fig. 21.15** The arrangement of deciduous enamel organs (identified by the Palmer-Zsigmondy system) at 17 weeks on the dental lamina of a lower jaw quadrant. Arrow indicates developing permanent tooth.

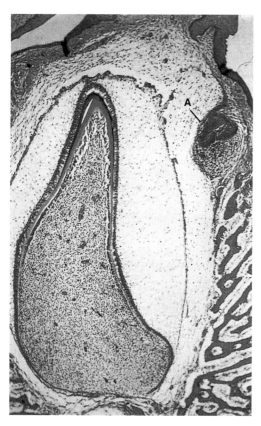

**Fig. 21.16** Late bell stage (appositional stage) of tooth development. Dentine matrix stained blue; enamel matrix stained red. A = permanent tooth (Masson's trichrome; ×60).

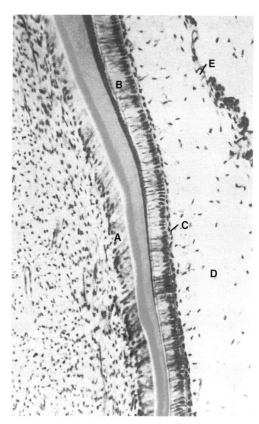

**Fig. 21.17** High-power view of a region of a tooth germ at the late bell stage to show enamel and dentine formation. A = odontoblasts; B = ameloblasts; C = stratum intermedium; D = stellate reticulum; E = external enamel epithelium; dentine matrix stained green; enamel matrix stained red (Masson's trichrome; ×130).

enamel organs. In deciduous teeth, these lingual downgrowths give rise to the tooth germs of the permanent successors and first appear alongside the incisors at about 5 months in utero. In enamel organs of permanent teeth, however, these downgrowths eventually disappear. Behind the deciduous second molar, the dental lamina grows backwards to bud off successively the permanent molar teeth. The first permanent molar appears at about 4

months in utero, the tooth bud for the second permanent molar appears about 6 months after birth, while that for the third permanent molar appears at about 4–5 years after birth.

Figure 21.17 provides a high-power view of a region of a tooth germ at the late bell stage to show enamel and dentine formation commencing at the tips of future cusps (or incisal edges). Under the inductive influence of developing ameloblasts (pre-ameloblasts), the adjacent mesenchymal cells of the dental papilla become columnar and differentiate into odontoblasts. The odontoblasts then become involved in the formation of predentine and dentine. The presence of dentine then induces the ameloblasts to secrete enamel.

## TRANSITORY STRUCTURES

During the early stages of tooth development, three transitory structures may be seen: the enamel knot, enamel cord and enamel niche.

## ENAMEL KNOT

The enamel knot (Fig. 21.18) is a localized mass of cells in the centre of the internal enamel epithelium. Characteristically, the enamel knot forms a bulge into the dental papilla, at the centre of the enamel organ. It was once thought that the enamel knot played a role in the formation of crown pattern by outlining the central fissure. However, the enamel knot soon disappears and seems to contribute cells to the enamel cord (see below). Although transitory, recent studies of the enamel knot suggest it may represent an important signalling centre during tooth development. Unlike adjacent cells, those within the enamel knot are non-proliferative and produce molecules associated with signalling in other sites. Such molecules include bone morphogenetic proteins (e.g. BMP-2 and BMP-7),

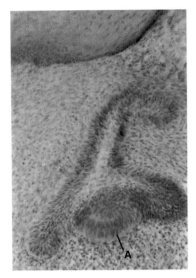

**Fig. 21.18** The enamel knot (A) (H & E; ×120).

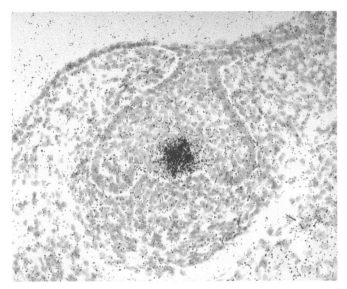

**Fig. 21.19** Localization of Fgf-4 mRNA (red stain) in a cap stage (E14) lower molar tooth by in-situ hybridization. Intense expression can be seen in the enamel knot. To aid interpretation of gene expression using $^{35}$S-labelled in-situ hybridization, both dark and bright field images were taken. Silver grains in the dark field image were selected, coloured red and then superimposed on to the bright field image (×120). Courtesy of T. Aberg.

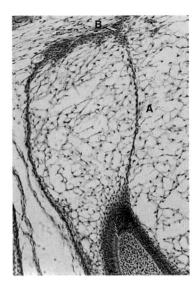

**Fig. 21.20** The enamel cord (A). B = enamel navel (Masson's trichrome; ×120).

fibroblast growth factor, p21 (cyclin-dependent kinase inhibitor), Shh (sonic hedgehog) and transcription factors (e.g. Msx1) (Fig. 21.19). The disappearance of the enamel knot by the bell stage may be associated with apoptosis.

## ENAMEL CORD

The enamel cord (Fig. 21.20) is a strand of cells seen at the early bell stage of development, that extends from the stratum intermedium into the stellate reticulum. When present, the enamel cord overlies the incisal margin of a tooth or the apex of the first cusp to develop (primary cusp). When it completely divides the stellate reticulum into two parts, reaching the external enamel epithelium, it is termed the enamel septum. Where the enamel cord meets the external enamel epithelium, a small invagination termed the enamel navel may be seen. The cells of the enamel cord are distinguished from their surrounding stellate reticulum cells by their elongated nuclei. It has been suggested that the enamel cord may be involved in the process by which the cap stage is transformed into the bell stage (acting as a mechanical tie) or that it is a focus for the origin of stellate reticulum cells.

## ENAMEL NICHE

The enamel niche (Fig. 21.21) is seen where the tooth germ appears to have a double attachment to the dental lamina (the lateral and medial enamel strands). These strands enclose the enamel niche, which appears as a funnel-shaped depression containing connective tissue. The functional significance of the enamel niche is unknown. The enamel cord and the double attachment of the tooth germ around the enamel niche were once regarded as evidence supporting the view that the complex crown form of mammalian teeth evolved from fusion of a number of individual, simpler elements. However, this view is not now accepted.

There is conflicting evidence as to when, and where, nerve fibres first appear during tooth development. It has been reported that nerve fibres are

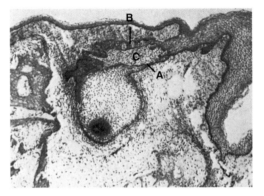

**Fig. 21.21** The enamel niche (C). A = lateral enamel strand; B = medial enamel strand (H & E; ×40).

present in the immediate vicinity of presumptive dental epithelium at the very earliest stage of tooth induction and subsequently form a plexus below the dental papilla at the cap stage. From such plexuses, the nerves spread into the dental follicle as it develops. Penetration of nerves into the dental papilla occurs with the onset of dentinogenesis. The nerve fibres associated with blood vessels are presumed to be autonomic; others lying free within the papilla are presumed to be sensory. However, the innervation of the dental papilla remains rudimentary until after birth and may be fully developed only after the tooth has erupted. Controversy also remains concerning the role of neuronal cells and neurotrophins in tooth development. Recent work indicates that, although nerve fibres seem not be required for odontogenesis, the pattern of localization of neurotrophins (and their associated receptors) does suggest a role for neural-like cells – perhaps related to the neural crest derivation of the dental mesenchyme. However, in transgenic animals where neurotrophins and their receptors are not expressed, tooth development is not affected.

## BLOOD SUPPLY

Small blood vessels invade the dental papilla at the early bell stage. They are also evident in the dental follicle in close association with the external enamel epithelium. Although vessels may lie in invaginations of the external enamel epithelium, they never penetrate the stellate reticulum.

## EPITHELIAL–MESENCHYMAL INTERACTIONS DURING TOOTH DEVELOPMENT

Tooth development (odontogenesis) is a very complex process involving many growth factors and transcription factors to ensure an ordered, and controlled, development for both individual tooth germs and the whole dentition. Epithelial–mesenchymal interactions are particularly in evidence and require signalling between the two major components of the tooth germ, one derived from the oral epithelium and one from the underlying mesenchyme. The tooth germ can be readily manipulated experimentally and therefore has been used not only to investigate the processes involved in odontogenesis but also as a useful model for understanding epithelial–mesenchymal interactions in general. Increasingly, the main purpose of research into odontogenesis is being seen in the context of tooth 'regeneration' for clinical dentistry. By understanding early odontogenic signals, it may eventually be possible to engineer dental tissues from stem cells. Although many problems await, arriving at such techniques to allow for tooth regeneration would undoubtedly revolutionize dentistry.

## INITIATION OF TOOTH DEVELOPMENT

Techniques have been developed whereby it is possible to dissect out, and recombine, mammalian epithelium and mesenchyme in different combinations before there are any signs of tooth development. Tissue recombination experiments have shown that the epithelium lining the first pharyngeal (branchial) arch has 'odontogenic potential' as, when first arch epithelium is combined with first arch mesenchyme, tooth germs form. However, with the reciprocal experiment, no tooth germs develop when the epithelium from the second arch is combined with first or second arch mesenchyme (instead, bone and cartilage develop). The potential for first arch epithelium to initiate tooth development only exists in the very early stages of odontogenesis. Thereafter, when first arch mesenchyme is combined with

second arch epithelium (which, as stated above, does not initiate odontogenesis), tooth germs are formed. This suggests that, after initiation by the oral epithelium, the 'control' of tooth development passes to the mesenchyme. This view is supported by research into the role of the enamel organ and the papilla at the cap stage of development (see page 307).

Many investigations have been conducted into the role of neural crest cells (ectomesenchyme) in odontogenesis and there is much evidence from both non-mammalians and mammalians showing that the mesenchyme within a tooth germ is derived from the neural crest. It has also been shown that cranial neural crest cells taken from their site of origin (near the developing neural tube), and before their migration into the pharyngeal arches, can produce tooth germs when combined with first arch epithelium (Fig. 21.22) but not when combined with second arch epithelium or epithelium from other sites (Fig. 21.23). Thus, it seems that the neural crest tissue migrating into the first arch is 'unspecified' and requires an interaction with the oral epithelium before it becomes odontogenic. Thus, the oral epithelium is instructive.

## MECHANISMS RESPONSIBLE FOR SPECIFYING THE TOOTH-FORMING ZONES IN THE ORAL REGION AND FOR CONTROLLING TOOTH NUMBER

The transcription factor Pitx2 is selectively expressed in the oral epithelium from the earliest stages of oral cavity formation and its expression is thereafter restricted to dental epithelium. As with a broad range of other tissues, Sonic hedgehog (Shh) is a major determinant of (or at least marks) the sites at which teeth develop. *Shh* gene expression is restricted to the dental epithelium at sites of tooth development and also appears to be involved in epithelial mesenchymal interactions. As Shh increases cell proliferation, restriction of expression to tooth-forming regions is important and seems to be accomplished by interactions with Wnt-signalling molecules. Indeed, Wnt helps maintain boundaries between tooth-forming areas and non-tooth-forming regions. The importance of Wnt/7b signalling can also be seen from experiments where its activity is inhibited, leading to the arrest of tooth morphogenesis at an early stage. Conversely, where

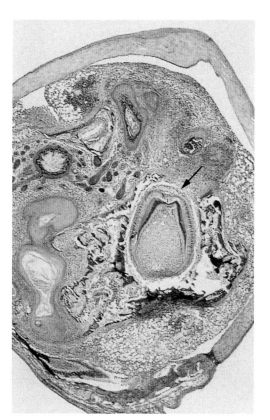

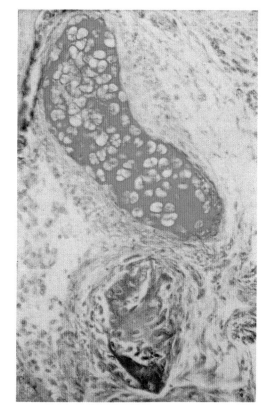

Fig. 21.22 The result of culturing premigratory cranial neural crest with oral epithelium. Note the developing tooth (arrowed) (Masson's trichrome; ×65). From Lumsden AGS 1988 Spatial organisation of the epithelium and the role of neural crest cells in the initiation of the mammalian tooth germ. *Development* 103(suppl): 155–169.

Fig. 21.23 The result of culturing premigratory neural crest with limb epithelium. Teeth do not develop; only islands of bone and cartilage (Masson's trichrome; ×200). From Lumsden AGS 1988 Spatial organisation of the epithelium and the role of neural crest cells in the initiation of the mammalian tooth germ. *Development* 103(suppl): 155–169.

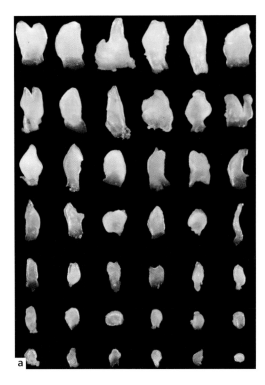

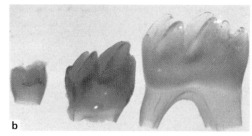

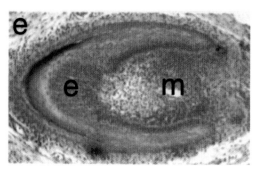

**Fig. 21.25** Chick 'tooth-like structure' formed by recombining chick mandibular epithelium (e) with chick skin mesenchyme (m) and culturing for 2 days (×80). From Chen Y et al 2000 Conservation of early odontogenic signalling pathways in Aves. *Proceedings of the National Academy of Sciences of the United States of America* 97: 10044–10049.

**Fig. 21.24** (a) 42 mineralized teeth of various sizes collected from one developing molar tooth in a mouse in which Wnt signalling was sustained. (b) The three molars present in normal mouse controls (×13). From Jarvinen E et al 2006 Continuous tooth generation in mouse is induced by activated epithelial Wnt/β-catenin signalling. *Proceedings of the National Academy of Sciences of the United States of America* 103: 18627–18632.

Wnt signalling is stimulated (by stabilizing β-catenin) in the oral epithelium, it results in the production of dozens of extra teeth. In the molar region of mice, these supernumerary teeth are in the form of unicuspid cones (Fig. 21.24) and this has been interpreted as evidence of a direct role for Wnt signalling in the formation of supernumerary enamel knots. It has also been suggested that the retention of Wnt signalling may account for the continuous succession of teeth in non-mammalian vertebrates.

An additional way of restricting Shh signalling activity involves the upregulation of its receptor, Patched (Ptc1) in excess of the Shh ligand and this mechanism has been found in the non-tooth-forming areas (the diastema region of rodents).

The *Pax9* and *Msx1* genes appear to be required to enable the tooth germ to progress beyond the bud stage, as absence of the gene arrests the tooth germ at the bud stage.

Some important information concerning the mechanisms responsible for specifying tooth–forming zones has arisen from study of 'hen's teeth'. The absence of teeth in modern birds has given rise to the phrase 'as rare as hen's teeth'. However, the topic also provides a stimulus to research into epithelial–mesenchymal interactions. Because the ancestors of birds had teeth, the question arises as to whether there is any latent potential in either the epithelium and/or mesenchyme of birds to form teeth and whether this potential can be unlocked. Research has shown that a number of growth and transcription factors are expressed during tooth development in mammals are present in the oral epithelial and mesenchymal tissues of chick (e.g. *Fgf8*, *Pitx2*, *Barx1* and *Pax9*). However, other factors are missing, such as *Shh*, *Bmp4*, *Msx1* and *Msx2*. When *Bmp4* protein is added exogenously to chick mandibles, it induces the expression of *Msx1* and *Msx2* in the mesenchyme. When chick epithelium is cultured with chick dorsal skin mesenchyme that does contain *Bmp4*, tooth-bud-like structures are produced (Fig. 21.25).

Experiments have been undertaken in which chick neural crest is replaced by mouse neural crest (Fig. 21.26). The resulting mouse/chick chimeras produce tooth germs (Fig. 21.27) up to the stage of the initial formation of organic matrix. This matrix is regarded as a dentine matrix, as the odontoblast-like cells produce dentine sialoprotein and nestin. This experiment indicates that mouse neural-crest-derived mesenchymal cells

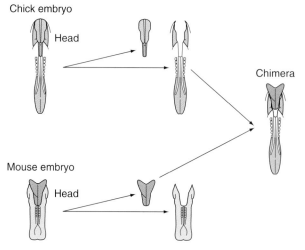

**Fig. 21.26** Diagram of the experimental procedure of mouse neural tube transplantation into chick host embryos for the creation of a chick/mouse chimera that has an abnormal head morphology. From Mitsiadis TA, Caton J, Cobourne M 2006 Waking up the sleeping beauty: recovery of the ancestral bird odontogenic program. *Journal of Experimental Zoology (Molecular and Developmental Evolution)* 306B: 227–233.

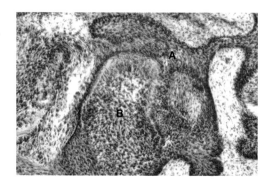

**Fig. 21.27** 'Chick tooth' derived from the chick/mouse chimera experiments shown in Fig. 21.26 at the bell stage. The epithelial enamel organ (A) is chick-derived and the dental papilla (B) is mouse-derived. The blue staining represents initial dentine matrix (Masson's blue trichrome; ×63). Courtesy of Dr T.A. Mitsiadis.

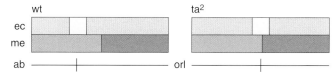

**Fig. 21.28** Model of alteration in the inductive interactions in wild-type chicks (wt) and ta² jaw leading to the initiation of teeth in the ta² mutant. In the wild type, a regional signalling centre is localized in the epithelium (yellow) by the interaction between Fgf8, Bmp4 and Shh signalling. This signalling centre demarcates the boundary between the oral and aboral epithelium (vertical mark on horizontal ab–orl line). This epithelial signalling centre does not overlie oral mesenchyme (purple) competent to make appendage structures. In the ta² mutant, early changes in Fgf8, Bmp4 and Shh signalling lead to medial positioning of the forming oral/aboral boundary such that the signalling centre and underlying competent mesenchyme are juxtaposed, permitting initiation of tooth developmental programmes. ec = ectoderm; me = mesenchyme; ab = aboral; orl = oral epidermis. From Harris MP, Hasso SM, Ferguson MWJ, Fallon JF 2006 The development of Archosaurian first-generation teeth in a chicken mutant. *Current Biology* 16: 371–377.

in avian oral epithelium have the ability to induce the avian oral epithelium and thus initiate the avian tooth developmental programme. That the teeth fail to mineralize properly and produce enamel is not surprising, as the chick genome appears to lack the genes associated with the production of enamel matrix.

A recent experiment that sheds further light on why modern birds lack teeth relates to a chick mutant known as 'talpid' (ta²). This is an autosomal recessive mutation that has serious consequences for the development of many organ systems. However, this mutant also uniquely exhibits the development of simple, unmineralized, tooth-like structures in the jaws. In explanation, from analysis of the distribution of growth and transcription factors (Fig. 21.28), it can be seen that a responsive mesenchyme is present in the normal (wild-type) situation that is displaced away from the responsive epithelium above, whereas in the mutant talpid the responsive mesenchyme is displaced to lie directly beneath the responsive epithelium.

## MECHANISMS RESPONSIBLE FOR SPECIFYING TOOTH TYPE AND TOOTH SHAPE (MORPHOGENESIS)

Early experiments were designed to answer the question posed by investigators: which of the two components is more important for inducing morphogenesis and histogenesis – the enamel organ or the dental papilla? Such experiments involved interchanging the epithelial and mesenchymal components between different developing teeth (incisors and molars) and with tissues from non-dental regions. The results indicated that, at the cap stage of tooth development, the principal organizer is the dental papilla, in terms of both morphogenesis and histogenesis. The result of culturing dental papilla mesenchyme with epithelium from the developing foot pad (Fig. 21.29) is normal tooth development, illustrating the importance of the dental papilla. On the other hand, if the enamel organ of a tooth is cultured with mesenchyme from the developing foot pad (Fig. 21.30), tooth development does not occur. Similar experiments have been conducted to determine whether the enamel organ or the dental papilla determine tooth shape. Such experiments involve separating and recombining enamel organ and papilla at the cap stage. Should an incisor enamel organ be combined with a molar papilla, the resulting tooth is molariform. Furthermore, if a molar enamel organ is combined with an incisor papilla, the resulting tooth is incisiform. Thus, as for histogenesis, the dental papilla is the dominant tissue determining tooth shape at the cap stage.

From the above experiments, research has progressed to try to understand the molecular mechanisms involved in morphogenesis. The underlying control of such patterning is based upon the hypothesis that, as in other parts of the body (such as the vertebral column), patterning is related to

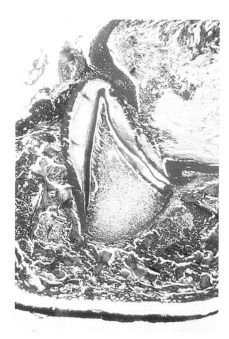

**Fig. 21.29** The result of culturing dental papilla mesenchyme with epithelium from the developing foot pad. A normal tooth develops (Masson's trichrome; ×40). From Kollar EJ, Baird GR 1970 Tissue interactions in embryonic mouse tooth germs II. The inductive role of the dental papilla. *Journal of Embryology and Experimental Morphology* 24: 173–186.

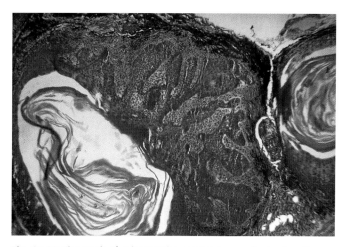

**Fig. 21.30** The result of culturing the enamel organ of a tooth with mesenchyme from the developing foot pad. Note the absence of tooth development (Masson's trichrome; ×75). Courtesy of Professor E. Kollar and the editor of the *Journal of Embryology and Experimental Morphology*.

the spatially restricted expression of homeobox genes in the ectomesenchyme of the developing jaws (referred to as the odontogenic homeobox code). These genes contain DNA-binding proteins that regulate gene transcription, thus controlling the expression of other genes necessary for the development of a particular structure, in this case a tooth. Accordingly, the group of homeobox genes expressed in the presumptive incisor region will dictate that incisiform teeth develop here, while the group of homeobox genes expressed at the back of the tooth row (in the presumptive molar region) will specify molariform teeth. For this hypothesis to be tenable, an important prerequisite is to establish that the presumptive incisor and molar regions do indeed contain some difference in their homeobox gene array and this feature has been demonstrated. It is known that the neural crest cells for the mesenchyme of the first pharyngeal arch express non-Hox homeobox genes, including *Msx1*, *Msx2*, *Dlx1*, *Dlx2*, *Barx1* and *Alx3*. Different combinations of these homeobox genes appear to instruct the tooth germ with respect to its tooth type. Thus, the neural-crest-derived mesenchyme in the incisor region expresses *Msx1* (but not *Barx1*) while

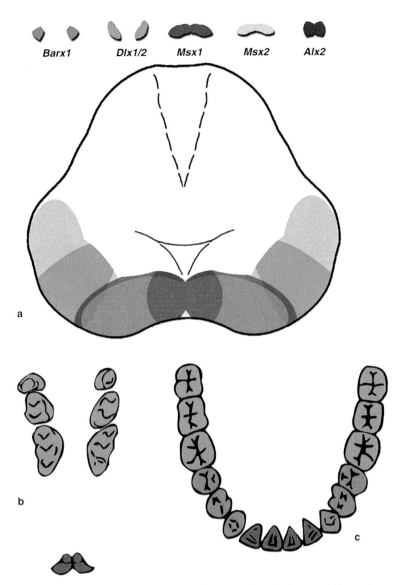

**Fig. 21.31** Schematic diagrams to show the mesenchymal odontogenic homeobox gene code. (a) Diagram illustrating the lower jaw of the mouse. Note the overlap (orange) between the domains of *Msx1* (red) and *Msx2* (yellow). (b) Model representing the mouse dentition. Note that molars develop from cells expressing *Barx1* and incisors from cells expressing *Msx1*, *Msx2* and *Alx3*. (c) Model representing the human dentition. It is predicted that incisors develop from cells expressing *Msx1*, *Msx2* and *Alx3*, canines and premolars from cells expressing *Msx1* and *Msx2* and molars from cells expressing *Barx1*. Courtesy of Professor P.T. Sharpe and the editor of *Bioessays*.

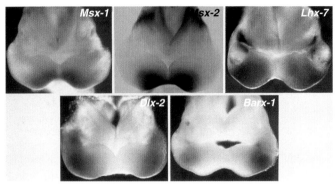

**Fig. 21.32** Whole-mount in-situ hybridization to show localization of homeobox genes (the darkly 'staining' regions) for the developing mandible. Courtesy of Professor P.T. Sharpe.

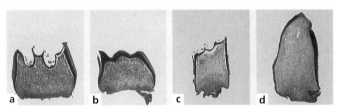

**Fig. 21.33** The results of experiments to transform teeth from incisor to molar shape following downregulation of *Msx1* and upregulation of *Barx1* in incisors. (a) Control section of normal molar. (d) Control section of normal incisor. (b, c) Sections from incisor teeth showing change to molar shape following upregulation of *Barx1* in the mesenchyme (×25). From Tucker AS, Matthews KL, Sharpe PT 1998 Transformation of tooth type induced by inhibition of BMP signaling. *Science* 282: 1136–1138.

neural-crest-derived mesenchyme in the molar region expresses *Barx1* (but not *Msx1*) (Figs 21.31, 21.32). As with other systems of early development and differentiation, temporal factors mean that there is only a narrow window of opportunity to successfully manipulate the homeobox genes. The difference in distribution of homeobox genes between the incisor and molar regions is at least consistent with the odontogenic homeobox code hypothesis. Evidence to support the importance of such molecules in initiating tooth development can be seen in transgenic mice where, for example, an absence of the homeobox gene *Msx1* results in tooth development being arrested at the bud stage. Similarly, early mesenchyme isolated from the overlying epithelium can still continue to develop in tissue culture if molecules such as BMPs and FGFs are added to the medium.

The odontogenic homeobox code can be considered in the light of a 'field model hypothesis' where each tooth germ starts the same but different concentrations of morphogens (e.g. growth factors) in the local environment are responsible for producing different tooth types. The patterning of the dentition has been shown to be related to the polarity of the epithelium. This epithelial polarity is thought to be associated with expression

of FGF-8 and BMP-4 growth factors. Accordingly, FGF-8 (with FGF-9) is expressed in the future molar region, whereas BMP-4 is expressed in the future incisor region. In relation to the homeobox genes, FGF-8 stimulates expression of *Barx1* and *Dlx2* and BMP4 stimulates *Msx1* and *Msx2* but inhibits *Barx1*.

One way of assessing the 'field model hypothesis' is to try to change the odontogenic homeobox code and determine whether the shape of a developing tooth can be altered. In this context, it is possible to culture early incisor tooth germs and absorb the Bmp produced by the epithelium (so that it does not switch on *Msx1* in the underlying mesenchyme cells). This is achieved by placing on the epithelial surface very small beads soaked in noggin protein, which is a Bmp antagonist. In this situation, not only is *Msx1* downregulated in the mesenchyme but *Barx1* (normally only present in the molar region) is seen to be expressed. When such tooth germs are then transplanted in vivo to renal capsules and allowed to continue to develop, multicuspid teeth with a molariform rather than an incisiform morphology can be produced (Fig. 21.33). The odontogenic homeobox code therefore would explain the formation of different tooth homologies.

There is also evidence that the odontogenic homeobox code differs in the mandibular and maxillary regions. This is based upon the observation that, when *Dlx1* and *Dlx2* gene expression is disrupted, mandibular molars still developed but not maxillary molars.

In contrast to the 'field model hypothesis', a 'clonal model hypothesis' has been put forward to explain tooth form. Accordingly, the tooth type is prespecified (probably at the original site of the neural crest cells) and is not dependent on the environment within the jaws. An experiment in which the possible contribution of the jaw environment was assessed required the removal of the dental lamina in the developing molar region, together with the surrounding mesenchyme. This very early, and undifferentiated, tooth germ (which would have given rise to the first molar) was then cultured in a site well away from the jaws. A tooth germ of the first molar at the cap stage of development removed from an embryo and transplanted

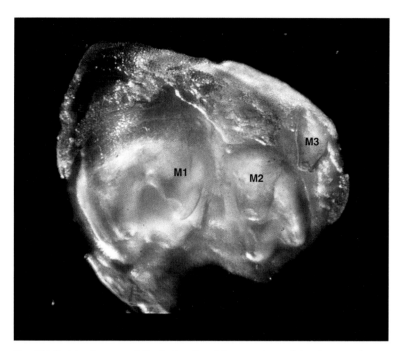

**Fig. 21.34** A tooth germ of the first molar at the cap stage of development has been removed from an embryo and transplanted for culture in a different site. Note the development of first (M1), second (M2) and third molars (M3) (Alizarin red whole-mount; ×10). From Lumsden AGS 1988 Spatial organisation of the epithelium and the role of neural crest cells in the initiation of the mammalian tooth germ. *Development* 103(suppl): 155–169.

for culture at a different site was seen to continue to develop normally and the remaining second and third molars also developed (Fig. 21.34). This finding is consistent with the idea that a series of related structures can form by budding off from a single precursor and that the differences between the individual structures (e.g. size and crown complexity) result from the increasing age of the tooth-budding region as it grows distally from the jaw (rather than from local environmental factors in the jaws). This 'clonal model hypothesis' could explain the successionary tooth formation of the second and third molars.

The formation of the specific shape of a tooth (including the formation of cusps) is signalled during the bud and cap stages of tooth development. Particular significance in morphogenesis has recently been placed on the presence of the enamel knot (Fig. 21.19). The shape of the enamel organ (producing the shape of the crown of the tooth) relates to the pattern of folding seen within the internal enamel epithelium and/or the forces present on either side of it. The enamel knot is thought to play a role in this morphogenesis as it is associated with each main cusp that develops and as it possesses molecules seen in other patterning situations. The enamel knot is under the direction of signals emanating from the underlying mesenchyme, Bmp4 stimulating the expression of *p21* (an inhibitor of cell proliferation) to produce the enamel knot. The enamel knot itself also expresses signalling molecules (FGF-4, Shh and BMPs and Wnt growth factors). Shh in particular is involved in the formation of the cap stage of the tooth germ, regulating cell survival at the tip of the enamel organ as it changes from the bud to the cap. Indeed, the survival of the enamel knot is a balance between growth and apoptosis (Fgf4 for growth, Bmp4 for apoptosis).

## THE NATURE OF THE INDUCTIVE MESSAGE

During tooth development, 'messages' pass between the epithelium and mesenchyme to produce changes of increasing complexity (i.e. differentiation) within the cell layers. The term 'induction' is used to describe the effect that one cell layer has on another. It has clearly been shown that bioactive signalling molecules in the form of small proteins pass between the epithelium and mesenchyme and usually have important interactions

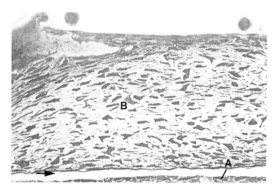

**Fig. 21.35** The enamel organ (A) and dental papilla mesenchyme (B) cultured on either side of a porous membrane (pore size 0.1 μm) (arrowed). No differentiation has occurred and cell processes do not pass through the membrane (Toluidine blue; ×70). Courtesy of Professor I. Thesleff and the editor of the *Journal of Embryology and Experimental Morphology*.

with the receptors on the cell membrane. These interactions set off a series of intracellular cascades that regulate gene expression and change the behaviour of the cell. It can still be instructive to refer to early experiments designed to investigate the nature of the inductive message. Indeed, three main hypotheses were put forward to explain how information leading to induction might be transferred between epithelium and mesenchyme:

1. A chemical substance (short-range hormone) is produced by one cell layer and diffuses across the narrow intervening space to be taken up and cause induction in the other cell layer.
2. Induction is triggered by direct cell-to-cell contact and does not involve a diffusible molecule.
3. Induction is due to the presence of the initial extracellular matrix, a thin layer situated between the epithelium and mesenchyme and comprising the basal lamina and adjacent region. The extracellular matrix has a complex composition, consisting of collagen (mainly type IV but possibly some type I and III), proteoglycans and glycoproteins.

To assess which of the three hypotheses is likely to provide the correct explanation for reciprocal control of differentiation, experiments have been undertaken in which the epithelial and mesenchymal components are dissected out and separated at the early bell stage, before any significant degree of cytodifferentiation. They are then recombined for tissue culture, but with a porous membrane placed between; the size of the pores in the membrane can be varied to ascertain the point at which both ameloblasts and odontoblasts differentiate. As molecules can readily diffuse through a pore size just less than 0.2 μm, the absence of differentiation seen in Figure 21.35 appears to argue against hypothesis 1 above (a diffusible chemical substance). The lack of differentiation with pores less than 0.2 μm coincides with both the absence of the extracellular matrix and with the absence of cell processes invading the porous membrane. Thus, either cell-to-cell contact or the extracellular matrix could be implicated in differentiation. Differentiation of the enamel organ and dental papilla are seen when pore size is 0.6 μm and cell processes are evident passing through the micropores (Fig. 21.36). However, as specialized cell contacts between differentiating odontoblasts and ameloblasts does not appear to occur in vivo (although the processes do come very close together), it is likely that the extracellular matrix may have an important role in induction. The extracellular matrix itself is a product of both the epithelial and the mesenchymal cells.

Evidence indicating the importance of the extracellular matrix in the inductive process can be obtained from the following experiments. First, drugs are available that can inhibit the formation of specific components of the extracellular matrix: for example, lathyrogens interfere with cross linking of collagen. When added to tissue culture medium, these drugs

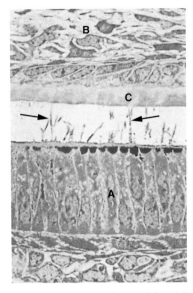

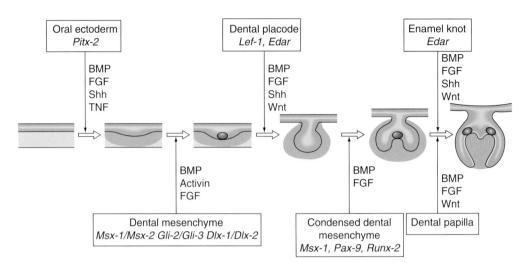

**Fig. 21.36** The enamel organ (A) and dental papilla mesenchyme (B) cultured on either side of a porous membrane (pore size 0.6 μm). C = predentine; cell processes from odontoblasts passing through pores are arrowed (Mallory's; ×45). Courtesy of Professor I. Thesleff and the editor of the *Journal of Embryology and Experimental Morphology*.

**Fig. 21.37** Model of the molecular regulation of tooth development from initiation to crown morphogenesis. Interactions between epithelial (green) and mesenchymal tissues (blue) are mediated by signal molecules (BMP = bone morphogenetic proteins; FGF = fibroblast growth factors; Shh = sonic hedgehog; TNF = tumour necrosis factor). These signals operate throughout development and regulate the expression of genes in the responding tissues (shown in boxes). Signalling centres (red) appear in the epithelium reiteratively and secrete locally many different signals that regulate morphogenesis and tooth shape. Courtesy of Professor I. Thesleff.

inhibit differentiation of the tooth germ. Second, isolated pieces of extracellular matrix will produce histological signs of differentiation in internal enamel epithelial cells of the enamel organ. It is conceivable that, in relation to the physical properties of the initial extracellular matrix, this matrix provides a surface for attachment of cells or enables interactions between bioactive molecules that induce early differentiation.

## CONCLUDING REMARKS

The experiments described above indicate that successful tooth development depends on complex reciprocal interactions between the dental epithelium and underlying mesenchyme. They also show that, initially, the epithelium from the first pharyngeal arch is instructive on the underlying neural-crest-derived ectomesenchyme. At a later stage, however, this instructive capacity is transferred to the mesenchyme, which can then induce epithelium of non-first-arch origin to help form a tooth germ. Signals involving bioactive molecules (such as transcription factors, growth factors, cytokines, etc.) are produced in a specific spatial and temporal sequence and the cascade of events results in a tooth consisting of the appropriate tissues and of an appropriate shape.

As mentioned earlier, a considerable number of genes and growth factors are expressed during early tooth development. A database has been established by the University of Helsinki (http://honeybee.helsinki.fi/toothexp) to allow comparisons of the expression patterns as a starting point for experimental studies. This database presently describes the expression at different stages of tooth development of growth factors, receptors, signalling molecules, transcription factors, intracellular and extracellular molecules and plasma membrane molecules. For growth factors, for example, a variety of BMPs, FGFs, Shh and TGFs are expressed at different stages of development. Epidermal growth factor appears to be expressed only during the bell stage of development. Neurotrophins, which are growth factors promoting neuronal growth, are also expressed at various developmental stages. Recent research has suggested that the dental epithelium signals to the underlying mesenchymal cells via Bmps (particularly Bmp2 and Bmp4), and Fgfs. Consequently, mesenchymal cell proliferation and condensation are stimulated and the expression

in the mesenchyme of syndecan and tenascin are upregulated (syndecan is a cell-surface heparan sulphate proteoglycan that binds to tenascin, probably influencing cell condensation). Bmps also induce the expression in the mesenchyme of *Msx1* and *Msx2* homeobox gene transcription factors.

Particular attention has been paid to the earliest stages of tooth development to help determine the biological mechanisms responsible for switching on the cascade of events for tooth development. As previously mentioned, the activation of non-Hox homeobox genes is of crucial importance at this time. These genes contain DNA-binding proteins that regulate gene transcription, thus controlling the expression of other genes necessary for the development of a particular structure, in this case a tooth. To date, the precise functions of such homeobox genes are not known, but they may be assumed to regulate the production of molecules important in morphogenesis (such as growth factors, factors controlling cell division and apoptosis, cell-surface receptors, integrins and cell adhesion molecules and cytoskeletal elements). The complexity of the topic is partly indicated in Figure 21.37 (this figure contains just a selection of the molecules known to be present in the developing tooth and their number is frequently being added to). Evidence to support the importance of such molecules in initiating tooth development can be seen in transgenic mice where, for example, deletion of the homeobox genes such as *Msx1* and *Pax9* results in tooth development being arrested at the bud stage. Similarly, early mesenchyme isolated from the overlying epithelium can still continue to develop in tissue culture if molecules such as BMPs and FGFs are added to the medium. Consideration also needs to be given as to how the forces are generated during morphogenesis.

## CLINICAL CONSIDERATIONS

Although much is known about normal tooth development, many details await investigation and it is hardly surprising, therefore, that we know relatively little about the changes in the tooth germ that lead to the range of congenital tooth abnormalities generally recognized. Clearly, disturbance of the epithelial–mesenchymal interactions can markedly disturb tooth development. Also, splitting of a tooth germ or joining of adjacent germs can be responsible for some of the variations in tooth numbers and shape. Trauma and infection of the deciduous predecessors have also been implicated in the malformation of the permanent teeth. Malformations of teeth can occur in the deciduous or permanent dentition, although they are more common in the permanent dentition. This may reflect the stable environment of the child before birth.

Malformations of teeth can be related to variations in size, in shape, in number, or in structure and many of these are illustrated on pages 54, 55.

Macrodontia refers to an enlarged tooth (see Fig. 2.167) and microdontia to a very much reduced size. Microdontia may accompany clefts of the lip or palate, Ehlers–Danlos syndrome, hypopituitary disorders and ectodermal disorders. A frequent variation in shape is the peg-shaped maxillary lateral incisor (see Fig. 2.166). Gemination refers to a situation where there is partial cleavage of a tooth germ (see Figs 2.168–2.169). Fusion occurs where there is union of two adjacent germs. In both germination and fusion, the appearance can suggest a 'double' tooth. However, in fusion the total number of teeth is one less than normal. Concrescence is the fusion of teeth at the roots. Abnormal tooth shapes (such as Hutchinson's incisors and mulberry molars) can result from congenital syphilis (Figs 21.38, 21.39).

Anodontia refers to a complete absence of teeth and this condition is very rare and may be found in some cases of ectodermal dysplasias. More commonly in ectodermal dysplasia a few teeth are present (Fig. 21.40).

Where just one or two teeth are absent (hypodontia), the most frequently affected teeth are the permanent third molars, then the permanent maxillary second incisors, followed by the second premolars. Having seen the important part played by certain transcription factors during tooth formation (pages 307–309), it is not surprising to find in both mice and humans that an absence of teeth has been associated with mutations in *Pax1* and *Msx1* genes.

Hyperdontia is an increase in tooth number, either by the appearance of supernumerary teeth (not having normal morphology – see page 54) or supplemental teeth (having normal morphology). A 'mesiodens' in the middle of the maxilla is an example of a supernumerary tooth (see Fig. 2.165). Figure 21.41 illustrates a very rare situation with a large number of supernumerary teeth and one supplemental tooth. In cleidocranial dysplasia, a condition caused by mutations in *Cbfa1*, many of the teeth may remain unerupted (see Fig. 26.55). In addition, there may be a number of supernumerary teeth.

During tooth development, components of the enamel organ may undergo abnormal proliferation to form a tumour-like mass of hard tissue called an odontome. An odontome may be symptomless or may be associated with a localized swelling. It may be found in the anterior region of the maxilla, where its presence may prevent eruption of an anterior tooth (Fig. 21.42), or it may also be encountered in the posterior region of the jaws, where it may prevent a posterior tooth from erupting (Fig. 21.43). When the odontome is comprised of many small, discrete, simple, tooth-like structures (denticles), each containing the normal arrangement of

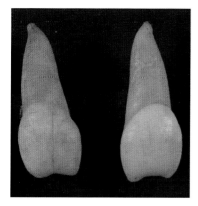

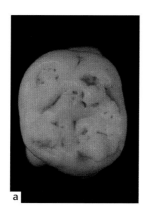

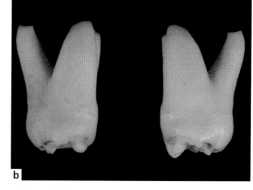

**Fig. 21.38** Maxillary permanent first incisors from a patient with congenital syphilis, showing a barrel-shaped outline and notched edge ('Hutchinson's incisors'). Courtesy of the Royal College of Surgeons of England.

**Fig. 21.39** Maxillary permanent molar teeth from a patient with congenital syphilis. (a) Occlusal view and (b) side view, both showing projections on the crown surface ('mulberry molars'). Courtesy of the Royal College of Surgeons of England.

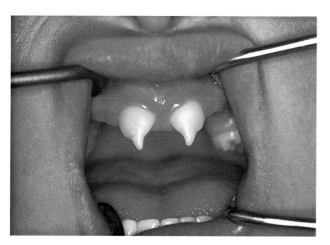

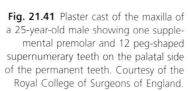

**Fig. 21.40** Ectodermal dysplasia showing absent teeth and conically shaped teeth. Courtesy of Dr P. Smith.

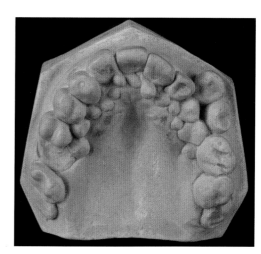

**Fig. 21.41** Plaster cast of the maxilla of a 25-year-old male showing one supplemental premolar and 12 peg-shaped supernumerary teeth on the palatal side of the permanent teeth. Courtesy of the Royal College of Surgeons of England.

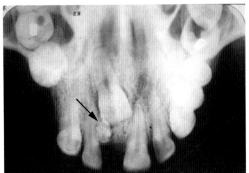

Fig. 21.42

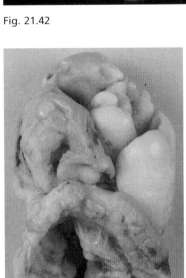

Fig. 21.44

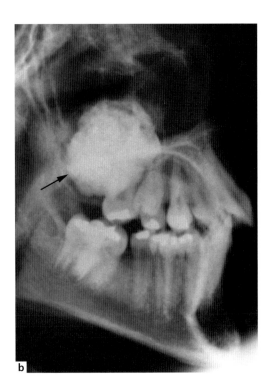

Fig. 21.43

**Fig. 21.42** Maxillary occlusal radiograph showing the presence of an odontome (arrow) whose presence has prevented the eruption of the underlying permanent first incisor. Courtesy of Professor D. Smith.

**Fig. 21.43** (a) 11-year-old patient in whom the maxillary first left permanent molar has failed to erupt because of the presence of an odontome. (b) Lateral radiograph of the patient in (a) showing the presence of a large odontome (arrow) associated with the non-eruption of the maxillary first left permanent molar. Courtesy of Dr J.D. Harrison.

**Fig. 21.44** Compound odontome removed from a patient showing a number of well defined, tooth-like structures of different shapes and sizes. Courtesy of the Royal College of Surgeons of England.

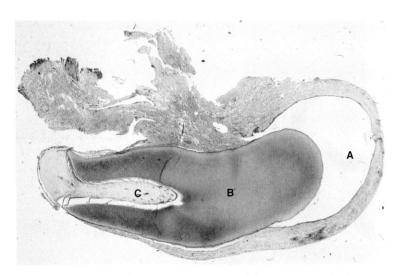

**Fig. 21.45** Micrograph of a single denticle dissected from a compound odontoma showing normal distribution of dental tissues. A = enamel space; B = dentine; C = dental pulp (Demineralized section; H & E; ×12). Courtesy of Dr J.D. Harrison.

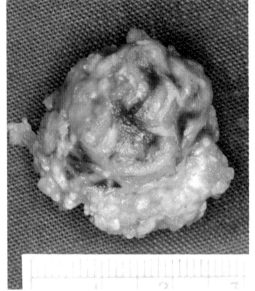

**Fig. 21.46** Complex odontome removed from a patient revealed as a calcific mass. There is a low degree of morphodifferentiation compared with the compound odontome seen in Fig. 21.44. Courtesy of Dr J.D. Harrison.

dental tissues, it is referred to as a compound odontome (Figs 21.44, 21.45). Where the calcified mass bears no resemblance to rudimentary teeth and the dental tissues are arranged haphazardly, it is termed a complex odontome (Figs 21.46, 21.47). Complex odontomes are said to be more common in the molar region of the mandible.

An invaginated odontome also occurs and was originally termed 'dens in dente' ('tooth within a tooth') (Fig. 21.48). This results either from

downward proliferation of a portion of the internal enamel epithelium of the enamel organ into the dental papilla or from retarded growth of part of the tooth germ. It presents on the fully erupted tooth as an extremely deep pit and most commonly affects the permanent maxillary second incisor. The full range of dental tissues (including cementum and bone from incorporation of the dental follicle) may be associated with the 'infolded' organ.

**Fig. 21.47** Micrograph of complex odontome. (a) Low power (×10). (b) High power (×45). There is a lack of morphodifferentiation. Areas occupied by enamel (A) appear empty when enamel is fully calcified or contain enamel matrix (darker purple staining) when maturation is incomplete. B = dentine; C = dental pulp; D = odontogenic epithelium present as irregular proliferations in the form of sheets and trabeculae of cells and duct-like structures. Courtesy of Dr J.D. Harrison.

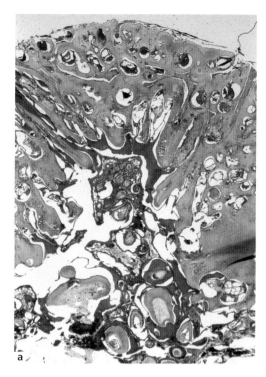
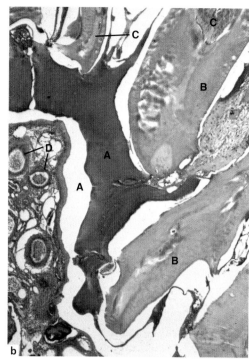

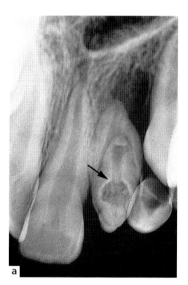
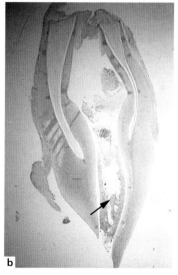

**Fig. 21.48** Dens in dente (arrows) seen radiographically (a) and in a histological section (b) (H & E). Courtesy of Dr J. Potts.

Conditions producing abnormalities in enamel and dentine, such as amelogenesis imperfecta, dentinogenesis imperfecta and hypomineralized teeth, are covered in the chapters concerned with development of those tissues (Chs 22 and 23).

As with other systems in the body, the first tentative steps have been undertaken with the ultimate aim of tissue engineering a complete tooth to replace those lost to the ravages of dental caries and periodontal disease. The obstacles to success are formidable. It would seem most desirable to obtain the epithelial and mesenchymal components required from the patient concerned rather than from another source as this would at least eliminate the problems of tissue rejection. At present, suitable mesenchymal stem cells may be provided from bone marrow, whereas a source for epithelial stem cells is less obvious. If suitable cells are available and seeded on an appropriate matrix, will any enamel and dentine formed be capable of being moulded into the specific morphology of the tooth type required and have the complex three-dimensional microstructure of the normal tissue? This will also involve generating the full thickness of the tissues, which, in real life, takes a number of years. If a suitable crown is ever produced, will it be followed by the successful development of the root of the tooth, a process that again normally takes several years to achieve? If a complete tooth is eventually engineered, will it be capable of erupting and then be maintained in an appropriate position in the mouth to enable it to function? Also, will it maintain an attachment to alveolar bone by a viable and functional periodontal ligament? These are certainly formidable challenges to be overcome, bearing in mind the apparent success that can now be confidently expected from the less complicated procedure of providing dental implants (see page 221).

Amelogenesis (enamel formation) is under genetic control. The features that enamel confers on the tooth, such as size, shape and colour, are inherited. Even susceptibility to caries is passed on. Defects in the genes encoding enamel result in inheritable malformations of enamel such as amelogenesis imperfecta.

The tooth begins its programmed development as a localized interaction between an area of oral epithelium and underlying mesenchymal cells, many of which have been derived from the neural crest. These epithelial–mesenchymal interactions during the early stages of tooth development are discussed in Chapter 21. The process is a continuous one but is most readily described in stages that represent snapshots of the developing tooth's growth and differentiation at different points. The names for these stages, bud, cap and bell, describe the morphology of the epithelial component of the developing tooth that becomes the enamel organ. Each of these stages is described in detail in Chapter 21. The innermost cell layer of the enamel organ, the internal enamel epithelium, deposits and later modifies the enamel. The other components of the enamel organ, the stratum intermedium, the stellate reticulum and the external enamel epithelium, play important supportive roles. The original descriptions we have of the developing tooth were derived from histological studies using stains of low specificity. More precise molecular techniques have contributed more detailed data that are sometimes difficult to reconcile with older hypotheses on the development of the tissue. For example, the use of the polymerase chain reaction technique, which allows the recognition of mRNA formed by transcription but present before translation, shows that the mRNA for two enamel proteins (tuftelin and amelogenin) are present in the cells of the internal enamel epithelium some time before there is any recognizable morphodifferentiation. This indicates that protein synthesis is going on at a much earlier stage than that suggested by histological studies.

In a single developing tooth, amelogenesis will be present at different stages. When enamel is being formed, the ameloblasts at different locations in the internal enamel epithelium will be at different stages of the enamel-forming process but, by the time enamel formation is complete, each ameloblast will have completed a similar life cycle. Different tooth types form enamel at different times, at different rates and with different final morphological outcomes.

Following the epithelial–mesenchymal interactions described in Chapter 21, amelogenesis and dentinogenesis occur almost simultaneously but as distinctly different processes. The site where they both begin is the enamel–dentine junction. Amelogenesis is a complex process and an understanding of it is best approached by providing an initial brief overview, followed by a more focused and detailed description.

Following the epithelial–mesenchymal interactions at the future enamel–dentine junction that constitute the presecretory stage of amelogenesis, crystal formation then begins on the enamel side of the enamel–dentine junction within an organic matrix formed by the ameloblasts and continues as the ameloblasts move away from the junction. The crystals become long ribbons arranged parallel to each other in bundles that, because of the presence of a Tomes process at the secretory surface of the ameloblast, form the enamel prisms (or rods). They grow in length but not in width at this stage. The final length of the crystals, and thus the thickness of the enamel, is determined by how long the ameloblasts lay down protein matrix. This is the secretory stage. Once the full width of the immature enamel is laid down, approximately half of the ameloblasts die and the rest shorten, stop producing matrix and then begin to degrade the matrix and selectively reabsorb much of it. This is the transition stage. The face of the ameloblast that has secreted the matrix becomes ruffled and continues the degradative process and reabsorbs almost all the remaining matrix. As this is happening, more mineral is being added to the sides of the crystals, such that they reach their final size and the enamel reaches its final level of mineralization. This is the maturation stage, which lasts for 3–4 years. The final step is the postmaturation stage, during which the enamel organ degenerates and eruption begins.

## LIFE CYCLE OF THE AMELOBLAST

The ameloblast carries out enamel formation in five stages: presecretory, secretory, transition, maturation and postmaturation. The major changes associated with each stage are summarized in Table 22.1 and Figure 22.1.

## PRESECRETORY STAGE

The odontoblasts of the developing dental pulp initiate dentine matrix formation prior to the beginning of amelogenesis. They produce collagen that is formed into bundles that point towards the cells of the internal enamel epithelium which are, at this point, known as pre-ameloblasts.

**Table 22.1** *Features associated with the five main stages of amelogenesis*

| Presecretory | Secretory | Transition | Maturation | Postmaturation |
|---|---|---|---|---|
| Cytodifferentiation: differentiation of ameloblasts | Initial layer of aprismatic enamel formed | Ameloblasts shorten, 50% die | Cycling of ruffled and smooth-ended ameloblasts | Enamel organ degenerates |
| Morphodifferentiation: bell stage including formation of the enamel knot | Ameloblasts develop Tomes processes | Vascular invagination of the enamel organ | Final degradation and withdrawal of matrix | Enamel coverings established |
| Resorption of the basal lamina of the internal enamel epithelium | Matrix secretion to final thickness | Re-formation of ameloblast basal lamina | Crystal growth continues to completion | Eruption |
| Epithelial–mesenchymal interactions | Initiation and continuation of mineralization to 30% by weight | Cessation of matrix secretion | Final third of mineralization after protein removal complete | Exposure to oral environment and posteruptive changes |
| | Crystallite elongation | Continued matrix degradation | | |
| | Matrix degradation | Selective matrix withdrawal | | |
| | Development of prismatic structure | | | |

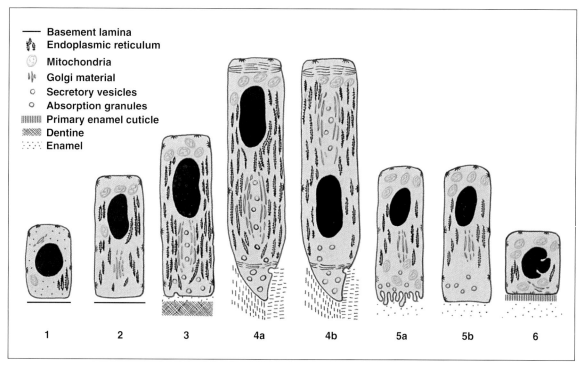

**Legend:**
— Basement lamina
Endoplasmic reticulum
Mitochondria
Golgi material
○ Secretory vesicles
○ Absorption granules
Primary enamel cuticle
Dentine
Enamel

1    2    3    4a    4b    5a    5b    6

**Fig. 22.1** The life cycle of an ameloblast. The cells of the internal enamel epithelium (1) start to differentiate, beginning at the future enamel–dentine junction of the cusp tip. The differentiating cell (2) is characterized by a reversed polarity; the cell becomes columnar and the nucleus moves to that part of the cell furthest from the dentine. Secreting organelles are formed and the end of the cell adjacent to the dentine becomes the site for secretion. At the next stage (3), the cell secretes the initial enamel component of the enamel–dentine junction. This thin layer will be continuous with the inter-rod enamel of the later formed tissue. As the cell retreats, the secreting pole becomes morphologically distinct as a pyramidal Tomes process (4a). Crystallites are formed at both surfaces of the process. The proximal region between two processes, deep in the junctional regions, always secretes ahead of the more distal region so that pits surrounded by inter-rod enamel are formed. These are then filled, giving the prism configuration to the tissue. Simultaneous secretion of both organic material and mineral continues until the full thickness of the tissue is formed. In this secreting phase, two appearances of ameloblasts can be distinguished by the position of the nuclei within the cell: high (4a) and low (4b). At the beginning of secretion, half the cells are in each form. Towards the end of secretion, most of the high nuclei have moved to a low position, effectively increasing the areas of the ameloblast cells as the surface of forming enamel increases. When the full thickness of enamel has formed, ameloblasts lose the secretory extension, the Tomes process (5a). Up to 50% of them die and are phagocytosed by others in the layer. The maturation phase lasts two to three times longer than the secretory phase. During the maturation phase there is a regular, repetitive modulation of cell morphology between a ruffled (5a) and a smooth (5b) surface apposed to the enamel. Once the maturation changes are complete, the cells regress in height (6). At this stage, they serve to protect the enamel surface during eruption and later will contribute to form the junctional epithelium.

The presecretory stage includes all activities of the future ameloblast before the secretion of the main component of the enamel matrix. This stage has two principal features: differentiation of the pre-ameloblasts and formation and subsequent resorption of a basal lamina. The morphological changes to the enamel organ as a whole are described in detail in the section on tooth development (Ch. 21). Here, the focus will be on the cells of the internal enamel epithelium. During the bell stage, the cells of the internal enamel epithelium (Fig. 22.2) have ceased to divide and have differentiated into committed enamel-forming cells, the ameloblasts. This differentiation begins at the future cusp tips or incisal margins and progresses cervically. During this phase, the ameloblasts differentiate from cuboidal into columnar cells over 60 μm in height and 2–4 μm in width. The cell becomes polarized as the nucleus and mitochondria stay close to the end of the cell that is in contact with the stratum intermedium. These columnar cells are pre-ameloblasts (Figs 22.3, 22.4).

Before any dentine is laid down the early differentiating ameloblasts (Fig. 22.1) possess a large ovoid nucleus, several mitochondria and a small Golgi apparatus close to the stratum intermedium end of the cell. In the cytoplasm adjacent to the dental papilla (which will become the dental pulp), rough endoplasmic reticulum is present, with many free ribosomes, mitochondria and vesicles. Pinocytotic invaginations of the cell membrane are also found here. Adjacent cells of the internal enamel epithelium are linked by terminal bars at their proximal (near the stratum intermedium) and distal (near the dental papilla) ends. A basal lamina separates the pre-ameloblast from the dental papilla. This lamina marks the position of the future enamel–dentine junction. Very shortly after morphological changes have begun in the internal enamel epithelium, parallel changes begin in

the adjacent mesenchymal cells of the dental papilla that are differentiating into odontoblasts (Figs 22.5, 22.6). This differentiation is controlled by the cells of the internal dental epithelium that release growth factors (particularly members of the transforming growth factor (TGF)β family) which can be deposited in the basal lamina, from where they are released by proteolytic enzymes. Once the odontoblasts of the dental papilla have differentiated, the basal lamina separating them from the pre-ameloblast disappears as the first layer of dentine matrix is laid down (Fig. 22.6). The pre-ameloblasts release enzymes by exocytosis that degrade the basal lamina and then resorb the degradation products by endocytosis. For a brief period following the degradation of the basal lamina, the future ameloblasts and odontoblasts are in intimate contact, allowing inductive signalling to occur between them. The odontoblasts are the first cells to lay down matrix and this provides the signal for the ameloblasts to begin secretion. The odontoblasts produce non-collagenous proteins as well, in particular dentine sialophosphoprotein (DSPP). A small amount of DSPP is also contributed by the pre-ameloblasts. This initial matrix defines the enamel–dentine junction. Before any mineralization begins, the pre-ameloblasts secrete enamel proteins on top of the dentin matrix, some of which diffuses through the matrix and is taken up by the odontoblasts. Immediately after this initial enamel matrix is laid down, the basal lamina of the pre-ameloblasts disappears and cell processes extend into irregularities on the adjacent predentine surface. Crystallites form in the enamel matrix within these irregularities in contact with the ameloblast. The pre-ameloblast cell processes shrink back towards the cell body as the crystallites lengthen. The surface of the first-formed dentine, once it has mineralized, becomes covered with a very thin layer of enamel into

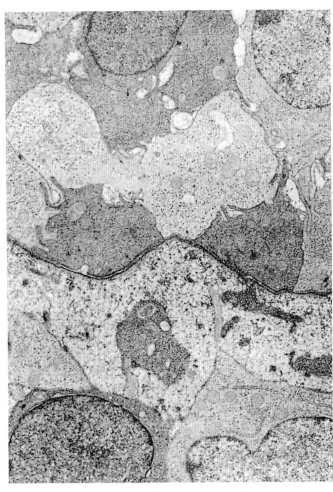

**Fig. 22.2** TEM showing the undifferentiated cells of the internal enamel epithelium. No secretory specialization is yet evident (×4800). Courtesy of Dr T. Sasaki and Karger Press.

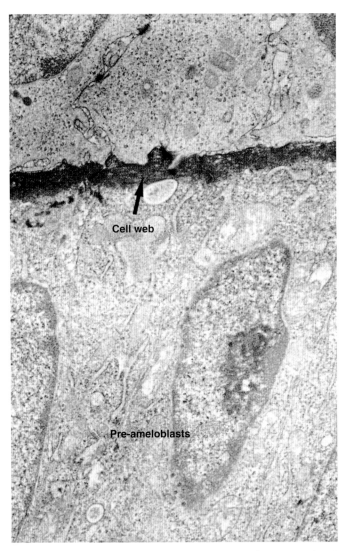

**Fig. 22.3** TEM showing pre-ameloblasts. Rough endoplasmic reticulum is evident and the terminal cell web is clearly stained (×5350). Courtesy of Dr T. Sasaki and Karger Press.

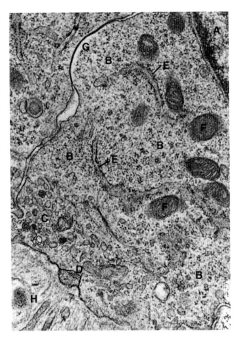

**Fig. 22.4** TEM illustrating the distal cytoplasm of an early differentiating ameloblast. A = nucleus; B = free ribosomes; C = vesicles; D = pinocytotic invagination; E = rough endoplasmic reticulum; F = mitochondria; G = gap junction; H = dental papilla (×21000). Courtesy of Dr E. Katchburian.

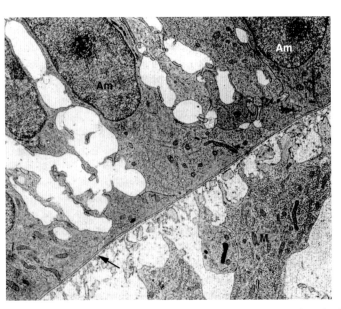

**Fig. 22.5** TEM showing ameloblasts (Am) in contact with mesenchymal cells of the dental papilla (M). A basal lamina (arrow) is still present (×500). Courtesy of Dr Z. Skobe and the CRC Press.

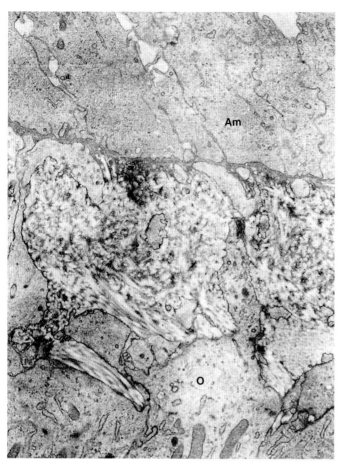

**Fig. 22.6** TEM showing dentine matrix formation by odontoblasts (O) preceding the secretion of enamel by ameloblasts (Am) (×5000). Courtesy of Dr Z. Skobe and the CRC Press.

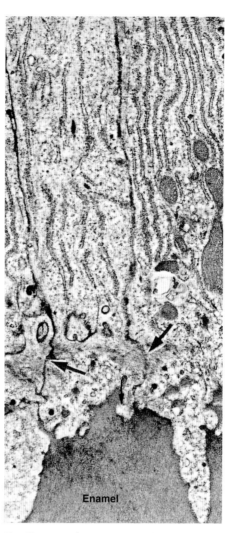

**Fig. 22.7** TEM demonstrating cell junctions proximal to Tomes processes, junctional complexes (arrows) and intracellular tonofilaments (×7500). Courtesy of Dr T. Sasaki and Karger.

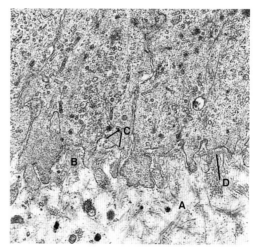

**Fig. 22.8** TEM showing the distal end of a late-differentiating ameloblast. A = forming dentine; B = invagination in ameloblast; C = coated pits; D = degenerating lamina (×15600). Courtesy of Dr E. Katchburian.

which some odontoblast processes extend, forming enamel spindles (see page 118). This initial enamel is aprismatic, as there are no sudden changes in crystal orientation due to the absence of a Tomes process on the pre-ameloblast. In this aprismatic enamel, the crystallites appear to lie in random orientations. The final part of the enamel formed at the surface of the crown is also aprismatic, but in this region the crystallites are arranged uniformly parallel to each other.

In the terminally differentiated pre-ameloblast, the nucleus is in the end of the cell adjacent to the stratum intermedium with mitochondria between it and the cell membrane. The rough endoplasmic reticulum, Golgi apparatus and secretory vesicles enlarge and come to lie between the nucleus and the end of the cell adjacent to the dental papilla, the pole from which enamel matrix will later be secreted. This redistribution of organelles is known as a reversal of polarity. The pre-ameloblasts are joined to each other at the stratum intermedium end by desmosomes, forming the proximal terminal web (Fig. 22.3). A similar distal terminal web will develop a little later at the secretory end of the cells (Fig. 22.7). The pre-ameloblasts are approximately 40 μm long and 2–4 μm wide. The pre-ameloblasts bulge into the stellate reticulum, perhaps to gain the advantage of increased surface area in absorbing precursors. At their distal end following the onset of dentinogenesis, the cell membrane becomes irregular with many projections and pits (Fig. 22.8). Vesicles and vacuoles appear in the cytoplasm. These changes may, in part, be associated with the removal of the basal lamina.

## SECRETORY STAGE

At the beginning of the secretory phase, the ameloblasts have become long, columnar cells over 60 μm in height and 2–4 μm in width, with their nuclei at the basal end (away from the forming enamel). Following the deposition

of the initial, thin, aprismatic enamel, a cone-shaped process, Tomes process, forms at the distal, secretory end of the ameloblasts (Figs 22.9–22.11). The shape of Tomes processes is responsible for the prismatic structure of enamel. There appears to be a relationship between ameloblast size and prism pattern (see Fig. 7.10). It is usually found that pattern 3 prisms are made by the largest ameloblasts and pattern 2 by the smallest. With the development of the Tomes process, the shape of the mineralizing front changes to a 'picket fence' arrangement (Figs 22.11–22.13). If the

**Fig. 22.9** Demineralized section of developing enamel showing the cone-shaped Tomes process (arrow) at the distal end of each ameloblast.
A = ameloblast; B = enamel matrix; C = dentine; D = stratum intermedium; E = terminal bar apparatus running through the ameloblast layer (Toluidine blue; ×1000). Courtesy of Dr D.W. Whittaker.

**Fig. 22.10** Section showing rat secretory ameloblasts. Nu = nuclei; TP = Tomes processes, En = forming enamel (×1000). Courtesy of Dr T. Sasaki and Karger.

**Fig. 22.11** TEM showing advanced secretory ameloblasts with their Tomes processes (A). B = developing enamel; C = interpit 'prongs' (×6000). Courtesy of Dr A. Boyde and Springer-Verlag.

**Fig. 22.12** The relationship between Tomes processes and enamel prism formation. The enamel of the core of the prism and the prism boundary/inter-rod regions differ largely in the orientation of crystallites. This is determined by the shape of the Tomes process. In human enamel, prisms are clearly seen, though at some points in the 'tail' of the prism the boundary between prismatic and interprismatic is lost (see Figs 7.11 and 7.63). Each prism is formed by a single ameloblast but four contribute to each interprismatic region. The prism boundary areas of enamel are formed first, giving the developing enamel front a pit-like surface appearance.

**Fig. 22.13** Fractured enamel with intact secretory-stage ameloblasts adhering to the forming enamel surface. Tomes processes (T) are clearly seen and appear triangular. Courtesy of Dr Z. Skobe.

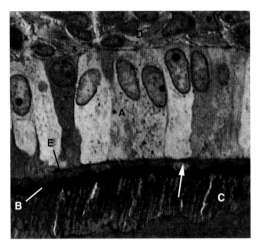

Fig. 22.9

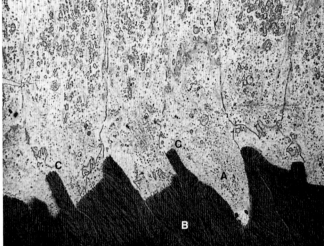

Fig. 22.11

Fig. 22.10

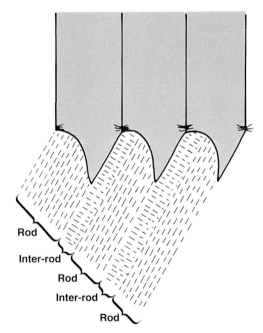

Fig. 22.13

Rod
Inter-rod
Rod
Inter-rod
Rod

Fig. 22.12

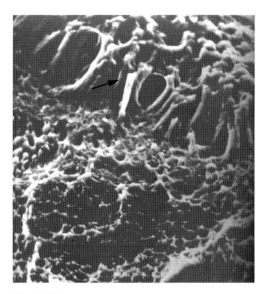

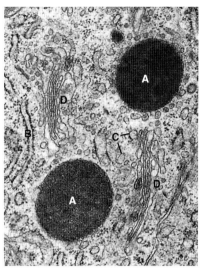

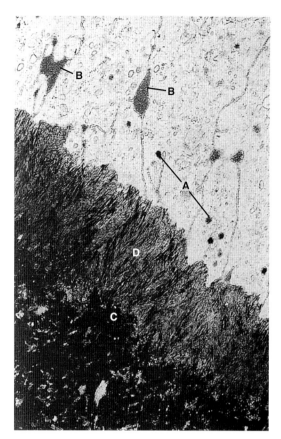

Fig. 22.14

Fig. 22.15

**Fig. 22.14** SEM of surface of developing enamel. At the top (arrow), some ameloblasts have been retained at the surface. Below where others have been lost, the developing enamel surface shows a series of pits previously occupied by the Tomes processes of the ameloblasts (×500). Courtesy of Dr R.P. Shellis.

**Fig. 22.15** TEM showing the synthetic and secretory apparatus in a secretory ameloblast. A = secretory granules; B = rough endoplasmic reticulum; C = Golgi vesicles; D = Golgi apparatus (×30 500). Courtesy of Dr E. Katchburian.

**Fig. 22.16** TEM showing early enamel formation. A = secretory vesicles; B = secreted matrix between ameloblasts; C = dentine; D = early enamel (×1500). Courtesy of Dr E. Katchburian.

Fig. 22.16

ameloblasts are pulled away from the surface, the mineralizing front presents a honeycomb appearance, the pits in the surface being occupied by the Tomes processes (Figs 22.13, 22.14). This appearance is reminiscent of the enamel surface following etching with certain acids (e.g. Fig. 7.63). Ameloblasts are joined to each other by a terminal bar apparatus (web) distally at the base of the Tomes processes (Fig. 22.9). This appearance of a linear structure is produced by the alignment of junctional complexes consisting of desmosomes and tight junctions. The tonofilaments associated with the desmosomes pass, for a short distance, into the cell and form an incomplete septum between the Tomes processes and the rest of the ameloblast. The junctions of the terminal web apparatus are zonular (encircling the cell) and effectively separate the environment of the developing enamel from the interior of the enamel organ such that all secretion and modification of the matrix occurs via the Tomes processes. Junctions at the basal end of the ameloblasts, adjacent to the stratum intermedium, are macular and provide mechanical union without the same isolation of the microenvironment. There are other isolated junctions between ameloblasts at other levels, particularly gap junctions, that may synchronize the activity of the cells. Interpit 'prongs' develop between the growing and elongating Tomes processes (Figs 22.10–22.12). The prongs between the processes deposit enamel matrix first, to form walls that represent the periphery of the prisms (and interprismatic regions) and that delineate pits or depressions in the enamel that are occupied by Tomes processes. The Tomes processes then infill the central pits as the ameloblasts retreat to form the main core of the enamel prism. The ameloblasts therefore have two main secretory sites.

The basic enamel matrix proteins are assembled in the endoplasmic reticulum and carried by transitional vesicles to the Golgi apparatus where glycosylation and sulphation take place before packaging into electron-dense secretory granules 0.25 μm in diameter (Fig. 22.15) The secretory granules are transported along microtubules towards the Tomes process of the cell.

As the ameloblasts shift from the presecretory to the secretory stage, there is a marked aggregation of vesicles (some containing stippled material) at the distal end of the ameloblast (Fig. 22.16). The material contained within the vesicles represents the organic matrix of the enamel. The contents of the vesicles are discharged into the extracellular space, both at the distal end of the cell and between the cell membranes of adjacent ameloblasts (Fig. 22.16). As the enamel matrix is secreted, the ameloblasts are pushed (or move) outwards away from the dentine surface (Fig. 22.17). Within this organic matrix, the initial hydroxyapatite crystallites of the

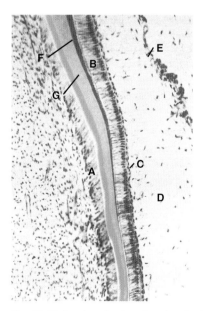

**Fig. 22.17** Demineralized section showing the initial stage of enamel formation. A = odontoblasts; B = ameloblasts; C = stratum intermedium; D = stellate reticulum; E = external enamel epithelium; F = developing enamel; G = developing dentine; (Masson's trichrome; ×80).

enamel appear almost immediately, before the matrix is 50 nm thick, so that a distinct zone of unmineralized matrix analogous to predentine or osteoid is never seen in enamel (Fig. 22.16). The first-formed crystallites are thin and needle-like and much smaller than the crystallites in mature enamel. They begin as thin ribbons, 10–15 nm wide and 1–2 nm in thickness. The enamel mineral is a carbonated calcium hydroxyapatite but differs from pure hydroxyapatite by including $HPO_4^{2-}$, $CO_3^{2-}$, $Na^+$, $F^-$ and other ions in its lattice. During development, enamel crystallites form and are aligned perpendicular to the distal surface of the ameloblasts. The mechanism(s) responsible for this alignment is not understood but it may be due to the organization of the organic matrix, the concentration gradients of the crystallite ions, the presence of microvilli at the cell membrane or the contributions due to ameloblast movement. The crystallites appear as flattened hexagons when viewed in cross-section. The crystallites extend in length, still aligned perpendicular to the surface and parallel to other crystallites forming at the same cell surface. The enamel crystallites that elongate around the tip of the Tomes process form the region of the prism core. Crystallites extending from where the ameloblasts are joined to each other form the region at the prism boundary. There is a clear border between prism core and prism boundary as part of the ameloblast is non-secretory. Prism core and prism boundary enamel are identical except for the orientation of the crystallites. The prism core crystallites are parallel to the long axis of the prism; the prism boundary deviate from this by up to 40–65°. Four ameloblasts contribute to the formation of a single prism and each ameloblast is involved in the development of four prisms. Nonetheless, there are the same number of prisms as there are ameloblasts.

Enamel prisms elongate incrementally. Each daily increment leads to a cross-striation (see page 112). Approximately every 7 days (range 6–10), prominent cross-striations produce the appearance of an enamel stria. Apart from the initial striae over the cusps and incisal ridges, these striae end on the surface of the enamel as perikymata (see pages 114, 115). The amount of enamel formed daily varies but it is approximately the same in all teeth forming at the same time. In teeth whose enamel is mineralizing at birth, there is an exaggerated incremental line, the neonatal line (see page 115).

The secretory phase ends once the full thickness of enamel matrix has been laid down. The Tomes process retracts so that the distal end becomes flat (Fig. 22.18) and a final, thin layer of aprismatic enamel is formed at the surface. However, this layer may be incomplete as prism end markings may sometimes be seen in the covering investments of newly erupted enamel or in enamel from areas that have been protected from attrition (see page 124). The crystallites in surface aprismatic enamel all run parallel to each other. The signalling mechanisms that determine when and where in the tooth the secretory process is turned on or off are unknown.

## THE TRANSITION STAGE

The enamel that is deposited initially has a high content of water and protein; a low content of mineral and is porous. The process that converts this young, immature enamel to fully mineralized enamel is termed maturation. Enamel maturation is carried out by the same cells that secreted the primary matrix, the ameloblasts, but in a very changed form. The period in which the ameloblasts change from a secretory to a maturation form is the transition stage. During this phase, enamel secretion stops and much of the matrix is removed. A reduction in height of the ameloblasts signals the onset of the transition. The number of ameloblasts is reduced by as much as 50% by apoptosis (programmed cell death). In those ameloblasts that remain, the organelles associated with protein synthesis (e.g. the rough endoplasmic reticulum and the Golgi apparatus) are reduced by autophagocytosis. The enamel organ becomes invaginated by blood vessels, and the cells of external enamel epithelium, stellate reticulum and stratum intermedium become covered with microvilli. However, blood vessels do

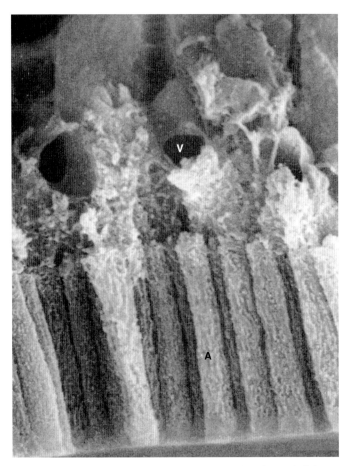

**Fig. 22.18** SEM showing flat-ended ameloblasts (A) at the end of the secretory phase. V = venule. (×1000). Courtesy of Dr Z. Skobe and the CRC Press.

not directly penetrate into the stellate reticulum, which is avascular. The blood vessels thus lie close to, but not in contact with, the proximal end (base) of the ameloblasts (Fig. 22.19).

## Enamel proteins

As one of the main processes in the maturation of enamel is the removal and modification of the initially formed proteinaceous matrix, it is necessary here to discuss the composition of the immature enamel matrix:

Proteins and peptides account for less than 1% of the weight of mature enamel but 25–30% of early developing enamel. Developing enamel matrix during the early secretory stage is almost entirely proteinaceous. They are unique proteins, different from any other protein in the body. Developing enamel contains two main groups of proteins: the amelogenins comprise 90–95% and the non-amelogenins comprise the remaining 5–10% (Fig. 22.19). Following the process of maturation, the majority of the amelogenin proteins are degraded and removed so that, in mature enamel, the remaining 1% by weight of protein is comprised mainly of non-amelogenin proteins. Although the precise functions of the enamel proteins have yet to be determined, mutations in their genes are associated with disturbances in enamel structure. A list of some possible functions of enamel proteins is given in Table 22.2.

As enamel matrix is secreted extracellularly and away from the ameloblast surface, it must convey within its unique protein structure the necessary information to direct mineralization to produce the complex microanatomy of human enamel. Of particular importance is the nucleation of the hydroxyapatite crystals, their controlled growth and their relative orientation to form prismatic enamel. Study of the functions of the enamel proteins is made difficult by the large number of amelogenin- and non-amelogenin-related proteins. This is due to a combination of three features:

**Enamel proteins**

- Mature
  - Tuft
    - Peptides
      - Others
- Immature
  - Enamelins (non-amelogenin) (anionic enamel proteins)
    - Ameloblastin
      - Tuftelin
        - Proteinases
          - Sulphated
            - Derived
  - Amelogenins
    - Multiple alternatively spliced proteins

**Fig. 22.19** Classification of enamel proteins. Redrawn from Fincham et al 2000 In: Teaford et al (eds) *Development, function and evolution of teeth*, with permission of Cambridge University Press.

**Table 22.2** *Some of the main enamel proteins and their possible functions*

| Protein | Function |
|---|---|
| Dentine sialophosphoprotein | Initiation of mineralization |
| Amelogenin, non-amelogenin | Mineral ion binding as crystallite |
| | Control of crystallite growth |
| Ameloblastin | Determination of prismatic pattern |
| Tuftelin, ameloblastin | Cell signalling |
| Breakdown products | Control of secretion |

1. Following their initial secretion, enamel proteins undergo a series of complex degradative changes carried out by various proteolytic enzymes. This results in the accumulation of many smaller enamel proteins and peptides.
2. The presence of alternative RNA splicing of the mRNA transcript results in the same amino acid sequence being present at either end of the molecule but with deficiencies occurring in the middle.
3. The amelogenin gene occurs on both the X and Y sex chromosomes, producing slightly different proteins: the amelogenin gene on the X chromosome has 106 base pairs while that on the Y chromosome has 112 base pairs. However, the male-specific proteins represent only a minor proportion of the total enamel protein. The functional significance of this sexual dimorphism is not known but it has forensic implications as the sex of an individual could be determined from viable nuclear material derived from the relatively well protected pulps of dead individuals by detecting the nature of the amelogenin gene.

### Amelogenin enamel proteins

The newly secreted major amelogenin molecule (before any processing) is a 25 kDa protein. It is a hydrophobic, proline-rich molecule that also has high levels of histidine, glutamine and leucine (Fig. 22.20). It is broken down by proteolytic cleavage with increasing depth of enamel and is absent from the inner layer of enamel. The parent 25 kDa form is broken down to a 20 kDa molecule and further processing leads to the accumulation of 13, 11 and 5 kDa amelogenins (Fig. 22.21). The 5 kDa molecule is a tyrosine-rich amelogenin peptide (TRAP). It is relatively insoluble and builds up near the end of the secretory stage of amelogenesis. The 13 and 11 kDa moieties are relatively soluble.

The breakdown of amelogenin (presumably enzymatic) commences soon after secretion of the enamel matrix occurs and continues throughout the secretory stage of enamel formation. The question arises as to whether this degradation is merely to remove the matrix and allow the enamel crystallites to enlarge, or whether some or all of the smaller molecules have specific functions in the development of enamel structure. For example, TRAP is thought to be important in crystal growth

Amelogenins are hydrophobic and tends to aggregate or 'clump'. When added to enamel matrix, they do not form a discrete appositional band, as

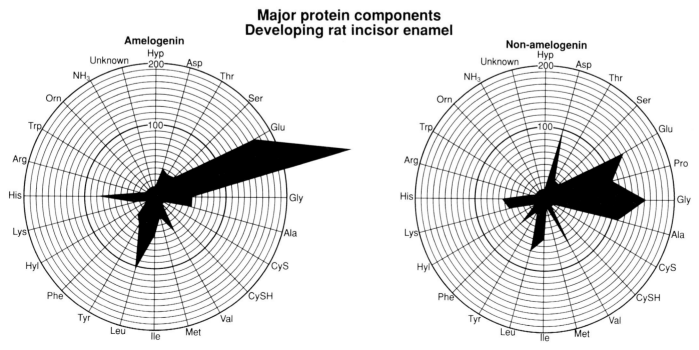

## Major protein components
## Developing rat incisor enamel

**Fig. 22.20** 'Rose' diagram showing the composition of the proteins in developing rat incisor enamel. Courtesy of Professor C. Robinson.

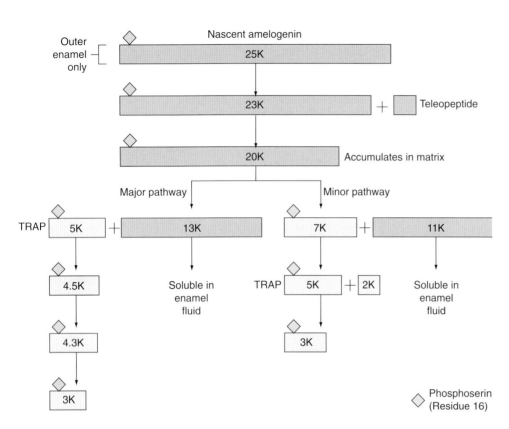

**Fig. 22.21** Diagram showing various stages in the degradation of native amelogenin enamel protein. From Robinson C, Brookes SJ, Shore RC, Kirkham J 1998 The developing enamel matrix: nature and function. *European Journal of Oral Science* 106(suppl); 282–291.

do the matrix proteins of dentine and bone. Instead, they spread throughout the whole developing enamel thickness. The resultant matrix is a gel through which molecules and ions can spread readily, a property of considerable significance in the production of large crystals. Folding of the molecule may permit protein–protein interactions between carboxyl and amino-terminal domains, resulting in self-assembly and the formation of minute nanospheres, having a diameter of about 20 nm. It has been proposed that the first crystals of enamel are formed between the spheres. Evidence in support of this view is that the initial thin enamel crystals are also spaced approximately 20 nm apart. Subsequently, the controlled extracellular degradation of the amelogenin proteins results in a reduction in the size and arrangement of the nanospheres, allowing for a later controlled increase in both the width and thickness of the enamel crystals in the deeper enamel layers.

### Non-amelogenin enamel proteins

These comprise about 10% of the protein of mature enamel. Because of their relatively low concentrations, they are not as well characterized as the amelogenins and their precise functions are unknown. Among the non-amelogenins to be considered are the enamelins, ameloblastin, tuftelin, proteases, sulphated enamel proteins and the derived proteins (Fig. 22.19). Like the amelogenins, examination of the non-amelogenins is complicated by the presence of alternative splicing and their degradation to form smaller molecules. Their degradation would appear to be undertaken by the same enzymes as that for the amelogenins.

### Enamelins

The glycine-rich parent molecules are the largest enamel proteins, having molecular weights of 142 ND and 89 kDa (Fig. 22.20). They are found in the outermost layer of newly secreted enamel but are soon broken down to smaller moieties having molecular weights of 30–40 kDa and 13–17 kDa. The lower-weight enamelins have been shown to be phos-phorylated glycoproteins rich in proline, glycine, glutamine and aspartine. Enamelins are primarily located in the prism cores. They can form aggregates with other proteins in the organic matrix and, being seen in the region of the enamel–dentine junction, are postulated by some to control the growth of enamel crystals by an inhibitory action.

### Ameloblastin (amelin, sheathlin)

The two transcripts of this nascent protein produced by alternative splicing are rich in proline, glycine and leucine and have a molecular weight of 62 kDa. The protein is located initially in the region of the prism core near secretory ameloblasts, while smaller breakdown products (e.g. 13–17 kDa fractions) are found at the prism boundary. For this reason, some have ascribed to it a function in the generation of prism structure. The gene for ameloblastin is located on chromosome 4. As ameloblastin-null mice produce defective enamel and their secretory ameloblasts are seen to become separated from the developing enamel surface, losing their polarity, this suggests that ameloblastin may play a role in cell adhesion. Ameloblastin is also produced by the epithelial root sheath during root formation and this is discussed further on page 347.

### Tuftelin

The parent protein(s) in this group is rich in glutamic and aspartic acid and has a molecular weight in the range of 58–66 kDa. Alternative slicing also occurs in the case of these proteins. A gene has been located on chromosome 1. As this is one of the earliest proteins to be produced, both before the amelogenin proteins and before the ameloblasts have differentiated, it has been suggested that one of its early functions is as a signalling molecule during epithelial/mesenchymal interactions. Its presence at the enamel–dentine junction has implicated this protein(s) as possibly being involved as a nucleator at the commencement of initial enamel mineralization.

Following maturation, some protein remains in the region corresponding to the enamel tufts (see Figs 7.55, 7.58, 7.59). Here it is referred to as tuft protein. Its relationship to tuftelin and/or its degraded products is unclear, although it appears to contains less proline and more leucine.

### Sulphated enamel proteins

These represent acidic enamel proteins that are present in small amounts and appear to be degraded within about 1–2 hours after their secretion. Their function is unknown.

### Proteolytic enzymes

Also present in developing enamel are low concentrations of proteinases and metalloproteinases, including enamelysin (whose cleavage products accumulate as the hydroxyapatite crystals lengthen) and kallikrein 4 (also known as enamel matrix serine proteinase). Alkaline phosphatase activity is also present. The activity of these enzymes peaks in early maturation when most of the enamel protein is lost.

### Serum-derived products

There are some proteins present in developing enamel that are not secreted by ameloblasts but are derived from serum. Because of their affinity for hydroxyapatite, these proteins are absorbed into the developing enamel. The major serum protein identified in developing enamel is albumin, which has the property of inhibiting mineral growth.

### Amelotin

This is a recently discovered protein produced by ameloblasts at the maturation stage, therefore being expressed later than other enamel proteins. As it is more often associated with basal laminae, it may play a role in cell adhesion. Its gene occupies chromosome 4.

## MATURATION STAGE

Once the entire thickness of the enamel has formed it is structurally complete, with all the morphological features of mature enamel. Newly formed enamel is 65% water, 20% organic material and 15% inorganic hydroxyapatite crystals by weight. The process by which the enamel changes into its final form is termed maturation. During maturation, enamel crystallites increase in width and thickness with a consequent reduction in intercrystallite space.

Ameloblasts move calcium, phosphate and carbonate ions into the matrix and remove water and degraded enamel matrix proteins from it. The protein content of the tissue is reduced from about 30% to about 1%. The removal of matrix occurs as the crystallites expand from their early average dimensions of 1.5 nm thick to their mature thickness of 25 nm. The degradation of the enamel matrix by serine proteases released from the enamel organ seems to precede the mineral gain. At this initial stage, the space caused by enamel matrix loss is occupied by water, with the enamel becoming more porous.

The ameloblasts undergo further morphological changes. The Tomes process is lost and the organelle content reduced. The remaining organelles congregate at the distal end of the cell where the plasma membrane infolds to form a striated border (Figs 22.22, 22.23). The ameloblast is then described as being 'ruffle-ended'. This morphology alternates with that of the 'smooth-ended' ameloblast, in which the striated border is absent (Fig. 22.24). Modulation between the two forms occurs about five to seven times during maturation. This modulation may indicate alternation between resorptive and secretory phases of activity. The cyclical changes in ameloblast morphology seem to be linked to at least two aspects of maturation:

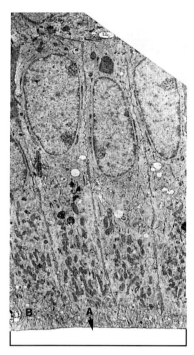

**Fig. 22.22** TEM of demineralized section showing the appearance of ruffle-ended ameloblasts during maturation phase of amelogenesis. A = enamel space; B = striated border. The Tomes process has been lost. The mitochondria are grouped in a basal cluster. The rough endoplasmic reticulum is much reduced (×2700).

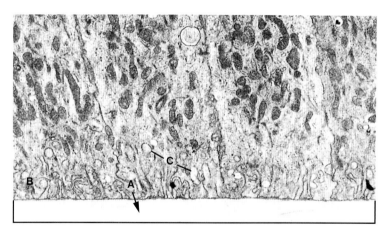

**Fig. 22.23** High-power view of Fig. 22.22, showing ruffled border of ameloblast during the maturation stage. A = enamel space; B = striated (ruffled) border; C = resorptive vesicles (×6700).

- the movement of calcium ions: in the ruffled-ended form, this movement may be actively controlled, whereas in the smooth-ended form calcium ions may move only by diffusion (and hence few would enter the enamel)
- local pH changes: physiologically normal pH favouring mineralization (ruffle-ended) would alternate with mildly acidic conditions handicapping mineralization (smooth-ended). The ameloblasts may induce these pH cycles by modulating bicarbonate levels.

A third process in maturation, lowering the molecular weight of enamel proteins by a group of proteinases resident in the enamel matrix, may be continuous rather than cyclical. The ameloblasts (which may produce the enzymes) do not control rate of this digestion although they do resorb and degrade its end products. These protein changes may, by an unknown mechanism, affect mineralization. Simple removal of the protein, increases the relative mineral content. The final one-third of the mineralization process goes on after virtually all protein has been removed. The increase in

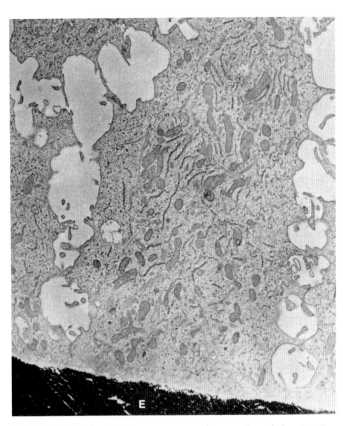

**Fig. 22.24** TEM showing the appearance of a smooth-ended maturation ameloblast. At this stage the cells lack a distinct terminal web distally. E = enamel (×7000). Courtesy of Dr Z. Skobe and the CRC Press.

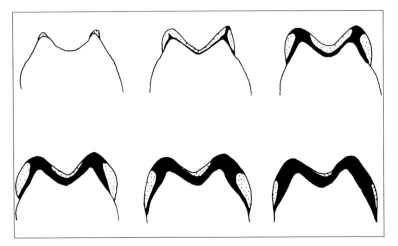

**Fig. 22.25** Pattern of mineralization during maturation, as mapped out by microradiography of ground sections. Stippled areas represent initial enamel deposition. Black areas show the pattern that increased mineralization follows during maturation. Once the full thickness of enamel is formed in any area, maturation commences. Initial deposition and maturation can thus occur at the same time. Mineralization during maturation follows a different pattern from initial deposition. Commencing at cusps, it passes to the enamel–dentine junction and along the junction before continuing throughout the more superficial regions.

mineral density begins over the cusp tips and progresses cervically (Fig. 22.25).

## POSTMATURATION STAGE

Once maturation of the enamel is complete, the ameloblasts become flattened (Figs 22.26, 22.27), except sometimes in the depths of fissures where they may remain columnar (Fig. 8.3). A thin, amorphous layer of protein, the primary enamel cuticle, separates the cells from the enamel. At the ultrastructural level, this has the appearance of a basal lamina and it may

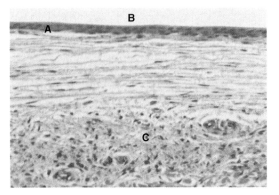

**Fig. 22.26** Demineralized section showing the position and morphology of the reduced enamel epithelium (A) covering the unerupted tooth. B = enamel space; C = connective tissue of the dental follicle (H & E; ×160).

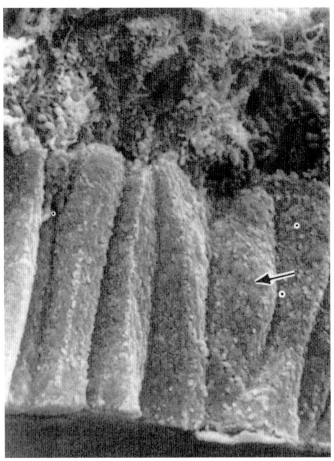

**Fig. 22.27** SEM showing the appearance of reduced ameloblasts. The bulge indicated by the arrow may be the result of multiple nuclei, which are sometimes seen in these cells (×2000). Courtesy of Dr Z. Skobe and the CRC Press.

represent either material extruded from the enamel during maturation or may be the last secretory product of the ameloblast. The cells themselves contain hemidesmosomes at their interface with the basal lamina applied to the enamel surface. The remnants of the enamel organ merge with the flattened ameloblasts to constitute the reduced enamel epithelium. The primary enamel cuticle together with the reduced enamel epithelium form Nasmyth's membrane (see page 123) and, during eruption, protects the enamel surface. The fluoride content of the enamel may be greater in teeth that have longer duration periods of eruption. It is not known whether the remaining cells of the enamel organ are active in this respect or not. Once the tooth has erupted into the oral cavity, the surface layer shows increasing mineralization through interaction with saliva (posteruptive maturation).

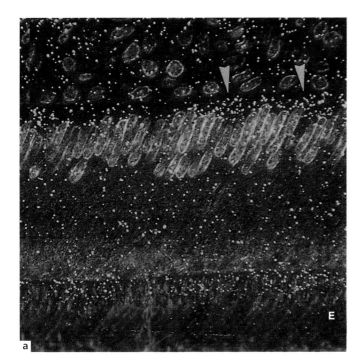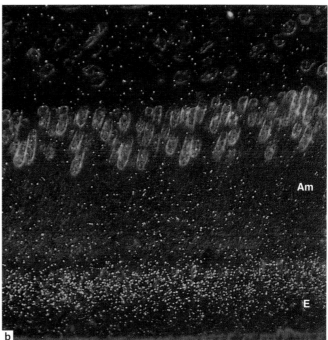

**Fig. 22.28** An autoradiographically labelled histological section viewed in dark field showing the movement of calcium through the ameloblast layer. Labelled calcium-45 autoradiographs showing the movement of calcium (white dots) through ameloblasts. Am = ameloblasts; E = enamel. The tissue (rat) in (a) was taken 30 seconds after the injection of the radioactive calcium. The arrows indicate the accumulation of calcium in the proximal ameloblast adjacent to the stellate reticulum. The tissue in (b) was taken 10 minutes after injection when most of the calcium has become incorporated into the enamel (×400). Courtesy of Dr Y. Takana and the editor of *Connective Tissue Research*.

## MINERALIZATION

There are a number of possible sources for the calcium that mineralizes the enamel matrix. The precise pathway and transport mechanism is unclear, although some elements of the process have been determined.

Calcium reaches the matrix principally via the enamel organ (rather than the dental papilla). It travels, possibly predominantly, by an extracellular route, although there is also evidence for a transcellular route (Figs 22.28, 22.29). There may be an active transport mechanism utilizing carriers in the cell membranes of the ameloblasts, or the calcium may flow passively from high concentrations in the blood plasma to low concentrations in the enamel matrix. The ameloblast layer has a limited and variable but controlled permeability to ions. This property is attributed to the proximal rather than distal cell junctional complexes. It may control the access not only to calcium ions but also to other significant ions, particularly fluoride.

Specific initiators of enamel mineralization have not been convincingly identified. The first-formed enamel at the enamel–dentine junction is less well organized than the bulk of mature enamel in terms of crystallite size and morphology, and is aprismatic. On the basis of this disordered morphology, it has been suggested that crystallite growth and possibly nucleation are directed by the enamel protein tuftelin. It has also been suggested, but not demonstrated, that initial nucleation may occur in dentine and cross the enamel–dentine junction. Matrix vesicles, which may participate in the onset of mineralization in some parts of the dentine, have not been reported in developing enamel. It has been proposed that the amelogenins are capable of self-assembling into minute spheres (nanospheres), between which the first crystallites of enamel are formed. The initial crystallites form as a precipitate from the matrix that is supersaturated with hydroxyapatite. Initially, crystallites may grow by the fusion of nucleation sites but once the prismatic structure is established crystallites are enlarged preferentially in length rather than in width.

The matrix can control crystallite growth by two basic mechanisms: 1) by breaking down protein in a controlled pattern to provide the space for new crystallite deposition and 2) by modulating the effect of inhibitory

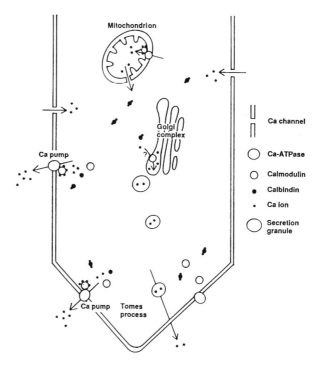

**Fig. 22.29** Model showing the proposed intracellular movement of calcium in the ameloblasts. Courtesy of Dr T. Sasaki and Karger.

molecules. The first could be achieved by the formation, in the matrix, of appropriately oriented microchannels with the same dimensions as the crystallites, and in which crystallites would form at the growing end of the prism. After the maturation phase, the role of the matrix proteins is largely ended as virtually all the protein has been lost and what remains is replaced with tissue fluid. The matrix proteins are actually removed long before crystallite growth ends. The degraded matrix proteins accumulate in the extracellular space around the ameloblasts and, by inhibiting further activity, could control and limit the thickness of enamel deposited.

## DEVELOPMENT OF THE PRISMATIC STRUCTURE

The increase in mineral during maturation follows a different pattern from the initial deposition. The first-formed enamel at what will be the enamel–dentine junction is laid against newly calcified dentine by flat-ended ameloblasts. It is aprismatic and initially contains small crystallites (10–15 nm wide, 1–2 nm thick and approximately 20 nm apart). The initial crystallites form as a precipitate within the matrix that is supersaturated with hydroxyapatite. Crystallites form and grow while close to the cell membrane of the Tomes process. They grow by the deposition of ions on the crystallite faces. As the ameloblasts retreat, they form pyramidal Tomes processes at their distal ends and the enamel formed thereafter is prismatic. As crystallites grow in length, they also increase in thickness and width and this continues until crystallites contact each other. Thus formed, the crystallite is a long, tapering pyramid with its apex at the enamel–dentine junction. After maturation, the crystallite is rod shaped and of uniform size along its length (about an average of 26 nm thick × 68 nm wide) and runs from the enamel–dentine junction to the surface. Enamel matrix is deposited in a non-homogeneous form. Amelogenins become located primarily within the prism, non-amelogenins more at the periphery of the prisms. The material secreted from the Tomes process forms the core of the prisms, while that secreted from distal to the terminal web forms the peripheral parts of the prisms (prism boundaries). Enamel crystallites form at right-angles to the face of the cell (see Fig. 22.12) and thus there is considerable variation in crystallite orientation within a prism. In human enamel, the crystals in the head of the prism are approximately parallel to the long axis of the prism but in the tail deviate from this direction by 60° (see page 109). The path of the retreating ameloblasts determines the arrangement of prisms. Viewed longitudinally, the path of a human ameloblast seems to be in an approximately straight line from the enamel–dentine junction to the enamel surface. However, viewed transversely the path is seen to be sinusoidal. Thus, the different directions traced out by different layers of ameloblasts is responsible for producing the appearance of Hunter–Schreger bands in mature enamel (see page 111).

Towards the end of enamel formation, the Tomes process is lost, such that the last formed layer of enamel, like the first, is aprismatic. In this layer, all the crystals are perpendicular to the surface and parallel to each other.

## INCREMENTAL LINE FORMATION

Various structural lines and patterns have been described in enamel, and have been attributed to the rhythmic and incremental activity of the ameloblasts. Cross-striations appear as lines about 2.5–6mm apart (see page 112). They are due to a diurnal rhythm in enamel prism growth. The enamel striae (see page 113) follow the contours of the developing crown and have been considered to be incremental (analogous to growth lines in trees), and may result from changes in the direction of enamel prisms. It seems more likely that the striae represent a boundary between groups of prisms formed by different cohorts of ameloblasts. In human enamel, about seven rows of ameloblasts are generated each week at the cervical loop and the resulting prisms will extend around the crown. Each group of ameloblasts will have a somewhat different orientation from the adjacent group and the boundary between the two could constitute a striation. The striae successively outline the position of the mineralizing enamel front. They do not reach the surface over the tips of the cusps or incisal edges (see Fig. 7.33). As the daily increments of enamel are smaller towards the end of enamel formation, the striae are closer together towards the cervical margin. As there are on average about seven cross-striations between successive striae (range 6–10), the striae are thought to represent approximately weekly incremental lines (circaseptan). One theory to account for their presence suggests that, superimposed on the normal

24-hour daily rhythm, there is another rhythm of about 27 hours. The two would coincide about every 7 days, resulting in the presence of striae.

Recent studies based on careful quantification of incremental lines have provided information concerning the rates of enamel formation along the length of the crown. These are illustrated in Figures 22.30 and 22.31 and show that crown formation is non-linear and slows towards the cervix in

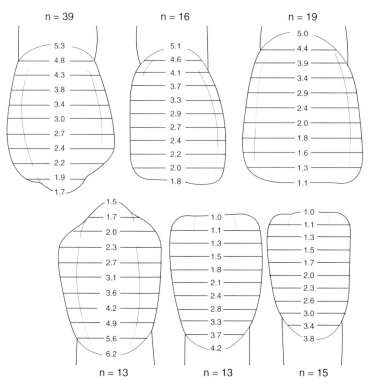

**Fig. 22.30** Mean estimates for chronological ages of enamel formation in anterior teeth. The right anterior quadrant of the mouth is depicted as viewed clinically by an observer. Each height of each tooth type is divided into 10 equally spaced zones. The age of appearance of the enamel at the incisal edge is considered coincident with the completion of cuspal enamel, when the first enamel stria reaches the surface. The mean age at completion of each zone of enamel formation is shown in years rounded up or down to one decimal place. Redrawn with permission from Reid DJ, Dean MC 2000 The timing of linear hypoplasias on human anterior teeth. *American Journal of Physical Anthropology* 113: 135–139.

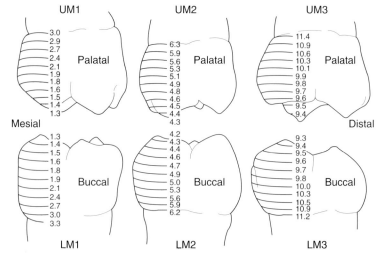

**Fig. 22.31** Mean estimates for chronological ages of enamel formation in molars. Each height of each tooth type is divided into 10 equally spaced zones. The age of appearance of the enamel at the incisal edge is considered coincident with the completion of cuspal enamel, when the first enamel stria reaches the surface. The mean age at completion of each zone of enamel formation is shown in years rounded up or down to one decimal place. Redrawn with permission from Reid DJ, Dean MC 2005 Variation in modern human enamel formation times. *Journal of Human Evolution* 50: 329–346.

all teeth. Also, there is no relation between tooth crown height and the total time taken to form enamel.

## MOLECULAR ELEMENTS OF AMELOBLAST DIFFERENTIATION

As well as describing amelogenesis in morphological and biochemical terms, it is now possible, thanks to the techniques of molecular biology, to describe the patterns of expression of many regulating, inducing and signalling molecules. The expression of a certain molecule at a particular stage of development suggests, but does not establish, a role for that molecule in amelogenesis. Experimental approaches involve deleting or over-expressing the factor under investigation and documenting the changes that occur in order to define its function with conviction. Current knowledge is fragmentary and, although increasing rapidly, a coherent and comprehensive account of the molecular mechanisms of amelogenesis is some time away. What follows is a summary of the fragments that have been found to date.

## GENE TRANSCRIPTION

Virtually all cells contain the DNA sequences (genes) that encode for enamel production. Gene regulation determines which genes are active and is the property of a class of DNA-binding proteins. Gene expression can be controlled at every step from the gene to the final functional protein. Much of the control is exercised at the stage of transcription when mRNA is produced on the DNA template. RNA is synthesized with an RNA polymerase acting in concert with transcription factors, while binding to a promoter site on the DNA. The mRNA thus formed may be modified and edited. The final mRNA, while sliding through a ribosome and acting via translational RNA, results in the assembly of polypeptides. Multiple, often different, polypeptides are conjugated into proteins, sometimes combined with polysaccharides, and given a physical configuration as they pass through the intracellular tubular pathway of the endoplasmic reticulum and Golgi apparatus. This process results most often in proteins bound in vesicles for export. The determination of which vesicles are released and when is related to intracellular signals that may be genetically programmed or may be produced in response to an external signal acting on a cell membrane receptor.

The above description of protein synthesis is generic. Only some of the factors involved in gene expression in the ameloblast are known. Homeobox genes encode for transcription factors and thus regulate transcription. Msx-2 is the product of a homeobox gene expressed in the pharyngeal (branchial) arches and in the early stages (bud) in the epithelium but not at later stages in the mesenchyme. It localizes in the enamel knot region and is possibly a regulator of morphogenesis (see page 303). Egr-1 is a transcription factor thought to regulate cell destiny in developing teeth. Its expression shifts back and forth between epithelium and mesenchyme and it is briefly expressed in the polarized ameloblasts before any matrix is produced.

At the molecular level, most information relates to the gene encoding for the enamel matrix protein amelogenin. Various forms of amelogenin may be produced by post-transcriptional modification of the mRNA and each form may have a different role in amelogenesis.

## MEMBRANE RECEPTORS

In developing tissues, cells differentiate and change their activities usually in response to an external signal. Receptor molecules on the cell surface recognize and bind signalling molecules that may, for example, be growth factors or extracellular matrix molecules. There are several families of receptor molecules. One of the integrin family of cell surface receptors, β5, is upregulated in the internal enamel epithelium during the cap stage after being expressed in the mesenchyme during the bud stage. It is then downregulated as the ameloblast differentiates. Receptors for fibroblast growth factors (FGFs) and epidermal growth factors (EGFs) are also present in the internal enamel epithelium of the bud stage but are downregulated during the cap stage. EGF expression returns to the ameloblast in maturation.

## INTRACELLULAR RECEPTORS

Some signalling molecules act on receptors that are within the cytoplasm of the cell. Cellular retinoic-acid-binding proteins transmit the signals of retinoic acid. They are expressed in the developing tooth wherever there are high rates of cell proliferation. One of these proteins (CRABP I) appears to be expressed by secretory, but not maturation-stage, ameloblasts. Growth hormone receptor is also intracellular, but appears only on the differentiating ameloblast. It seems to be related to pre-ameloblast proliferation. Vitamin D receptors have also been identified during differentiation.

## CLINICAL CONSIDERATIONS

Defects in enamel formation are common. Estimates vary from 8% to 80% of the population as having at least one affected permanent tooth. Over 100 different conditions have been identified. A group of hereditary conditions known as amelogenesis imperfecta (Fig. 22.32) affects only enamel. These are relatively common. Estimates of their prevalence range from 1 in every 14 people to 1.4 per 1000 depending upon type. Three groups of amelogenesis imperfecta are recognized, based on the phase of amelogenesis affected: 1) hypoplastic, in which the enamel is of normal colour but thin and grooved or pitted; 2) hypocalcified, in which the mineralization is poor and the enamel is dark and chips easily; and 3) hypomaturation, in which the enamel is dark, mottled and chips easily. Other hereditary conditions (including systemic metabolic disorders) in which enamel is thin and pitted also affect other tissues (e.g. mucopolysaccharidosis), while systemic ectodermal/epidermal disorders (e.g. epidermolysis bullosa) have many subtypes (including hypoplastic enamel among many more serious

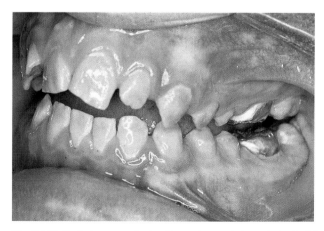

**Fig. 22.32** Teeth from a patient with amelogenesis imperfecta. In this example the enamel is of apparently normal appearance in many of the teeth but seriously abnormal in the first molars, where much of the enamel has chipped off exposing the underlying dentine. The underlying dentine is usually normal and restorative procedures, especially crowns, can be used to maintain the dentition. Courtesy of Dr M. Ignelzi.

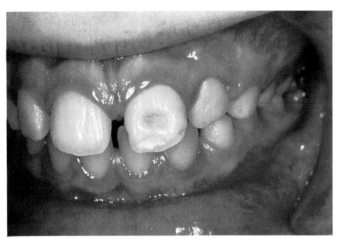

**Fig. 22.33** Tooth with enamel defect caused by trauma. This child had a blow to the maxillary left deciduous incisor that damaged the developing permanent tooth sufficiently to result in a localized defect in enamel formation. This produced a pit, seen on the facial surface of the tooth when erupted. Courtesy of Dr M. Ignelzi.

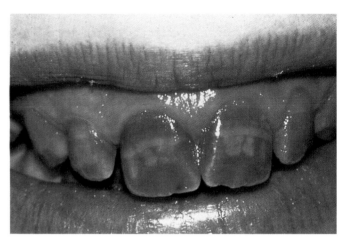

**Fig. 22.35** Teeth stained as a result of tetracycline administration. This is an extreme example of tetracycline staining: the entire enamel (and dentine) has become pigmented. As the staining is built into the structure of the tooth, bleaching procedures do not usually greatly improve the appearance of these teeth. Crowns or, more conservatively, veneers, will do so. Courtesy of Dr M. Ignelzi.

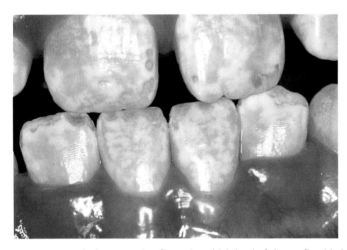

**Fig. 22.34** Teeth demonstrating fluorosis. A high level of dietary fluoride has resulted in much of the enamel becoming opaque in patches, giving a 'mottled' appearance. Courtesy of Dr M. Ignelzi.

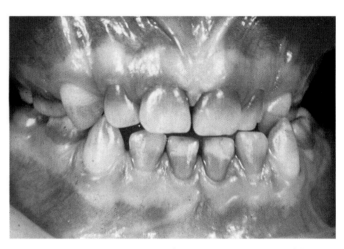

**Fig. 22.36** Teeth showing haemoglobin pigmentation. Haemoglobin residues released during Rhesus factor incompatibility are taken up by the developing teeth, resulting in a brown stain. Because of effective screening this is now a rare occurrence. Courtesy of Dr M. Ignelzi.

features). Localized trauma can result in disturbances in enamel formation in individual teeth (Fig. 22.33).

The most obvious clinically important dietary factor that affects enamel development is fluoride. Ingestion of levels above 5 parts per million results in fluorosis, characterized by the presence of a diffuse white opacity of variable extent. In severe cases, the fluoritic areas may be brown and pitted (Fig. 22.34). The principal change is a subsurface hypomineralization of varying extent.

Febrile diseases can disturb amelogenesis for the term of the illness and result in a band of poorly formed enamel. Some drugs, the best known being the tetracyclines, may affect amelogenesis. Tetracycline is incorporated into the developing enamel and results in a band of brown enamel (Fig. 22.35). When Rhesus factor incompatibility results in erythroblastosis fetalis, haemoglobin residues are incorporated into developing enamel, resulting in a brown pigmentation of the teeth (Fig. 22.36).

Dentine formation begins when the tooth germ has reached the bell stage of development. The enamel organ is fully formed, with the internal enamel epithelium differentiated and poised to secrete enamel matrix, although no enamel has yet been laid down. By convention, the dental papilla becomes the dental pulp once dentinogenesis has begun.

Dentinogenesis and amelogenesis show some common features as well as some significant differences. Among the most obvious are:

- The forming cells, odontoblasts and ameloblasts, are columnar in shape with the obvious features of protein-secreting cells (e.g. rough endoplasmic reticulum, Golgi complex).
- The forming cells both produce processes, although the odontoblast process is left behind in the dentine to occupy the tubule. The Tomes process of the ameloblast remains at the mineralizing enamel front and is related to the prismatic structure.
- The organic matrix of dentine is principally collagen, which is little changed during formation. However, the matrix of enamel is comprised of unique proteins that undergo degradation and are largely lost during the maturation of enamel. In this manner, enamel reaches a higher degree of mineralization and its crystals are larger.
- There is a lag period between the initial deposition of dentine matrix and its mineralization so that there is always a layer of predentine at the dentine–pulp interface. Enamel matrix is mineralized immediately so there is no equivalent 'pre-enamel' layer.
- Dentine is formed throughout life. Enamel is not and is fully formed prior to eruption, although some posteruptive maturation occurs in the surface layers as a result of ionic exchange with saliva.
- Whereas enamel has a more or less uniform structure, dentine shows more variation to produce regions such as the mantle, granular and hyaline layers.
- Being reactive, dentine can respond to external stimuli, producing sclerotic dentine, dead tracts and tertiary dentine.

- Dentinogenesis and amelogenesis both show evidence of phasic formation in the presence of short- and long-period incremental lines.
- There are reciprocal interactions between enamel- and dentine-forming cells during development.

Dentine formation follows a specific anatomical pattern. It begins where cusps will later be formed and continues uniformly down the slopes of the cusps and the walls of the crown to the cervical loop. This is coronal dentine. Root dentine then forms as the root sheath extends and odontoblasts differentiate on its pulpal surface. The length of the root is genetically determined and implemented, presumably, by halting the extension of the root sheath. Dentinogenesis continues and the thickness of dentine increases steadily until at a predetermined point it slows down dramatically and secondary dentine is deposited slowly. This is an age-related change, as is the simultaneous formation of peritubular dentine. Environmental factors may also affect the deposition of peritubular dentine, although this is not entirely clear.

Dentinogenesis is a continuous process, but can be, for descriptive purposes, subdivided into five stages:

- Differentiation of the odontoblasts
- Deposition of organic matrix
- Mineralization and modification of the organic matrix
- Peritubular and secondary dentine formation
- Tertiary dentine formation in response to injury.

## DIFFERENTIATION OF THE ODONTOBLASTS

The cells that will form the dentine differentiate from the ectomesenchyme of the dental papilla and are of neural crest origin (Fig. 23.1). The process of differentiation and the properties of the differentiated cells have been

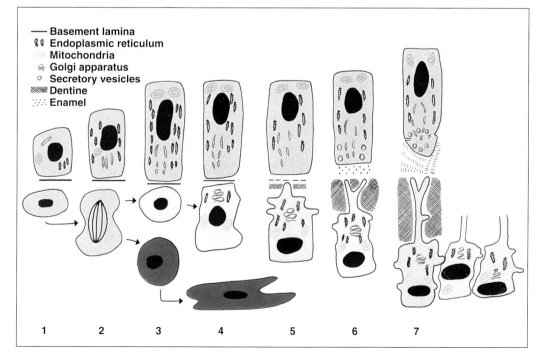

—— Basement lamina
ℓℓ Endoplasmic reticulum
Mitochondria
Golgi apparatus
Secretory vesicles
Dentine
Enamel

1   2   3   4   5   6   7

**Fig. 23.1** Life cycle of the odontoblast (lower cell line) related to that of the ameloblast (upper cell line). 1 = Ameloblast begins to differentiate first. 2 = Peripheral ectomesenchymal cells divide, with some daughter cells migrating below the odontoblast layer. 3 = Acting on a signal from the ameloblast, the pre-odontoblasts begin to differentiate. 4 = Synthetic organelles increase in size and number, especially the Golgi apparatus and rough endoplasmic reticulum. 5 = Nucleus moves basally as the cell becomes polarized. A number of odontoblast processes begin to form. One odontoblast process becomes enlarged and begins to secrete matrix. 6 = The odontoblast retreats as matrix is laid down, leaving behind a single main process. Once a narrow layer of matrix is laid down mineralization commences. 7 = Once the first layer of dentine is laid down the differentiated ameloblast begins to deposit matrix.

studied in detail by experiments recombining samples of dental papilla cells and cells from the oral ectoderm in co-culture. In addition, there have been extensive molecular observations describing the nature and sequence of gene expression in the differentiating cells. Odontoblasts express not only the genes responsible for production of the unique dentine matrix proteins but perhaps also those responsible for the morphology of the completed tooth, determining whether it is a molar, canine or incisor (morphogenetic genes – see pages 303, 310).

## EPITHELIAL–MESENCHYMAL INTERACTIONS

The differentiation of the odontoblast does not occur in isolation. Neural crest cells from the appropriate location do not differentiate to form dentine unless they come into contact with the dental epithelium. Differentiation is initiated and controlled by a series of epithelial signals. The primary enamel knot is a signalling centre that forms at the tip of the epithelial tooth bud. It is fully developed and recognizable in the cap stage and expresses at least 10 different signalling molecules belonging to the BMP, FGF, Hh, and Wnt families. In molar teeth, secondary enamel knots appear in the enamel epithelium at the sites of the future cusps. They also express several signalling molecules, and their formation precedes the folding and growth of the epithelium. The differentiation of odontoblasts always starts from the tips of the cusps, and therefore, it is conceivable that some of the signals expressed in the enamel knots may act as inducers of odontoblast differentiation. It requires temporospatially regulated epigenetic signalling. There is also an interaction in the opposite direction. Cell–cell signalling pathways and their target nuclear factors have been identified as key mediators of the progressively complex exchange of information between ectoderm and ectomesenchyme. The constantly changing direction of the reciprocal signalling and cell responses between ectoderm and ectomesenchyme enables cells to monitor their relative spatial positions and differentiated states continuously. Oral ectoderm, although differentiated into enamel epithelium, does not deposit enamel matrix until dentine deposition has started.

The basement membrane of the dental epithelium plays a major role both as a substrate and as a reservoir of signalling molecules. Time-limited changes in the composition of the basement membrane occur coincident with odontoblast differentiation. These changes include expression and localization of laminin, chondroitin-containing proteoglycans and enamel proteins. Although not strictly components of the basement membrane, fibronectin and decorin also accumulate at the distal pole of the differentiating cell. It is not known which, if any, of these changes initiate or control differentiation. Other, as yet unknown, factors may pass through the membrane too quickly to have been detected.

Growth factors are biological molecules that can control growth and repair in cells. A number, particularly those belonging to the transforming growth factor (TGF) family, insulin-like growth factor (IGF) and bone morphogenic protein (BMP) have been found in the internal enamel epithelium during the differentiation of odontoblasts. Some of these have been shown to affect, under some conditions, the development and behaviour of odontoblast-like cells maintained in culture. These cultured cells can be shown to express some of the membrane receptors for these molecules. Growth factors play an important role in the development of many tissues. While it is not currently known which are significant and what their precise role is in odontoblast differentiation, interesting hypotheses are being tested. These include the proposal that TGFβ family members, which are trapped then released from the basement membrane of the internal enamel epithelium, act on the pre-odontoblasts and, via a series of intervening steps, modulate the expression of genes involved in the assembly of the cytoskeleton. The cytoskeleton is of pre-eminent importance in the relocation of intracellular organelles and in being associated with changes in the morphology of the cell. Members of the TGF family

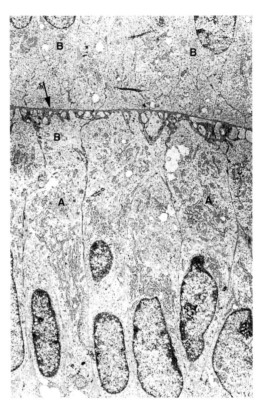

**Fig. 23.2** TEM of the interface between odontoblasts (A) and ameloblasts (B) just before the deposition of matrix. The arrow indicates the basement membrane of the ameloblasts (×38 000). Courtesy of Dr P. Glick.

may also be involved in the withdrawal of the cells that will become odontoblasts from the mitotic cycle.

## MORPHOLOGICAL CHANGES IN ODONTOBLASTS DURING DIFFERENTIATION

The morphologically discernible differentiation of the odontoblast begins with the dental papilla cells adjacent to the deepest invagination(s) of the internal enamel epithelium, beneath what will become the cusps or incisal margins. The pre-odontoblast (the cell left in contact with the basement membrane of the internal enamel epithelium after the last division of the neural crest (ectomesenchymal) cells has no well developed organelles nor a specific orientation. This changes rapidly. The cells increase in size (hypertrophy) and the nucleus comes to lie in the basal part of the cell, that furthest from the internal enamel epithelium (Fig. 23.2). The Golgi complex becomes pronounced and positioned above the nucleus. The rough endoplasmic reticulum increases in size and becomes flattened parallel to what is becoming the long axis of the cell. The elongation and polarization of the cell is accompanied by a redistribution of the intracellular skeletal proteins actin, vinculin and vimentin as well as new expression of nestin and cytokeratin. Changes also occur in the membrane of the cell including increased expression of the protein that binds fibronectin.

Many small cell processes extend from the differentiating odontoblast. Most of these are directed towards the basement membrane of the internal enamel epithelium. As differentiation proceeds, the number of processes is reduced and one large process will dominate, although some smaller processes will remain and link the odontoblasts to each other and to underlying cells in the pulp. Cell-to-cell junctions, particularly between odontoblasts but also linking odontoblasts to subodontoblastic cells, increase in number. Tight, gap and macula adherens (desmosomes) junctions occur. It is likely that some of the signals that coordinate the activities of the odontoblasts pass through the gap junctions that allow the passage of small molecules from cell to cell, although synchrony may also (or alternatively) be achieved by response to a common external signal.

Differentiation of the odontoblasts occurs in a specific temporospatial pattern, beginning under what will become the cusp tip or incisal margin and progressing rootwards. The control of this progression may lie either in the ability of the internal enamel epithelium to induce changes sequentially or in the competence of the pre-odontoblasts to act on a signal that is uniformly available. Current evidence suggests the latter, although these possibilities are not mutually exclusive.

## DEPOSITION OF DENTINE MATRIX

Once fully differentiated, the odontoblast begins to secrete its characteristic organic matrix, the components of which are listed in Table 23.1. Both collagen I and phosphophorin precursors are found within the endoplasmic reticulum, the Golgi complex and secretory granules, although they are not found together within the same compartments. Phosphophorin is localized within the tubular endoplasmic reticulum, round-shaped transitional vesicles, the Golgi complex and in narrow asymmetric secretory granules. These asymmetric secretory granules are abundant in the odontoblastic process boundary. Collagen I was localized within rosette form endoplasmic reticulum compartments, the Golgi complex and large, distinctive secretory granules. Collagen I is deposited at the cell–predentine boundary phosphophorin (as dentine phosphoprotein) by the process. The matrix thus formed consists primarily of type I collagen fibrils with dentine phosphoprotein (DPP) as the second most abundant constituent. This and dentine sialoprotein (DSP), are secreted not only by odontoblasts but also during the early stages of dentinogenesis by the pre-ameloblasts of the internal enamel epithelium.

Both DPP and DSP were thought to be unique to dentine and not found in bone. DSP has now been reported in alveolar bone, cellular cementum, osteocytes, cementocytes and their matrices. It has also become clear that DSP and DPP are formed from the proteolysis of a single parent molecule, dentine sialophosphoprotein.

It has been postulated that DPP has a significant role in dentine mineralization. DSP may also have a role, although less important, in mineralization. It has also been suggested that DPP is involved in signalling during epithelial–mesenchymal interactions. Many other proteins (such as glycoproteins and proteoglycans) are added to the matrix. In the first-formed dentine (mantle dentine), some of the matrix components may be contributed by dental pulp cells beneath the odontoblasts. The odontoblast is still undergoing the late stages of differentiation as the first layer of dentine matrix is being deposited. Numerous cytoplasmic processes rapidly resolve into a single large process. As it is formed by odontoblasts that are still differentiating and because other cells appear to contribute to its formation, mantle dentine in the crown (and possibly the hyaline and granular layers in the root) is of somewhat different structure and probably composition than the bulk of the matrix (Fig. 23.3).

The type I collagen fibres that are laid down initially lie at right angles to the future dentine–enamel junction. In sections of harshly fixed tissue stained with silver, these fibres take on a 'corkscrew' appearance (Fig. 23.4).

Once the initial mantle layer has been laid down, the bulk of the primary circumpulpal dentine is laid down in a regular incremental pattern. This

**Table 23.1** *Components of organic dentine extracellular matrix*

| Collagens | Enamelysin |
|---|---|
| Type 1 | |
| Type 1 trimer | |
| Type V | |
| Type III (?) | |
| Type VI | |
| | |
| **Proteoglycans** | **Lipids** |
| Decorin (PG II) | Phospholipids (phosphatidylcholine, |
| Biglycan (PG I) | phosphatidylethanolamine |
| Other chondroitin 4-sulphate- | Cholesterol |
| containing proteoglycans | Cholesterol esters |
| Dermatan sulphate proteoglycans | Triacylglycerols |
| Keratan sulphate (?) | |
| Perlecan | |
| | |
| **Glycoproteins/sialoproteins** | **Serum-derived proteins** |
| Osteonectin | α2HS-glycoprotein |
| Dentine sialoprotein(s) (DSPs) | Albumin |
| Bone sialoprotein | Immunoglobulins |
| Osteopontin | |
| Bone acidic glycoprotein 75 | |
| Syndecan 2 | |
| | |
| **Phosphoproteins** | **Growth factors** |
| Dentine phosphoproteins (DPPs) | TGFβs |
| Dentine matrix protein 1 | Chondrogenic inducing factor |
| γ-Carboxyglutamate-containing | Bone morphogenic proteins (BMPs) |
| proteins | Fibroblast growth factors (FGFs) |
| Osteocalcin | Insulin-like growth factors (IGFs) |
| Matrix Gla protein | |
| Amelin-1 (transient expression) | |

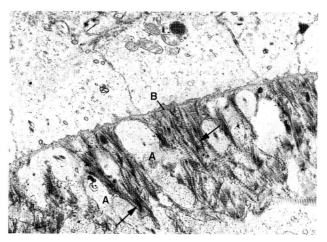

**Fig. 23.3** TEM showing early dentine matrix formation. The basement membrane of the ameloblasts (B) is still present. Some components may cross the basement membrane from the ameloblasts. The odontoblasts initially have multiple processes (A). Note initial collagen fibrils are oriented perpendicular to enamel–dentine junction (arrows) (×9500). Courtesy of Dr P. Glick.

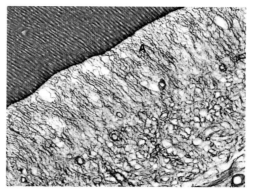

**Fig. 23.4** Micrograph of a demineralized section showing 'corkscrew' fibres (of von Korff) (A). These are thought to be the first-formed type I collagen fibres whose orientation differs from those laid down later. Harsh fixation makes them curly and the deposition of silver makes them appear thick. They are thus an artefact but one based on a real difference between the structure of mantle and the later formed dentine (Silver stain; ×200).

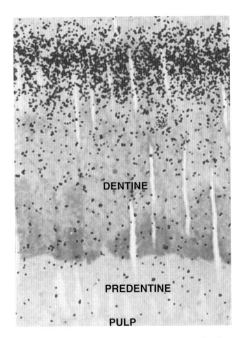

**Fig. 23.5** Light microscope radioautograph of dentine formation 4 days after injection of ³H-proline. A labelled band (silver grains) approximately the same width as the predentine is clearly seen, demonstrating the incremental nature of matrix deposition (Iron haematoxylin stain; ×560). Courtesy of Drs H. Warshawsky and K. Josephsen and the editor of the *Archives of Oral Biology*.

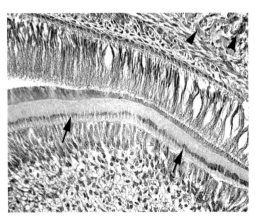

**Fig. 23.6** Localization of phosphophorin at the mineralization front (arrows) and in the odontoblast cells (×250). Courtesy of Dr A. George and the editors of *Cell Tissue Organs*.

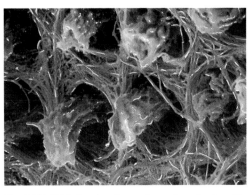

**Fig. 23.7** SEM showing the surface of predentine. The collagen fibrils (brown) form an interlacing network perpendicular to the odontoblast process (blue) (×4000). Courtesy of Professor L. Fonzi.

pattern can be followed by observing the distribution of injected radio-labelled amino acids (Fig. 23.5). The synthetic pathways followed in the cell are those well established for the production of proteins and complex molecules that include proteins. The release of the various matrix components, however, can follow differing pathways. Type I collagen is released primarily from the odontoblast cell body as it moves inwards. Thus, the odontoblast is always closely juxtaposed to the unmineralized predentine. Dentine phosphophorin, on the other hand, is released primarily from the odontoblast process a short distance from the cell body, consistent with its important role in mineralization (see below) and allowing it to bypass some of the predentine (Fig. 23.6).

Once the mantle layer is formed, the remaining type I collagen is laid down with its fibres approximately parallel to the pulp dentine border. Minor, but coincident, changes in orientation about every week (20 μm) could be responsible for the long-period incremental lines (Andresen lines – see page 141).

The deposition of new organic matrix proceeds at a pace similar to that of mineralization, such that there is always a layer of unmineralized matrix, the predentine, on the pulpal surface of the tissue (Fig. 23.7). Collagen is secreted at the cell border, apparently primarily by the cell body of the odontoblast. The odontoblast process secretes the other non-collagenous proteins such that a complex of collagen and non-collagenous proteins is formed at the junction of the predentine and calcified dentine, the mineralization front (Fig. 23.8). The phosphophorins and other non-collagenous proteins bind to the collagen; the phosphophorins bind in a highly specific manner at the 'e' band in the gap region of the type I fibrils.

What controls the secretory activity of the odontoblast is unclear. The rate of secretion varies, following both short-term (diurnal) and long-period rhythms. Serious systemic disturbances (such as birth and disease) can slow or stop it. Dentine seems to be less vulnerable to dietary deficiencies than bone. Presumably much of its activity is genetically predetermined. Once the odontoblast is separated from the internal enamel

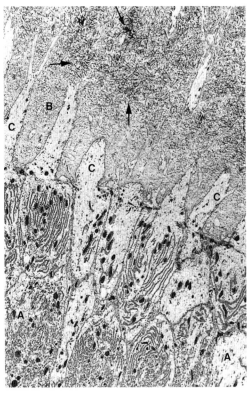

**Fig. 23.8** TEM showing dentine matrix formation (B) and mineralization. The outer matrix is mineralizing (arrows), initially with small groups of crystals. The odontoblasts (A) have a single large process (C) (×6500). Courtesy of Dr P. Glick.

epithelium, the effect of other cell populations is unknown. The rate of dentine deposition can be altered (increased) by injury to the nerves supplying the pulp. Much of this effect could be explained as secondary to changes in blood flow or (in erupted teeth) as a result of a loss of sensory activity that might lead to greater wear on the teeth. However, proteins unique to synapses (synapsin and synaptotagmin) have been detected within dentinal tubules in regions where axons enter dentinal tubules (Fig. 23.9). It is thus possible that, in some areas at least, efferent nerve activity may have an effect on matrix secretion. The effect would probably be on secretion rather than synthesis as the synaptic proteins are absent from around the odontoblast cell body.

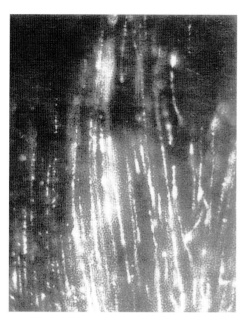

**Fig. 23.9** Immunofluorescence micrograph of inner dentine close to the pulp horn stained with a labelled antibody for synaptotagmin, a protein characteristic of synapses. Its presence (white staining) and distribution in a pattern similar to nerves suggest that intradentinal nerves may be releasing a transmitter (Immunohisto-  ·  chemistry; ×400). Courtesy of T. Norlin, M. Hilliges and L. Brodin and the editor of the *Archives of Oral Biology*.

## MINERALIZATION OF DENTINE

Dentine mineralization is a complex and controversial subject. Of the five mineralized tissues (bone, calcified cartilage, cementum, dentine and enamel), the process in enamel is unique, involving a protein matrix not found elsewhere and a two-step accumulation of mineral. In the remaining collagen-containing tissues, the process is similar but with sufficient diversity to make the structure and properties of the tissues different. The questions that are posed about mineralization in general, and mineralization in dentine in particular, include:

- What initiates mineralization? The first layers of dentine matrix are unmineralized but when it reaches a certain width mineralization begins and progresses at the same rate as matrix formation.
- Where does the mineral that is deposited come from? Is it transported by odontoblasts or present in the extracellular fluid?
- What controls the rate of mineralization?
- Are the dentine crystals initially deposited at their more or less final size or do they grow?
- Are the crystals deposited in the extracellular fluid or on the fibrillar collagen of the matrix?
- Is mineralization merely the addition of crystals to the organic matrix or does the matrix undergo changes during the deposition of mineral?
- Can variations in the mineralization process explain some of the structural features of dentine such as mantle dentine, interglobular dentine, incremental lines and peritubular dentine?
- Does the mineralization of secondary and tertiary dentine differ from that of primary dentine?
- How does intrapulpal mineralization (pulp stones) occur?
- Does the remineralization of dentine following exposure to acids or dental caries follow the same process as the original mineralization of the tissue?
- Are defects in mineralization a component of dentine dysplasias?

Although several hypotheses have been put forward to explain dentine mineralization and several factors may contribute to the overall process, the key element in initiating and controlling mineralization is clearly the odontoblast. It produces the matrix that becomes mineralized. It controls the transport and release of calcium ions. It determines the presence and distribution of the matrix components that can initiate and modulate the process. Mineralization only occurs when odontoblasts are present.

The data from which one can attempt to develop a coherent account of dentine mineralization have been accumulated from a variety of sources; histological and histochemical studies, biochemical analyses of the tissue at various stages and in vitro studies either of odontoblast-like cells or pulpal tissue maintained in culture. Molecular biological (genetic expression) data directly related to mineralization are scarce, although, as mineralization is so closely linked to matrix formation, the body of work available from this is highly relevant. In any experimental study the data generated are obviously related to the techniques used and no single approach can provide a complete description of a complex process. Some data from bone studies have been extrapolated to dentine.

## MINERALIZATION OF CIRCUMPULPAL DENTINE

Odontoblasts actively transport calcium ions to the mineralization site (Fig. 23.10). Although the precise intracellular mechanisms are not completely understood, serum calcium is taken up by the odontoblast and accumulates in the distal body and process, much of it bound to organelles rather than in the cytosol (intracellular fluid). High concentrations of calcium ions are toxic to cells but the odontoblast seems to be protected against this. Although some calcium ions reach the dentine by an extracellular pathway this is probably not the major route. The intracellular route (Fig. 23.11) of calcium transport actively controls the level in the mineralizing area and maintains calcium ion concentrations that are not in equilibrium with body fluids.

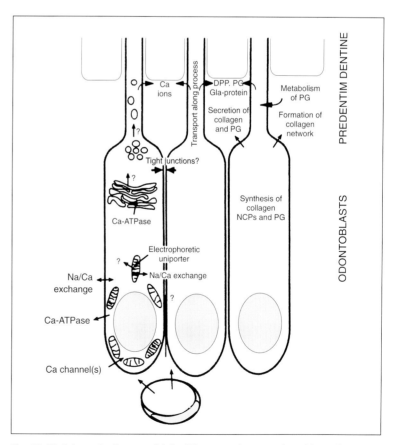

**Fig. 23.10** Schematic diagram of fully differentiated active odontoblasts showing different calcium ion transport mechanisms (left side of figure) as well as putative transport routes for the dentine matrix macromolecules (right side of figure). Courtesy of Dr A. Linde and the editor of the *International Journal of Developmental Biology*.

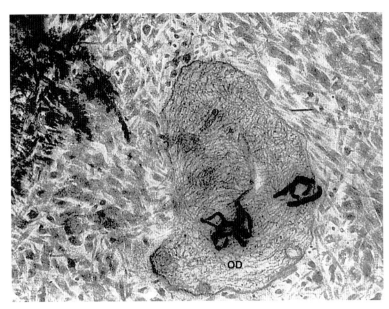

**Fig. 23.11** TEM autoradiograph showing an odontoblast process (OD) near the predentine–dentine junction 30 minutes after intravenous infusion of $^{45}$Ca. Note the silver grains representing this Ca over the cytoplasm of the process. The black zone at the top left corner represents mineralizing dentine (×30000). Courtesy of Drs R.M. Frank and N. Nagai and the editor of *Cell and Tissue Research*.

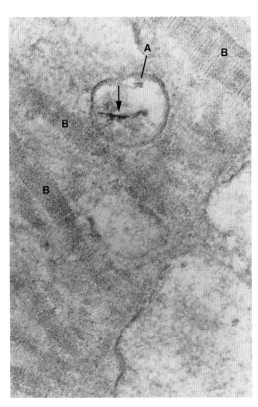

**Fig. 23.12** TEM showing a matrix vesicle consisting of a membrane (A) around fluid containing a crystal (arrow) among recently deposited collagen fibrils (B) (×70000). Courtesy of Dr P. Glick.

Evidence that has accumulated over about the past 20 years suggests that the calcium transported by the odontoblasts becomes a crystalline mineral in the dentine by deposition on to a template formed by type I collagen fibrils and is largely under the control of the predominant non-collagenous protein in dentine, DPP.

DPP is highly anionic and thus able to bind calcium. Changes in conformation of the protein allow it to bind increasing numbers of calcium ions, allowing the formation and growth of a crystal. In high concentrations, DPP inhibits crystal formation. Thus, by controlling the release and level of DPP, the odontoblast can control the initiation of mineralization and the rate of deposition.

Mineral crystals first appear in the hole zone formed by the quarter-stacking of the collagen molecules. The collagen triple helices are stacked in parallel with overlapping regions and spaces between adjacent molecules. Ultrastructurally, the bulk of the dentine mineral is on the surface of the dentine collagen.

The evidence that DPP is involved in the initiation and growth of mineral includes its distribution. DPP is absent from non-mineralized matrix and concentrated at the mineralization front (Fig. 23.6). In vitro, it can be shown to bind calcium, induce hydroxyapatite nucleation and control crystal growth. It is absent from the dentine of patients with dentinogenesis imperfecta.

The postulated role of DPP in mineralization may be summarized as:

1. Transport of ions to the mineralization front
2. Aggregation of collagen fibres
3. Location of nucleation to specific regions of the collagen fibril surface
4. Stabilization and orientation of the formed crystal.

Although DPP gets the most attention as the master of mineralization, other proteins have mineralizing characteristics in vitro but, given their low concentrations and more limited properties, it is difficult to say how much these other proteins may contribute to the mineralization of dentine.

*Osteonectin* is a phosphorylated glycoprotein produced by the odontoblast and present in human dentine. In vitro, it can inhibit the growth of hydroxyapatite crystals and promote calcium and phosphate binding to collagen.

*Osteopontin* is a phosphorylated protein capable of promoting mineral formation in dentine.

*Bone sialoprotein*, another phosphorylated glycoprotein, is found in early mineralizing dentine and in peritubular dentine.

*Dentine sialoprotein* (DSP), the other non-collagenous protein unique to dentine and the dental pulp, is a non-phosphorylated glycoprotein found predominantly in predentine and thus unlikely to be significantly involved in mineralization.

*Chondroitin sulphates 4 and 6* are present around the collagen fibrils (together with phospholipids) throughout dentine and predentine. Their properties can vary depending on whether they are in solution (as they are in the predentine) or adsorbed on to collagen (as in mineralizing dentine). In predentine, they may play a role in transport and diffusion and act as hydroxyapatite inhibitors, whereas in dentine they may promote hydroxyapatite initiation. The concentration of chondroitin sulphate decreases as mineralization proceeds.

## OTHER PROCESSES POSSIBLY INVOLVED IN THE INITIATION OF MINERALIZATION

When dentine mineralization is initiated, two other processes have been implicated in addition to, or in place of, the DPP-mediated nucleation on collagen fibrils. Cell budding or cell fragmentation to form 'matrix vesicles' occurs in what will become mantle dentine. Membrane-bound organelles (30–200 nm) are formed, containing a variety of enzymes (including alkaline phosphatase) that lead to a concentration of phosphate ions within the vesicle. Mineral crystals develop within the vesicles (Fig. 23.12). As these are the only crystalline structures present very early in mantle dentine formation, they have been credited with an initiating role in mineralization. Similar matrix vesicles have been implicated in the initial mineralization of bone and calcified cartilage. Mineralizing material can accumulate within cells including the odontoblast process. As the odontoblast process retreats, cell debris may remain and form a nidus

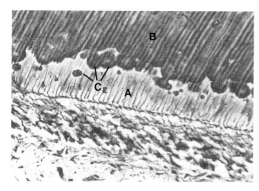

**Fig. 23.13** Demineralized section showing the region of mineralizing dentine. A = predentine; B = mineralized dentine; C = calcospherites (H & E; ×230).

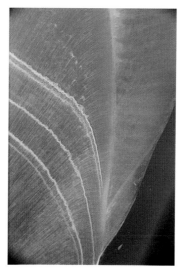

**Fig. 23.16** Ground section of a tooth viewed with fluorescent light. The incremental nature of mineralization is demonstrated in an individual who has been treated with tetracycline. Tetracycline binds to the mineral as it is deposited and is represented by the bright yellow lines, indicating that the patient has had multiple injections of the antibiotic. The irregularity of the line indicates both calcospheritic and linear patterns of mineralization. This can lead to the discoloration of teeth, and the use of tetracycline should be avoided during the period of tooth development. Tetracycline also fluoresces under ultraviolet light (Ground section, fluorescent light; ×5). Courtesy of Dr B.A.W. Brown.

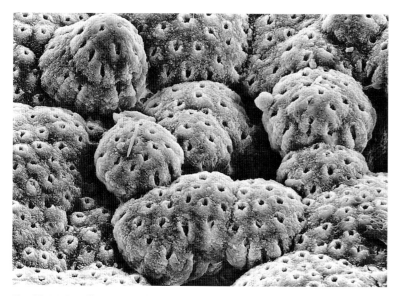

**Fig. 23.14** SEM illustrating calcospherites at the mineralizing front. In this preparation all the organic material (including the predentine) has been removed by hypochlorite to reveal the underlying mineralized dentine (×1500). Courtesy of Professor M.C. Dean.

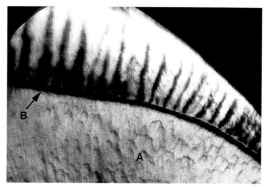

**Fig. 23.17** Ground section of a tooth viewed in polarized light. Calcospherites (A) are distributed widely in circumpulpal dentine. The changes in crystal orientation at the boundary of the original crystallites differ and differentially block the polarized light. In single-phase light at this orientation the mantle layer completely blocks transmission and thus appears black (B) (×25).

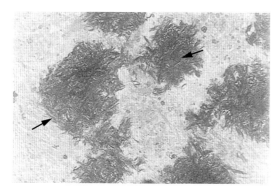

**Fig. 23.15** Calcospherites (arrowed) at the mineralizing front of dentine (TEM; ×1450).

for mineralization. The presence of matrix vesicles is limited to mantle dentine.

As matrix deposition and mineralization continue, there will always be a zone of mineralization discernible histologically (Fig. 23.13). The mineralizing front often appears irregular: in some areas, mineralization appears to progress linearly by apposition on to previously mineralized areas, while in others it seems to occur in spheres that eventually fuse (Figs 23.14, 23.15). In yet other situations, mineralization is a combination of the two (Fig. 23.13). These mineralization patterns can be visualized when the mineralizing front is highlighted by the antibiotic tetracycline (Fig. 23.16).

Owing to the complex biochemical changes occurring at the mineralizing front, it often stains differently and has been referred to as intermediate dentine.

The pattern of calcospherite formation is common throughout dentine. It is possible that some form around matrix vesicles, especially in the first-formed mantle dentine, but the widespread nature of the calcospherites and the rarity of matrix vesicles suggest that such a pattern of accretion also occurs around centres of initial mineralization that form on collagen fibrils. Failure of such calcospherites to fuse may result in the appearance of 'interglobular' dentine, often seen in peripheral dentine (see page 139). In calcospherites, the crystallites are arranged in a radiating pattern and, despite complete mineralization of the dentine, their outline can still be discerned using polarized light (Fig. 23.17). The size and shape of the calcospherites generally varies in different regions (Fig. 23.18).

## FORMATION OF ROOT DENTINE

The basic process of root dentinogenesis does not differ fundamentally from coronal dentinogenesis. Such differences as do occur are in the early stages such that the histological appearance of the peripheral dentine differs between crown and root. These are, presumably, due to differing contributions in terms of control and content from the internal enamel epithelium of the crown, which will go on to form enamel, and the epithelial root sheath, which, after initiating radicular dentinogenesis, does not undergo further differentiation but fragments. Initial collagen deposition does not begin in the root immediately against the basal lamina of the epithelial cells of the root sheath. The space between the initial collagen and the epithelial cells becomes filled with an amorphous ground substance and a fine, fibrillar, non-collagenous matrix secreted by the root sheath comprising, in part, enamel-like proteins. These elements form a hyaline layer of approximately 10 μm. In the past, this has been described as a component of either dentine or cementum; it is discussed further on pages 138, 139. The initial collagen fibres deposited in the root lie approximately parallel to the cementum–dentine junction. This contrasts with the mantle dentine in the crown, where the collagen fibres are deposited perpendicular to the enamel–dentine junction. Radicular odontoblasts differ slightly from those in the crown, developing several fine branches that loop in umbrella fashion (Fig. 23.19). This gives rise to the appearance of the granular layer (of Tomes), although this may, in part, be due to the presence of many small, unmineralized interglobular areas. The loss of continuity of the epithelial cells as the root sheath breaks down results in larger numbers of interglobular areas and, possibly, also in the incorporation of some epithelial remnants in the peripheral dentine. Radicular dentine forms at a slightly slower rate than coronal dentine. Its pattern of mineralization is similar, although its initial calcospherites are smaller and its interglobular areas more numerous. In general, root mineralization proceeds as a continuation of that in the crown although, in multirooted teeth, separate isolated areas of mineralization may occur. Unusually, there is evidence that the first-formed root dentine undergoes delayed mineralization compared with the root dentine formed a little later; this may be related to its bonding with the cementum (see pages 138–140).

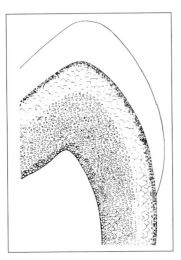

**Fig. 23.18** The distribution of calcospherites in dentine. Most calcospherites are spherical. However, many have an arcade shape, such that the round apex of the arcade is directed towards the outer surface of the dentine and the opening is directed towards the pulp. The size varies considerably: the arcade variety tends to be larger than the spherical variety. The size and shape of the calcospherites seem to be governed by the rate of dentine formation and by the rate at which new calcospherites are initiated. There is a fairly consistent pattern of distribution within the tooth. In the mantle dentine of the crown, in the hyaline layer of the root and in the superficial circumpulpal dentine the calcospherites are small, spherical and closely packed. In the middle region of the circumpulpal dentine they are larger, more widely spaced and arcade-like in form (although the region tends to be free of calcospherites towards the root apex). The inner half to two-thirds of the circumpulpal dentine contains spherical calcospherites. Courtesy of Dr R.P. Shellis and the publishers of *The companion to dental studies*, vol 2, Blackwell, Oxford.

## PERITUBULAR AND SECONDARY DENTINE FORMATION

### PERITUBULAR (INTRATUBULAR) DENTINE

Peritubular dentine (see page 132) consists of small crystals in an amorphous (non-fibrillar) matrix consisting of glycoproteins, proteoglycans, lipids, osteonectin, osteocalcin and bone sialoprotein. Despite the difference in composition, there is structural continuity between the peritubular and intertubular dentine.

The composition of the peritubular dentine suggests that it is a product of the odontoblast and plasma proteins that have diffused along the cell membrane. Evidence that it is physiological rather than a result of degeneration or retreat of the odontoblast includes:

- the presence of small tubules in it representing where lateral processes of the odontoblast once were
- the occasional finding histologically of odontoblast processes surrounded by peritubular dentine
- the occurrence in two species, the elephant and opossum, of peritubular dentine formation preceding intertubular dentine formation (Fig. 23.20).

Although much is known about the composition of peritubular dentine and a reasonable description of its origin has been established, little is known about either the signal that initiates the onset of tubular occlusion

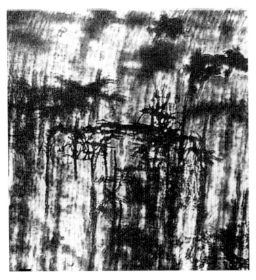

**Fig. 23.19** Ground section of root showing evidence of looping and branching of dentine tubules in the granular layer of the root. In this preparation, the dentinal tubules have become filled with a silver stain and the tissue has been examined in a thicker than normal section. While this obscures much fine detail by superimposition, it does allow some insight into the three-dimensional arrangement. The peripheral terminations of several tubules may be seen, and a profuse branching in three dimensions can be distinguished. Above the tubules in focus are others below the plane of focus. Here, it may be seen how this arrangement could contribute to the appearance of the granular layer (Silver stain; ×490).

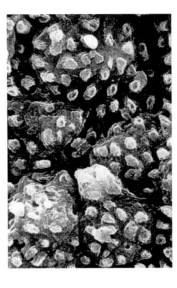

**Fig. 23.20** SEM of anorganic preparation of the surface of mineralizing dentine in the opossum. Projecting localized white zones of peritubular dentine are visible, which therefore are forming (in this species) before the adjacent intertubular dentine (×1000). Courtesy of N. Azevedo and M. Goldberg and the editor of the *Journal de Biologie Buccale*.

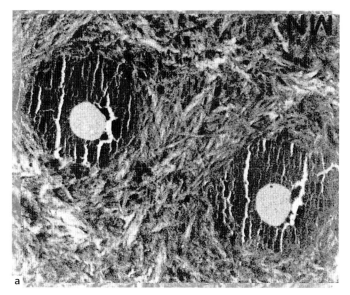
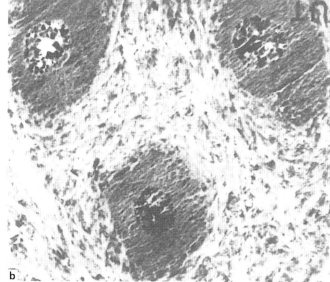

Fig. 23.21

**Fig. 23.21** Peritubular dentine (a) and sclerotic dentine (b). In sclerotic dentine, a second form of crystal formation, whitlockite, can fill in the tubules within, but distinct from, the peritubular dentine (TEM; ×10 000). Courtesy of Dr T. Fusayama and the editor of the *Journal de Biologie Buccale*.

**Fig. 23.22** Confocal microscope image showing apoptotic (dying) cells in the subodontoblastic region (SO) of the coronal pulp (CP). The cells have been fluorescently labelled (white) with a stain unique for dying cells (×60). Courtesy of J.-C. Franquin and the editor of the *European Journal of Oral Science*.

**Fig. 23.23** Demineralized transverse section of a cat canine 30 days after denervation viewed with a fluorescence microscope. The animal was injected with tetracycline at the time of denervation. The arrowed line shows the dentine that has incorporated the tetracycline. Regular secondary dentine has formed after this point at a rate faster than in non-denervated teeth. The increase in rate is transient and, by 180 days postdenervation, the amount of secondary dentine deposited in control and operated teeth is the same. P = dental pulp; AB = alveolar bone (×10). Courtesy of L. Olgart and the editor of the *European Journal of Oral Sciences*.

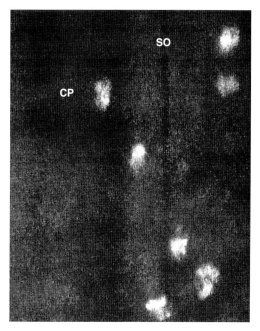

Fig. 23.22

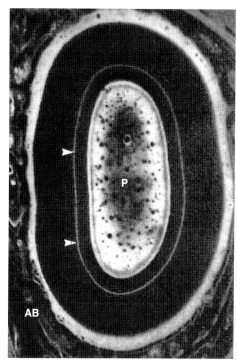

Fig. 23.23

or what controls its rate of deposition. It would seem likely that age is the principal factor. The degree of tubular occlusion (as measured by the presence of translucent dentine, particularly in the root) can be used to determine the age of teeth and is applied in forensic circumstances. Peritubular dentine formation does not seem to be related to outside stimuli as it is found in unerupted teeth. The rate of tubular occlusion by peritubular dentine formation beneath dental caries is little different from that in intact teeth. Tubules directly beneath caries can become occluded, but this is thought to be due to the reprecipitation of mineral during the demineralization process that characterizes dental caries (Fig. 23.21). In older teeth, peritubular dentine formation is usually most pronounced near the root apices, remote from areas of attrition or caries. Until more detail is known about the switching of odontoblast production from intertubular to peritubular it is best attributed to a preprogrammed genetic trigger.

## SECONDARY DENTINE

As noted earlier in this chapter, the original odontoblasts form secondary dentine that, like peritubular dentine, seems to be a preprogrammed age change rather than a response to external activity. Part of this may be attributed to apoptosis (Fig. 23.22). As the pulp volume decreases with continuing dentine deposition, odontoblasts die. Over a 4-year period, the odontoblast population may be reduced by 50%. This dramatic reduction in numbers also presumably leads to the change in direction of the tubules, establishing a contour line (see page 141).

Experimental denervation results in increased secondary dentine formation (Fig. 23.23). This may be mediated by changes in blood flow, although a direct trophic effect is possible. It is not known whether the innervation has an influence physiologically on the formation of either primary or secondary dentine.

## TERTIARY DENTINE FORMATION IN RESPONSE TO INJURY

The nature and severity of stimuli that reach the dental pulp vary over a considerable range. Dental caries will induce inflammation and may lead to necrosis. Protecting the pulp and encouraging it to recover after caries has been removed is a principal aim of restorative dentistry. Tertiary dentine is the tissue that is laid down in response to a stimulus of any kind. It is a response rather than an age change. Tertiary dentine takes one of two forms depending on the severity of the stimulus. If the stimulus is mild and the original odontoblasts remain alive they will lay down a tubular form of tertiary dentine, *reactionary dentine*. If the stimulus is more severe and sufficient to kill the original odontoblasts, new odontoblasts will differentiate from pulpal stem cells and lay down another form of tertiary dentine, *reparative dentine*, which is atubular and bone-like.

One important difference between the activity of these new odontoblasts and those involved in primary and secondary dentine formation is that the new cells do not form dentine phosphophorin. This molecule, apparently so important to the production of primary dentine, seems to have no role in the making of tertiary dentine. The effect of signalling molecules, especially TGFβ and BMPs, may be important in tertiary dentine formation. One hypothesis suggests that members of the TGFβ family present in dentine and predentine may be released by acids produced during the progress of dental caries and diffuse through the dentine to stimulate activity in the original odontoblasts or induce the differentiation of new odontoblasts from stem cells. The difference in response could be related to differences in the nature, amount and direction of the signalling molecules.

## CLINICAL CONSIDERATIONS

Serious systemic disease occurring during the period of tooth development can result in the disturbance of both matrix formation and its mineralization, which would usually be reflected in both the dentine and the enamel that were forming at the time. There are two groups of inherited defects that are limited to dentine, dentinogenesis imperfecta types I and II (Figs 23.24, 23.25) and dentine dysplasia types I and II. Both dysplasias result in incomplete obliteration of the pulp chamber with histologically abnormal root dentine (dentine dysplasia I has irregular, sparse tubules; type II aberrantly oriented tubules). Type I but not type II causes stunted roots.

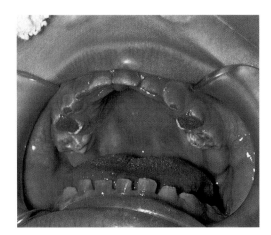

Fig. 23.24

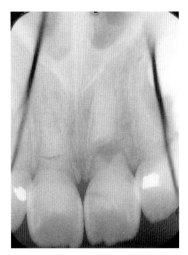

Fig. 23.25

**Fig. 23.24** A patient with dentinogenesis imperfecta. The teeth are malformed and are dark because of the absence of pulp chambers and the consequent loss of translucency. The enamel is normal but flakes off as it is only weakly attached to the dentine. In this example the enamel from the first molars has been lost. Courtesy of M. Ignelzi.

**Fig. 23.25** An intra-oral radiograph of the upper central incisors from a patient with dentinogenesis imperfecta. There are no pulp chambers or root canals. Both central incisors have fractured because of their great fragility. Courtesy of M. Ignelzi.

Both forms of dentinogenesis imperfecta result in similar changes but in addition the morphology of the tooth crown is bulbous. The types are distinguished by type I occurring as part of a more widespread connective tissue disease, osteogenesis imperfecta. In all these disorders the odontoblasts seem to be incompletely developed and it is possible that the production of dentine phosphophorin is defective.

At the bud stage of tooth germ development a region of more densely packed mesenchymal cells becomes evident around the developing enamel organ (Fig. 24.1). All the cells that form the dental papilla are derived from the neural crest (ectomesenchyme) and have migrated from their position by the pharyngeal arches. Cells from other sources are not able to induce tooth formation (see Ch. 21). The first pharyngeal arch, the future mandible, is populated by neural crest cells originating from the caudal midbrain and rostral hindbrain. The frontonasal process, giving rise to much of the future maxillae, is colonized by neural crest cells originating in the forebrain. Neural crest cells are more densely packed than the surrounding mesenchyme, are separated by relatively little extracellular matrix and are rapidly dividing This mass of cells expands around the tooth bud (see Fig. 21.6). Once the bud-stage enamel organ invaginates to become the cap stage, the cells and matrix within the invagination are recognized as the dental papilla (Fig. 24.2). During growth of the tooth germ, although undifferentiated, the expansion of the dental papilla exerts a morphogenetic effect on the enamel organ (see page 310). The mesenchymal cells

surrounding the developing enamel organ externally form the dental follicle that will give rise to the periodontal ligament and supporting tissues of the tooth (see Ch. 25). As the enamel organ surrounding the dental papilla enlarges and enters the bell stage (Fig. 24.3), the cells within the dental papilla undergo cytodifferentiation into a peripheral layer of odontoblasts and a central mass of fibroblasts. This change is induced by signals originating in the internal enamel epithelium (see Ch. 23). Immature dendritic antigen-presenting cells appear in and around the odontoblast layer at an early stage (Fig. 24.4). Once the odontoblasts have begun to lay down dentine, the dental papilla becomes, by convention, the dental pulp. The small, undifferentiated, ectomesenchymal cells of the dental papilla are packed closely together with little intercellular material content relative to that in the mature tooth. They are stellate in shape with a relatively large nucleus and little cytoplasm. As the pulp develops, the cytoplasmic component of these central cells expands and synthetic organelles appear. The material the organelles produce is released into the extracellular space and forms fine collagen fibres that are embedded in an amorphous ground substance. Coarse fibre bundles appear only at about the time that the tooth reaches maturity. In the early stages of pulpal development, the ground substance has a high glycosaminoglycan content relative to that of the mature tooth. The level of glycosaminoglycans increases until the time of eruption and then decreases. The chondroitin sulphates are the main glycosaminoglycans present during pulp development, with only a minor quantity of hyaluronan. This balance is reversed in the mature pulp. Not all cells undergo differentiation, a proportion remaining as

**Fig. 24.1** A developing enamel organ at the early bud stage (A), with a condensation of mesenchymal cells (B) around it (Masson's trichrome stain; ×80).

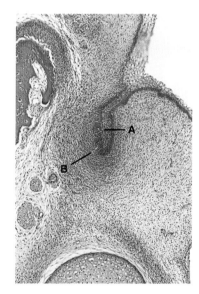

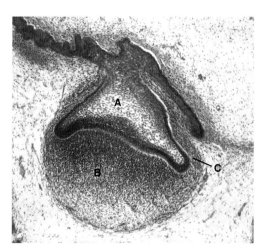

**Fig. 24.2** An enamel organ at the cap stage of development (A) surrounding the mesenchymal cells of the dental papilla (B). The tooth germ is surrounded by the developing dental follicle (C) (H & E; ×80). Courtesy of Professor M.M. Smith.

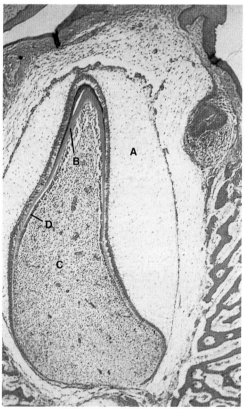

**Fig. 24.3** A developing tooth at the late bell stage of development (appositional phase). A = enamel organ; B = developing dentine; C = dental papilla; D = odontoblast layer (Masson's trichrome; ×55).

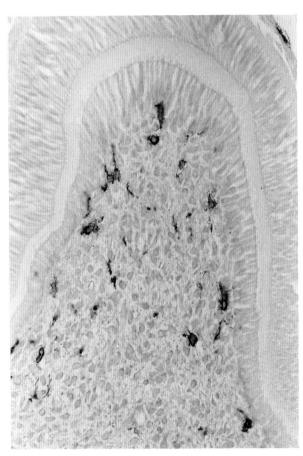

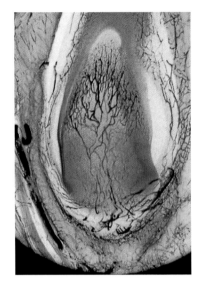

Fig. 24.5

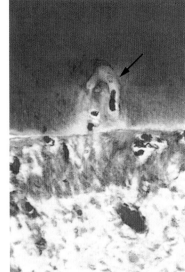

Fig. 24.7

**Fig. 24.4** Dark-staining dendritic cells in the periphery of the developing pulp (rat molar, post-natal day 1, immunohistochemistry; ×300). Courtesy of Drs E. Tsuruga, Y. Sakahura, T. Yajima and N. Shide and the editor of *Histochemistry and Cell Biology*.

undifferentiated mesenchymal cells retaining the potential to differentiate in later life.

Dentinogenesis then progresses by the processes described in Chapter 23 but at the same time differentiation continues as the enamel organ extends as Hertwig's epithelial root sheath and determines the final morphology of the space (pulp chamber and root canals) that the dental pulp will occupy. The actions and interactions of the dental follicle (outside the epithelial root sheath), the epithelial root sheath and the dental papilla result in the formation of cementum (described in Chapter 25) on the surface of the developing root dentine. Once the full length of the root is established the developmental stage of the dental pulp can be considered complete. However, dentine deposition will continue throughout life. A cell-rich zone develops beneath the odontoblast layer at the time of eruption. It arises by the migration of more central cells rather than by local cell division. A cell-free zone may be evident in the crown of the tooth at the time of eruption, although some believe this may be a fixation artefact. The dental pulp retains the potential to differentiate new odontoblasts from stem cells and deposit reparative forms of dentine (see page 159) in response to dental caries.

## BLOOD SUPPLY

Vascularization of the developing pulp starts during the early bell stage, with small branches from the principal vascular trunks of the jaws entering the base of the papilla. Of these small pioneer vessels, a few become the principal pulpal vessels, enlarge and run through the pulp towards the cuspal regions. Here the vessels give off numerous small branches, which form a bed of venules, arterioles and capillaries in the subodontoblast and odontoblast layers (Fig. 24.5). The vascularity of the odontoblast layer

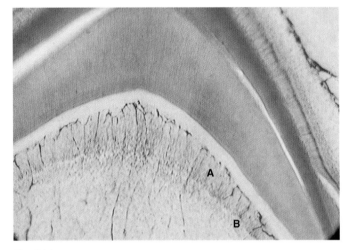

Fig. 24.6

**Fig. 24.5** The vascular pattern within the dental papilla at the late bell stage of development. The vascular system has been perfused with Indian ink (H & E; ×40). Courtesy of Dr D. Adams.

**Fig. 24.6** The vascular plexuses beneath the developing cusp. A = odontoblast layer; B = subodontoblastic plexus. The vascular system has been perfused with Indian ink (H & E; ×100). Courtesy of Dr D. Adams.

**Fig. 24.7** A capillary looping (arrow) into developing dentine (Masson's trichrome; ×20).

increases as dentine is progressively laid down, probably as the result of the odontoblasts migrating inwards through the vascular bed (Fig. 24.6). Eventually, some capillaries are found immediately next to the predentine surface, occasionally looping into the developing dentine (Fig. 24.7). The time and pattern of development of lymphatics in the pulp has not yet been established. The mature pulp contains macrophages, pericytes and lymphoid cells that probably enter the pulp with the blood vessels.

## NERVE SUPPLY

Trigeminal nerve branches enter the mandibular and maxillary processes well before the first appearance of tooth primordial and project to future sites of tooth formation. The dental follicle becomes innervated as soon as it appears during the cap stage of tooth development. However, axons do not enter the dental pulp until dentinogenesis and amelogenesis are well under way. Thus, the innervation of the pulp is delayed in comparison to neighbouring tissues. This seems to be due to the presence at this stage of nerve-repelling molecules. Molecules stimulating neurite growth, including nerve growth factor and brain-derived neurotrophic factor, are expressed in the periphery of the developing dental pulp in the odontoblast layer (Fig. 24.8) but these neurotrophins do not exert their effect in the early stages. The first fibres to enter the developing pulp become located close to the blood vessels. These nerves, although anatomically part of the sensory nervous system, play an important role via axon reflexes in controlling blood flow.

The sympathetic innervation follows later and is restricted largely to the radicular pulp as it supplies the smooth muscle of arterioles whose presence is limited largely to the radicular pulp. A large number of nerves enter the pulp before root formation, but the final pattern, including the formation of the subodontoblastic plexus (of Raschkow), is not established until root formation is complete. In the crown, particularly at the cusps, some sensory fibres insinuate themselves between the odontoblasts and enter dentinal tubules. This is an active process and not a merely a trapping of these axons during progressive dentine deposition.

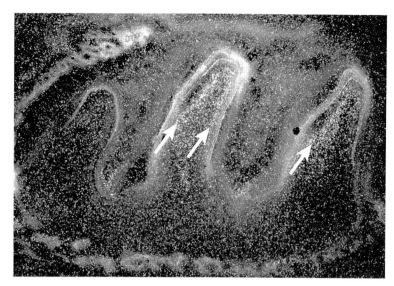

**Fig. 24.8** Labelled nerve growth factor (NGF) in the periphery of the developing dental pulp (Rat molars 2 days post-natal). Messenger RNA for NGF has been radioactively labelled by in-situ hybridization and viewed under dark field illumination. Under these conditions mineralized tissue appears as a bright solid (arrows) and NGF mRNA as bright granules (×20). Courtesy of Dr C. Nosrat and the editor of the *European Journal of Oral Science*.

Root development proceeds some time after the crown has formed and involves interactions between three components: 1) the dental follicle, 2) a structure derived from the cervical loop region of the enamel organ (see page 301) called the epithelial root sheath (of Hertwig) and 3) the dental papilla. The onset of root development coincides with the axial phase of tooth eruption.

Single and multirooted teeth are formed in the manner shown in Figure 25.1. Soon after the crown has completed its formation, the external and internal enamel epithelia at the cervical loop of the enamel organ form a double-layered epithelial root sheath (see Fig. 25.3) that proliferates apically to map out the shape of the future root. The primary apical foramen at the growing end of the epithelial root sheath may subdivide into a number of secondary apical foramina by the ingrowth of epithelial shelves from the margins of the root sheath (arrowed region in Fig. 25.1b,c) that subsequently fuse near the centre of the root. The number and location of these epithelial shelves correspond to the number and location of the definitive roots of the tooth, and may be under the inductive control of the dental papilla. It has been suggested that the ingrowth of the epithelial shelves takes place along paths of low vascularity.

When a permanent tooth first erupts into the mouth, only about two-thirds of the length of the root is formed. A wide, 'open' root apex is present in these situations, surrounded by a thin, regular knife-edge of dentine (Fig. 25.2). It takes about 3 more years for root completion in a permanent tooth to occur and about 1½ years for root completion in a deciduous tooth. At this time, only a narrow pulp opening exists. The addition of root increments may result in the appearance of fine lines running transversely around the root. Root extension is of the order of 5–10 µm per day.

During root development (Fig. 25.3), growth of the **epithelial root sheath** occurs to enclose the **dental papilla**, except for an opening at the base (the primary apical foramen). Beneath the dental papilla, the epithe-lial sheath usually appears angled to form the root diaphragm. Unlike the cervical loop region in the enamel organ of the crown, there is no stellate reticulum or stratum intermedium between the two epithelial layers of the root sheath. As the cervical loop region is the site of the stem cell niche (see page 301), its replacement by the epithelial root sheath may be related to the disappearance of Notch protein in the epithelium and growth factors

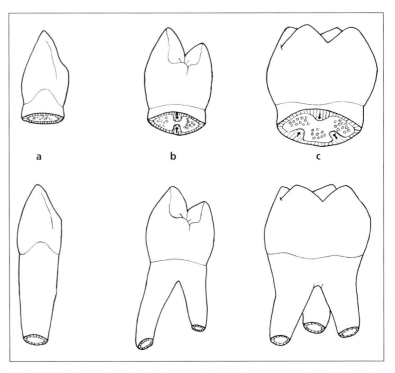

**Fig. 25.1** The formation of a single-rooted tooth (a), a two-rooted tooth (b) and a three-rooted tooth (c). Small red circles indicate vascular concentrations.

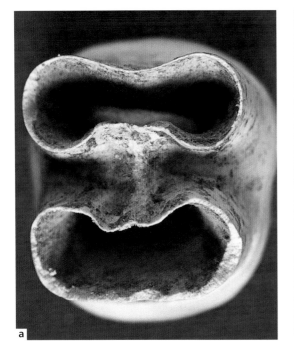

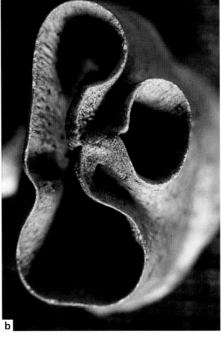

**Fig. 25.2** Apices of developing roots. (a) Two-rooted tooth. (b) Three-rooted tooth.

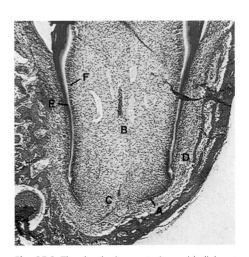

**Fig. 25.3** The developing root. A = epithelial root sheath; B = dental papilla; C = primary apical foramen; D = dental follicle; E = developing root dentine; F = odontoblast layer (H & E; ×32).

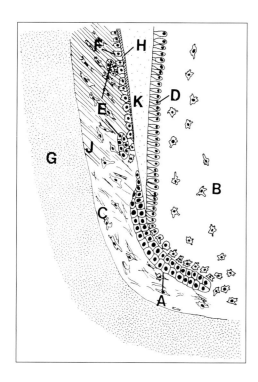

**Fig. 25.4** Schematic drawing of the developing root. A = epithelial root sheath; B = dental papilla; C = dental follicle; D = odontoblasts; E = epithelial rests; F = cementoblasts; G = developing alveolar bone; H = developing cementum; J = developing periodontal ligament; K = root dentine.

**Fig. 25.5** The apical region of the developing root, periodontal ligament and alveolus. A = epithelial root sheath; B = dental papilla; C = odontoblasts; D = dentine of root; E = predentine layer; F = cementoblasts; G = developing cementum; H = developing alveolar bone; I = inner investing layer of dental follicle; J = outer layer of the dental follicle; K = intermediate layer of dental follicle. Arrow indicates oblique orientation of follicular tissue with formation of cementum (H & E; ×150).

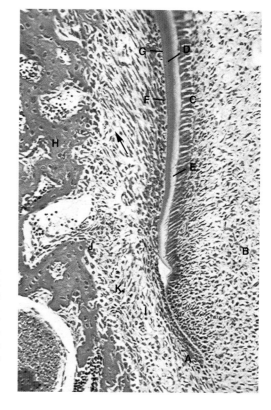

(e.g. fibroblast growth factor, FGF) in the adjacent mesenchyme. The localized retention of such factors may help explain the occasional presence of stellate reticulum and stratum intermedium in the root, giving rise to areas of enamel (enamel pearls) on the root surface (see Fig. 7.66). The **dental follicle** lies external to the root sheath and forms cementum, periodontal ligament and (probably) alveolar bone.

In the region of the root diaphragm, the epithelial root sheath is seen as a continuous sheet of tissue sandwiched between the undifferentiated mesenchyme of the dental papilla internally and the dental follicle externally (Fig. 25.4) and separated from both by a basement membrane. Above the root diaphragm, towards the developing crown, the cells of the internal layer of the epithelial root sheath induce the peripheral cells of the dental papilla to differentiate into odontoblasts. Following the onset of dentinogenesis in the root, the epithelial cells of the root sheath lose their continuity, becoming separated from the surface of the developing root dentine. The mesenchymal cells of the dental follicle adjacent to the root dentine now differentiate into cementoblast-like cells and cementogenesis commences with the formation of acellular (primary) cementum. There is evidence, however, that epithelial cells of the sheath may also differentiate into the first-formed cementoblast-like cells. The epithelial remnants are retained and subsequently form the epithelial rests seen in the periodontal ligament (see Fig. 12.46).

Figure 25.5 shows the apical region of the developing root, periodontal ligament and alveolus. The tissues of the dental follicle in the developing root have been described as comprising three layers (see also Fig. 21.10). Adjacent to the epithelial root sheath is the inner investing layer of the dental follicle, which is thought to be derived from ectomesenchyme (neural crest). Adjacent to the developing alveolar bone is the outer layer of the dental follicle, which is separated from the inner layer by an intermediate layer. Unlike the tissues of the inner layer, the outer and intermediate layers are said to be mesodermal in origin; their cells contain few cytoplasmic organelles and the extracellular compartment appears relatively featureless. Cells of the inner layer of the dental follicle differentiate into the cementoblasts that form an initial layer of cells on the surface of the root dentine. In primary (acellular) cementum, the collagen is of the extrinsic fibre type, being derived from the periodontal ligament

and passing into the cementum roughly perpendicular to the surface (see page 172). The cementoblasts associated with acellular cementum, therefore, contribute little material towards the extracellular matrix of the tissue. Later, with the formation of cellular (secondary) cementum, the cementoblasts form a more distinctive layer of cuboidal cells that secrete collagen parallel to the surface, forming the matrix of the cementum (intrinsic fibre cementum). Once cementogenesis has begun, cells of the remaining dental follicle become obliquely oriented along the root surface and show an increased content of intracellular organelles, becoming the fibroblasts of the periodontal ligament. These fibroblasts secrete collagen of the periodontal ligament into the extracellular compartment. This collagen will become embedded as Sharpey fibres into the developing acellular cementum at the tooth surface and into the developing bone at the alveolar surface.

There has been controversy concerning the connective tissue immediately beneath the developing root apex. Initially called the **cushion hammock ligament**, this connective tissue was described as a fibrous network with fluid-filled interstices, with attachments on either side to the alveolar wall. It was thought to provide a resistant base so that forces produced by the growing root were prevented from causing bone resorption and were resolved into an eruptive force. This view is no longer held, as the thin fibrous membrane seen in this site is not attached to alveolar bone but merges at the sides with the fibres of the developing periodontal ligament. The structure is more correctly termed the **pulp-limiting membrane** (Fig. 25.6). It does not appear to be directly involved in tooth eruption as its surgical removal (together with the developing root apex) does not affect tooth eruption.

It has been suggested that changes in vascular permeability in the connective tissues around the apex of the developing root can be related to eruptive behaviour. Dense accumulations of tissue fluid (effusions) have been envisaged beneath the growing roots of erupting teeth. Furthermore, when radioactive fibrinogen was injected intravascularly, the radioactive label became incorporated rapidly into the effusions, supporting the view that they are vascular in origin. As effusions were seen most prominently when the growing root was situated close to the base (fundus) of the bony tooth socket/ crypt, it has been suggested that they might force the root

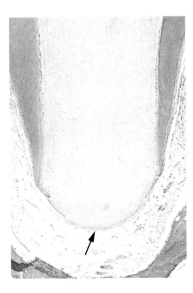

**Fig. 25.6** The pulp-limiting membrane (arrowed) (Mallory's trichrome; ×30). Courtesy of Dr D. Adams.

and bone apart and thereby contribute to eruption and enable further root growth. The vascular hypothesis of eruption is considered further on page 364.

## FORMATION OF COLLAGEN FIBRES WITHIN THE PERIODONTAL LIGAMENT

A generalized view of the development of the collagen fibres of the periodontal ligament is shown in Figure 25.7. One major difference in fibre formation exists between teeth with or without predecessors: in the latter (i.e. deciduous teeth and permanent molars) the principal fibre groups develop earlier than in the former (i.e. permanent incisors, canines and premolars). This is illustrated in Figure 25.8. To visualize the difference, Figure 25.9 shows an erupting permanent molar (of a marmoset, *Callithrix*

*jacchus*) just emerging into the oral cavity where it can be seen that the coronal half of the periodontal ligament is composed of well formed, obliquely orientated, principal collagen fibre bundles. In contrast, the bulk of the periodontal ligament of an erupting permanent premolar (of a squirrel monkey, *Saimiri sciureus*) (Fig. 25.10) lacks significant numbers of organized principal collagen fibre bundles passing from tooth to alveolar bone.

It appears, therefore, that collagen fibres may not be well organized during eruption in some groups of teeth, and this is significant if it is believed that collagen fibres have an important role in the generation of tractional forces during eruption (see page 363). However, there are species differences in the ontogeny of principal collagen fibres. In some animals, the fibres associated with succedaneous teeth do pass between tooth and bone as the tooth erupts into the oral cavity. For example, in a permanent canine (of the ferret, *Mustela putorius*) erupting into the oral cavity, the principal collagen fibres are seen passing from tooth to bone (Fig. 25.11). This contrasts with the development of the primate periodontal ligament shown in Figure 25.10. However, in this permanent canine tooth the collagen fibres are not as well organized (in terms of thickness and orientation) as those for the fully erupted tooth illustrated in Figure 25.12.

There is some evidence of a change in the obliquity of the principal collagen fibres, and in their dimensions, as the tooth reaches its functional position. The inclination of the oblique fibres has been reported to decrease, while the principal fibres are said to thicken with function. However, there may again be species differences.

Qualitative differences in the type of collagen present during the development of the periodontal ligament have been reported. Thus, type VI collagen appears to be absent from the ligament during the main axial eruptive phase but present when the tooth has fully erupted. Type XII collagen similarly appears only after the tooth has erupted. It is of interest to note that this pattern for type XII collagen is recapitulated on the pressure side of the periodontal ligament following orthodontic loading and remodelling of the ligament.

**Fig. 25.7** Summary of the development of collagen fibres of the periodontal ligament. (1) Fine brush-like fibres are first seen emanating from cementum (C). Only a few fibres project from the alveolar bone (B) and extend into the unorganized collagenous elements that occupy the broad central zone of the developing periodontal ligament. (2) Sharpey fibres, thicker and more widely spaced than those of cementum, emerge from the bone to extend towards the tooth and appear to unravel as they arborize at their ends. The closely spaced, cemental fibres are still short, giving the root a brush-like appearance. (3) The alveolar fibres extend further into the central zone to join the lengthening cemental fibres. (4) With occlusal function, the principal fibres become classically organized, thicker and continuous between bone and cementum. Redrawn with permission from Grant DA, Berwick S 1972 The formation of the periodontal ligament. *Journal of Periodontology* 43: 17–25.

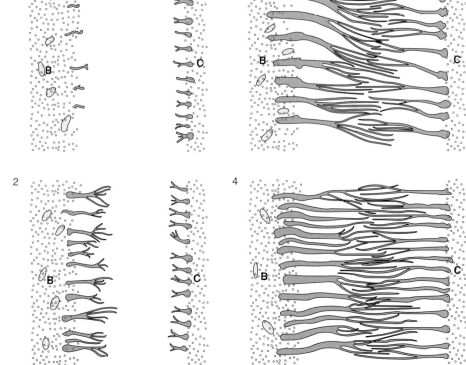

**Fig. 25.8** A comparison of the development of the principal periodontal ligament collagen fibres between primary (left) and succedaneous teeth (right). (1) Before eruption, the dentogingival and oblique periodontal fibres are well developed in the permanent molar. In the permanent premolar, however, only the dentogingival fibres are organized, the developing periodontal ligament being composed of loosely structured collagenous elements. (2) As the tooth emerges into the oral cavity, the periodontal ligament of the permanent molar is well differentiated, the oblique fibres being the most conspicuous. However, at this stage in the permanent premolar only the fibres in the region of the alveolar crest are becoming organized. In the periodontal ligament itself, although collagen fibres are developing, they do not yet span the periodontal space. (3) On reaching occlusion, the fibre groupings in the cervical region of the permanent molar now become organized. In the permanent premolar, while the fibre groups cervically appear prominent, those in the apical part of the root appear relatively undeveloped. (4) After a period in function, the fibres of both the permanent molar and premolar show the classical organization of the principal fibres. Redrawn with permission from Grant DA, Bernick S, Levy BM, Dreizen S 1972 A comparative study of periodontal ligament development in teeth with and without predecessors in marmosets. *Journal of Periodontology* 43: 162–169.

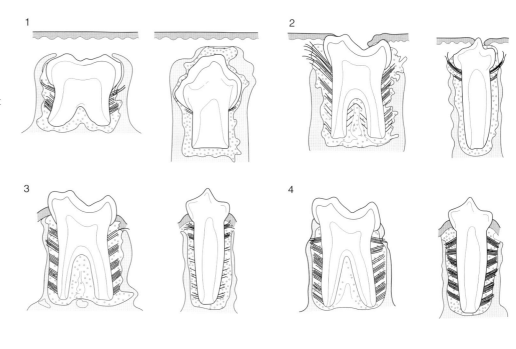

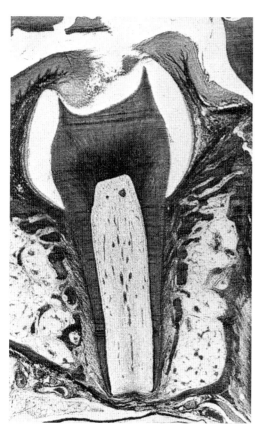

**Fig. 25.9** Erupting permanent molar (of a marmoset, *Callithrix jacchus*) just emerging into the oral cavity. Note the presence of periodontal ligament fibres (Mallory's trichrome; ×15). From Grant DA, Bernick S, Levy BM, Dreizen S 1972 A comparative study of periodontal ligament development in teeth with and without predecessors in marmosets. *Journal of Periodontology* 43: 162–169.

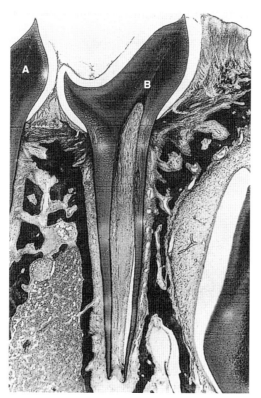

**Fig. 25.10** Erupting second premolar (of a squirrel monkey, *Saimiri sciureus*) just emerging into the oral cavity (B). A = erupted first premolar. Note the absence of periodontal ligament fibres (Mallory's trichrome; ×35). Redrawn with permission from Grant DA, Berwick S 1972 The formation of the periodontal ligament. *Journal of Periodontology* 43: 17–25.

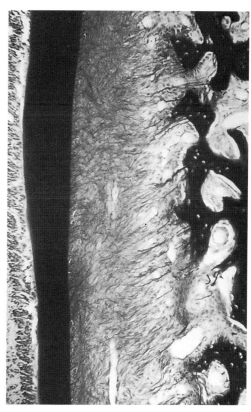

**Fig. 25.11** Principal collagen fibres associated with an erupting permanent canine (of the ferret, *Mustela putorius*) as it emerges into the oral cavity (Aldehyde fuchsin and van Gieson; ×150).

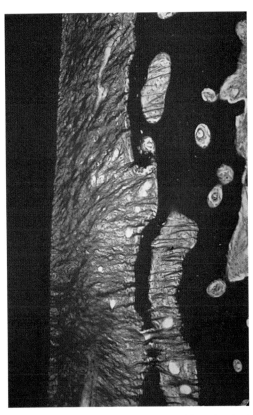

**Fig. 25.12** Well differentiated collagen fibres for the fully erupted permanent canine of the ferret (*Mustela putorius*) (Aldehyde fuchsin and van Gieson; ×130).

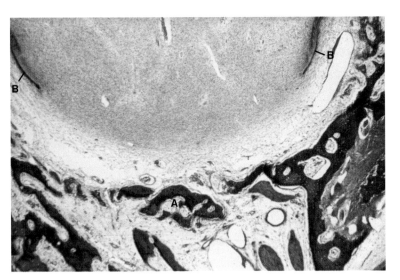

**Fig. 25.13** Apical region of an erupting tooth showing little evidence of bone deposition at the base of the socket (A). B = Epithelial root sheath (Masson's blue trichrome stain; ×25).

Some changes occurring in the ground substance during root formation are considered on pages 186, 187.

## DEVELOPMENT OF THE CELLS OF THE PERIODONTAL LIGAMENT

Prior to root formation, the cells of the dental follicle have the characteristics of undifferentiated fibroblasts, containing few cytoplasmic organelles. With the onset of root formation, the cells show an increase in cytoplasmic organelles, especially those associated with protein synthesis and secretion, and extracellular spaces begin to fill with collagen and ground substance.

The cells of the dental follicle give rise to cementoblasts, fibroblasts and osteoblasts of the periodontal ligament. There is evidence that cells from the apical region of the dental papilla migrate around the epithelial root sheath and supplement the number of cells in the dental follicle. Cells may also migrate into the developing periodontal ligament from the endosteal spaces of the adjacent alveolar bone.

During the formation of the root and periodontal ligament, there is obviously a dramatic increase in the number of connective tissue-forming cells (i.e. cementoblasts, fibroblasts and osteoblasts). Stem cells exist within the region to allow for this, perhaps lying in a perivascular location. It is not clear whether the three main cell types all arise from a common stem cell or whether each type has its own specific stem cell.

There appear to be few structural differences between fibroblasts in the developing periodontal ligament of erupting teeth and those associated with fully erupted teeth. However, changes during eruption have been reported for the non-fibrous extracellular matrix elements and the vascularity of the periodontal ligament (see pages 186, 187 and 364, 365).

In addition to the main connective tissue-forming cells, osteoclasts also appear in the developing periodontal ligament at the alveolar bone surface, allowing bone to remodel in association with tooth eruption (and bone

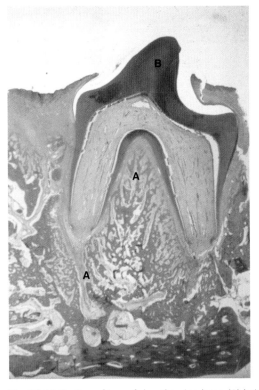

**Fig. 25.14** Section of jaw of dog showing bone (A) being deposited beneath the erupting premolar tooth (B) (H & E; ×5). Courtesy of Dr S.C. Marks Jr.

growth). As the tooth erupts, there is little evidence of any significant bone deposition at the base of the socket (i.e. beneath the developing root – Fig. 25.13), resorption often being prominent at this site. Thus, bone deposition at this site is precluded as a cause of tooth eruption. There are species differences, however, bone deposition being found beneath the erupting permanent premolars of dogs (Fig. 25.14). The different patterns of bone activity in different species may relate to the distance a tooth has to erupt: if the distance is much greater than the length of the root then bone deposition is clearly necessary to maintain the normal dimensions of the periodontal ligament at the root apex of the tooth. Remodelling of alveolar bone other than at the base of the socket may also be seen during eruption and this can be related to the relocation of the teeth during jaw growth and to the establishment of occlusion.

## DEVELOPMENT OF THE NEUROVASCULAR ELEMENTS

Prior to eruption, nerve fibres can be demonstrated in the pulp, but few are present within the lower part of the dental follicle that will form the periodontal ligament. With root formation and subsequent eruption, nerves adjacent to the bone grow into the periodontal ligament, usually accompanying blood vessels, to establish its innervation. These initial nerves are autonomic. It would seem that the sensory innervation is not established until the ligament is fully organized following eruption.

Blood vessels in the forming periodontal ligament seem to be derived from two main sources. Blood vessels enter from the periapical area and pass upwards within the ligament and form anastomoses with vessels entering from the adjacent developing alveolar bone. As the tooth erupts it receives vessels from the adjacent gingiva. In the case of permanent teeth, connections also develop with the periodontal ligament of the overlying deciduous teeth. There is evidence that differences may be present in the periodontal vessels of erupting and fully erupted teeth, in that the number of fenestrated capillaries is greater in erupting teeth (see pages 364–365).

## CEMENTOGENESIS

Cementogenesis will be considered in terms of the formation of acellular (primary) cementum and then of cellular (secondary) cementum (see Ch. 11). There may be differences between the cells forming each type of cementum. Our understanding is clouded by species differences, resulting in problems in terminology, particularly with regard to structures at the cementum–dentine interface (see page 140).

As for the crown, the hard tissues that comprise the root (i.e. cementum and dentine) develop under the control of epithelial–mesenchymal interactions (see pages 305–310). However, unlike that of the crown, the epithelial component involved in root formation retains a simpler morphology, rapidly loses its continuity with adjacent cells and is not evident as a conspicuous layer during initial cementum formation. Although it was once thought that its function was primarily to induce the formation of root odontoblasts, present evidence also indicates that the epithelium has an important role in cementogenesis. As the aim of periodontologists is now not only to halt the ravages of periodontal disease but also to try to regenerate the tissues lost, there has been a resurgence of interest in how cementum forms. It is only through a thorough understanding of this process that clinical strategies can be developed to encourage the regeneration of new cementum, alveolar bone and periodontal ligament.

## ACELLULAR (PRIMARY, AEFC) CEMENTUM

Once the crown has fully formed, the internal and external enamel epithelia proliferate downwards as a double-layered sheet of somewhat flattened epithelial cells, the epithelial root sheath (of Hertwig) that maps out the shape of the root(s) (Figs 25.1, 25.5 and 25.15). The process of cementogenesis is initiated at the cervical margin and extends apically as the root grows downwards. The cells of the epithelial root sheath, in contrast to those of the enamel organ during enamel formation, do not enlarge during this inductive stage. The epithelial root sheath is separated by a basal lamina on both of its surfaces from the adjacent connective tissues of the dental follicle and dental papilla. The epithelial root sheath induces the adjacent cells of the dental papilla to differentiate into odontoblasts. As these odontoblasts initially retreat inwards, they synthesize and secrete the organic matrix of the first-formed root predentine, comprising ground substance and some collagen fibrils. Although some collagen fibrils are oriented perpendicular to the surface, others are aligned more obliquely. This may explain why this first-formed layer can be later distinguished from the rest of the root dentine using polarized light (see Fig. 9.37). As

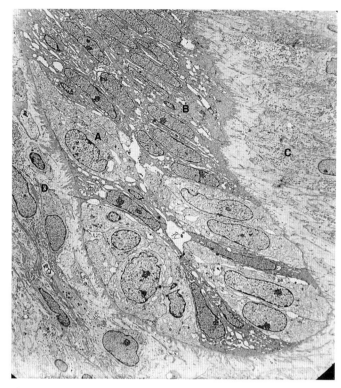

**Fig. 25.15** TEM illustrating epithelial root sheath in developing root. A = outer layer of epithelial root sheath; B = inner layer of epithelial root sheath; C = differentiating odontoblasts; D = dental follicle (×2000). From Bosshardt DD, Selvig KA 1997 Dental cementum: the dynamic tissue covering of the root. *Periodontology 2000* 13: 41–75.

the odontoblasts also do not leave behind an odontoblast process in this initial few microns of tissue (Fig. 25.16), its structureless (and later glass-like) appearance is responsible for the term 'hyaline layer' that is given to this (approximately 10 μm) layer once it is mineralized.

The epithelial root sheath is in contact with the initial predentine layer for only a short distance before the continuity of its cells is lost. The presence within the epithelial root sheath cells of organelles, such as endoplasmic reticulum, Golgi material and mitochondria, indicates that the cells are capable of the synthesis and secretion of bioactive molecules that may play an important role in root formation. There is evidence that the epithelial root sheath cells secrete enamel-related protein(s) into the collagenous matrix of the hyaline layer at the cementum–dentine boundary. Thus, the hyaline layer is formed by contributions from both the odontoblast and epithelial root sheath layers. The enamel-related protein(s) has been identified as amelogenin (Fig. 25.17), although there is some dispute as to whether another enamel-related protein, ameloblastin, is also present. Difficulties in solving this dispute relate to the small amount of protein present and to problems of cross-reactivity of antibodies. The function of such enamel-related proteins is unclear but may concern epithelial–mesenchymal interactions involving the induction of odontoblasts and cementoblasts, and/or the process of mineralization. During the subsequent mineralization of cementum and the hyaline layer, the enamel-related protein(s) is lost, although remnants may be retained in the granular layer of the root dentine (Fig. 25.18).

The cause of fenestration of the epithelial root sheath is not known, but it may not simply be due to programmed epithelial cell death (apoptosis). Fibroblast-like cells of the adjacent dental follicle pass through the fenestrations and come to lie close to the surface of the, as yet, unmineralized hyaline layer (Fig. 25.19). These cells, which represent cementoblasts associated with the formation of acellular cementum, appear to secrete collagen fibrils. At their deep surface, these fibrils intermingle with those of the hyaline layer, subsequent mineralization of this zone producing a firm bond between dentine and cementum: at their superficial surface these

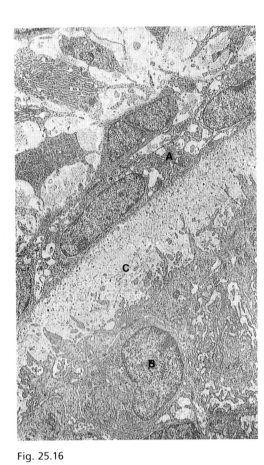

Fig. 25.16

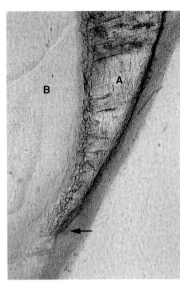

Fig. 25.17

**Fig. 25.16** TEM of early stage in root formation. The first-formed matrix (C) lies between the newly differentiated odontoblasts (B) and the epithelial root sheath cells (A). This matrix receives contributions from both the odontoblast and epithelial cell layers. It lacks major processes from the odontoblasts and forms the hyaline layer (×5000). Courtesy of Dr P.D.A. Owens.

**Fig. 25.17** Immunohistochemistry showing presence of enamel-like proteins (stained brown – arrow) at the surface of the developing root. This represents a frozen ground section through a premolar root using an antibody against amelogenin. A = dentine; B = pulp (×100). Courtesy of Professor L. Hammarström.

**Fig. 25.18** Immunohistochemistry showing presence of enamel-like proteins (brown staining – arrow) in interglobular dentine (×100). From Hammarstrom L 1997 Enamel matrix, cementum development and regeneration. *Journal of Clinical Periodontology* 24: 658–668.

**Fig. 25.19** TEM showing a fibroblast-like cell (A) from dental follicle with cytoplasmic processes lying close to the unmineralized external surface of initial root dentine layer. B = coronal termination of intact inner enamel epithelial cell of epithelial root sheath; C = portion of odontoblast cell (×6250). From Bosshardt DD, Selvig KA 1997 Dental cementum: the dynamic tissue covering of the root. *Periodontology 2000* 13: 41–75.

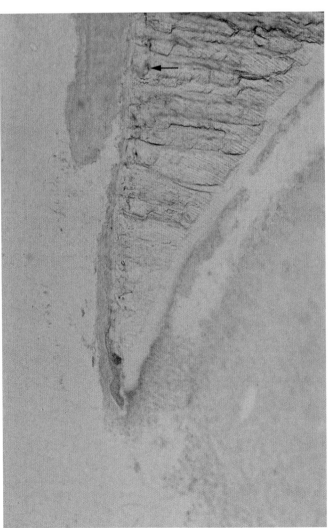

Fig. 25.18

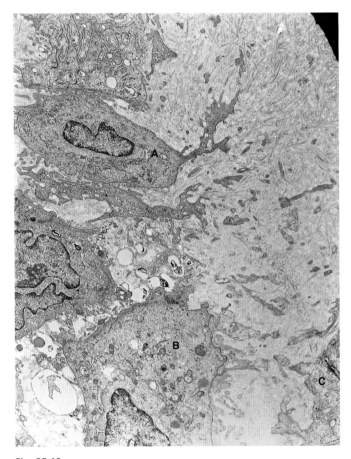

Fig. 25.19

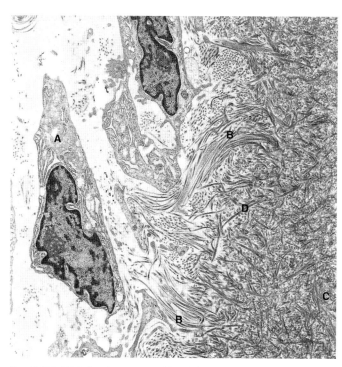

**Fig. 25.20** TEM showing cementoblast (A) at root surface secreting collagen fibrils that form a fibrous fringe (B) that intermingles with the as yet unmineralized outer region of the root predentine (C). D = site of future dentine–cementum junction and, adjacent to it, the hyaline layer (×5800). From Bosshardt DD, Selvig KA 1997 Dental cementum: the dynamic tissue covering of the root. *Periodontology 2000* 13: 41–75.

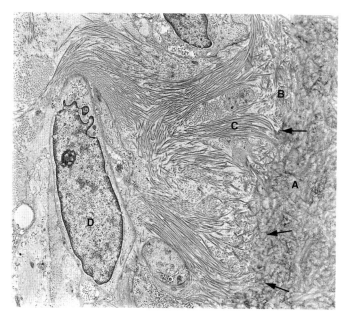

**Fig. 25.21** TEM showing the external mineralization front (arrows) of the outermost root dentine (A) has now extended outwards to reach the fibrillar dentine–cementum junction (B). The dentine is now almost completely covered by the cementum matrix in the form of a fibrous fringe (C). D = cementoblast (×570). From Bosshardt DD, Selvig KA 1997 Dental cementum: the dynamic tissue covering of the root. *Periodontology 2000* 13: 41–75.

fibrils form a 'fibrous fringe' extending perpendicularly into the periodontal space for about 10–20 μm (Fig. 25.20). These fibroblast-like cells of the dental follicle do not form a conspicuous layer on the developing root surface and may retreat and mingle with adjacent fibroblasts of the periodontal ligament.

As the newly differentiated odontoblasts at the periphery of the pulp migrate inwards (centrifugally) beyond the hyaline layer, they start to trail behind them their odontoblast processes. Initially, there is much branching and looping of these processes in the future granular layer (of Tomes), after which the odontoblast processes become more regular in the region of the circumpulpal dentine.

Mineralization of the first-formed dentine of the hyaline layer occurs within matrix vesicles. Unlike the crown, this does not initially occur at the outermost surface of the hyaline layer, but a few microns within it. From this initial centre, mineralization spreads both inwards towards the pulp and outwards towards the periodontal ligament (centrifugally).

Thus, the outermost part of the hyaline layer undergoes delayed mineralization (Fig. 25.21). This is visualized by the V-shaped configuration at the extreme apical edge of the developing root, showing continuity of the unmineralized predentine layer at the periphery of the pulp with the unmineralized part of the hyaline layer at the outer root surface (Fig. 25.22). A similar configuration is evident when the mineralizing front is highlighted following administration of the antibiotic tetracycline (Fig. 25.23).

During the next phase of development in the formation of acellular cementum, the delayed mineralization front in the hyaline layer gradually spreads outwards (centripetally) until this layer is fully mineralized and then continues on into the first few microns of the fibrous fringe secreted by the fibroblast-like cells of the dental follicle. (Fig. 25.24). In this manner, the first few microns of acellular cementum are firmly attached to the root dentine. At this stage, the collagen fibres in the adjacent periodontal ligament are oriented more parallel to the root surface and have not yet gained an attachment to the fibrous fringe (Fig. 25.25). The stages

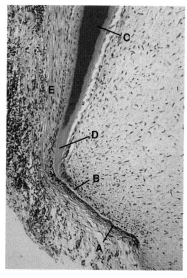

Fig. 25.22

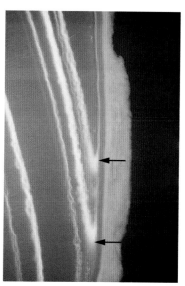

Fig. 25.23

**Fig. 25.22** Section of the developing root of extracted tooth. A = epithelial root sheath; B = differentiating odontoblasts at the periphery of the dental papilla; C = matrix of mineralized dentine (red); D = unmineralized predentine (pale blue) continuous around root apex with first-formed but as yet still unmineralized matrix on outer surface of dentine (corresponding to hyaline layer); E = dentine follicle, which will give rise to periodontal ligament (Masson's trichrome, ×100).

**Fig. 25.23** Fluorescent micrograph of ground longitudinal section of tooth of a patient who had received multiple injections of the antibiotic tetracycline. The antibiotic is incorporated into tissues mineralizing at the time of the injection. There is continuity at the edge of the section where the original predentine recurves upwards at the site of the hyaline layer (arrows), similar to the situation seen in Fig. 25.22. Courtesy of Dr R. O'Sullivan.

in formation of acellular (AEFC) cementum are summarized in Figure 25.26.

As with bone, the early stage of acellular cementum formation results in the secretion by the associated cementoblasts of various non-collagenous proteins (e.g. osteopontin, cementum-attachment protein,

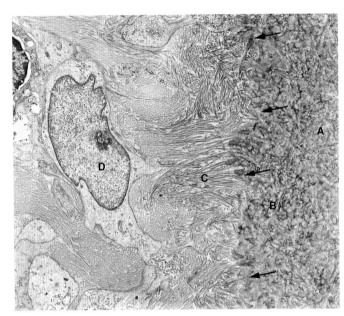

**Fig. 25.24** TEM showing the mineralization front in the developing root extending from the dentine (A) across the dentine–cementum junction (B) and into the base (arrowed) of the fibrous fringe of the cementum (C). D = cementoblast (×6250). From Bosshardt DD, Selvig KA 1997 Dental cementum: the dynamic tissue covering of the root. *Periodontology 2000* 13: 41–75.

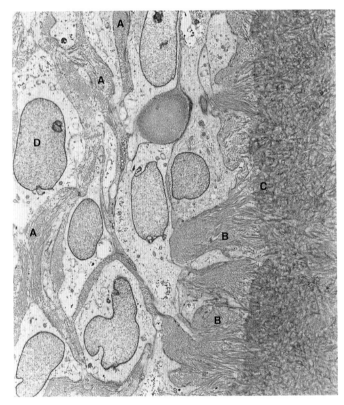

**Fig. 25.25** TEM of developing root showing fibres in the developing periodontal ligament (A) running parallel to the root surface with little attachment to the cementum fibres (B), which are perpendicular to the root surface. C = dentine–cementum junction, beneath which would lie the hyaline layer; D = fibroblast of periodontal ligament. The mineralization front extends from the dentine across the dentine–cementum junction to involve the base of the cementum fibres (×4300). From Bosshardt DD, Selvig KA 1997 Dental cementum: the dynamic tissue covering of the root. *Periodontology 2000* 13: 41–75.

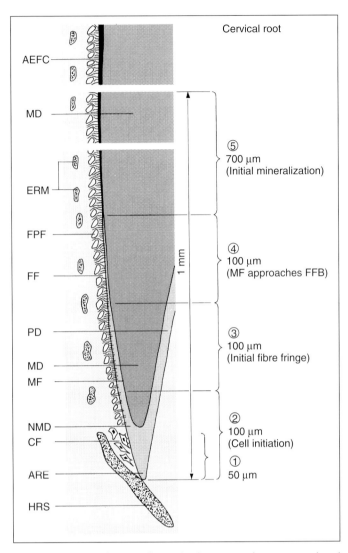

**Fig. 25.26** The initial stages of root development on human premolars developed to 50–60% of their final root length. 1. Fibroblasts contact root/predentine and become committed. 2. Fibroblasts start to form and attach collagen fibrils. 3. Initial fibrous fringe with maximum fibre density is established. 4. Cell/fibrous fringe meshwork is established and the mineralization front approaches the base of the fibrous fringe. 5. Mineralization front progresses into initial fibrous fringe. AEFC = acellular extrinsic fibre cementum; ARE = advancing root edge; CF = committed fibroblasts; ERM = epithelial cell rests of Malassez; FF = collagenous fibrous fringe; FPF = fibrous-fringe-producing fibroblasts; HRS = Hertwig's epithelial root sheath; MD = mineralized dentine; MF = mineralization front; NMD = non-mineralized dentine or predentine; PD = predentine. Courtesy of Professors H.E. Schroeder and D.D. Bosshardt and the editors of *Cell and Tissue Research*.

bone sialoprotein), cytokines and growth hormones (Fig. 25.27a). The precise roles of such molecules await clarification but they may be involved in processes such as chemoattraction, cell attachment, cell growth and differentiation, and mineralization. It has also been suggested that these (and other) molecules play a role in bonding the cementum to the outer surface of the root dentine. Their importance may be indicated by reference to a pathological condition in which osteoclasts are deficient. In this condition (leading to a type of osteopetrosis), where there is a failure of production of bone sialoprotein by cells at the root surface, root formation is grossly interfered with (Fig. 25.27b). As epithelial cell rests have also been shown to express a number of bioactive molecules (e.g. glycosaminoglycans, osteopontin, cytokines, growth hormones, matrix metalloproteinases), the question arises as to whether they play an additional role in cementogenesis.

The subsequent development of acellular cementum involves:

- its slow increase in thickness
- the establishment of continuity between the principal collagen fibres of the periodontal ligament with those of the fibrous fringe at the surface of the root dentine
- continued slow mineralization of the collagen at the root surface.

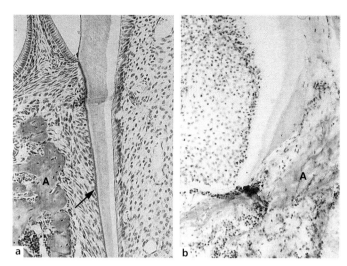

**Fig. 25.27** (a) Decalcified longitudinal section of mouse molar using immunohisto-chemical techniques to localize the presence of bone sialoprotein (red). Positive staining is seen at the developing cementum surface (arrow) and throughout the alveolar bone (A). (H & E; ×100). (b) Similar section from an osteopetrotic mouse lacking macrophage-colony-stimulating factor: the root is stunted in its development and the cementum lacks bone sialoprotein, although this molecule is still present in alveolar bone (A). D'errico JA et al 1995 Models for the study of cementogenesis. *Connective Tissue Research* 33: 9–17.

It is only with the establishment of continuity between periodontal ligament fibres and those of the initial fibrous fringe projecting from the acellular cementum that the tooth can be properly supported within the socket. There may be a considerable difference in the timing of the establishment of this support between deciduous and succedaneous teeth (see page 344). Thus, for permanent teeth, this attachment may not occur until after the tooth has erupted into the mouth, when about two-thirds of the root has formed and the acellular cementum may only be about 10 μm thick. Thus, the acellular cementum lining the root before this time (which may be considered in years) could be considered as acellular **intrinsic** fibre cementum.

Once periodontal ligament fibres become attached to the surface of the cementum layer, the cementum may be classified as acellular extrinsic fibre cementum (Fig. 25.28). It increases slowly and evenly in thickness throughout life at a rate of about 2 μm per year. Although the cementoblasts may not form a distinctive and recognizable layer of cells that can be distinguished from adjacent cells of the periodontal ligament (Fig. 25.28), some cells lying between the perpendicularly oriented periodontal fibre bundles may become more cuboidal (Fig. 25.29). The cementoblasts contain small amounts of the intracellular organelles associated with protein synthesis and secretion and probably contribute to the formation of the ground substance surrounding the collagen. Presumably, secretion is polarized at the surface of the cells adjacent to the cementum surface and, together with the slow rate of formation, ensures that the cells are not entombed by their own secretion.

Mineralization of the cementum matrix does not appear to be controlled by its cells as matrix vesicles have not been observed at its surface. It may be that the presence of hydroxyapatite crystals in the adjacent dentine initiates mineralization in cementum. The adjacent periodontal ligament fibroblasts, which are rich in alkaline phosphatase, may play a role in mineralization, as does the presence of non-collagenous proteins, such as bone sialoprotein, in the vicinity of its surface (Fig. 25.27). Mineralization proceeds very slowly in a linear fashion and, as with bone but unlike dentine, calcospherites are not observed in cementum. Owing to the slow progress of mineralization, there is usually no evidence of a layer of precementum associated with acellular cementum homologous to that in forming dentine (predentine) and bone (osteoid). When mineralization of initial root dentine is interfered with (as following the

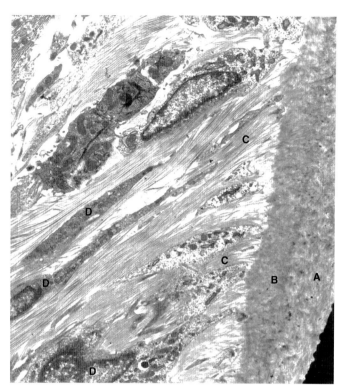

**Fig. 25.28** TEM of decalcified root surface showing formation of acellular extrinsic fibre cementum. A = dentine; B = cementum; C = Sharpey fibres; D = cells of periodontal ligament. Note the absence of a definite layer of cementoblasts (×3500). Courtesy of Professor M.M. Smith.

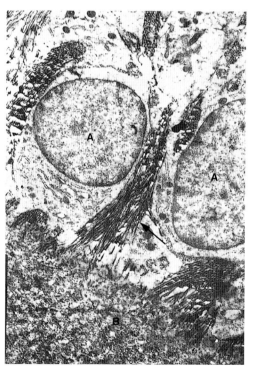

**Fig. 25.29** TEM of decalcified root surface forming acellular extrinsic fibre cementum (B). Between the Sharpey fibres (arrow), the cells (cementoblasts, A) are more cuboidal (×5000).

administration of drugs known as bisphosphonates), there is inhibition of cementogenesis.

Cementogenesis occurs rhythmically, periods of activity alternating with periods of quiescence. Structural lines may be visible within the tissue, indicating the incremental nature of its formation. The periods of decreased activity are associated with these incremental lines (see page 172), which are believed to have a higher content of ground substance and mineral and a lower content of collagen than the adjacent cementum. These lines may also reflect changes in crystallite orientation. The periodicity of the incremental lines is not known but, using refined preparation techniques allied to digital graphics, it has recently been suggested that they might be annual and can be used to age individuals. As acellular cementum is formed very slowly, the incremental lines are closer together than corresponding lines seen in cellular cementum that is deposited more rapidly.

The precise origin of the fibroblast-like cells at the surface of acellular cementum is not clear. They may be derived from the cells of the investing layer of the dental follicle. However, there is also evidence suggesting that they may be derived from epithelial root sheath cells as a result of epithelial/mesenchymal transformation. This is based on studies showing that cells having the morphological features of cementoblasts: 1) at the electron microscope level contain tonofilaments as well as the intracellular organelles for protein synthesis and secretion, are linked by desmosomes and have a collagenous matrix in the intercellular spaces; and 2) in immunohistochemical studies react positively to both cytokeratins (characteristic of epithelial cells) and vimentin (characteristic of mesenchymal cells).

Epithelial cell rests may sometimes be trapped within cementum. Cementum that contains cell inclusions near the cementum–dentine junction has been referred to as **intermediate cementum** and occurs principally in the apical half of the roots of molar teeth (see page 176). Epithelial cells may occasionally lie in the same lacunae as cementocytes and the two types of cell may be connected by desmosome-like structures. More deeply lying epithelial cells undergo apoptosis.

## ACELLULAR AFIBRILLAR CEMENTUM

Acellular afibrillar cementum may be deposited as a thin layer overlying enamel at the cervical margin of the tooth. One explanation for this presumes that the reduced enamel epithelium overlying and protecting this cervical enamel in an unerupted tooth is damaged or lost. The adjacent connective tissue cells of the dental follicle could then come into contact with the enamel surface, where they are induced to form cementoblasts. These cells then secrete a matrix (probably consisting of non-collagenous proteins but lacking collagen fibrils) that calcifies. A similar type of layer has also been shown to occur experimentally in animals when the reduced enamel epithelium has been surgically removed from unerupted teeth. A similar layer can also be induced on top of enamel by enamel matrix alone.

## CELLULAR (SECONDARY, CIFC) CEMENTUM

Following the formation of acellular cementum in the cervical portion of the root, cellular cementum appears in the apical region of the root at about the time the tooth erupts. Cellular cementum is also formed in the furcation area of the cheek teeth. This type of cementum is associated with an increase in the rate of formation of the tissue. The early inductive changes associated with the development of odontoblasts and dentine appear to be similar to those described for acellular cementum. However, following the loss of continuity of the epithelial root sheath, large basophilic cells are seen to differentiate from the adjacent cells of the dental follicle against the surface of the root dentine (or acellular cementum). These cells form a more distinct cuboidal layer of cementoblasts adjacent to the root surface. They generally possess more cytoplasm and more cytoplasmic processes than the cells associated with the formation of acellular cementum. The basophilia at the light microscope level corresponds to roughened endoplasmic reticulum at the ultrastructural level (Fig. 25.30). This indicates that the cementoblasts secrete the collagen (together with ground substance) that forms the intrinsic fibres of the cellular cementum (CIFC). These fibres are oriented parallel to the root surface and do not extend into

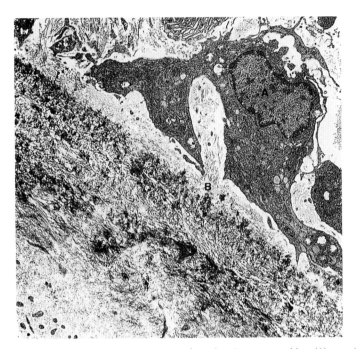

**Fig. 25.30** TEM of decalcified root surface showing cementoblast (A) associated with the formation of cellular cementum. The cell is typically more irregular in morphology and contains larger amounts of the intracellular organelles associated with protein synthesis and secretion (such as endoplasmic reticulum). B = precementum (×4000). Courtesy of Dr P.D.A. Owens.

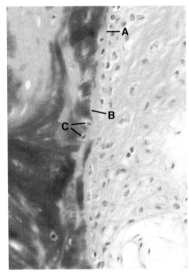

**Fig. 25.31** Section of decalcified root surface showing cellular cementum formation. A = cementoblasts; B = precementum; C = cementocytes becoming incorporated into the cementum matrix (Masson's trichrome; ×230).

the periodontal ligament. Associated with the increased rate of formation, a thin unmineralized precementum layer (about 5 μm thick) will be present on the surface of cellular cementum (Fig. 25.31). Mineralization in the deeper layer of the precementum occurs in a linear manner but, overall, this type of cementum is less mineralized than acellular cementum. As in bone, the multipolar mode of matrix secretion by the cementoblasts and its increased rate of formation results in cells becoming incorporated into the forming matrix and these are converted into cementocytes. Unlike bone, cementocytes lying deeply within cementum may be non-viable and this is likely to occur when their distance from the surface exceeds that required for the diffusion of nutrients.

As the chemical composition of acellular and cellular cementum differs, it is assumed that this reflects differences in the secretory activity of the cells involved. Thus, dentine sialoprotein, fibronectin and tenascin, as well as a number of proteoglycans (e.g. versican decorin and biglycan), are present in cellular cementum but not acellular cementum. This may be

**Table 25.1** *Possible phenotypical differences between cementoblasts associated with acellular and cellular cementum*

| Cementoblasts from acellular cementum | Cementoblasts from cellular cementum |
|---|---|
| Identifiable for only a short time | Identifiable for longer period |
| Fibroblast-like morphology | Osteoblast-like morphology |
| Derived from epithelial root sheath | Derived from mesenchyme |
| Express cytokeratin | Do not express cytokeratin |
| Do not express osteocalcin | Express osteocalcin |
| Do not express receptors for parathormone | Express receptors for parathormone |
| Do not express TGFβ and IGF | Express TGFβ and IGF |
| Do not react with E11 antibody | React with E11 antibody |

E11 antibody = a marker reacting with osteoblasts and young osteocytes; IGF = insulin-like growth factor; TGF = transforming growth factor.

related to the presence of cementocytes, as many of the proteoglycans are located at the periphery of the lacunae and canaliculi.

The incorporation of cementocytes, as with the osteocytes of bone, necessitates the generation of new cementoblasts from stem cells/precursors within the periodontal ligament. Progenitor cells are present within the periodontal ligament, particularly around blood vessels, and must migrate through the periodontal ligament to the cementum surface. Some of these cells may represent true stem cells, having the characteristics of both self-renewal and multilineage differential potential. Other cells having the power to differentiate into cementoblasts may migrate in from the stroma of the adjacent alveolar bone.

Incremental lines will be present in cellular cementum but, because of the increased rate of formation, are more widely spaced than in acellular cementum. The stages in the formation of cellular intrinsic fibre cementum are illustrated in Figure 25.32.

Cellular cementum is usually present as the intrinsic fibre type (see Ch. 11). This type of cementum does not act in a supportive role as no Sharpey fibres from the periodontal ligament are inserted into it. However, most commonly in the apical and the furcation areas of human cheek teeth, this type of cementum alternates with layers of acellular extrinsic fibre cementum to form what is called cellular mixed stratified cementum (see Fig. 11.18a). The layers may be present in various combinations and in various thicknesses. When a layer of acellular extrinsic fibre cementum is covered by a layer of cellular intrinsic fibre cementum, there must be a functional change as the Sharpey fibres over the affected portion of the root will largely be detached from the root surface. Conversely, when cellular intrinsic fibre cementum is covered by a layer of acellular extrinsic fibre cementum, Sharpey fibres will gain an attachment to the tooth.

An additional type of cementum is cellular mixed fibre cementum. In this variety, the normal cellular intrinsic cementum does give attachment to some extrinsic fibres arising from the periodontal ligament (see Fig. 11.19).

As mentioned for acellular cementum, the precise origin of the cells in the dental follicle associated with the formation of cellular cementum awaits clarification. The possibility exists that different cell populations are responsible for the formation of the two types of cementum. Evidence is building up to suggest that the cells associated with acellular and cellular cementum do show different phenotypes; some of these are listed in Table 25.1. If this suggestion is correct then, during the formation of cellular mixed stratified cementum, there is a switch from one formative cell to another. Because of the similarity between osteoblasts and cementoblasts, it has been suggested that stem/progenitor cells primarily associated with alveolar bone could migrate into the periodontal ligament and provide a source of new cementoblasts.

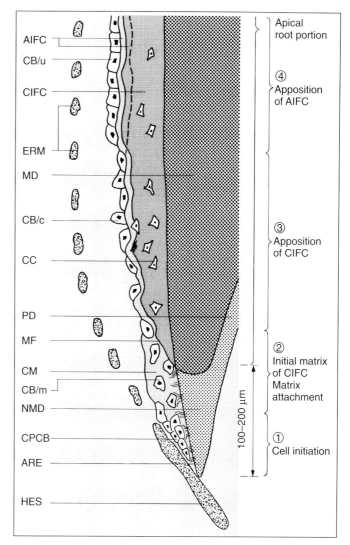

**Fig. 25.32** The initial stages of cellular intrinsic fibre cementum (CIFC) formation on human premolars developed to about 75% of their final root length.
1. Committed clone of precementoblasts contacts root predentine and produces first matrix fibrils. 2. Cementoblasts form initial collagenous matrix attached to predentine. 3. First-formed and mineralized CIFC (including cementocytes) grows by apposition. 4. CIFC is covered with a layer of acellular intrinsic fibre cementum. AIFC = acellular intrinsic fibre cementum; CB/u = cementoblasts with unipolar matrix production; ERM = epithelial cell rests of Malassez; MD = mineralized dentine; CB/c = cementoblasts with potential to become cementocytes; CC = cementocytes; PD = predentine; MF = mineralization front; CM = initial cementum matrix; CB/m = cementoblasts with multipolar matrix production; NMD = non-mineralized dentine or predentine; CPCB = committed precementoblasts; ARE = advancing root edge; HES = Hertwig's epithelial root sheath. Courtesy of Professors H.E. Schroeder and D.D. Bosshardt and the editors of *Cell and Tissue Research*.

## ALVEOLAR BONE DEVELOPMENT

The mandible and maxillae develop intramembranously. Thus, in a fibrocellular condensation, a centre of ossification appears in which osteoblasts lay down first-formed embryonic or woven bone. As the teeth develop, bone extends from the developing mandible and maxillae to surround and protect the teeth, forming the alveolus (see Fig. 19.5). The alveolus is separated from the developing enamel organ by the dental follicle (see Fig. 21.10). To accommodate the growing tooth germs, the lamellae of the developing alveolar bone undergo resorption on the inner wall of the alveolus (indicated by Howship's lacunae) while, on the outer wall of the alveolus, bone is deposited (indicated by osteoblasts lining an osteoid seam). The developing teeth therefore come to lie in a trough of bone. Later, the teeth become separated from each other by the development of interdental septa.

With the onset of root formation, interradicular bone develops in multi-rooted teeth. As in other sites, the collagen fibres in the newly formed alveolar bone have a more variable diameter and lack a preferential orientation, giving the bone a matted (basket weave) appearance when viewed in polarized light. This immature bone, termed woven bone, has larger and more numerous osteocytes than adult bone. It is formed more rapidly and has a higher turnover rate. Woven bone is subsequently converted to fine-fibred adult lamellar bone. The source of the cells forming alveolar bone is uncertain although some have suggested that it may be from neural crest cells of the investing layer of the dental follicle (see Fig. 21.10).

During crown formation, relocation of the tooth germ within the growing jaws may be associated with appropriate patterns of resorption and deposition on the internal surfaces of the alveolar bone. With the onset of tooth eruption, the bone overlying the tooth undergoes resorption to provide a pathway of eruption (see pages 359, 360). In addition, as the tooth erupts and the jaws increase in size, bone deposition is prominent in the region of the alveolar crest. The predominant activity in the fundus of the socket is one of bone resorption, except for teeth whose eruptive pathway is greater than the length of the root (see page 346). On occasions where bone deposition is seen lining the alveolus, it may be related to relocation of the erupting tooth within the growing jaws. Sharpey fibres from the periodontal ligament become attached to the wall of the alveolus during tooth eruption, although the timing is related to whether the tooth is of the primary or secondary dentition (see page 344). The bone of the alveolar wall may then be referred to as bundle bone (see page 218).

## COMPARISON OF ALVEOLAR BONE AND CEMENTUM

Having described aspects of the formation of cementum and alveolar bone and with previous knowledge of their structure (see Chs 11 and 13), it is possible to compare and contrast some of their principal features. In comparing alveolar bone and cellular cementum:

- Both tissues have a similar composition, being comprised of an inorganic component of small hydroxyapatite crystals and an organic component consisting principally of type I collagen fibres and a smaller non-collagenous component. However, the non-collagenous component may be distinguished by the presence of specific components (e.g. cementum has unique cementum attachment protein).
- Both tissues have a lag phase in the mineralization such that the surface is lined by a layer of unmineralized matrix, the osteoid and precementum layers.
- Both alveolar bone and cellular cementum display three similar cell types: osteocytes/cementocytes, osteoblasts/cementoblasts and osteoclasts/odontoclasts. However, compared with osteocytes, cementocytes are scattered less uniformly within cementum and their canaliculi are preferentially oriented towards the periodontal ligament (see Fig. 11.11).
- Bone remodelling is continuous throughout life and osteoclasts are always evident. In cementum, resorption is a rarer and more localized event and the presence of odontoclasts is much less common.
- Unlike cementum, alveolar bone contains blood vessels, nerves and marrow spaces.
- Osteocytes may be arranged circumferentially as Haversian systems around central haversian vessels. The orientation of collagen fibres in this situation is more complex than in cementum (see Fig. 13.7).
- The initial mineralization of bone involves matrix vesicles, whereas initial mineralization of cementum does not, and this may be the result of the prior presence of mineralized dentine.

- When exposed to similar orthodontic loading, alveolar bone will resorb preferentially.

When alveolar bone is compared with acellular cementum:

- unlike alveolar bone, because of its slower rate of formation, acellular cementum lacks the presence of a precementum layer and the presence of any cementocytes
- alveolar bone and acellular cementum both have Sharpey fibres from the periodontal ligament inserted into them, providing attachment for the tooth. In acellular cementum, however, these extrinsic fibres form the sole source of collagen, there being few, if any, intrinsic fibres.

Considerable information exists concerning epithelial–mesenchymal interactions in the crown, particularly concerning the roles of transcription factors, cytokines and growth hormones (see pages 305–310). Far less is known about the presence and functions of such molecules during root formation. However, molecules such as the transcription factors Msx2 and Dlx2, bone morphogenetic proteins, epidermal growth factor and transforming growth factor (TGF)β have all been identified during the epithelial–mesenchymal interactions associated with root development. Their importance can be seen from experiments in which inhibition of the activity of bone morphogenetic protein in transgenic mice results in root abnormalities.

## EXPERIMENTAL STUDIES RELATING TO ROOT DEVELOPMENT

Experiments have shown that, when a tooth germ at the early bell stage is dissected from the jaw, it is surrounded by the inner investing layer of the dental follicle (thought to be of neural crest/ectomesenchyme origin; see page 301). When the tooth germ is transplanted in this condition, the investing layer has the capacity to give rise to all the investing tissues (i.e. cementum, periodontal ligament and bone). This, however, does not preclude a contribution to the periodontium in vivo from the outer part of the dental follicle. When the dental follicle cells are excluded and the enamel organ and dental papilla alone are transplanted to an ectopic site, there is regeneration of the investing layer of the dental follicle and formation of cementum and the root-related periodontal ligament, but no formation of alveolar bone. Combined with other studies, this indicates that dental papilla mesenchymal cells in the region of the root apex, in addition to being a source of odontoblasts, provide an important source of cells that migrate out into the dental follicle and may give rise to cells such as cementoblasts and periodontal fibroblasts.

That the epithelial root sheath is important in the differentiation of root odontoblasts is indicated by experimental recombinations between isolated epithelial root sheath cells and dental papilla cells. Such studies demonstrate that root dentine will form only in the presence of the epithelial root sheath. One question that arises relates to whether the presence of root dentine alone is sufficient to induce dental follicle cells to become cementoblasts, or whether the epithelial root sheath contributes to the process. This has been tested by experimental recombinations of slices of root dentine and dental follicle cells with and without the presence of epithelial root sheath cells. Although a cementum-like tissue is formed on root dentine in both cases, this tissue separates relatively easily from the dentine in the absence of epithelial root sheath cells. This supports the view that the epithelial root sheath plays an important role in early cementogenesis in firmly uniting the cement and dentine together via the presence of the hyaline layer. This may relate particularly to its secretion of enamel-related proteins.

## CLINICAL CONSIDERATIONS

## ENAMEL PEARLS

These are small isolated spheres of enamel that are occasionally found on the root surface, especially towards the cervical margin, They are particularly common in the root bifurcation area (Fig. 25.33, see also Fig. 7.66) but may also occur at lower levels (Fig. 25.34), usually (but not always) in interradicular regions. It is thought that, in the region affected, stellate reticulum and stratum intermedium develop between the internal and external enamel epithelia of the root sheath.

Enamel pearls may provide a site for the accumulation of plaque if exposed in the mouth.

## HYPOPHOSPHATASIA

Hypophosphatasia is a condition in which there is reduced activity of tissue non-specific alkaline phosphatase. It is a rare autosomal recessive disease in which there is a marked deficiency in the presence of both acellular and cellular cementum. The lack of attachment of periodontal ligament fibres to the residual cement is associated with premature loss of the deciduous teeth. In such patients, any orthodontic treatment is likely to be accompanied by the premature loss of any permanent teeth required to be moved.

## REGENERATION FOLLOWING CHRONIC PERIODONTAL DISEASE

The most important clinical condition affecting the periodontal ligament is chronic inflammatory periodontal disease, in which toxic products are released by dental plaque lying in the gingival crevice. Interacting with

the host's defence mechanisms, these products result in the destruction and loss of periodontal ligament tissue and adjacent alveolar bone. Such a process leads to the formation of a periodontal pocket and a vicious circle is established. The loss of attachment tissue may expose the root of the tooth in the mouth and, with increasing mobility, the tooth may eventually be lost. When treating such a condition, the dental surgeon may consider two types of outcome: 1) to **repair** the existing condition so that the disease progresses no further (usually involving surgical removal of diseased tissue) or 2) to attempt to **regenerate** the lost tissues, restoring the bone, periodontal ligament and cementum to its original dimensions, including the reattachment of new periodontal ligament fibres to both the cementum and bone. The cementum tissue required to regenerate is acellular extrinsic fibre cementum in order to provide attachment to the periodontal fibres. To attempt to regenerate the attachment tissues, a detailed understanding of how each tissue develops normally is required, particularly the manner in which the cementum layer bonds firmly to the root dentine.

One common complication following surgery is the tendency for the junctional epithelium to proliferate rapidly downwards to cover the root surface, thereby preventing periodontal ligament fibres from fully attaching to cementum. Following periodontal surgery and the removal of diseased tissue, a variety of methods of conditioning the root surface have been described that claim to improve the degree of reattachment of periodontal ligament fibres. Such methods include root planing and acid etching of the surface using various solutions (e.g. citric acid or EDTA).

Following initial periodontal surgery, the connective tissue of the wound may be repopulated by the gingiva growing down and/or by the periodontal ligament growing up. Present opinion suggests that the best result is achieved when the wound is repopulated by cells of the existing periodontal ligament. Although both connective tissues may appear to be similar, they differ in several respects, which may be important to the final outcome (Table 25.2). For this reason, surgical techniques have been adopted to exclude the gingival tissues from the deeper part of the wound by placing a tissue barrier (resorbable or non-resorbable) over the alveolar crest. This is thought to aid 'guided tissue regeneration', such that the wound is repopulated primarily by periodontal ligament connective tissue.

Bioactive molecules (e.g. growth factors, cytokines and non-collagenous proteins such as bone sialoprotein, cementum-attachment protein, osteopontin) are important during the induction of periodontal cells (osteoblasts, cementoblasts and fibroblasts). Some of these molecules (e.g. bone

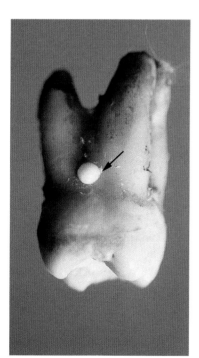

Fig. 25.33

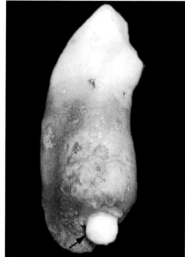

Fig. 25.34

**Fig. 25.33** An enamel pearl located near the root bifurcation area (arrow). Courtesy of Dr C. Franklyn.

**Fig. 25.34** An enamel pearl located near the root apex. Courtesy of the Royal College of Surgeons of England.

Table 25.2 *Some features distinguishing fibroblasts from gingiva and periodontal ligament*

|  | Gingiva | Periodontal ligament |
|---|---|---|
| Collagen type III | 9% | 20% |
| Collagen turnover | 5 weeks | 1 week |
| Cell volume | 8% | 40% |
| Ground substance | More | Less |
| Alkaline phosphatase | Less | More |
| Contractile proteins | Less | More |
| Prostaglandin release (in response to histamine) | More | Less |
| Collagen production | Less | More |
| Proliferation rates | Lower | Higher |
| Collagen/Fibronectin positive | 57% | 99% |

(the last four rows bracketed as: in vitro)

morphogenetic protein) have been placed in suitable carriers within wounds and are claimed to improve the degree of periodontal ligament regeneration. However, difficulties encountered in interpreting results from such studies relate to the fact that the concentrations of the growth factor used far exceed physiological levels and it is difficult to determine how long the factor is retained in an active form at the site. In addition, although reparative cementum may be formed, it may not be firmly attached to the root and may give little functional attachment to Sharpey fibres. The placement of bone grafts into areas of bone loss following periodontal disease has also been claimed to improve the degree of periodontal ligament regeneration.

During normal development, the epithelial root sheath is important in the differentiation of root odontoblasts, as indicated by experimental recombinations between isolated epithelial root sheath cells and dental papilla cells. These studies demonstrate that root dentine will form only in the presence of the epithelial root sheath. Similar experimental recombinations of slices of root dentine and dental follicle cells, with or without epithelial root sheath cells, indicate that the epithelial root sheath cells play an important role in early cementogenesis by firmly uniting the cement and dentine via the presence of the hyaline layer. Emphasis has been placed on the findings that epithelial root sheath cells secrete enamel-related proteins that may be important in cementogenesis, although the amount secreted and their significance is in dispute. Nevertheless, it has been reported that treating the surgically cleaned root surface of periodontally affected teeth with enamel matrix derivatives (obtained from porcine enamel and commercially available as Emdogain) has a positive effect on periodontal regeneration (Fig. 25.35). The particular beneficial ingredient in such a preparation has not been specifically identified, as additional components such as growth factors may also be present.

Researchers are now applying the principles of tissue engineering to determine the feasibility of assembling a construct in the laboratory that could be placed against a surgically prepared root surface and that would be able to regenerate cementum, periodontal ligament and alveolar bone in a functional setting. For this to succeed, appropriate stem/precursor cells will need to be seeded in a suitable three-dimensional scaffold incorporating any necessary growth factors and signalling molecules. Using nanotechnology, it might be possible to seed on the root surface selected precursor cells with a phenotype associated with cells forming acellular cementum, while precursor cells adjacent to the bone surface would have a phenotype associated with osteoblasts. The centrally positioned cells would have a phenotype of periodontal fibroblasts and be able to produce the necessary collagen fibre bundles The construct would have to be immunocompatible with the patient, the cells used perhaps being stem cells derived from the patient. Some of the growth factors and signalling molecules could be provided by the cells themselves if they had undergone genetic manipulation.

## ASSESSMENT OF CLINICAL STUDIES

There is an extensive literature involving both animal and human studies that assesses the value of the experimental procedures outlined above on the outcome of periodontal surgery. For animal experimentation, an important question is how closely the 'model' resembles human chronic inflammatory periodontal disease. In particular, how are we to evaluate the conclusions reached by these studies in attempting to improve surgical outcomes? For example, there are many papers indicating that etching of the root surface improves the chances of reattaching periodontal ligament fibres to the tooth.

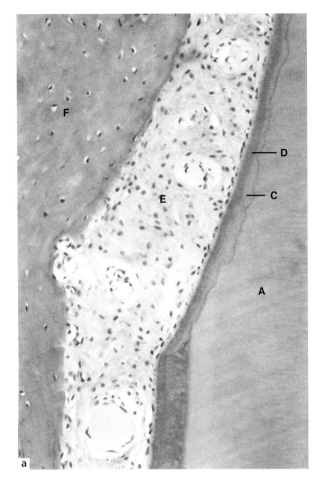
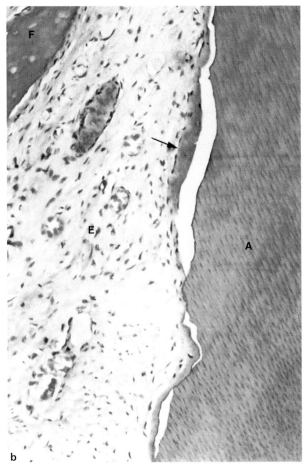

**Fig. 25.35** Experimental cavities in the roots of lateral mandibular incisors of a monkey. The incisors were gently extracted and the experimental cavities were made by means of a round burr under constant irrigation with physiological saline. Porcine enamel matrix was then applied in one of the cavities (a) after which the incisor was immediately replanted. The other incisor (b) served as control and nothing was placed in the cavity of this tooth before it was replanted. Eight weeks after the replantation, the cavity (a), where enamel matrix had been placed, is covered by a layer of acellular cementum. The cavity in the control tooth, (b), is covered by a cellular hard tissue poorly attached to the dentine (arrow) (H & E; ×150). A = dentine; B = original acellular cementum; C = new, regenerated acellular cementum; D = new cellular reparative cementum; E = periodontal ligament; F = bone. From Hammarstrom L 1997 Enamel matrix, cementum development and regeneration. *Journal of Clinical Periodontology* 24: 658–668.

## Cochrane reviews

Cochrane reviews are publications aiming to provide the best available information concerning healthcare interventions. Their stated aim is to critically appraise the evidence for and against the effectiveness and appropriateness of treatments associated with clinical trials. Meta-analyses, in which data from studies are combined, have been used to test the assumption of similarity between studies (homogeneity) and the possible effects of bias (or other variables) on the outcome. The complete reviews are published in the *Cochrane Library*, available on the worldwide web. As such analytical methods are highly developed in Cochrane reviews, they act as part of the quality assurance process of research. Cochrane reviews have been published in relation to aspects of periodontal regeneration.

Cochrane reviews have shown that the size of the difference between regenerative techniques and non-regenerative (conventional) surgery might be influenced in part by bias in patient selection and/or operator or examiner blinding. Indeed, the analyses show that apparently similar types of patient and procedure give rise to wider variations in treatment outcomes than would be expected by chance. Although there is some evidence suggesting the possible role of bias in this variability, it could also be related to severity of disease, presence of plaque and surgical skill, although there is a paucity of information about these factors. In consequence, care should be taken about citing only the summary meta-analysis value from systematic reviews.

Publication bias could be inflating the difference between test and control groups, with a tendency towards more frequent publication of studies with positive outcomes than those showing no difference between groups. Another limitation of the data presented in the systematic reviews is the measurement of effectiveness or success of treatment employed in the studies. This is almost always based on determining any change in pocket depth by clinical probing. However, the relationship between changes in probing measurements and true patient benefits (such as tooth retention) is not clear. It is also noteworthy that such changes may not reflect histological regeneration.

To date, the Cochrane reviews related to periodontal surgery indicate that surgery combined with guided tissue regeneration, enamel matrix proteins or bone allograft appears to result in improved clinical outcomes compared with surgery without such adjuncts. Heterogeneity between studies in these analyses was usually substantial, with a range of treatment outcomes ranging from favourable to unfavourable. The degree of unpredictability is also highlighted by the calculation of the numbers needed to treat (NNT) value. This statistic indicates how many individuals would need to be treated to achieve a defined benefit. For two systematic reviews, the NNT was based upon the chance of the regenerative surgery achieving at least 2 mm more probing attachment gain than conventional surgery. This threshold was used both because it should represent a greater change than measurement error and also for convenience, as this threshold is often reported in the primary trials. The NNT for enamel matrix proteins was 6. This means that for every six patients treated, one will gain this degree of advantage over conventional surgery and five will not. For guided tissue regeneration, the NNT was 8. Root conditioning with citric acid, EDTA or tetracycline was shown not to be an effective treatment.

In view of the potential impact of bias and variability on these results, it is reasonable to conclude that, comparing the benefit of surgery with adjuncts over conventional surgery, both the size and the predictability of achieving a benefit are uncertain.

Description of the development of the dentitions requires consideration of the processes of tooth eruption and of the development of occlusion post-eruptively. Three distinct phases of tooth development can be recognized that ultimately lead to the establishment of the full dentition. First, there is a phase termed the pre-eruptive phase, which starts with the initiation of tooth development and ends with the completion of the crown (see Ch. 21). Second, there is the phase of tooth eruption (prefunctional phase), which begins once the roots commence to form. Third, after the teeth have emerged into the oral cavity, there is a protracted phase concerned with the development, and maintenance, of occlusion (the functional phase).

## TOOTH ERUPTION

Eruption is the process whereby a tooth moves axially from its develop-mental position within the alveolar crypt of the jaw into its functional position within the oral cavity. It is a remarkable event in that nowhere else in the body does a developing organ (in this case a tooth) leave the confines of its developing intrabony location. Although the definition of eruption provided above suggests that eruption is entirely a developmental process, there is no evidence to suggest that eruption entirely ceases once a tooth meets its antagonist in the mouth, and outward axial movements occurring during the functional phase may also be eruptive movements (i.e. overeruption following removal of the antagonist tooth in the opposite jaw and compensatory eruption relating to attrition). It is sometimes sug-gested that the eruptive forces that are generated during the prefunctional (intraosseous) phase and functional (supraosseous and supragingival) phase are produced by different mechanisms. However, there is no exper-imental evidence to support this view and it seems hardly likely from basic biological principles that similar axial eruptive movements would require two separate mechanisms.

Throughout the pre-eruptive phase of tooth development, there is con-centric growth of the tooth within its follicle without any active bodily movement in a direction indicating eruption towards the oral cavity (Fig. 26.1). For a permanent mandibular second molar, there are two stages of active eruption (Fig. 26.2): the first stage occurs between 6 and 12 years when the tooth emerges into the mouth; a later second stage occurs at about 16 years in association with the adolescent growth spurt.

While the main direction of the eruptive force is axial (i.e. related to the long axis of the tooth), movement also occurs in other planes, accounting for tilting and drifting. Eruption rates of teeth are greatest at the time of crown emergence. Rates also differ according to tooth type. Permanent maxillary first incisors are reported to erupt at about 1 mm/month; the rates for mandibular second premolars have been determined to be about 4.5 mm in 14 weeks. For permanent third molars, where space is available, erup-tion rates of 1 mm in 3 months have been recorded. In crowded dentitions, however, the eruption rate may be less than 1 mm in 6 months. The rate of eruption represents a balance between forces tending to move the tooth into the mouth (eruptive force) and forces tending to prevent this move-ment (resistive force). Resistance may be produced by overlying soft tissues and alveolar bone, the viscosity of the surrounding periodontal ligament/dental follicle, and occlusal forces. Thus, changes in the rate of tooth movement may be brought about by changes in either the eruptive forces and/or the resistive forces. At present, little is known about the nature, source and magnitude of either the eruptive or resistive forces

(although only relatively small forces exerted by a spring are sufficient to stop a tooth erupting). Furthermore, it is not known whether the forces are of the same nature and magnitude at various stages of the eruptive cycle.

Although eruption commences at the time the root of the tooth begins to form, a growing root is not required for eruption to proceed (see page 363). The molecular events associated with the initiation of eruption are not well understood. There is evidence that epidermal growth factor (EGF) may be required and that there might also be an involvement of transform-ing growth factor α. Furthermore, macrophage colony-stimulating factor (MCSF) can induce tooth eruption. However, these growth factors can have different effects on different tooth types (incisor versus molar teeth). It has been proposed that bone deposition at the base of the developing

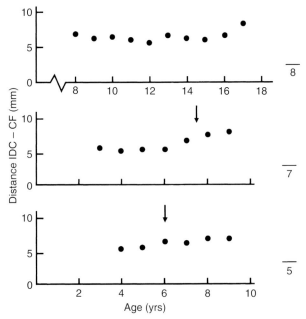

**Fig. 26.1** Graphs plotting the mean distance from the mandibular canal (IDC) (regarded as a fixed point) to the centre of developing crowns of teeth during their pre-eruptive phase (CF). The upper graph is for a permanent mandibular third molar, the middle graph is for a permanent mandibular second molar, the lower graph is for a mandibular second premolar. Arrows indicate age at crown completion. Courtesy of Dr B.G.H. Levers.

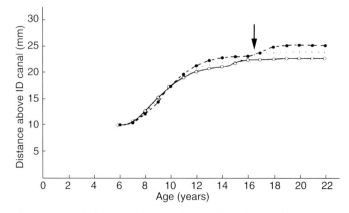

**Fig. 26.2** Graph showing the mean distance from the mandibular canal (ID canal) to the occlusal surface for a permanent mandibular second molar during its eruption. Note the adolescent growth spurt (arrow). Courtesy of Dr B.G.H Levers.

root can initiate eruption and move the tooth axially. This is most obviously seen at the bases of erupting premolar teeth of dogs (see Fig. 25.14). However (and as mentioned on page 346), for most species there is little evidence of bone deposition beneath the base of the erupting tooth (see Fig. 25.13), resorption often being evident. The different patterns of bone activity in different species may relate to the distance a tooth has to erupt: if the distance is much greater than the length of the root, then bone deposition is clearly necessary to maintain the normal dimensions of the periodontal ligament at the root apex of the tooth.

Undoubtedly, whatever initiates tooth eruption, and whatever generates the force(s) of eruption, remodelling of the alveolus is required to accommodate eruptive movements and to allow the tooth to move through the bone (via an eruptive pathway) towards the oral cavity. This will involve a complex and very well regulated process that recruits mononuclear cells

that, in turn, form osteoclasts for the resorption of the overlying alveolar bone (Fig. 26.3). The evidence indicates that the complex signalling process occurs within and between the dental follicle and the tooth germ (Figs 26.4, 26.5). Recruitment of mononuclear cells to the dental follicle around the erupting tooth seems to require macrophage-colony stimulating factor (MCSF) and/or monocyte chemotactic protein (MCP)-1. The genesis of osteoclasts additionally involves inhibition of osteoprotegerin synthesis and increased receptor activator for NF-κB ligand (RANKL). From the tooth germ, signalling from the stellate reticulum of the enamel organ also appears to have a role in regulating eruption. This signalling seems to occur via parathyroid-hormone-related protein and interleukin-1α. EGF and TGFβ1 can also enhance the recruitment of mononuclear cells and osteoclastogenesis. Osteoblasts may influence the process of osteoclastogenesis through signalling via the RANKL/OPG pathway (see page

**Fig. 26.3** (a) The alveolar bone (A) above the crown of an erupting tooth (B) is being resorbed by multinucleated osteoclasts (C) derived from the dental follicle. (b) High-power view of (a) showing osteoclasts (arrows) resorbing overlying alveolar bone. Courtesy of Dr T. Arnett.

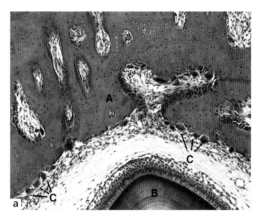
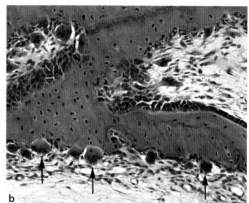

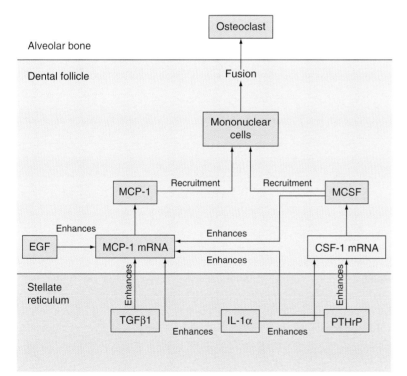

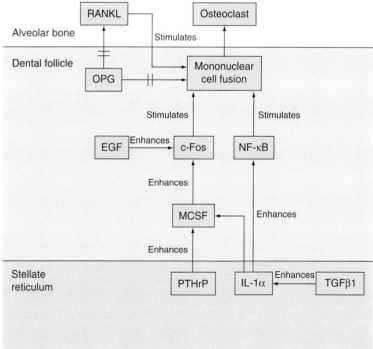

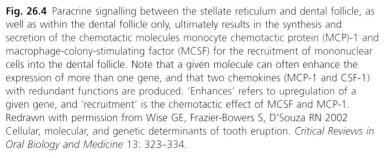

**Fig. 26.4** Paracrine signalling between the stellate reticulum and dental follicle, as well as within the dental follicle only, ultimately results in the synthesis and secretion of the chemotactic molecules monocyte chemotactic protein (MCP)-1 and macrophage-colony-stimulating factor (MCSF) for the recruitment of mononuclear cells into the dental follicle. Note that a given molecule can often enhance the expression of more than one gene, and that two chemokines (MCP-1 and CSF-1) with redundant functions are produced. 'Enhances' refers to upregulation of a given gene, and 'recruitment' is the chemotactic effect of MCSF and MCP-1. Redrawn with permission from Wise GE, Frazier-Bowers S, D'Souza RN 2002 Cellular, molecular, and genetic determinants of tooth eruption. *Critical Reviews in Oral Biology and Medicine* 13: 323–334.

**Fig. 26.5** Possible signalling cascades that may promote the fusion of the mononuclear cells recruited to the dental follicle. Both MCSF and receptor activator of nuclear factor kappa B ligand (NF-κB or RANKL), are known to promote osteoclast formation, whereas osteoprotegerin (OPG) inhibits this by preventing cell-to-cell signalling. The downstream products of the transcription factors c-Fos and NF-κB that promote osteoclast formation are not yet known. The crossed arrows with crosses (⫣→) reflect inhibition of gene expression, whereas other arrows reflect enhancement of gene expression or stimulation of cell fusion. Redrawn with permission from Wise GE, Frazier-Bowers S, D'Souza RN 2002 Cellular, molecular, and genetic determinants of tooth eruption. *Critical Reviews in Oral Biology and Medicine* 13: 323–334.

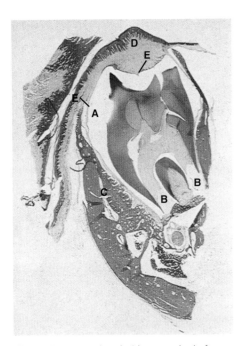

**Fig. 26.6** An erupting deciduous molar before its emergence into the oral cavity. A = enamel space; B = developing roots; C = developing alveolar crypt; D = oral mucosa and overlying connective tissue; E = reduced enamel epithelium (Decalcified, transverse section through the jaw; H & E; ×4).

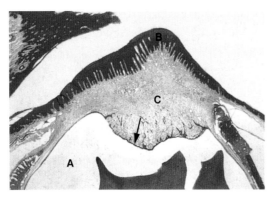

**Fig. 26.7** The soft tissues overlying the enamel space (A) of an erupting tooth. B = oral epithelium; C = connective tissue between developing tooth and oral epithelium. Arrow indicates the reduced enamel epithelium (H & E; ×10).

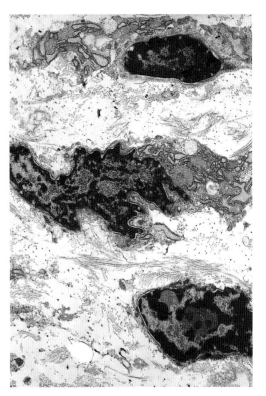

**Fig. 26.8** Fibroblasts in the connective tissue overlying an erupting tooth showing evidence of degeneration (TEM; ×10 000).

214). Recent evidence indicates that an osteoblast transcription factor termed Cbfal (Runx2) might regulate tooth eruption and that this molecule is also expressed by the cells of the dental follicle. Note that the signalling pathways described suggest that there is a redundancy of function (e.g. both MCSF and MCP-1 act as chemokines for the recruitment of mononuclear cells to the dental follicle). Defects in bone resorption may therefore prevent eruption.

As a tooth approaches the oral cavity, there are marked changes in the overlying soft tissues. The enamel surface is covered by the reduced enamel epithelium, which is a vestige of the enamel organ. Figure 26.6 shows an erupting deciduous molar before its emergence into the oral cavity and Figure 26.7 a higher-power view of the soft tissues overlying the enamel space of an erupting tooth. As the tooth erupts, the outer cells of the reduced enamel epithelium proliferate into the connective tissue between the cusp tip and the oral epithelium. It has been suggested that these proliferating epithelial cells secrete enzymes that degrade collagen. Reduced enamel epithelial cells may also be concerned with the removal of breakdown products resulting from resorption of connective tissue. Depolymerization of the non-fibrous components of the extracellular matrix has been detected in the connective tissue overlying erupting teeth. Although a relationship between the degeneration of the connective tissue and the pressure exerted by the underlying erupting tooth has not been established, ischaemia is thought to be a contributory factor. That pressure alone is not entirely responsible is indicated by the finding that there is always evidence of some new collagen formation in this region.

Many of the fibroblasts in the connective tissue overlying an erupting tooth cease fibrillogenesis, actively take up extracellular material (as evidenced by intracellular collagen profiles – see pages 188–189) and synthesize acid hydrolases. Eventually, the nuclei become pyknotic and the cells degenerate (Fig. 26.8).

The development of the dentogingival junction during the eruption of a tooth is shown diagrammatically in Figure 26.9. As the tooth approaches

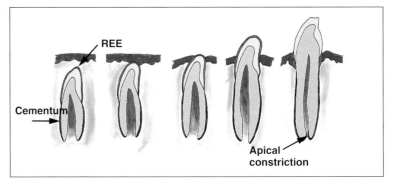

**Fig. 26.9** Diagrammatic representation of the development of the dentogingival junction during the eruption of a tooth. REE = reduced enamel epithelium (green). Red outline delineates oral epithelium.

the oral epithelium, the cells of the outer layer of the reduced enamel epithelium and the basal layer of the oral epithelium actively proliferate and eventually unite. The epithelium covering the tip of the tooth then degenerates at its centre, enabling the crown to emerge through an epithelium-lined pathway into the oral cavity. Further emergence of the tooth results from active eruptive movements and passive separation of the oral epithelium from the crown surface. When the tooth first erupts into the mouth, the reduced enamel epithelium is attached to the unerupted part of the crown, thus forming an epithelial seal – the junctional epithelium (see pages 328–340). It is generally believed that the reduced enamel epithelial component of the junctional epithelium is eventually replaced by oral epithelium. With continued eruption, as more of the crown is exposed, a gingival crevice is formed. An erupting tooth about to emerge into the oral cavity through an epithelium-lined pathway as a result of fusion of the oral epithelium and the reduced enamel epithelium is shown in Figure 26.10.

For the eruption of a permanent tooth, where there is a deciduous predecessor (i.e. excluding the permanent molars), the roots of the deciduous tooth must be resorbed to allow for shedding. Initially, each deciduous

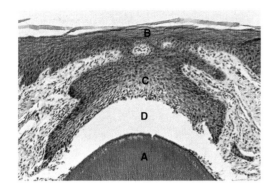

Fig. 26.10

**Fig. 26.10** An erupting tooth (A) about to emerge into the oral cavity through an epithelium-lined pathway as a result of fusion of the oral epithelium (B) and the reduced enamel epithelium (C) D = enamel space. (H & E; ×12). Courtesy of Professor A.G.S. Lumsden.

**Fig. 26.11** Buccolingual section through an erupted deciduous canine (A) and its erupting successor (B). C = gubernacular canal (Decalcified section; H & E; ×4).

**Fig. 26.12** Buccolingual section through a resorbing deciduous tooth (A) and its erupting successor (B). Arrows indicate multinucleated odontoclasts (Decalcified section; Masson's trichrome; ×70).

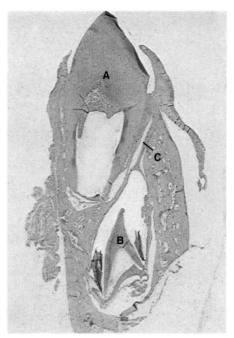

Fig. 26.11

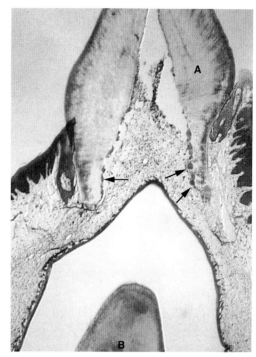

Fig. 26.12

tooth and its developing permanent successor share a common alveolar crypt, the permanent tooth germ being situated lingually to the developing deciduous tooth (see Fig. 21.16). With continued growth, this relationship changes and the permanent tooth comes to lie near the root apex of the deciduous tooth within its own bony crypt. Note that the alveolar crypt of the permanent tooth shown in Figure 26.11 is not complete, there being the opening of a canal in its roof through which the dental follicle of the tooth germ communicates with, and is attached to, the overlying oral mucosa. This canal has been termed the gubernacular canal (see page 362).

The appearance of a resorbing deciduous tooth above its erupting successor is illustrated in Figure 26.12. During the early eruptive stages of the permanent tooth, the bone separating it from its deciduous predecessor is resorbed. Following this, resorption of the hard tissues of the deciduous tooth takes place by the activity of multinucleated osteoclast-like cells termed odontoclasts. The vascular, resorbing tissue has been termed the resorbing organ of Tomes.

For a deciduous incisor or canine, root resorption initially occurs on the lingual surface adjacent to the developing permanent tooth (Fig. 26.11). With subsequent movement and relocation of the teeth in the growing jaws, the developing permanent tooth comes to lie directly beneath the deciduous tooth and further resorption occurs from the apex. For a deciduous molar, root resorption often commences on the inner surfaces where the permanent premolars initially develop. The premolars later come to lie beneath the roots of the deciduous molar and further resorption occurs from the root apices. The shift in position of the deciduous tooth relative to the permanent successor may account for the intermittent nature of root resorption.

The initiation of root resorption may be an inherent developmental process or it may be related to pressure from the permanent successor against the overlying bone or tooth. To assess which of these explanations is correct, permanent tooth germs have been surgically removed, when it was seen that resorption of the deciduous predecessors still occurred, although this was delayed. These findings are also consistent with the clinical observation that shedding of a deciduous tooth still occurs, but is retarded, where the successor is congenitally absent or occupies an abnormal position within the jaw.

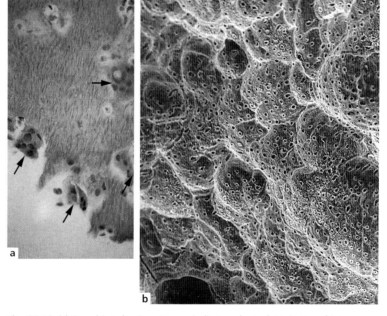

**Fig. 26.13** (a) Resorbing dentine. Arrows indicate odontoclasts in Howship's lacunae (H & E; ×215). (b) SEM of the resorbing surface of a deciduous tooth showing Howship's lacunae. Within the lacunae, dentinal tubules are seen as small circular openings (Anorganic specimen; ×400). Courtesy of Professor S.J. Jones and Springer-Verlag.

It has been suggested that increased masticatory loads affect the pattern and rate of deciduous tooth resorption. Indeed, it has been shown that, if deciduous teeth are splinted following the removal of the developing permanent teeth, there is less root resorption than that seen with removal of the permanent teeth alone.

Resorbing dentine is illustrated in Figure 26.13. Multinucleated osteoclast-like cells (odontoclasts) lie within resorption lacunae (Howship's lacunae, Fig. 26.14). Odontoclasts, like osteoclasts, differentiate from circulating monocyte-like cells. They are vacuolated and have long cytoplasmic processes. In an electron micrograph, the cytoplasmic projections form a brush border with the tooth surface. The odontoclasts have an abundance of ribosomes and a large number of mitochondria.

Howship's lacunae in resorbing teeth tend to be larger and more spherical than lacunae in bone.

Resorption of deciduous teeth is not a continuous process. During rest periods, reparative tissue may be formed, leading to a reattachment of the periodontal ligament. The tissue of repair is cementum-like and the cells responsible for its formation are similar in appearance to cementoblasts (see page 177). If the repair process prevails over the resorption, the tooth may become ankylosed to the surrounding bone, with loss of the periodontal ligament (Fig. 26.14). Ankylosis may also be caused by trauma or infection of a tooth. Ankylosis is discussed further on page 375.

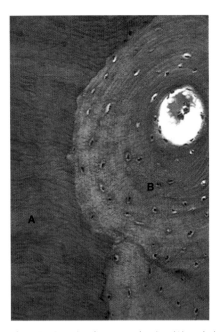

**Fig. 26.14** Fusion between dentine (A) and alveolar bone (B) in an ankylosed tooth (Decalcified section viewed in blue light; × 150). Courtesy of Dr B.G.H. Levers.

A specialized feature associated with the erupting permanent tooth is the presence of a gubernacular canal (Fig. 26.11). The gubernacular canal contains the gubernacular cord. The cord is composed of a central strand of epithelium (derived from the dental lamina) surrounded by connective tissue. The connective tissue is organized into inner and outer layers. Collagen fibres of the inner layer show greater organization and run mainly parallel to the long axis of the epithelium. In the outer layer, the collagen fibres are fewer and less organized. Differences between the layers can also be discerned with respect to the vasculature, the vessels in the outer layer being larger. During eruption, the gubernacular cords decrease in length but increase in thickness and become less dense. Surgical removal of the cord does not prevent eruption of the permanent tooth.

## MECHANISMS OF TOOTH ERUPTION

All tissues within the vicinity of the tooth thought capable of generating a force have, at one time or another, been implicated in the eruptive process. The theories advanced to explain the mechanism of tooth eruption can be divided into two main groups. One view suggests that the tooth is pushed out as a result of forces generated beneath and around it, by alveolar bone growth, root growth, blood pressure/tissue fluid pressure or cell proliferation. Alternatively, the tooth may be pulled out as a result of tension within the connective tissue of the periodontal ligament.

Many of the experiments conducted to elucidate the eruptive mechanism have required the use of the continuously growing incisors of rats and rabbits. This is because of the ease of experimentally manipulating the teeth, the continuous eruption of the teeth, and the rapid rates of eruption that can be as high as 1 mm per day. Figure 26.15 shows the distribution of tissues in the continuously growing rat incisor. Because of what is perceived as the specialized nature of a tooth of continuous growth compared to the tooth of limited growth found in the human dentition, some researchers have questioned the use of the rodent incisor and have

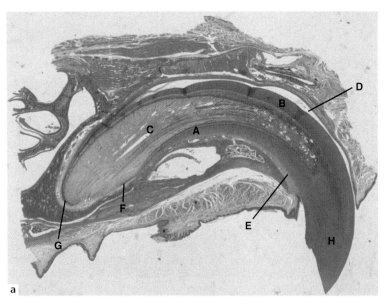
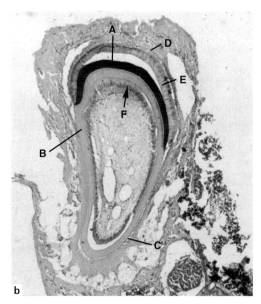

**Fig. 26.15** (a) The continuously growing maxillary rat incisor, showing the distribution of tissues. In essence, this tooth represents root tissue (i.e. dentine and cementum, A) on its lingual side and crown tissue (i.e. dentine and enamel, B) on its labial side. C = dental pulp; D = enamel space. On the lingual side of the tooth, a true periodontal ligament (E) passes from the cementum to the alveolar bone, while connective tissue intervenes labially between (although it is not attached to) the enamel surface and the alveolar bone. In the region of the proliferative 'root' apex, structures homologous with an epithelial root sheath (F) and an enamel organ (G) continually produce new dental tissues to compensate for attritional loss. In the laboratory rat, incisor teeth in occlusion erupt at a rate of about 400 μm/day (impeded eruption rate). If the teeth are cut out of occlusion, their eruption rate attains levels of about 1 mm/day (unimpeded eruption rate). To prevent pulp exposure during continuous incisor eruption, secondary dentine (H) is continually deposited beneath the incisal edge (H & E; ×8). (b) Cross-section of the mandibular incisor of a rat. The developing enamel matrix (A) is limited to the labial surface of the tooth. The remainder of the dentine (B) is covered by a very thin layer of cementum. A true periodontal ligament (C) is only present in association with the cementum-covered component of the tooth. A loose connective tissue (D) separates the enamel from the surrounding socket wall. E = Ameloblast layer; F = odontoblast layer. (Masson's trichrome; ×40). (a) Courtesy of Dr M. Robins.

suggested that the results of experiments on such teeth cannot be extrapolated to human teeth. However, teeth of continuous growth evolved from teeth of limited growth and, on basic biological principles, modification to existing systems and mechanisms would be expected rather than radically alternative mechanisms. Importantly, there are more similarities between the teeth than differences and, in this respect, the results of experiments/studies on the eruption of teeth of continuous and limited growth show remarkable convergence of viewpoint (e.g. that eruption requires a force generated by the surrounding connective tissues (i.e. dental follicle or periodontal ligament) that does not require a tractional force pulling the tooth towards the oral cavity).

Although no one theory to explain the generation of eruptive force(s) is yet supported by sufficient experimental evidence, the brief review that follows will show that the eruptive mechanism: 1) is a property of the periodontal ligament (or its precursor, the dental follicle); 2) does not require a tractional force pulling the tooth towards the mouth; 3) is multifactorial in that more than one agent makes important contributions to the overall eruptive force; and 4) could involve a combination of fibroblast activity (although the evidence to date remains poor) and vascular and/or tissue hydrostatic pressures.

## ROLE OF THE PERIODONTAL LIGAMENT IN ERUPTION

Experiments involving root resection or root transection of the continuously growing incisors of rodents (or rabbits) indicate that the periodontal ligament is the probable source for the generation of the forces responsible for eruption. Root resection involves the surgical removal of the proliferative odontogenic tissues at the base of the continuously growing incisor; root transection involves cutting the incisor into proximal and distal portions. Both surgical procedures result in a situation where the tooth (or the distal segment following transection) remains merely as a fragment attached to the jaw by a periodontal ligament but without the possibility of root growth and with degeneration of the pulp. Furthermore, there can be no contribution to eruption from bone growth as none occurs at the base (fundus) of the socket. The resected and transected incisors continue to erupt to the point where they are exfoliated from the socket. That the movement in these surgically prepared teeth is eruptive-like and not an artefactual exfoliation is indicated by experiments that show that the resected rodent incisor changes its rate of eruption in response to factors/drugs that similarly affect the rate of eruption in normal incisors.

Although the periodontal ligament is implicated in the generation of the eruptive force, experiments show that, for teeth of limited growth, this property can be undertaken by its precursor, the dental follicle. When a developing unerupted premolar tooth is surgically removed and replaced with a metal replica, the replica will 'erupt', provided that the dental follicle is retained. This experiment confirms that rootless teeth (both experimentally produced and clinically observed) can erupt and that the eruptive mechanism is present in a connective tissue (periodontal ligament or dental follicle) that need not gain a direct attachment to the tooth.

Investigation into the eruptive behaviour of the continuously growing lathyritic incisor confirms that the eruptive force is unlikely to involve a tractional element that pulls the tooth towards the oral cavity. Lathyrogens are drugs that specifically inhibit the formation of collagen cross-links, thereby disrupting the fibre network in the periodontal ligament. Compared with controls, eruption rates of lathyritic rodent incisors are unaffected, provided that occlusal forces (which could traumatize the already weakened ligament) are reduced by regular trimming of the tooth to the gingival level. Thus, the lathyrogen experiments support the experiments on rootless teeth (of non-continuous growth) and indicate that traction of collagen fibres is not required to effect eruption. Further evidence against a tractional eruptive force comes from study of the development of the periodontal ligament (see page 344), which indicates that teeth can erupt in the absence of well developed periodontal fibres. These studies also disprove the theory that contraction of periodontal collagen fibre is responsible for generating the eruptive force.

Although the opinion is held that the force effecting eruption is derived from a single source (i.e. a prime mover), it is conceivable that more than one agent contributes to the overall force. That eruption is multifactorial is evident when considering the variety of processes that must be involved to produce and sustain eruption. Indeed, four processes seem to be necessary.

- First, there must be the mechanism itself that generates the eruptive forces.
- Second, there are processes whereby eruptive forces are translated into eruption by movements through the surrounding tissues (e.g. overcoming the resistance of the tissues to eruption).
- Third, eruption must be sustained by processes that enable the tooth to be supported in its new position.
- Fourth, eruption occurs alongside a process of remodelling of the periodontal tissues to maintain the functional integrity of the system.

Experiments support the view that eruption is multifactorial; on the basis of study of the interactions of various drugs/hormones known to influence eruption, they suggest that there are at least two factors involved – a cortisone-sensitive factor and a cortisone-insensitive factor. A study of eruption rates in rodent incisors showed that, when a drug is given that severely retards eruption (in this case the antimitotic drug cyclophosphamide), the remaining component of eruption is no longer affected by cortisone administration (which would normally produce a marked increase in eruption). Although it is possible to interpret these data in other ways, additional experiments show that the recovery of eruption following root resection (perhaps due to the removal of abnormal tissues at the base) also has both cortisone-sensitive and cortisone-insensitive phases.

Having established that the connective tissues around the developing tooth are most likely to be the source of the eruptive mechanism, two major systems have been implicated in the generation of the eruptive force. One view holds that the force is produced by the activity of periodontal fibroblasts through their contractility and/or motility; the other that vascular and/or tissue hydrostatic pressures in and around the tooth are responsible for eruption.

Whatever the system implicated in the eruptive mechanism, the evidence should be judged according to the following five criteria:

1. The proposed system must be capable of producing a force under physiological conditions that is sufficient to move a tooth in a direction favouring eruption.
2. Experimentally induced changes to the system should cause predictable changes in eruption.
3. The system requires characteristics that enable it to sustain eruptive movements over long periods of time.
4. The biochemical characteristics of the system should be consistent with the production of an eruptive force.
5. The morphological features associated with the system should be consistent with the production of an eruptive force.

### Periodontal fibroblast motility/contractility hypothesis

A role for the periodontal ligament fibroblasts in eruption is based upon the notion that these cells can exert a tractional force on to the tooth through the collagen network or through cell-to-cell contacts. This is in some ways analogous to the events occurring during wound contraction, which are thought to be the result of activities of specialized cells termed myofibroblasts. However, the periodontal ligament differs markedly from granulation tissue, and there is considerable evidence against the requirement for a tractional eruptive force acting through the periodontal collagen network (see page 363). Reviewing the evidence in terms of our prescribed criteria, there is at present nothing to indicate that the fibroblasts can exert a force under physiological conditions sufficient to move a tooth in a direction favouring eruption. Neither has it been possible to devise procedures to affect selectively periodontal fibroblast activity in vivo to assess whether the experimental procedures have predictable effects on eruption. It has been shown that the drug colchicine, by its known disturbance of intracellular microtubules, reduces cell motility and this might explain the drug's significant retardatory effect on eruption. However, colchicine influences more than just cell migration (for example, it also affects connective tissue turnover). To date, the evidence relating to the fibroblast activity hypothesis relies almost entirely upon consideration of the morphology of the fibroblasts (criterion 5 above) and upon the possible characteristics of the system that would sustain the eruptive forces over long periods of time (criterion 3 above).

When periodontal fibroblasts are cultured on plastic, they assume the appearance and behaviour of migratory cells. They have a highly elongated shape with numerous, highly polarized arrays of microtubules and microfilaments. Their motility in vitro ceases with colchicine. When periodontal fibroblasts are cultured in a collagen gel, they generate tension by their contractility and assume the appearance of myofibroblast-like cells (i.e. fibroblasts with some of the properties of smooth muscle cells, a feature of fibroblasts in granulation tissue). During their contractile phase, these cells possess thick cell coats, considerable amounts of microfilamentous material dispersed throughout the cytoplasm, numerous cell contacts resembling gap junctions and occasional crenulated (folded) nuclei, but little rough endoplasmic reticulum. Their contraction in vitro is inhibited when drugs interfering with microfilaments (e.g. cytochalasin) are added to the culture medium. In vivo, however, periodontal fibroblasts show features of neither migratory cells nor myofibroblasts. Instead, they tend to be rounded or flattened in outline without polarity of shape, have relatively little microfilamentous material (and then primarily as stress fibres beneath the cell membrane, a feature of cells generally exhibited 'after' migration/contraction), have only infrequent gap junctions (but more cell contacts in the form of simplified desmosomes), and contain considerable amounts of rough endoplasmic reticulum (see page 188). Thus, the periodontal fibroblast in vivo shows all the characteristics of a cell actively synthesizing and secreting protein rather than of a motile/contractile cell. Care must therefore be taken in extrapolating from the in vitro to the in vivo situation.

In terms of criterion 3 (above), there is evidence of sustained migration of periodontal fibroblasts in vivo. Studies where the nuclei of cells have been labelled with tritium-labelled thymidine indicate that periodontal fibroblasts move occlusally at a rate equal to that of eruption; if the eruption rate is increased there is a concomitant increase in the rate of migration. Although providing some evidence of a shift in the position of periodontal fibroblasts, such work does not in itself indicate whether the cells are moving actively to generate the force of eruption or whether they are merely being transported passively within the ligament, the eruptive force being generated by another mechanism.

Other morphological features of the periodontal fibroblasts argue against their involvement in the generation of the eruptive force. The presence of cell contacts (not a usual feature of fibroblasts in a mature connective tissue) might indicate that a force could be generated through cell-to-cell contacts. However, the contacts are simplified desmosomes and not the fibronexus usually seen for myofibroblasts in contracting wounds. Furthermore, many of the simplified desmosomes for periodontal fibroblasts are located at right angles to the long axes of the cells and they lack any recognizable microfilament bundles – arrangements that do not seem suited to transmit a tractional force directly through the cells themselves.

One way of assessing the contribution of the periodontal fibroblasts to eruption involves analysing quantitatively the structure of these cells in different periodontal ligaments and in teeth exhibiting different eruptive behaviours. The findings of studies using this approach also provide evidence against the periodontal fibroblast motility/contractility hypotheses. For example, there are no differences in the cells and their various organelles when periodontal fibroblasts in rapidly erupting and fully erupted teeth are compared.

## Periodontal vascular/tissue hydrostatic pressure hypothesis

An eruptive force might be generated via the periodontal vasculature either directly through blood pressure or indirectly by influencing periodontal tissue (hydrostatic) pressures. Whether acting directly or indirectly, the periodontal vascular hypotheses clearly do not require a tractional mode of activity within the periodontal tissues.

That vascular pressures can alter the position of a tooth in its socket is shown by the fact that a tooth moves ($0.4\ \mu m$) in synchrony with the arterial pulse. Furthermore, spontaneous changes in blood pressure have been shown to influence eruptive behaviour and, at death, when the arterial blood pressure is zero, eruption ceases. Therefore, there is some evidence that, without experimental intervention, vascular/tissue pressures can produce a force sufficient to move a tooth in a direction favouring eruption (criterion 1 above). Experimental alterations to the periodontal vasculature following the administration of vasoactive drugs or interference with the sympathetic vasomotor nerve supply also result in predictable changes in eruption-like behaviour (criterion 2 above). For example, using a sensitive displacement transducer, it is possible to continuously monitor eruptive behaviour. Following the administration of a hypotensive drug (e.g. hexamethonium), as a probable result of increased capillary and periodontal tissue hydrostatic pressures, there is a marked increase in the rates of extrusive, eruption-like movements. In addition, stimulation of the cervical sympathetic system results in cessation of eruption and significant intrusion of the tooth, probably as a result of vasoconstriction and decreased capillary and periodontal tissue pressures (once the stimulus is removed, eruption recommences).

To sustain eruptive movements according to the vascular hypotheses, it is necessary to postulate that periodontal tissue pressures are high, that there are pressure differentials along the periodontal ligament, and that changes in such pressures change eruptive behaviour (criterion 3 above). Indeed, there is evidence to support all three postulates. However, there remains debate as to whether periodontal tissue hydrostatic pressures are supra-atmospheric or subatmospheric.

To assess whether the biochemical composition of the periodontal ligament is consistent with the production of an eruptive force by 'vascular' means (criterion 4 above), analysis of the periodontal ligament proteoglycans at different stages of tooth development has shown that a proteoglycan, with possibly significant osmotic influences on the tissue, increases in quantity during the active phase of eruption (see Fig. 12.26).

Quantitative electron microscopy of the periodontal vasculature (criterion 5 above) has shown that, for both the degree of vasculature and the numbers of fenestrations on the capillaries, marked changes occur with different phases of eruption. For the non-continuously-growing molar of the rodent, the number of fenestrations is three times greater during eruption than after eruption. In addition, for the continuously growing incisor of the rodent, the fenestrations are relatively low in number near the alveolar crest (approximately $1 \times 10^6/mm^3$ of tissue) but are higher near the root base of the erupting tooth (approximately $4 \times 10^6/mm^3$), perhaps providing evidence for differential vascular activity along the periodontal ligament. Thus, while no single piece of evidence briefly reported here for a role in eruption of the vascular elements of the periodontal ligament is incontrovertible, the sum of the evidence does suggest that it could provide one factor in the multifactorial mechanism of eruption.

Some observations have been made on the rate of eruption of human teeth. Initially, there is a period of slow eruption when the crown is carried towards the oral mucosa. For permanent teeth, this period may take 2–4 years. A tooth erupts most rapidly as it enters the oral cavity, at which time the length of its root is about two-thirds complete. Eruption then slows as the tooth approaches the occlusal plane. Once the tooth has emerged into the oral cavity it may take 1–2 years to reach the occlusal plane. The emergence of the crown is partly due to axial movement of the tooth (active eruption) and partly due to retraction of the adjacent soft tissues (passive eruption). The maximum eruption rate occurs at the time of crown emergence (see page 358).

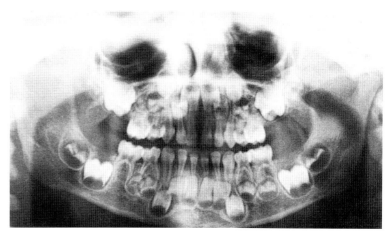

**Fig. 26.16** Dental age 4 years – orthopantomogram.

## DEVELOPMENT OF THE DENTITION AND OCCLUSION

Because no individuals are exactly alike, the times for tooth development shown in Table 26.1 are approximate. Variations of 6 months either way are not unusual, but the tendency is for teeth to erupt late rather than early. By and large, the development of the permanent dentition is more advanced in girls; there does not appear to be any sex difference in the development of the deciduous dentition. Ethnic differences also appear to exist.

As the sequence of development and eruption of teeth is under genetic control, and since chronological age is an unreliable guide to the progress of development of an individual child, dental age is a useful index of maturity, especially when used in conjunction with skeletal age. Dental age may be estimated clinically by a visual assessment of the stage of eruption of the dentition or, more satisfactorily, by a radiographic assessment of both the stages of development of the crowns and roots and the stages of eruption.

Orthopantomograms of the dentition at various ages are illustrated in Figures 26.16–26.22. Examples of jaws dissected to reveal the state of

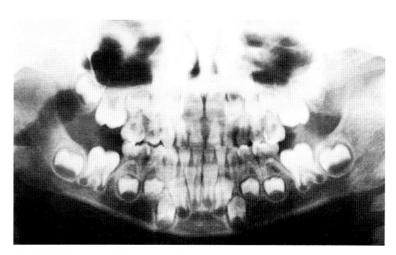

**Fig. 26.17** Dental age 5½ years – orthopantomogram.

**Table 26.1** *Chronology of tooth development and the order of eruption*

| Chronology of the deciduous dentition | | | | | Chronology of the permanent dentition | | | | |
|---|---|---|---|---|---|---|---|---|---|
| Tooth | First evidence of calcification (months in utero) | Crown completed (months) | Eruption (months) | Root completed (years) | Tooth | First evidence of calcification | Crown completed (years) | Eruption (years) | Root completed (years) |
| **Maxillary** | | | | | **Maxillary** | | | | |
| A | 3–4 | 4 | 7 | 1½–2 | 1 | 3–4 months | 4–5 | 7–8 | 10 |
| B | 4½ | 5 | 8 | 1½–2 | 2 | 10–12 months | 4–5 | 8–9 | 11 |
| C | 5 | 9 | 16–20 | 2½–3 | 3 | 4–5 months | 6–7 | 11–12 | 13–15 |
| D | 5 | 6 | 12–16 | 2–2½ | 4 | 1½–1¾ years | 5–6 | 10–11 | 12–13 |
| E | 6–7 | 10–12 | 21–30 | 3 | 5 | 2–2½ years | 6–7 | 10–12 | 12–14 |
| | | | | | 6 | Birth | 2½–3 | 6–7 | 9–10 |
| | | | | | 7 | 2½–3 years | 7–8 | 12–13 | 14–16 |
| | | | | | 8 | 7–9 years | 12–16 | 17–21 | 18–25 |
| **Mandibular** | | | | | **Mandibular** | | | | |
| A | 4½ | 4 | 6½ | 1½–2 | 1 | 3–4 months | 4–5 | 6–7 | 9 |
| B | 4½ | 4 | 7 | 1½–2 | 2 | 3–4 months | 4–5 | 7–8 | 10 |
| C | 5 | 9 | 16–20 | 2½–3 | 3 | 4–5 months | 6–7 | 9–10 | 12–14 |
| D | 5 | 6 | 12–16 | 2–2½ | 4 | 1¾–2 years | 5–6 | 10–12 | 12–13 |
| E | 6 | 10–12 | 21–30 | 3 | 5 | 1¼–2½ years | 6–7 | 11–12 | 13–14 |
| | | | | | 6 | Birth | 2½–3 | 6–7 | 9–10 |
| | | | | | 7 | 2½–3 years | 7–8 | 12–13 | 14–15 |
| | | | | | 8 | 8–10 years | 12–16 | 17–21 | 18–25 |

Unless otherwise indicated all dates are postpartum. The teeth are identified according to the Palmer-Zsigmondy system

All dates are postpartum. Teeth are identified according to the Palmer-Zsigmondy system

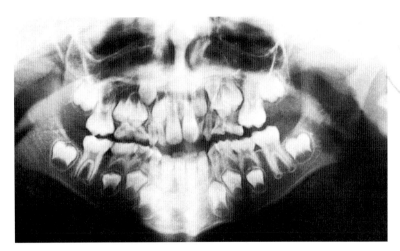

**Fig. 26.18** Dental age 7 years – orthopantomogram.

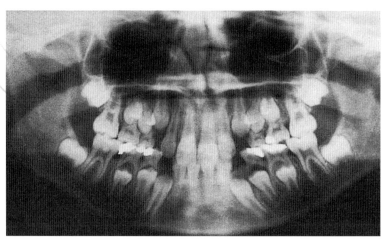

**Fig. 26.19** Dental age 9 years – orthopantomogram.

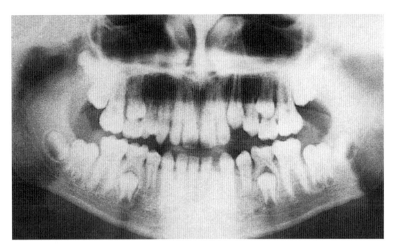

**Fig. 26.20** Dental age 11 years – orthopantomogram.

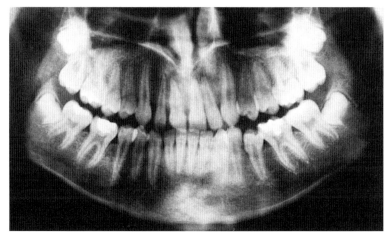

**Fig. 26.21** Dental age 14 years – orthopantomogram.

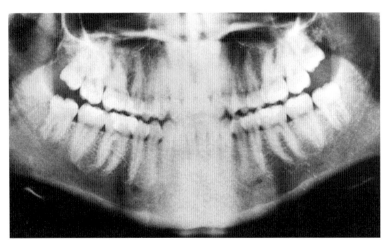

**Fig. 26.22** Dental age 19 years – orthopantomogram.

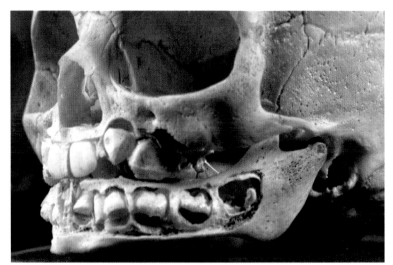

**Fig. 26.23** Dissected skull showing state of development of the teeth at 4 months. Teeth erupted – none; teeth unerupted – maxilla ABCDE6; mandible ABCDE6.

development of the teeth are illustrated in Figures 26.23–26.29. A longitudinal series of models taken from the same patient show the developing dentitions from birth to 22 years of age (Figs 26.30–26.42).

At birth, the oral mucosa over the developing alveoli is greatly thickened to form the maxillary and mandibular gum pads. They show a series of elevations, each of which corresponds to an underlying deciduous tooth. The elevations associated with the second deciduous molars do not, however, become prominent until the age of about 6 months (Fig. 26.43). The maxillary and mandibular gum pads rarely come into occlusion, the space left between them being increased in the anterior region and being occupied by the tongue. The maxillary gum pad overlaps the mandibular gum pad both buccally and labially, the overjet usually being considerable.

This reflects the small mandible. With normal growth, the anteroposterior position of the mandible will move forwards (and downwards) to match that of the maxilla during the mid-teenage years. Beneath the gum pads, there is generally considerable crowding of the developing teeth, especially the incisors. During the first year of life, however, the gum pads grow rapidly, especially in lateral directions, thus providing space for the developing teeth.

The maxillary and mandibular alveolar processes are not well developed at birth. Occasionally, a 'natal tooth' is present. This tooth is usually a supernumerary tooth (see page 311), formed by an aberration in the

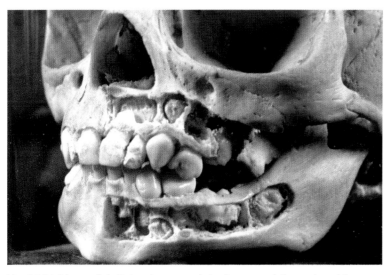

**Fig. 26.24** Dissected skull showing state of development of the teeth at 18 months. Teeth erupted – maxilla ABCD, mandible ABCD; teeth unerupted – maxilla 123E6, mandible 123E6.

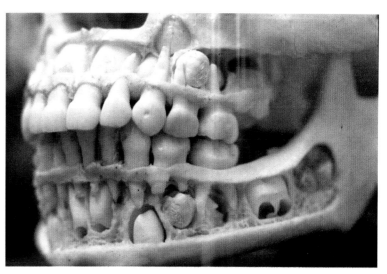

**Fig. 26.25** Dissected skull showing state of development of the teeth at 4 years. Teeth erupted – maxilla ABCDE, mandible ABCDE; teeth unerupted – maxilla 1234567, mandible 1234567.

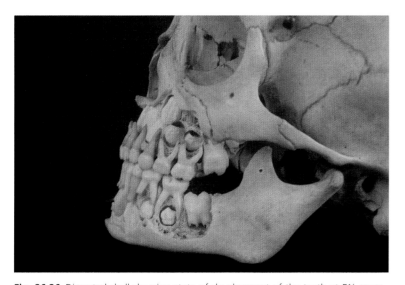

**Fig. 26.26** Dissected skull showing state of development of the teeth at 5½ years. Teeth erupted – maxilla ABCDE, mandible ABCDE; teeth unerupted – maxilla 1234567, mandible 123456(7). Courtesy of the Royal College of Surgeons of England.

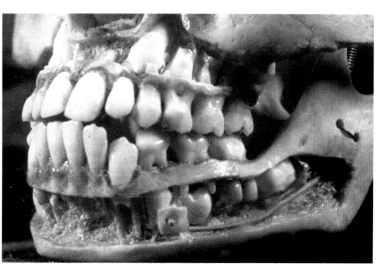

**Fig. 26.27** Dissected skull showing state of development of the teeth at 9 years. Teeth erupted – maxilla 12CDE6, mandible 123DE6; teeth unerupted – maxilla 3457, mandible 4567.

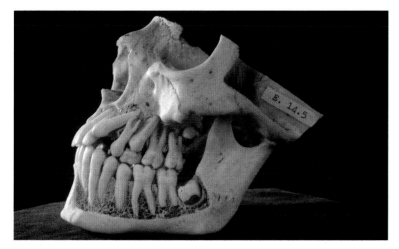

**Fig. 26.28** Dissected skull showing state of development of the teeth at 11 years. Teeth erupted – maxilla 1234E67, mandible 1234567; teeth unerupted – maxilla 58, mandible 8. Courtesy of the Royal College of Surgeons of England.

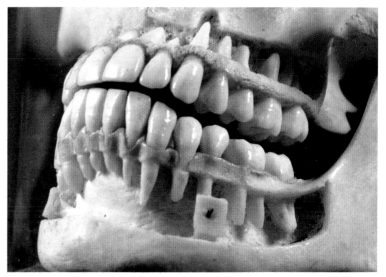

**Fig. 26.29** Dissected skull showing state of development of the teeth at 15 years. Note that the permanent third molars are not present in this skull. Teeth erupted – maxilla 1234567, mandible 1234567.

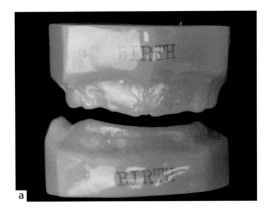

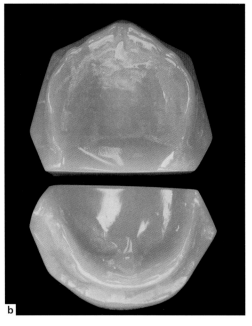

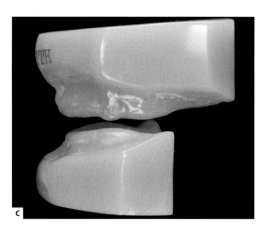

**Fig. 26.30** Models of dentition at birth.

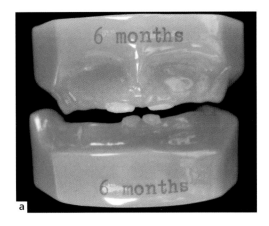

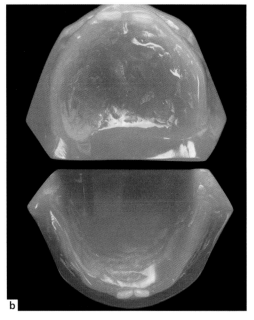

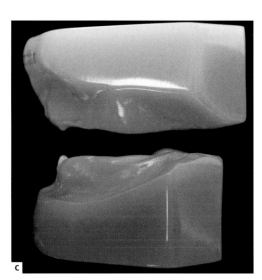

**Fig. 26.31** Models of dentition at 6 months.

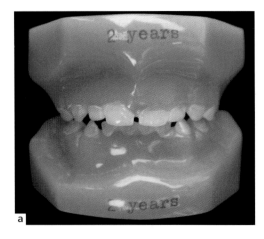

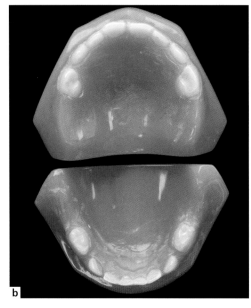

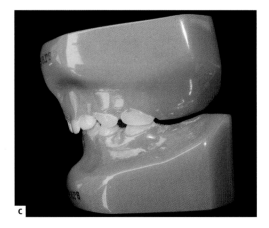

**Fig. 26.32** Models of dentition at 2 years.

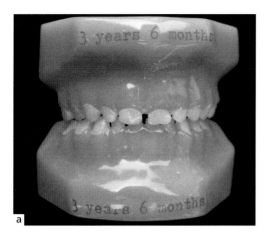
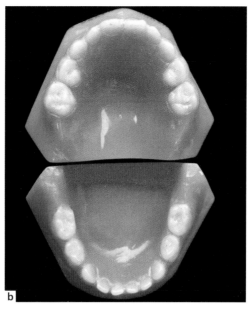
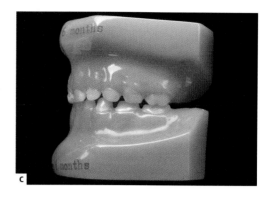

**Fig. 26.33** Models of dentition at 3 years 6 months.

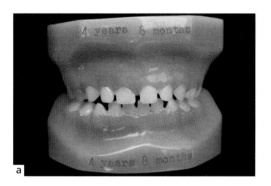
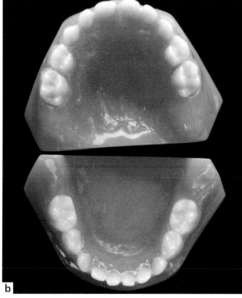
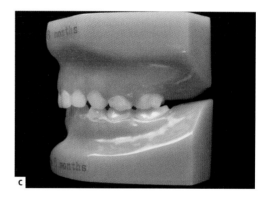

**Fig. 26.34** Models of dentition at 4 years 8 months.

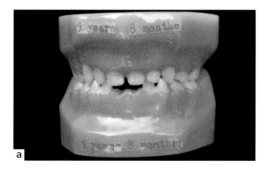
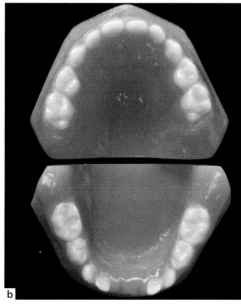
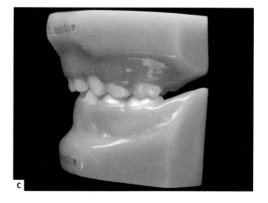

**Fig. 26.35** Models of dentition at 5 years 8 months.

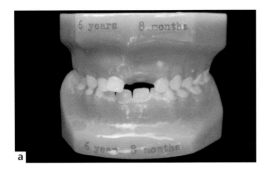

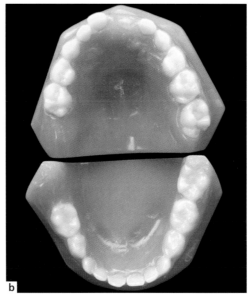

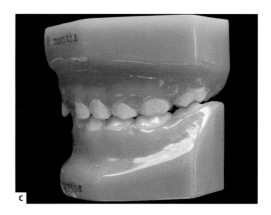

**Fig. 26.36** Models of dentition at 6 years 8 months.

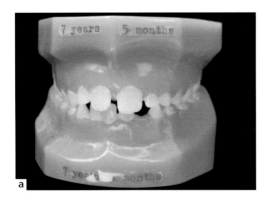

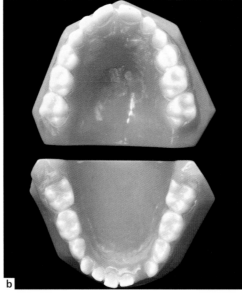

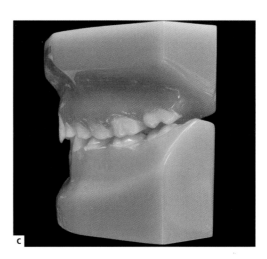

**Fig. 26.37** Models of dentition at 7 years 5 months.

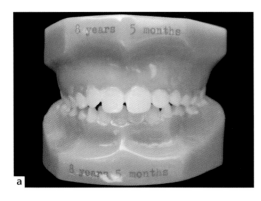

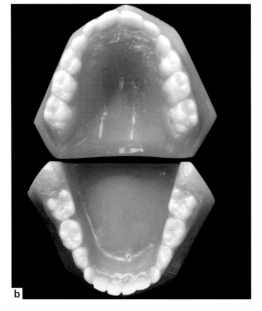

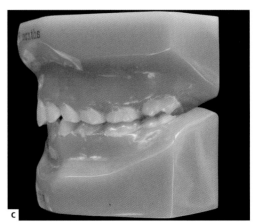

**Fig. 26.38** Models of dentition at 8 years 5 months.

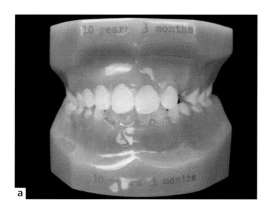
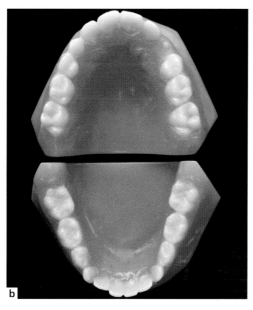
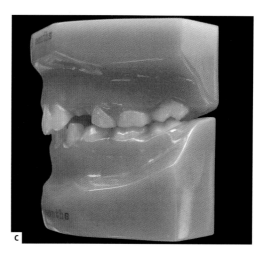

**Fig. 26.39** Models of dentition at 10 years 3 months.

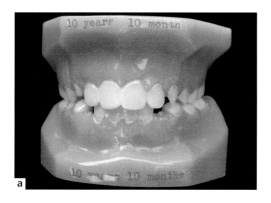
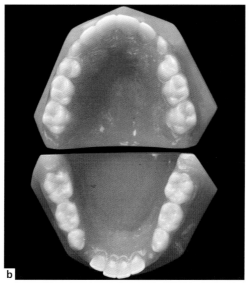
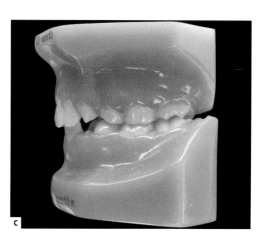

**Fig. 26.40** Models of dentition at 10 years 10 months.

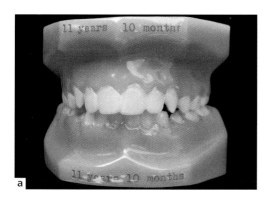
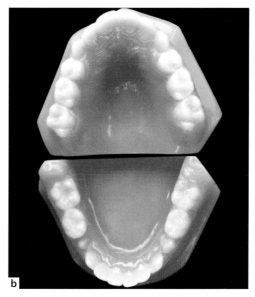
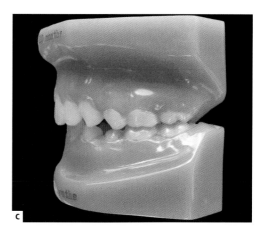

**Fig. 26.41** Models of dentition at 11 years 10 months.

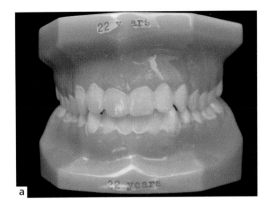

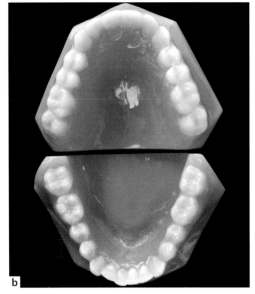

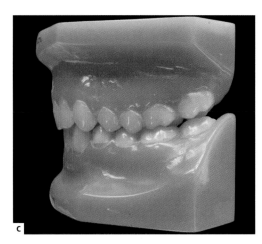

**Fig. 26.42** Models of dentition at 22 years.

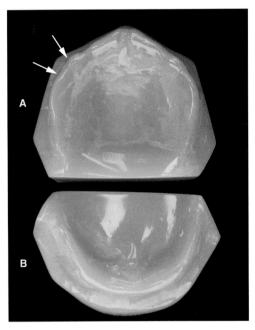

**Fig. 26.43** Dentition at birth, showing gum pads with swellings (arrows) beneath which deciduous teeth are developing. A = maxilla; B = mandible.

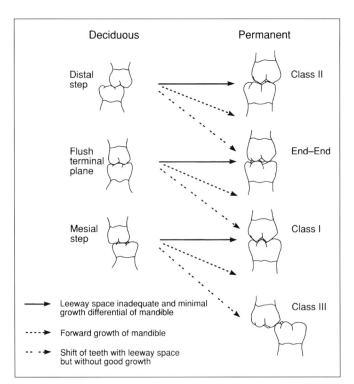

**Fig. 26.44** Occlusal relationships of the deciduous and permanent molars. Modified from Moyers RE 1988 *Handbook of orthodontics*. Year Book Medical Publishers, Chicago.

development of the dental lamina, but occasionally it is merely a very early, but otherwise normal, deciduous first incisor (see Fig. 26.48).

The deciduous teeth start to erupt at the age of 6 months and the deciduous dentition is complete by the age of 3 years. At this time, the occlusion of the deciduous dentition differs from that of the permanent dentition in the following respects (Fig. 26.33c):

- The incisors are more vertically positioned within the alveolus and are often spaced.
- The overbite is usually greater.
- There may be significant spacings distal to the mandibular canines and mesial to the maxillary canines (the anthropoid or primitive spaces).
- Although the anteroposterior relationships of the deciduous arches have not been adequately assessed, it appears that the distal edges of the maxillary and mandibular deciduous molars are flush and the mesiobuccal cusps of the maxillary first and second deciduous molars occlude in the buccal grooves of the mandibular first and second deciduous molars respectively.

Several changes occur in the deciduous occlusion before the appearance of the permanent teeth. These result from changes in the dental bases. As the dental arches become wider and longer, so the deciduous teeth become more spaced. Since there is a greater forward growth of the mandible than the maxilla, the lower arch moves forwards relative to the upper, so that an edge-to-edge incisor relationship is obtained. As a further consequence, the distal surfaces of the deciduous second molars may now show a slight mesial step from maxilla to mandible, the mesiobuccal cusp of the maxillary second deciduous molar lying distal to the buccal groove of the mandibular second deciduous molar. As the deciduous teeth approach the end of their functional life, they may show signs of considerable wear (the enamel of deciduous teeth being less mineralized and thinner than the enamel of permanent teeth – see page 14).

The occlusal relationships of the deciduous and permanent molars are shown in Figure 26.44. The flush terminal plane relationship is the usual relationship in the deciduous dentition. When the first permanent molars

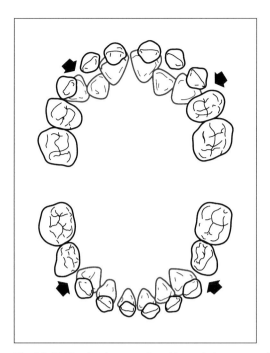

**Fig. 26.45** The developmental positions of the crowns of the permanent teeth (red) relative to the functional positions of the crowns of the deciduous teeth (black). Arrows point to the 'primate' spaces.

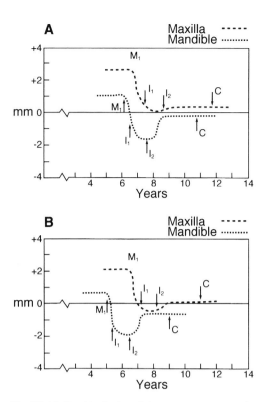

**Fig. 26.46** Graphic display of the average amount of space available within the dental arches for boys (A) and for girls (B). The arrows indicate the timing of eruption of the first molars (M1), first and second incisors (I1 and I2) and canines (C). Modified after Dr C.F.A. Moorrees and J.M. Chadha and *Angle Orthodontics*.

start to erupt, at about the age of 6 years, their relationship is determined by that of the primary molars. The molar relationship tends to shift at the time the second deciduous molars are shed and the adolescent growth spurt occurs. As shown in Figure 26.44, the change in molar relationship depends upon whether there is leeway space for tooth movement and upon mandibular growth.

After the age of 6 years, the dentition is said to be mixed, comprising both deciduous and permanent teeth. The first molars are the first permanent teeth to erupt. Initially, they have a cusp-to-cusp relationship (the flush terminal plane; Fig. 26.44), which is governed by the position of the deciduous second molars. The first molars take up their normal adult relationship once the deciduous second molars are shed. The permanent incisors erupt between the ages of 6 and 9 years. Since the permanent incisors are much larger than their deciduous predecessors, they are accommodated into the dental arches not just by utilization of the space left by the deciduous predecessors, but also by lateral growth of the alveolar arches and the greater proclination of the permanent incisors. In their developmental positions, the lateral incisors are overlapped by the first incisors, being positioned more palatally. As a rule, space is made for the second incisors as the first incisors erupt. However, should there be insufficient growth of the alveolus, the second incisors may continue to lie in their developmental, palatal positions (Fig. 26.45). Frequently, when the permanent incisors erupt, they fan out (incline distally) so that there may be a significant space or diastema between the first incisors. This appearance has been termed the 'ugly duckling' stage and is said to result from pressure on the roots of the permanent incisors from the developing permanent canines. The diastema usually closes following eruption of the permanent canines. The canines and premolars, which usually erupt between the ages of 9 and 12 years, are readily accommodated into the dental arches because the combined mesiodistal diameters of the deciduous canines and molars are generally greater than those of their permanent successors. Any leeway space that remains is usually taken up by forward movement of the first permanent molars. By the age of 12 years, all the deciduous teeth have been shed, to be replaced by permanent teeth, and henceforth the occlusion appears similar to that in the adult (see pages 36–38). Space is provided for the permanent molar teeth by continued growth and remodelling of the mandible and maxilla.

In Figure 26.45 note the lingual positioning of the permanent teeth (particularly for the maxillary lateral incisors). Spaces between the deciduous canines and the first molars for the mandible, and between the deciduous lateral incisors and canines for the maxillae, may be seen and are termed 'primate spaces', so named because they are most marked in the dentitions of primates. The primate spaces are usually seen from the time the teeth erupt. Developmental spaces between the incisors are often present at eruption but become larger as the child grows and the alveolar processes expand. Generalized spacing of the primary teeth is a requirement for proper alignment of the permanent incisors.

A graphic display of the average amount of space available within the dental arches is shown in Figure 26.46. Note that, for both sexes, the amount of space for the mandibular incisors is negative for about 2 years after their eruption. Thus, a small degree of crowding in the mandibular arch at this time is not unusual. The teeth erupt slightly earlier in girls than boys. In an individual, any discrepancy in eruption time greater than 6 months for a matching contralateral tooth should be investigated.

Although there is a tendency for the mandible to grow slightly further forward than the maxilla after the age of 12 years, usually there is no appreciable occlusal change. During the later stages of facial growth, there may be an accompanying uprighting of the incisors, with the result that they become more crowded. It has been suggested that mesial drift may take up any remaining space in the arches or even be responsible for some late crowding.

Once a tooth reaches its functional position, it is believed to occupy a position of equilibrium between the soft tissues of the cheeks and lips externally and the tongue internally (see Fig. 2.84).

## MESIAL DRIFT

The interproximal contact points of newly erupted and relatively unworn teeth cover only a small area. While attrition removes hard tissues at the

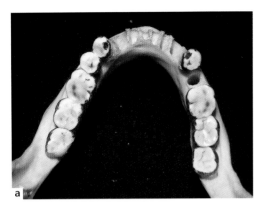

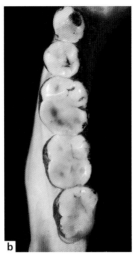

**Fig. 26.47** (a) Occlusal view of mandible with teeth showing evidence of considerable attrition. Because of mesial drift, the cheek teeth have maintained contact and the interproximal contact points are broad. (b) Higher-power view of cheek teeth with interproximal attrition and broad contact points as a result of mesial drift.

occlusal surfaces, it is also accompanied by wear of the interproximal surfaces of teeth. Even though this is accompanied by a reduction in the mesiodistal (anteroposterior) dimensions of the cheek teeth, the teeth maintain contact with each other because of a forward movement of the teeth known as mesial drift. This will result in the contact points meeting over a larger area (Fig. 26.47). It has been reported that, where the food is abrasive and there is considerable masticatory activity, the first permanent molar drifts approximately 4 mm in a mesial direction between the ages of 6 and 18 years. The mesial drift that occurs in these situations helps provide space for erupting mandibular third molars. The absence of an abrasive diet and the accompanying reduction in mesial drift associated with soft diets may account for the high occurrence of impacted mandibular third molars in some modern populations.

Four hypotheses have been postulated to account for mesial drift:

1. The mesial inclination of teeth produces a resultant force during biting that favours mesial drift.
2. The actions of certain jaw muscles, particularly the buccinator, 'propel' the teeth forwards.
3. Bone deposited preferentially on the distal surface of the sockets pushes the teeth mesially.
4. Contraction of the gingival connective tissues (especially the transseptal collagen fibres in the gingiva – see page 242) brings about mesial drift.

Concerning hypothesis 1, a detailed analysis of mesial drift would not indicate a direct relationship with the angulation of the teeth. Evidence against hypothesis 2 is the observation that mesial drift still occurs even when teeth are protected by an overlay that would prevent muscle contact. Bone activity is observed during mesial drift (hypothesis 3), but it is not possible to separate cause and effect. Although there is some evidence that damage to the gingiva retards mesial drift, there is little evidence that connective tissues contract in vivo. As with tooth eruption, the evidence might indicate that the mechanisms of mesial drift are multifactorial and involve the periodontal tissues.

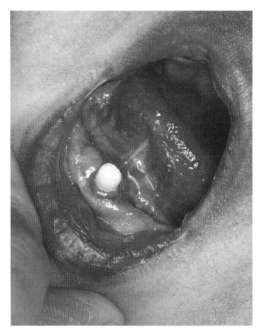

**Fig. 26.48** Mandibular left deciduous incisor erupted at birth, representing a natal tooth.

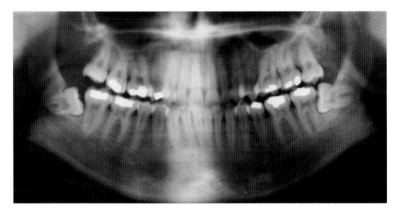

**Fig. 26.49** Orthopantomogram showing impacted mandibular third permanent molars.

## CLINICAL CONSIDERATIONS

One or more teeth may be present at birth and are referred to as natal teeth. They are common in the mandibular incisor region (Fig. 26.48). If they appear during the first month of birth they are called neonatal teeth. Natal teeth may be found in the anterior region of the maxilla in association with cleft lip/palate. They have only a small amount of root formed and are mobile. For this reason (together with difficulty associated with breast

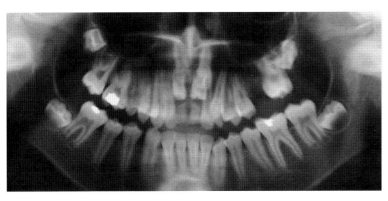

**Fig. 26.50** Orthopantomogram of a 14-year-old patient with two supernumerary teeth (small arrows) preventing the eruption of the two maxillary first permanent incisors (large arrows). Note the associated retention of the two maxillary first deciduous incisors.

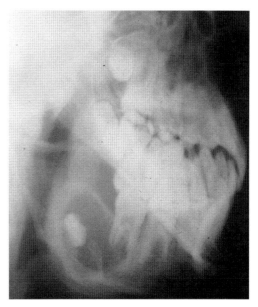

**Fig. 26.51** Lateral radiograph showing an unerupted mandibular third molar (arrow) surrounded by radiolucent dentigerous cyst. Courtesy of Professor J.D. Langdon.

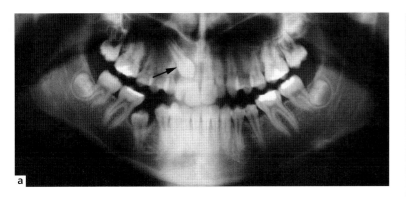

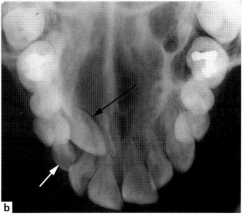

**Fig. 26.52** (a) Orthopantomogram of a 15-year-old patient with an unerupted maxillary permanent canine (arrow), above which is a retained deciduous maxillary canine. (b) Maxillary occlusal radiograph showing the unerupted maxillary permanent canine (large arrow) and the retained maxillary deciduous canine (small arrow).

feeding), they are often extracted. Permanent teeth may erupt early when their deciduous predecessors have been extracted prematurely because of dental caries. Early eruption of the whole dentition may be associated with a general hormonal disturbance such as hyperpituitarism or hyperthyroidism.

The most common eruptive disorders are delayed eruption (or non-eruption) of one (or more) permanent anterior maxillary teeth or the mandibular third molar(s). In the case of mandibular third molars, the reason is lack of space so that the tooth is impacted against the second permanent molar immediately in front (Fig. 26.49). If the crown of the impacted third molar is partially erupted, food debris may accumulate in the stagnation area between the overlying gum flap and the crown and may lead to an inflammatory reaction in the gingiva (pericoronitis). This may eventually spread to involve surrounding tissue spaces (see pages 76–80). If the tooth is malaligned, it may remain unerupted. Delayed eruption of maxillary permanent first incisors is most commonly due to obstruction by a supernumerary tooth (Fig. 26.50) or an odontome (see Fig. 21.42). Removal of the obstruction will allow for eruption with or without the aid of orthodontic appliances. In some cases, no obstruction is present and the occlusal margins of the anterior teeth can be seen just beneath the oral mucosa and yet the teeth refuse to erupt. In such cases, surgical exposure will usually be sufficient to allow eruption. Delayed eruption may also be

associated with teeth where the enamel organ has undergone a cystic change to form a dentigerous (eruption) cyst above its tooth, hence preventing its eruption (Fig. 26.51).

Because of its high developmental position within the maxilla, its malalignment and the presence of crowding within the dental arch, the maxillary permanent canine may be prevented from erupting into the dental arch and this is reflected in the retention of its deciduous predecessor (Fig. 26.52). Assuming such impacted teeth are favourably positioned, they may be drawn into the dental arch by suitably designed orthodontic appliances.

If the periodontal ligament is damaged, the root of a tooth may become fixed (ankylosed) to the adjacent alveolar bone. The deciduous tooth is then unable to move. Its position within the jaw remains constant so that, as height of the alveolar bone increases, the tooth appears to sink gradually below the level of the adjacent teeth. Such ankylosed teeth are referred to as 'submerged' teeth (Figs 26.53, 26.54). The submergence may continue to such an extent that the teeth become completely buried within bone. The cause of this condition is not always apparent, although there may be an association with trauma/inflammation. It may also affect permanent molars.

There are many human syndromic conditions that can disrupt eruption and these are shown in Table 26.2. Approximately 50% of these conditions

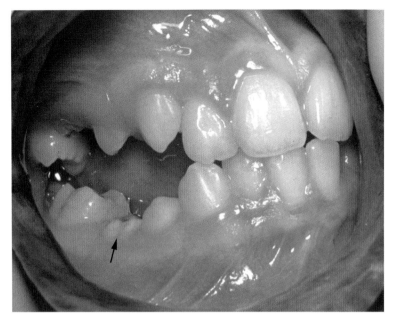

**Fig. 26.53** Patient with a submerging mandibular right deciduous second molar (arrow). Courtesy of Dr P. Smith.

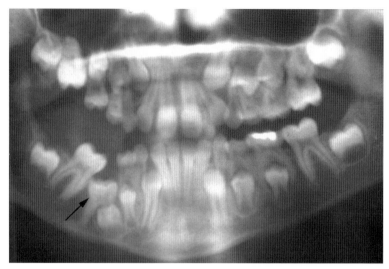

**Fig. 26.54** Orthopantomogram of patient with a submerging mandibular second deciduous molar (arrow) that will prevent the eruption of the second premolar beneath it. Courtesy of Dr P. Smith.

can now be attributed to a genetic defect. Note that 'primary failure of eruption' affects mainly permanent posterior teeth and refers to a localized failure with no other systemic involvement. It has been suggested that this condition is a defect of the eruption mechanism itself. However, the precise cause of the lack of eruption is presently unknown. As an example of a syndromic condition, Figure 26.55 represents an orthopantomogram of a patient with cleidocranial dysplasia (dysostosis). This syndrome is caused by a mutation in the *Cbfa1* gene (see page 212). The majority of teeth are unerupted and a number of supernumerary teeth may be encountered.

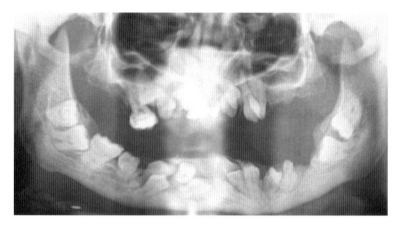

**Fig. 26.55** Orthopantomogram of patient with cleidocranial dysplasia (dysostosis). The majority of teeth are unerupted and may include supernumerary teeth.

**Table 26.2** *Genetic disorders of eruption*

| Syndrome/condition | Eruption phenotype | Genetic defect | Mode of inheritance |
|---|---|---|---|
| Cleidocranial dysplasia | Delayed eruption | Six different types of mutation in *PEBP2αA/CBFA1* | Autosomal-dominant |
| Osteopetrosis | Failure of eruption | *TRAF6* | Autosomal-recessive and -dominant forms |
| GAPO syndrome | Failure of eruption | Unknown | Autosomal-recessive |
| Osteopathia striata with cranial sclerosis | Failure of eruption in some cases | Unknown | Autosomal-dominant |
| Osteoglophonic dysplasia | Failure of eruption of 2° teeth | Unknown | Autosomal-dominant |
| Singleton–Merten syndrome | Dysplastic development with delayed eruption of 2° teeth | Unknown | Possibly autosomal-dominant |
| Aarskog's syndrome | Delayed eruption | *FGDY1* codes for Rho/Rac guanine nuclear exchange factor (involved with growth regulation) | X-linked recessive |
| Acrodysostosis | Delayed tooth eruption (23% of cases) | Unknown | Autosomal-dominant |
| Albright's hereditary osteodystrophy | Delayed eruption | Variety of mutations in *GNAS1* (G, protein) | Autosomal-dominant |
| Apert's syndrome | Delayed and ectopic eruption | Mutations in *FGFR2* gene | Autosomal-dominant |
| Chondroectodermal dysplasia (Ellis–van Creveld syndrome) | Delayed eruption, partial anodontia | Several mutations in the *EVC* gene | Autosomal-recessive |
| Cockayne's syndrome | Delayed eruption | *CSB* (*ERCC6*) gene (helicase) | Autosomal-recessive |
| De Lange's syndrome | Delayed eruption | Unknown (*SHOT* is candidate gene) | Possibly autosomal-dominant |
| Dubowitz's syndrome | Delayed eruption and hypodontia | Unknown | Possibly autosomal-recessive |
| Frontometaphyseal dysplasia (Gorlin–Cohen syndrome) | Delayed eruption and retained deciduous teeth | Unknown | Autosomal-dominant or X-linked recessive (debated) |
| Goltz's syndrome (focal dermal hypoplasia) | Delayed eruption and hypodontia with hypoplastic teeth | Unknown | X-linked dominant with lethality in hemizygous males |
| Hunter's syndrome | Delayed eruption | Variety of mutations in *IDS* (iduronate-2 sulphatase) gene | X-linked |
| Incontinentia pigmenti | Delayed eruption, hypodontia in 80% | Mapped to Xp11.2, rarely *IKK* gene | X-linked dominant, lethality in males |
| Killian's/Teschler–Nicola syndrome | Delayed eruption | Mosaic tetrasomy 12p in skin fibroblasts | Chromosomal aberration |
| Levy–Hollister syndrome | Delayed eruption of 1° teeth | Unknown | Autosomal-dominant |
| Maroteaux–Lamy mucopolysaccharidosis syndrome | Delayed eruption with small teeth | Variety of mutations in aryl sulphatase B (*ASB*) gene | Autosomal-recessive |
| Osteogenesis imperfecta syndrome type I | Delayed eruption, dysplastic teeth | *COL1A1* and *COL1A2* | Autosomal-dominant variable expressivity |
| Progeria syndrome (Hutchinson–Gilford syndrome) | Delayed eruption of 1° and 2° teeth and hypodontia of 2° teeth | DNA helicase, telomerase | Autosomal-recessive |
| Pyknodysostosis | Delayed eruption and occasional anodontia | Cathepsin K gene | Autosomal-recessive |
| Primary failure of eruption | Failure of 2° teeth to erupt partially or completely | Unknown | Unknown |

From Wise GE, Frazier-Bowers S, D'Souza RN 2002 Cellular, molecular, and genetic determinants of tooth eruption. *Critical Reviews in Oral Biology and Medicine* 13: 323–334.

# 27 Ageing and archaeological and dental anthropological applications of tooth structure

Ageing is a natural stage in the human life cycle and is a term usually applied to describe those who are 65 years and over. It involves a progressive decline in the ability to respond effectively to 'the stresses of a dynamic environment'. This leads to reduced function and increased vulnerability to pathological processes. Although it can be difficult to distinguish between normal ageing and superimposed disease, there are reliable and identifiable features of the ageing dentition which are not pathologies.

An understanding of the ageing of the human dentition is important as there will be in excess of 2 million people aged over 80 years by 2025 in the UK. In the USA, the corresponding figure is nearly 8 million. This has arisen because the average life expectancy has increased markedly in recent times. For example, in the UK at the beginning of the 20th century, the average life expectancy was approximately 50 years whereas today it is about 75 years. Elderly people will therefore form a significant proportion of persons seeking dental treatment. While the oral changes associated with ageing are not life-threatening, they can contribute to a diminishing quality of life. In evolutionary terms, it might be argued that the human permanent dentition was never expected to last beyond 40 years. However, given advances in dentistry, more and more people are able to maintain a reasonably healthy dentition throughout their lives.

There have been many theories of ageing. Much may come to be explained on a genetic basis (e.g. an association with telomeres of the chromosomes). Functional genomic technologies using microarrays are being employed to look at the expression and suppression of many genes involved in ageing. Indeed, about 20% of the human genome changes with an inadequate diet, although the reasons for this are unclear. This suggests that changes in the diets of elderly people, whether due to changes in eating habits, metabolic requirements or even a poorly functioning dentition, might accelerate the ageing process. The prospect of using stem-cell technology to routinely repair worn out and aged tissues is in the offing, assuming of course that ethical and societal objections are overcome.

Two of the most common age changes relate to changes in the characteristics of collagen and the loss of calcium in the skeleton. Consequently, one might expect that the teeth would also be adversely affected by such changes. However, enamel and dentine do not turnover or remodel and there is no loss of calcium from the dental tissues.

Although descriptions of the age changes in individual tissues have already been given, it is worthwhile bringing them together to highlight this important topic. Treatment protocols and procedures have to be adjusted when dealing with aged tissue in aged patients. Furthermore, as teeth and bones are the least destructible of human tissues, study of their remains has obvious forensic implications. Forensic odontology is a well-recognized, and important, speciality. The ability to date and age teeth and bones in their archaeological context has important scientific implications. Some of the basic principles of this topic will also be introduced.

## AGE CHANGES IN ENAMEL

One of the unique properties of enamel is that, after the tooth has erupted, it has no further contact with cells capable of repairing or remodelling it. It does, however, undergo changes immediately after eruption as the surface enamel comes into equilibrium with its environment. Both mineral and organic material may be adsorbed into the surface enamel. This results in the 'filling in' of prism boundaries such that the prismatic pattern is obscured. These are not age changes but related to initial appearance of the crown in the mouth. Further exchanges occur with age that will largely be determined by the properties of the biofilm (plaque) that develops on the surface, in particular from the bacteria that inhabit it. Pigmented or stained organic material comes to be included in the surface enamel. These and other factors, such as the progressive thickening of the underlying dentine, reduce translucency and contribute to the darkening of teeth with age. This can be reversed, temporarily and to a limited extent, by the use of bleaches that oxidize the organic material. The exchange of ions between the saliva and enamel continues throughout life, depending on the composition (especially the pH of the saliva) and the activities of the plaque microorganisms. In general, surface enamel that is not affected by caries will become slightly more mineralized. Some ions will be exchanged, most significantly fluoride (from the saliva). This may explain, at least in part, why enamel in older individuals has a reduced vulnerability to caries. The artificial presence of fluoride ions in saliva, whether from diet or toothpaste, will increase this affect. This movement of mineral elements into the enamel is applied in the remineralization of early enamel lesions. One other clinical consideration with surface enamel is whether its adhesion to restorative materials changes over time. From the data currently available, the bonding of adhesive materials to enamel does not appear to change with age.

In health, the deeper portion of enamel is well protected from environmental changes. It has been shown that some materials can pass through the dentine and into the innermost layer of enamel. This has been shown in animal studies using blood-borne dyes, but its biological significance is unknown. The extent of this penetration is reduced with age, but this is more likely to be due to changes in the thickness and composition of dentine than to changes in the enamel.

The thickness of enamel is reduced over time by both occlusal and interproximal attrition, although this is will vary with both diet and occlusion. Loss of enamel by abrasion and erosion will also increase with age. Toothbrush abrasion will lead to the loss of surface enamel. Thus, perikymata will disappear, although some may be retained in protected areas, such as interproximally.

## AGE CHANGES IN DENTINE

Unlike enamel, dentine is a living tissue and has a layer of cells on its inner surface that continues to be active throughout life. Two major changes in dentine are closely related to age. One is the formation of secondary dentine, which is tubular and whose tubules are continuous with those of the primary dentine. The demarcation of secondary from primary dentine is often visible as a line of Owen (see page 143), where there is a coincidence of a change in secondary curvatures. This coincides in time with the completion of root formation. Secondary dentine continues to be laid down throughout life and its thickness can be used to determine, approximately, the age of a tooth. The number of tubules in secondary dentine is reduced over time as the number of odontoblasts declines. As the surface area of the inner dentine is much less than the outer, the number of tubules per unit area is increased towards the pulp. The deposition of secondary dentine is of considerable clinical significance as it can, perhaps in concert with the formation of any tertiary dentine, reduce the size of the pulp chamber and root canals. Often the pulp chamber becomes completely occluded and the root canals reduced to a size only visible through a microscope. These changes make the endodontic treatment of older teeth a considerable challenge.

The second major change related to age is the infilling of the tubules by peritubular (more correctly termed intratubular) dentine. The difference in appearance and composition of peritubular dentine has been discussed elsewhere (see page 132). As the infilling of the tubules continues, dentine can become as translucent as glass (sclerotic or translucent dentine – see page 134). That peritubular dentine is an age change rather than a response to external irritation or injury is supported by two simple observations: 1) translucent dentine is found most abundantly in roots and 2) peritubular dentine is found in (older) unerupted teeth. The mechanism by which peritubular dentine is formed is a mystery. Whether it is the last product of a retreating odontoblast process or is produced by some form of precipitation only after the process has retracted, is unclear. The first hypothesis is supported, to some extent, by the occasional observation of odontoblast processes in tubules lined by peritubular dentine. The difficulty of preserving cellular structure in this tissue obscures a clear answer to this question. As for secondary dentine, the extent of translucent dentine is related to chronological age.

Tertiary dentine, whether reparative or regenerative, is not an age change but a response to injury.

## AGE CHANGES IN DENTAL PULP

The most obvious change in the dental pulp related to age is a progressive decrease in its size as secondary dentine is laid down. The number of odontoblasts declines in line with this by apoptosis such that, between the ages of 20 and 70 years, approximately 50% of the number of original odontoblasts are lost. The rest of the tissue undergoes a similar decline in cellularity.

As in other connective tissues, both the vascularity and the innervation of the pulp decline with age. Pulpal blood flow and the ability to respond to injury are reduced as is the apparent sensitivity of the dentine. This loss of sensitivity, however, is more likely to be due to the deposition of peritubular dentine and possibly secondary dentine than to a decline in pulpal innervation. It is often said that the pulp becomes more fibrous with age, although convincing evidence of this in healthy teeth is lacking. As the pulp is prone to artifactual changes, a number of phenomena, such as 'wheatsheafing' of the odontoblasts or 'reticulation', have been described that are not biological in origin.

Pulp stones are commonly found in the pulps of older individuals and their incidence is related to age. Their clinical significance is limited to the increase in the difficulty of endodontic procedures when pulp stones are present. Their presence is not, in itself, an indication for endodontic treatment.

## AGE CHANGES IN CEMENTUM

As cementum is deposited slowly throughout life, its thickness increases about threefold between the ages of 16 and 70, although whether this proceeds in a linear manner is not known. Cementum may be formed at the root apex in much greater amounts as a result of compensatory tooth eruption in response to attrition (wear) at the occlusal surface. Such hypercementosis (see Fig. 11.31) may cause problems during tooth extraction. Most roots of permanent teeth show small, localized areas of resorption and these are said to increase with age. The cause of this is not known but may be associated with microtrauma

Cementum is deposited rhythmically, resulting in incremental lines (of Salter; Fig. 11.13). Unlike enamel and dentine, the precise periodicity

between the incremental lines is a matter of controversy. Some studies claim that, with careful preparation of the specimen, it is possible to show that the lines represent annual increments and that teeth can be aged by counting the incremental lines within cementum. However, other studies do not support this view.

## AGE CHANGES IN THE PERIODONTAL LIGAMENT

Despite the obvious importance (both biologically and clinically) of investigating the effects of ageing on the periodontal ligament, our understanding of this subject is at present poor. There have been remarkably few studies concerned with the changing composition and functions of the periodontal ligament. Indeed, the effects of ageing upon the turnover rates of the extracellular matrix have yet to be assessed. Furthermore, most of the studies concerned with the structural aspects of the aged periodontal ligament have involved experimental animals, have been at the light microscope level and have been mainly qualitative.

Concerning cellular age changes, a decrease in cellularity has often been reported within the human periodontal ligament. In addition to a reduction in cell density, a decrease in the mitotic index has also been described and the suggestion has been made that the fibroblasts in the ageing periodontal tissues have longer 'lives' than those in younger tissues. Whether this cellular reduction affects stem cells awaits clarification. In terms of the cellular organelles, the fibroblasts of the aged periodontal ligament differ in three respects: the areas occupied by endoplasmic reticulum are significantly less; the areas occupied by intracellular collagen profiles are also less; both the numbers and sizes of intercellular contacts are significantly different (decreased numbers; increased size). Thus, the aged periodontal fibroblasts appear to have diminished protein synthesis and collagen degradative capabilities. Furthermore, the nature of cell–matrix and cell–cell interactions are markedly changed. Immunocytochemical investigation of the cytoskeletal components of periodontal ligament fibroblasts indicate that the aged cells express cytokeratin 19 in addition to vimentin (in younger tissues only vimentin is expressed). Cytokeratin 19 intermediate filaments have also been seen during the most active phase of tooth eruption. Its appearance in the aged periodontal ligament may be related to the increased rates of eruption-like movements reported for aged teeth, or it may reflect the diminished cell–matrix and cell–cell interactions deduced from quantitative electron microscopy.

It has been reported that fat cells appear within the aged human periodontal ligament. In addition, large, multinucleated fibroblastic cells have been seen in aged supracrestal periodontal connective tissues. Indeed, these cells accounted for more than 17% of the cells in this region. The multinucleated fibroblastic cells differ from osteoclasts in that they have considerable amounts of rough endoplasmic reticulum, a conspicuous Golgi complex and intracellular collagen profiles, and also possess multiple centrioles. It can be concluded, therefore, that these cells arise by cell fusion. That the cells are fibroblastic is shown by their uptake of tritiated proline and by acid phosphatase activity associated with phagolysosomes. Unlike neighbouring (mononuclear) fibroblasts, however, the cell membranes do not show the presence of alkaline phosphatase.

For the extracellular matrix of the periodontal ligament, changes due to ageing have been reported for both the collagen fibres and the ground substance. The earliest studies suggested that the amounts of soluble collagen and of 'acid mucopolysaccharides' decrease with age. From histological examination of the aged human periodontal ligament, results indicate that the main age change appears to be increased collagen fibrosis. More specifically, the principal collagen fibre bundles become thicker, the fibre groups seem to be broader and more highly organized, there are areas of hyalinization and there is a reduction in areas staining positive with Alcian blue. Furthermore, some of the fibres may become mineralized. In contrast, the number of periodontal ligament fibres is said by other researchers to decrease with age and there may be an age-dependent decrease in the rate of collagen synthesis. For the Sharpey fibre insertions, it has been found that the alveolar bone surface changes from smooth and regular with evenly distributed insertions of principal fibres in younger tissue into jagged and uneven with irregular fibre insertions in aged tissue.

An important feature of the ageing of a connective tissue relates to the changes that occur in collagen fibril diameters. For the periodontal ligament, however, there is disagreement as to the fate of the collagen fibrils with age. It has been claimed that the mean fibril diameter decreases by nearly 50% over the life span. However, several findings from quantitative electron microscopy have shown that there is little change in fibril diameters with age. Although in many connective tissues ageing effects can be attributed to alterations in elastin (rather than to the collagen), there is very little information concerning the effects of ageing on the elastic network of the periodontal ligament (including oxytalan). Furthermore, little is known about the changes that occur in the neurovascular elements of the ligament, although it has been reported that degenerative vascular changes can be discerned.

Unfortunately, there is almost no information concerning the effects of age upon the functions of the periodontal ligament. Nevertheless, it has been shown that human teeth become less mobile with age. This change might be related to increases in length of the root or to changes in the number and diameters of the principal fibres of the periodontal ligament. It has also been reported that the eruption rates (of the rat incisor) are markedly increased with age, the mechanism whereby the eruptive force is generated being a property of the periodontal ligament (see page 363).

Other studies on the effects of ageing on the periodontium have been concerned with the influence of inflammatory periodontal disease. Indeed, differentiation between age change and pathological change is imprecise and provides one of the fundamental problems in studying the pathogenesis of periodontal disease. It is well established that the prevalence of periodontitis increases with age. However, it is questionable whether periodontal changes are due to a disease process or an ageing process. Indeed, it has been found that periodontal age-related changes occur in gnotobiotic rats in the absence of inflammatory periodontal disease. In particular, gradual recession of alveolar bone occurs with increasing age. On the other hand, some clinicians are of the opinion that lack of oral hygiene is the most influential factor in periodontal destruction and that the effect of age is negligible when good oral hygiene is maintained. Nevertheless, it has been shown that many aged persons have considerable quantities of plaque yet do not develop periodontal destruction. On this basis, there is probably a multifactorial aetiology to the disease such that the influence of ageing cannot be overruled. The ageing of the periodontal ligament may have a bearing on other clinical problems. For example, orthodontic treatment is most often undertaken within the dentitions of teenagers or young adults, and it is probable that age is influential in the response of the periodontium (including alveolar bone) to orthodontic loads.

Overall, the evidence suggests that there is some degeneration of the periodontal ligament with age. However, some features (e.g. the lack of change for collagen fibril diameters) indicate that the reactions and mechanisms of this degeneration may differ markedly from other fibrous connective tissues. The relative paucity of studies on this topic is therefore to be regretted.

## AGE CHANGES IN ALVEOLAR BONE

The most clinically important age change in bones is osteoporosis, the loss of cancellous bone in the hip and vertebrae predisposing towards fracture. The lack of significant amounts of cancellous bone in the jaws has not allowed for osteoporotic changes to be established in these sites. As alveolar bone is maintained by the presence of teeth, tooth loss will be accompanied by atrophy of the associated alveolar bone.

When measurements are taken on radiographs to determine the distance from the cementum–enamel junction to the alveolar bone crest, the results indicate a loss of crestal bone with age, the general state of oral hygiene contributing only slightly to the effect.

The degree of mineralization of the mandible has been shown to be greater than that of other postcranial bones. There is also evidence of an increase in mandibular mineralization density with age. The aged mandible also exhibits highly mineralized cement lines and packets containing dead mineralized osteocytes. This increased mineralization density may account for the clinical perception that tooth extraction is more difficult in the elderly: better-mineralized bone is more resistant to bending. As no relationship could be established between the overall degree of tissue mineralization and the number, size or percentage of the tissue occupied by vascular (Haversian) canals, the possibility was raised that bone tissue at different sites may be regulated by intrinsically distinct local and systemic factors.

It is often stated that the healing rate of fractures is slower in the elderly. This could possibly be due to a reduction in the number of stem cells available in the aged population. Aspects of treatment using tissue engineering principles are discussed on pages 221, 222.

## AGE CHANGES IN ORAL MUCOSA

Overall, the detailed changes with ageing that occur within the oral cavity have not been well established and, because of regionalization, the findings for one type of oral mucosa may not necessarily be true for other regions.

With age, there is evidence of a thinning of the epithelium on the dorsal and lateral surfaces of the tongue, with less interdigitation at the epithelium–lamina propria interface. There is an increase in collagen content and a decrease in the number of taste fibres.

Although gingival recession may be associated with age, it is difficult to determine whether this is a direct effect or whether it is secondary to lack of oral hygiene or other oral features such as incorrect tooth brushing. Although little change in the epithelium of the gingiva has been reported with age, there is some evidence of an increase in collagen content in the lamina propria.

There is an increasing susceptibility to the appearance of precancerous and cancerous conditions in the oral epithelium with age. As a possible contributing factor, it has been found that there is a raised level of p53, the protein associated with DNA repair.

As saliva contributes to the health of the oral mucosa, any possible reduced flow in an ageing population, associated with the increased intake of drugs, may account for some of the age changes described in the oral mucosa.

## AGE CHANGES IN SALIVARY GLANDS

A wide range of age changes has been documented in salivary glands. These include a decrease in the amount of glandular tissue (over 50 years of age) and an increase in the amount of fibrous tissue, fat cells, inflammatory cells and oncocytes (see page 277). An increase in duct volume has also been described, although some of this increase may be due to shrinkage of acini giving the appearance of duct-like forms.

With such a significant loss of parenchyma (in both major and minor glands), it might be assumed that there would be a reduction in the amount of saliva produced in the aged population, giving rise to the clinical condition of xerostomia (dry mouth). However, in healthy, unmedicated individuals, this is not the case and this could be interpreted as the result of salivary glands being able to produce more saliva than is needed. The increase in the incidence of xerostomia in the ageing population is more likely to be a secondary effect related to the increased use of medication (many drugs depress salivary production and are anticholinergic – antidepressants, antihistamines).

## AGEING ISOLATED HUMAN TEETH

It is relatively easy to age a dentition of up to about 20 years of age. However, it is less easy on dentitions, and particularly on isolated teeth, in older specimens. Yet teeth may be the only parts of a body available for trying to identify and age specimens for forensic purposes. Thus, forensic odontology is an important speciality in forensic science. All the dental features described above that may change with age can be brought to bear in this task. Thus, one can estimate the amount of wear in enamel and dentine, one can X-ray the tooth and estimate the amount of dentine formation and the reduction in the size of the pulp cavity. If histological examination is possible, it may also be possible to estimate further features such as the amount of secondary and translucent dentine and the thickness of cementum. For each of a number of such features, one can give a score and, by deriving a total score for the tooth, look up an appropriate table and get an estimate of age. The single most reliable feature for age estimation appears to be the amount of translucent dentine in the root.

## ARCHAEOLOGICAL/DENTAL ANTHROPOLOGICAL IMPLICATIONS OF TOOTH STRUCTURE

Because of their durability, teeth and bones are usually the only remaining trace of humans and animals from the past. For this reason, much scientific study of hard tissues has been undertaken using a variety of innovative techniques to maximize what teeth can tell us about the past. Of particular interest is information concerning ageing, diet, climate and origins.

## AMINO ACID RACEMIZATION AND THE AGEING OF MINERALIZED TISSUE

Amino acids comprise the bulk of the organic matrix of bone and dentine (as collagen) and of enamel (as enamel proteins). Amino acids can exist in two different forms, a left handed form (levorotatory or L form) and a right handed form (dextrorotatory or D form). When first formed, the amino acids are invariably of the L form, but there is a slow transformation to the D form, and the changing ratio of D to L is the basis of a method for ageing archaeological and fossil material up to tens of thousands of years old. Indeed, it has also been applied on modern material to determine the age at death, although the rate of change following death is slower because of the lower temperature in the ground (compared to body temperature). This chemical method of determining age is known as amino acid racemization (AAR).

The two main amino acids used in AAR are aspartic acid and isoleucine. The L and D forms of aspartic acid (with one chiral centre in its structure) are known as enantiomers. For isoleucine, which has two chiral centres, the interconversion process is referred to as epimerization. For this analysis, the amino acids in the matrix of bone, dentine and enamel are separated and quantified by gas chromatography or high-pressure liquid chromatography.

Determining age by racemization has had somewhat limited use because of problems associated with methodology. For example, the rate of racemization depends on temperature, so that the thermal history of the sample needs to be known. In addition, the protein may be contaminated or may undergo denaturation depending on the surrounding pH. Thus, careful calibration must be undertaken using such methodology. Even within a dentition the D:L ratios may vary from tooth to tooth and from site to site in the same tooth. However, the method can be used in conjunction with other methods of estimating age, such as radiocarbon dating.

## DIET, CLIMATE AND ORIGINS

Some information concerning the diet of an animal can be obtained by studying the attrition patterns of teeth and, in the case of humans, by the presence of dental caries (indicating the consumption of a carbohydrate-rich diet). However, more detailed information relating to whether an animal has a mainly herbivorous or carnivorous diet, and even the type of the plant material eaten, can be determined from knowledge of the isotopes present in teeth and bones. An isotope is a variety of an element with a different number of neutrons. Interpretation of such data can additionally yield information about environmental factors, such as climate and place of origin. Because of the relative stability of the mineralized tissues, the information can be applied to specimens millions of years old. The most common isotopes studied are carbon, oxygen, nitrogen and strontium.

### Stable carbon isotopes

The stable isotopes of carbon are carbon-12 and carbon-13. Although present in only very small quantities in the atmosphere, they are incorporated into plants during photosynthesis. Herbivores eating such plants will incorporate the carbon isotopes in the amino acids of their structural proteins and in the carbonate present in hydroxyapatite crystals of their mineralized tissues. Thus, isotopic analysis of stable carbon isotopes in both the organic (collagen) and inorganic components (hydroxyapatite crystallites) of mineralized tissues will give a characteristic value that would indicate a chiefly plant diet. As isotope concentration is enriched by consumers as they pass between trophic levels, a carnivore feeding on herbivores will have its own distinctive isotope levels. Whereas collagen is derived only from dietary protein, the carbon present in hydroxyapatite crystals is derived from the whole diet.

In the manner of their photosynthesis, plants can be divided into two main groups. The majority of plants (95%) are known as C3 plants, as the first organic compound synthesized during photosynthesis contains three carbon atoms. C3 plants comprise trees, shrubs, flowering plants, rice, wheat, barley and potatoes and can exist in moist, colder climates. The second group constitutes C4 plants (5%), so called because the first organic compound synthesized during photosynthesis contains four carbon atoms. C4 plants are found in dry, arid regions and include maize, sugar cane and most tropical grasses. When both types of plant are available, animals may restrict themselves to C3 (browsers) or C4 (grazers) material. A key feature in the metabolism of the two groups is that they incorporate different amounts of carbon-13, C4 plants incorporating more. Isotope levels from herbivores selectively eating either C3 or C4 will differ. Intermediate levels will indicate a herbivore with a diet comprised of both types of plant. Carnivores eating the meat of land herbivores will have another distinctive isotope value. The identification of C4 plants in a diet would also indicate a dry, arid climate.

Stable carbon isotope values for marine plants differ from those of terrestrial plants. Marine herbivores will therefore have isotope levels that distinguish them from terrestrial herbivores, while carnivores feeding on the meat of marine herbivores will have isotope levels distinguishing them from land carnivores.

Analysing the ratios of carbon-12 and carbon-13 (using a mathematical formula involving a standard) in a sample of collagen from bone or dentine or from the carbonate in the mineral phase has provided much information concerning the nature of the diet of modern and archaeological/fossil material. As bone is widely used for analysis, consideration must be given to deleterious changes that occur within the tissue following burial (diagenesis) such as demineralization/remineralization. In this respect, the more stable enamel is especially useful to study, as the larger crystal size and the lack of porosity ensures it is more resistant to diagenesis.

As bone continually turns over, the isotope values may be considered as an overall representation of the last 10 years of the individual's life. Values associated with enamel indicate the diet at known periods in childhood and comparisons between different teeth in the same individual can indicate a change in diet during childhood.

The stability of teeth over time, particularly enamel, has allowed them to provide data on the diet of dinosaurs. The application of carbon isotope studies to humans has shown, for example, that early hominids such as *Paranthropus robustus*, unlike modern-day great apes (chimpanzees, gorillas and orang-utans) whose diet is almost totally associated with C3 plant material, ate a diet containing a small but significant component of C4 plant material (probably by eating the flesh of grass-eating animals). It has also been applied to determine the date at which early human populations in America first introduced the agriculture of maize, the only significant C4 crop grown by Native Americans.

## Stable nitrogen isotopes

As with carbon, the ratios of two stable nitrogen isotopes, nitrogen-15 and nitrogen-14, in the collagen of bone can be used to reveal dietary information. Herbivores feeding on legumes will have a different nitrogen-15 fingerprint from animals eating plants that derive their nitrogen from the soil. Stable nitrogen isotope values from bone collagen will also help differentiate carnivores from herbivores and marine from terrestrial feeders.

Nitrogen-15 values in the collagen of teeth and bones from birth onwards have been investigated in an attempt to determine the approximate time of weaning. This is based on the observation that breast-fed children have slightly higher nitrogen-15 levels in their collagen than their mothers. By observing a fall in nitrogen-15 values, weaning in a medieval population was found to occur at less than 1 year of age and to be relatively abrupt.

## Stable oxygen isotopes

Oxygen has two stable isotopes, oxygen-16 and the rarer oxygen-18. Water vapour evaporated from the ocean in clouds will fall as rain over the land, with the heavier isotope, oxygen-18, falling sooner and therefore being more common in the drinking water associated with a warmer tropical climate nearer the ocean. The lighter oxygen-16 will be given off later a further distance from the ocean and in colder climates towards the poles. Thus, the ratio of stable oxygen isotopes in water will vary according to latitude, water temperature and weather patterns. During the Ice Age, with so much water incorporated in the polar ice, rain everywhere would have had a higher concentration of oxygen-18. Reference isotope levels for the majority of regions of the Earth are known and are relatively stable with time, although corrective factors can be applied to take account of climatic changes.

The oxygen incorporated into the structure of the hydroxyapatite crystallite is ultimately derived from drinking water. Crystallites from enamel, being the most stable, would give precise information about the environment during the period of crown formation. Comparisons between the isotope values from different teeth in the same individual would also indicate any migration to areas with different isotope values. Indeed sampling across a section of enamel from a single tooth might provide

considerable information about an individual's movement during childhood. Dentine and bone, being slowly deposited throughout life, would provide information particularly concerning an individual's environment after the age of about 20 years. Similar information may also be extractable from mineral crystals in any dental calculus present around the teeth.

Analysis of stable oxygen isotopes has provided much important information in assessing collections of bodies in burial sites, when it is possible to distinguish 'locals' from 'foreigners'. An important example of the use of isotopic analysis in shedding light on human archaeology relates to the 'Iceman', estimated to have died about 5,200 years ago. His well-preserved, mummified remains were found in 1991 high up on an alpine glacier in the Otsal Alps (hence his nickname, Otzi), between Italy and Austria. The presence of the mountain results in distinct isotopic oxygen profiles for water occurring north and south of it. Analysis of the stable oxygen isotopes from both enamel and bone samples indicated that the Iceman had lived on the south side in Italy (having more of the heavier isotope). In addition, isotopic values also indicated that, having spent his childhood at a lower altitude, he had later migrated to higher ground.

## Stable strontium isotopes

As for carbon and nitrogen, strontium passes from the soil into plants and thence up the food chain. Strontium readily substitutes for calcium in the hydroxyapatite crystallite and is therefore present in relatively high amounts (100 ppm). It can provide information concerning aspects of the diet (for example, carnivores show a lower strontium : calcium ratio than herbivores). However, perhaps a more important application concerning strontium levels is to indicate the place of origin of a bone/tooth sample and possibly indicate any significant movement away from this site. The two stable isotopes of strontium used in such studies are strontium-87 and strontium-86. As the former isotope is created by the radioactive decay of rubidium, it can also be used for ageing specimens.

Strontium-87 : strontium-86 ratios provide a unique 'fingerprint' to the geology of an area. By matching such values locked up in the mineralized tissue of an individual with those of the surrounding land, light can be shed on the origin of an individual. Data from enamel crystallites provide information as to the whereabouts of an individual during early childhood, while those of adult bone and dentine, because of their continual formation, reflect their more recent site of occupation. Unlike the more resistant enamel, allowance must again be made when examining bone and dentine from archaeological/fossil specimens to account for diagenesis, associated with possible crystal dissolution and of absorption of strontium from the surrounding soil. Strontium analyses in material from burial sites can separate 'locals' from 'foreigners'.

An example of the use of strontium isotope analysis to human archaeology again relates to the 'Iceman' (see above). Oxygen isotope studies having shown him to originate on the Italian side of the Alps, stable strontium isotope analysis of tooth and bone samples pinpointed his origin to just a few valleys about 60 km from the site of the body.

## Lead

The presence of lead in mineralized teeth can be used to provide data similar to that of strontium when considering pre-metallurgical societies. However, once lead-containing artefacts were manufactured, such as drinking utensils and lead pipes, lead values rose and were a reflection of cultural habits. They could also be interpreted as an indication of class as, for example, only the rich in Roman society could afford to drink from pewter vessels (and therefore risk dying from lead poisoning!).

From the above account, it can be seen that analysis of mineralized tissues supports the contention that 'You are what you eat and you were what you ate'.

# Further reading

The following list provides students with some introductory references to allow them to seek further insights.

## ORAL ANATOMY, HISTOLOGY AND EMBRYOLOGY, CHAPTERS 1–6.

### Anatomy

Ash MM Jr 1993 Wheeler's dental anatomy, physiology and occlusion, 7th edn. Saunders, Philadelphia

Berkovitz BKB, Moxham BJ 2002 Head and neck anatomy: a clinical reference. Martin Dunitz, London

Bertilsson O, Strom D 1995 A literature survey of a hundred years of anatomical and functional lateral pterygoid muscle research. Journal of Orofacial Pain 9: 17–23

Burns RC, Herbranson EJ 2001 Tooth morphology and cavity preparation. In: Cohen S, Burns RC (eds) Pathways of the pulp, 8th edn. Mosby, St Louis, pp 179–229

Carrotte P 2003 Morphology of the root canal system. In: A clinical guide to endodontics. British Dental Association, London, pp 21–25

Christo JE, Bennett S, Wilkinson TM, Townsend GC 2005 Discal attachments of the human mandibular joint. Australian Dental Journal 50: 152–160

Evans BT, Wiesenfeld D, Clauser L, Curioni C 2002 Surgical approaches to the infratemporal fossa. In: Langdon JD, Berkovitz BKB, Moxham BJ (eds) Surgical anatomy of the infratemporal fossa. Dunitz, London, pp 141–180

Hillson S 1996 Dental anthropology. Cambridge University Press, Cambridge

Lang J 1995 Clinical anatomy of the masticatory apparatus and peripharyngeal spaces. Georg Thieme, Stuttgart

McDevitt WE 1989 Functional anatomy of the masticatory system. John Wright, Chichester

Orr C 2005a 12 steps to smile design. 1: Macroaesthetic elements. Aesthetic Implants 7 (vol.1): 16–22

Orr C 2005b 12 steps to smile design. 1: Macroaesthetic elements. Aesthetic Implants 7 (vol.2): 14–20

Osborn JW 1985 The disc of the human temporomandibular joint: design, function and failure. Journal of Oral Rehabilitation 12: 279–293

Plunkett DJ, Dysart PS, Kardos TB, Herbison GP 1998 A study of transposed canines in a sample of orthodontic patients. British Journal of Orthodontics 25: 203–208

Scott GR, Turner II, CG 1997 The anthropology of modern human teeth. Cambridge University Press, Cambridge

Standring S (ed) 2005 Gray's anatomy, 39th edn. Churchill Livingstone, Edinburgh

Tiwari RM 2002 Tumours and tumour-like disorders of the infratemporal fossa. In: Langdon JD, Berkovitz BKB, Moxham BJ (eds) Surgical anatomy of the infratemporal fossa. Dunitz, London, pp 125–140

Van Beek GC 1983 Dental morphology: an illustrated guide. John Wright, Bristol

Williams PL (ed) 1995 Gray's anatomy, 38th edn. Churchill Livingstone, Edinburgh

Woelfel JB, Scheid RC 1997 Dental anatomy: its relevance to dentistry, 5th edn. Williams & Williams, Baltimore

### Occlusion, radiography and functional anatomy

Brons R 1998 Facial harmony. Quintessence Publishing, London

Dawson PE 2007 Functional occlusion from TMJ to smile design. Mosby, St Louis

Ferrario VF, Sforza C, Lovecchio N, Mian F 2005 Quantification of translation and gliding components in human temporomandibular joint during mouth opening. Archives of Oral Biology 50: 507–515

Graber TM, Vanarsdall RL Jr 2000 Orthodontics: current principles and techniques, 3rd edn. Mosby, St Louis

Hannam AG, McMillan AS 1994 Internal organization in the human jaw muscles. Critical Reviews in Oral Biology and Medicine 5: 55–89

Huang BY, Whittle T, Murray GM 2005 Activity of inferior head of human lateral pterygoid muscle during standardised lateral jaw movements. Archives of Oral Biology 50: 49–64

Jacobson A, Caufield PW 1985 Introduction to radiographic cephalometry. Lea & Febiger, Philadelphia

McDonald F, Ireland AJ 1998 Diagnosis of the orthodontic patient. Oxford University Press, Oxford

McNeill C 1997 Science and practice of occlusion. Quintessence Publishing, Chicago

Miyashita K 1996 Contemporary cephalometric radiography. Quintessence Publishing, Tokyo

Murray GM, Phanachet I, Uchida S, Whittle T 2004 The human lateral pterygoid muscle. A review of some experimental aspects and possible clinical relevance. Australian Dental Journal 49: 2–8

Orchardson R, Cadden SW 1998 Mastication. In: Linden RWA (ed) The scientific basis of eating. Taste and smell, salivation, mastication and swallowing and their dysfunctions. Frontiers of Oral Biology Series 9. Karger, Basel, pp 76–121

Paster FA 1993 Colour atlas of dental medicine – radiology. Thieme, Stuttgart

Proffit WR, Fields HW Jr 2000 Contemporary orthodontics, 3rd edn. Mosby, St Louis

Thexton A 1998 Some aspects of swallowing. In: Harris M, Edgar M, Meghji S (eds) Clinical oral science. Wright, Oxford, pp 150–166

Thexton AJ, Crompton AW 1998 The control of swallowing. In: Linden RWA (ed) The scientific basis of eating. Taste and smell, salivation, mastication and swallowing and their dysfunctions. Frontiers of Oral Biology Series 9. Karger, Basel, pp 168–222

Valvassari GE, Masee MS, Carter BL 1995 Imaging of the head and neck. Thieme, Stuttgart

Whaites E 2007 Essentials of dental radiography and radiology, 4th edn. Churchill Livingstone, Edinburgh

## CHAPTERS 7–16

### Enamel

Boyde A 1989 Enamel. In: Oksche A, Volrath L (eds) Teeth. Handbook of microscopic anatomy, vol 6. Springer Verlag, Berlin, pp 309–473

Chadwick D, Cardew G (eds) 1997 Dental enamel. Ciba Foundation Symposium 205. Wiley, New York

Dean MC 2000 Incremental markings in enamel and dentine: what they can tell us about the way teeth grow. In: Teaford MF, Smith MM, Ferguson MWJ (eds) Development, function and evolution of teeth. Cambridge University Press, Cambridge, pp 119–130

Elliott JC, Wong FS, Anderson P et al 1998 Determination of mineral concentration in dental enamel from X-ray attenuation measurements. Connective Tissue Research 38: 61–67

Habelitz S, Marshall SJ, Marshall GW Jr, Balooch M 2001 Mechanical properties of human dental enamel on the nanometre scale. Archives of Oral Biology 46: 173–183

Palamara J, Phakey PP, Rachinger WA, Orams HJ 1989 Ultrastructure of spindles and tufts in human dental enamel. Advances in Dental Research 3: 249–257

Risnes S 1998 Growth tracks in dental enamel. Journal of Human Evolution 35: 331–350

Robinson C, Kirkham J, Shore R (eds) 1995 Dental enamel: formation to destruction. CRC Press, Boca Raton, FL

Sasaki T, Goldberg M, Takuma S, Garant P 1990 Cell biology of tooth enamel formation: functional electron microscopic monographs. S Karger, Basel

Shellis RP 1998 Utilization of periodic markings in enamel to obtain information on tooth growth. Journal of Human Evolution 35: 387–400

Shellis RP, Dibdin GH 2000 Enamel microporosity and its functional implications. In: Teaford MF, Smith MM, Ferguson MWJ (eds) Development, function and evolution of teeth. Cambridge University Press, Cambridge, pp 242–251

Von Koenigswald W, Sander PM (eds) 1997 Tooth enamel microstructure. AA Balkema, Rotterdam

White SN, Luo W, Paine ML et al 2001 Biological organization of hydroxyapatite crystallites into a fibrous continuum toughens and controls anisotropy in human enamel. Journal of Dental Research 80: 321–326

Xu HH, Smith DT, Jahanmir S et al 1998 Indentation damage and mechanical properties of human enamel and dentin. Journal of Dental Research 77: 472–480

## Enamel integuments

Carranza FA Jr 1996 Dental calculus. In: Carranza FA Jr, Newman MG (eds) Clinical periodontology, 8th edn. Saunders, Philadelphia, pp 150–160

Ferguson DB 1998 Oral biosciences, 2nd edn. Churchill Livingstone, Edinburgh, pp 159–175

Jin Y, Yip HK 2002 Supragingival calculus: formation and control. Critical Reviews in Oral Biology & Medicine 13: 426–441

Long NP, Mombelli A, Attstrom R 1998 Dental plaque and calculus. In: Linde J, Karring T, Long NP (eds) Clinical periodontology and implant dentistry, 3rd edn. Munksgaard, Copenhagen, pp 101–137

Marsh P, Martin MV 1999 Oral microbiology, 4th edn. Wright, Oxford

Newman HN 1977 Ultrastructure of the apical border of dental plaque. In: Lehner T (ed) The borderland between caries and periodontal disease, vol. 1. Academic Press, London, pp 73–103

Newman HN, Wilson M (eds) 1999 Oral biofilms in health and disease. Bioline, Cardiff

Rohanizadeh R, LeGeros RZ 2005 Ultrastructural study of calculus-enamel and calculus-root interfaces. Archives of Oral Biology 50: 89–96

Sawada T, Inoue S 2001 High resolution ultrastructural reevaluation of dental cuticle in monkey tooth. Journal of Periodontal Research 36: 101–107

Schupbach FG, Oppenheim FG, Lendenmann U et al 2001 Electron-microscopic demonstration of proline-rich proteins, statherin and histatins in aquired pellicles in vitro. European Journal of Oral Sciences 109: 60–68

Tan B, Gillam DG, Mordan NJ, Galgut PN 2004 A preliminary investigation into the ultrastructure of dental calculus. Journal of Clinical Periodontology 31: 364–369

## Dentine

Bjorndal L, Darvann T 1999 A light microscopic study of odontoblastic and non-odontoblastic cells involved in tertiary dentinogenesis in well-defined cavitated carious lesions. Caries Research 33: 50–60

Butler WT 1998 Dentin matrix proteins. European Journal of Oral Sciences 106(Suppl 1): 204–210

Butler WT, Ritchie HH, Bronckers AL 1997 Extracellular matrix proteins of dentine. In: Chadwick D, Cardew G (eds) Ciba Foundation Symposium 205. Wiley, New York, pp 107–115

Dean MC 1998 Comparative observations on the spacing of short-period (von Ebner's) lines in dentine. Archives of Oral Biology 43: 1009–1021

Dean MC, Scandrett AE 1996 The relation between long-period incremental markings in dentine and daily cross-striations in enamel in human teeth. Archives of Oral Biology 41: 233–241

Frank RM, Nalbandian J 1989 Structure and ultrastructure of dentine. In: Oksche A, Volrath L (eds) Teeth. Handbook of microscopic anatomy, vol 6. Springer Verlag, Berlin, pp 173–247

Gale MS, Darvell BW 1999 Dentine permeability and tracer tests. Journal of Dentistry 27: 1–11

Goldberg M, Boskey AL 1996 Lipids and biomineralizations. Progress in Histochemistry and Cytochemistry 31: 1–187

Goldberg M, Septier D, Lecolle S et al 1995 Lipids in predentine and dentine. Connective Tissue Research 33: 105–114

Goldberg M, Takagi M 1993 Dentine proteoglycans: composition, ultrastructure and functions. Histochemical Journal 25: 781–806

Holland GR 1994 Morphological features of dentine and pulp related to dentine sensitivity. Archives of Oral Biology 39(Suppl): 3S–11S

Kagayama M, Sasao Y, Sato H et al 1999 Confocal microscopy of dentinal tubules in human tooth stained with alizarin red. Anatomy and Embryology 199: 233–238

Marshall GW 1993 Dentin: microstructure and characterization. Quintessence International 24: 606–617

Marshall GW, Marshall SJ, Kinney JH, Balooch M 1997 The dentin substrate: structure and properties related to bonding. Journal of Dentistry 25: 441–458

Norlin T, Hilliges M, Brodin L 1999 Immunohistochemical demonstration of exocytosis-regulating proteins within rat molar dentinal tubules. Archives of Oral Biology 44: 223–231

Ohtsuka M, Saeki S, Igarashi K, Shinoda H 1998 Circadian rhythms in the incorporation and secretion of $^3$H-proline by odontoblasts in relation to incremental lines in rat dentin. Journal of Dental Research 77: 1889–1895

Rees JS, Jacobsen PH, Hickman J 1994 The elastic modulus of dentine determined by static and dynamic methods. Clinical Materials 17: 11–15

Smith AJ 2000 Pulpo-dentinal interactions in development and repair of dentine. In: Teaford MF, Smith MM, Ferguson MWJ (eds) Development, function and evolution of teeth. Cambridge University Press, Cambridge, pp 82–91

Sogaard-Pedersen B, Boye H, Matthiessen ME 1990 Scanning electron microscope observations on collagen fibers in human dentin and pulp. Scandinavian Journal of Dental Research 98: 89–95

Thomas GJ, Whittaker DK, Embery G 1994 A comparative study of translucent apical dentine in vital and non-vital human teeth. Archives of Oral Biology 39: 29–34

Tziafas D 1995 Basic mechanisms of cytodifferentiation and dentinogenesis during dental pulp repair. International Journal of Developmental Biology 39: 281–291

Yoshima M, Masada J, Uchida A, Ishida H 1989 Scanning electron microscope characterization of sensitive vs insensitive human radicular dentin. Journal of Dental Research 68: 1498–1502

## Dental pulp

Burke FM, Samarawickrama DY 1995 Progressive changes in the pulpo-dentinal complex and their clinical consequences. Gerodontology 12: 57–66

Byers MR, Narhi MV 1999 Dental injury models: experimental tools for understanding neuroinflammatory interactions and polymodal nociceptor functions. Critical Reviews in Oral Biology and Medicine 10: 4–39

Frank RM, Nalbandian J 1989 Stucture and ultrastructure of the dental pulp. In: Oksche A, Volrath L (eds) Teeth. Handbook of microscopic anatomy, vol 6. Springer Verlag, Berlin, pp 249–305

Franquin JC, Remusat M, Abou Hashieh I, Dejou J 1998 Immunocytochemical detection of apoptosis in human odontoblasts. European Journal of Oral Sciences 106(Suppl 1): 384–387

Fried K, Nosrat C, Lillesaar C 2000 Molecular signalling and pulpal nerve development. Critical Reviews in Oral Biology and Medicine 11: 318–332

Heyeraas KJ, Berggreen E 1999 Interstitial fluid pressure in normal and inflamed pulp. Critical Reviews in Oral Biology and Medicine 10: 328–336

Hildebrand C, Fried K, Tuiski F, Johansson CS 1995 Teeth and tooth nerves. Progress in Neurobiology 45: 165–222

Hillmann G, Geurtsen W 1997 Light-microscopical investigation of the distribution of extracellular matrix molecules and calcifications in human dental pulps of various ages. Cell and Tissue Research 289: 145–154

Jontell M, Okiji T, Dahlgren U, Bergenholtz G 1998 Immune defense mechanisms of the dental pulp. Critical Reviews in Oral Biology and Medicine 9: 179–200

Levin LG, Rudd A, Bletsa A, Reisner H 1999 Expression of IL-8 by cells of the odontoblast layer in vitro. European Journal of Oral Sciences 107: 131–137

Lohinai Z, Szekely AD, Benedek P, Csillag A 1997 Nitric oxide synthase containing nerves in the cat and dog dental pulp and gingiva. Neuroscience Letters 227: 91–94

Lukinmaa PL, Waltimo J 1992 Immunohistochemical localization of types I, V, and VI collagen in human permanent teeth and periodontal ligament. Journal of Dental Research 71: 391–397

Matthews B, Andrew D 1995 Microvascular architecture and exchange in teeth. Microcirculation 2: 305–313

Okabe E 1994 Endogenous vasoactive substances and oxygen-derived free radicals in pulpal haemodynamics. Archives of Oral Biology 39(Suppl): 39S-45S

Okiji T, Kosaka T, Kamal AM et al 1996 Age-related changes in the immunoreactivity of the monocyte/macrophage system in rat molar pulp. Archives of Oral Biology 41: 453–460

Olgart L 1996 Neural control of pulpal blood flow. Critical Reviews in Oral Biology and Medicine 7: 159–171

Pashley DH 1996 Dynamics of the pulpo-dentin complex. Critical Reviews in Oral Biology and Medicine 7: 104–133

Ranly DM, Thomas HF, Chen J, MacDougall M 1997 Osteocalcin expression in young and aged dental pulps as determined by RT-PCR. Journal of Endodontics 23: 374–377

Sasaki T, Garant PR 1996 Structure and organization of odontoblasts. Anatomical Record 245: 235–249

Sawa Y, Yoshida S, Ashikaga Y et al 1998 Immunohistochemical demonstration of lymphatic vessels in human dental pulp. Tissue and Cell 30: 510–516

Trowbridge HO, Kim S, Suda H 2001 Pulp development, structure and function. In: Cohen S, Burns RC (eds) Pathways of the pulp, 8th edn. Mosby, St Louis, pp 411–455

Woodnutt DA, Wager-Miller J, O'Neill PC et al 2000 Neurotrophin receptors and nerve growth factor are differentially expressed in adjacent nonneuronal cells of normal and injured tooth pulp. Cell and Tissue Research 299: 225–236

Yoshida S, Ohshima H 1996 Distribution and organization of peripheral capillaries in dental pulp and their relationship to odontoblasts. Anatomical Record 245: 313–326

## Cementum

Ababneh KT, Hall RC, Embery G 1999 The proteoglycans of human cementum: immunohistochemical localisation in healthy, periodontally involved and ageing teeth. Journal of Periodontal Research 35: 87–96

Bosshardt DD 2005 Are cementoblasts a subpopulation of osteoblasts or a unique phenotype? Critical Reviews in Oral Biology & Medicine. Journal of Dental Research 84: 390–406

Bosshardt DD, Selvig KA 1997 Dental cementum: the dynamic tissue covering the root. Periodontology 2000 13: 41–75

Diekwisch TG 2001 The developmental biology of cementum. International Journal of Developmental Biology 45: 695–706

Harrison JW 1995 Intermediate cementum. Development, structure, composition, and potential functions. Oral Surgery, Medicine and Pathology 79: 624–633

MacNeil RN, D'Errico JA, Ouyang H et al 1998 Isolation of murine cementoblasts: unique cells or uniquely-positioned osteoblasts? European Journal of Oral Science 106(Suppl 1): 350–356

Rex T, Kharbanda OP, Petocz P, Darendeliler MA 2005 Physical properties of cementum. American Journal of Orthodontics and Dentofacial Orthopedics 127: 177–185

Saygin NE, Giannobile WV, Somerman MJ 2000 Molecular and cell biology of cementum. Periodontology 2000 24: 73–98

Schroeder HE 1986 Cementum: structural aspects. In: Oksche A, Volrath L (eds) The periodontium. Handbook of microscopic anatomy, vol 5. Springer Verlag, Berlin, pp 81–128

Schroeder HE 1992 Biological problems of regenerative cementogenesis; synthesis and attachment of collagenous matrices on growing and established root surfaces. International Review of Cytology 142: 1–59

Schroeder HE 1993 Human cellular mixed stratified cementum: a tissue with alternating layers of acellular extrinsic and cellular intrinsic fiber cementum. Schweizer Monatsschrift für Zahnmedizin 103: 550–560

Suzuki M, Matsuzaka K, Yamada S et al 2006 Morphology of Malassez's epithelial rest-like cell in the cementum. Journal of Periodontal Research 41: 280–287

Van den Boss T, Handoko G, Niehof A et al 2005 Cementum and dentine in hypophosphatasia. Journal of Dental Research 84: 1021–1025

Weismann HP, Meyer U, Plate U, Hohling HJ 2005 Aspects of collagen mineralization in hard tissue formation. International Review of Cytology 242: 121–156

## Periodontal ligament

Bartold PM (ed) 2000 Connective tissues of the periodontium: research and clinical ramifications. Periodontology 2000 24: 9–269

Bartold PM, Narayanan AS 1998 Biology of the periodontal connective tissues. Quintessence, Chicago

Bartold PM, Narayanan AS 2006 Molecular and cell biology of healthy and diseased periodontal tissues. Periodontology 2000 40: 29–49

Beertsen W, McCulloch CAG, Sodek J 1997 The periodontal ligament; a unique, multifactorial connective tissue. Periodontology 2000 13: 20–40

Berkovitz BKB 2004 Periodontal ligament: structural and clinical correlates. Dental Update 31: 46–54

Berkovitz BKB, Moxham BJ, Newman HN (eds) 1995 The periodontal ligament in health and disease, 2nd edn. Mosby-Wolfe, London

Bosshardt DD 2005 Are cementoblasts a subpopulation of osteoblasts or a unique phenotype? Critical Reviews in Oral Biology and Medicine. Journal of Dental Research 84: 390–406

Chitakanon K, Sims MR 1994 Ultrastructural morphology of vascular endothelial junctions in periodontal ligament. Australian Dental Journal 39: 105–110

Cho MI, Garant PR 2000 Development and general structure of the periodontium. Periodontology 2000 24: 9–27

Everts V, Van der Zee E, Creemers L, Beetsen W 1996 Phagocytosis and intracellular digestion of collagen, its role in turnover and remodelling. Histochemical Journal 28: 229–245

Fiorellini JP, Kim DM, Ishikawa SO 2007 The tooth-supporting structures. In: Newman MG, Takei HH, Carranza FA (eds) Carranza's clinical periodontology, 10th edn. Saunders, London, pp 68–91

Foong K, Sims MR 1999 Blood volume in human bicuspid periodontal ligament determined by electron microscopy. Archives of Oral Biology 44: 465–474

Grzesik WJ, Cheng H, Oh JS et al 2000 Cementum-forming cells phenotypically distinct from bone-forming cells. Journal of Bone and Mineral Research 15: 52–59

Karimbux NY, Nishimura I 1995 Temporal and special expressions of type XII collagen in the remodelling periodontal ligament during experimental tooth movement. Journal of Dental Research 73: 313–318

Kirkham J, Robinson C, Spence J 1989 Site specific variations in the biochemical composition of healthy sheep periodontium. Archives of Oral Biology 34: 405–411

Lekic P, McCulloch CAG 1996 Periodontal ligament cell populations: the central role of fibroblasts in creating a unique tissue. In: Nanci A, McKee MD, Smith CE (eds) The biology of dental tissues. Anatomical Record 245: 327–341

Linde J, Karring T 1998 Anatomy of the periodontium. In: Linde J, Karring T, Long NP (eds) Clinical periodontology and implant dentistry, 3rd edn. Munksgaard, Copenhagen, pp 19–68

Maeda T, Ochi K, Nakura-Ohshima K et al 1999 The Ruffini ending as the primary mechanoreceptor in the periodontal ligament: its morphology, cytochemical features, regeneration and development. Critical Reviews in Oral Biology and Medicine 10: 307–327

Maruya Y, Sasano Y, Takahashi I, Kagayama M, Mayanagi H 2003 Expression of extracellular matrix molecules, MMPs and TIMPs in alveolar bone, cementum and periodontal ligaments during rat tooth eruption. Journal of Electron Microscopy 52: 593–604

Mavragani M, Brudvik P, Selvig KA 2005 Orthodontically induced root and alveolar bone resorption: inhibitory effect of systemic doxycycline administration in rats. European Journal of Orthodontics 27: 215–225

Moxham BJ, Berkovitz BKB 1995 The effects of external forces on the periodontal ligament. In: Berkovitz BKB, Moxham BJ, Newman HN (eds) The periodontal ligament in health and disease. Mosby-Wolfe, London, pp 215–241

Nagatomo K, Komaki M, Sekiya Y et al 2006 Stem cell properties of human periodontal ligament cells. Journal of Periodontal Research 41: 303–310

Nanci A, Bosshardt DD 2006 Structure of periodontal tissues in health and disease. Periodontology 2000 40: 11–28

Rincon JC, Young WC, Bartold PM 2006 The epithelial cell rests of Malassez – a role in periodontal regeneration? Journal of Periodontal Research 41: 242–252

Thilander B, Rygh P, Reitan K 2005 Tissue reactions in orthodontics. In: Grabner TM, Vanarsdall RL, Vig KWL (eds) Orthodontics: current principles and techniques. Mosby, London, pp 145–219

Wikesjo UME, Selvig KA (eds) 2000 Periodontal wound healing and regeneration. Periodontology 2000 19: 7–172

## Alveolar bone

Arnett TR 2003 Regulation of bone cell function by acid–base balance. Proceedings of the Nutrition Society 62: 511–520

Arnett TR 2007 Acid–base regulation of bone metabolism. International Congress Series 1297: 255–267

Arnett TR, Henderson B (eds) 1998 Methods in bone biology. Chapman & Hall, London

Arnett TR, Gibbons DC, Utting JC et al 2003 Hypoxia is a major stimulator of osteoclastic formation and bone resorption. Journal of Cellular Physiology 196: 2–8

Bilezikian JP, Raisz LG, Rodan GA (eds) 1996 Principles of bone biology. Academic Press, London

Boyde A 2003 The real response of bone to exercise. Journal of Anatomy 203: 173–189

Cope JB, Samchukov ML 2005 Craniofacial distraction osteogenesis: basic principles and clinical applications. In: Grabner TM, Vanarsdall RL, Vig KWL (eds) Orthodontics: current principles and techniques. Mosby, London, pp 1053–1096

Davies J, Turner S, Sandy JR 1998 Distraction osteogenesis – a review. British Dental Journal 185: 462–467

Favus MJ (ed) 1999 Primer on the metabolic bone diseases and disorders of mineral metabolism, 4th edn. Lippincott Williams & Wilkins, Philadelphia

Hall BK (ed) 1990 Bone. Vol 1. The osteoblast and osteocyte. Telford Press, Caldwell, NJ

Hall BK (ed) 1991 Bone. Vol 2. The osteoclast. CRC Press, Boca Raton, FL

Hughes FJ, Turner W, Belibasakis G, Martuscelli G 2006 Effects of growth factors and cytokines on osteoblast differentiation. Periodontology 2000 41: 48–72

Jones SJ, Taylor ML, Arnett TR, Boyde A 1995 The significance of the size of an osteoclast. In: Davidovitch Z (ed) Mechanisms of tooth eruption, resorption and replacement by implants. EBSCO Media, Birmingham, AL, pp 51–71

Meghji S, Sandy JR, Harris M 1998 Bone remodelling – cellular and biochemical aspects. In: Harris M, Edgar M, Meghji S (eds) Clinical oral science. Wright, Oxford, pp 85–97

Meghji S, Morrison MS, Henderson B, Arnett TR 2001 pH dependence of bone resorption: mouse calvarial osteoclasts are activated by acidosis. American Journal of Physiology, Endocrinology and Metabolism 280: E112–E119

Roberts WE 2005 Bone physiology, metabolism and biomechanics in orthodontic practice. In: Grabner TM, Vanarsdall RL, Vig KWL (eds) Orthodontics: current principles and techniques. Mosby, London, pp 221–292

Sasaki T 2003 Differentiation and functions of osteoclasts and odontoclasts in mineralised tissue resorption. Microscopic Research Techniques 61: 483–495

Schroeder HE 1986 Alveolar process and alveolar bone. In: Oksche A, Volrath L (eds) The periodontium. Handbook of microscopic anatomy, vol 5. Springer Verlag, Berlin, pp 129–170

Sodek J, McKee MD 2000 The molecular and cell biology of bone. Periodontology 2000 24: 99–126

Van der Plas A, Nijweide PJ 1992 Isolation and purification of osteocytes. Journal of Bone and Mineral Research 7: 389–396

Wang LC, Takahashi I, Sasano Y, Sugawara J, Mitani H 2005 Osteoclastogenic activity during mandibular distraction osteogenesis. Journal of Dental Research 84: 1010–1015

## Oral mucosa

Barrett AW, Sculley C 1994 Human oral mucosal melanocytes: a review. Journal of Oral Pathology and Medicine 23: 97–103

Barrett AW, Cruchley AT, Williams DN 1996 Oral mucosal Langerhans cells. Critical Reviews in Oral Biology and Medicine 7: 36–58

Barrett AW, Morgan M, Nwaeze G, Kramer G, Berkovitz BKB 2005 The differentiation profile of epithelium of the human lip. Archives of Oral Biology 50: 431–438

Berkovitz BKB, Barrett AW 1998 Cytokeratin intermediate filaments in oral and odontogenic epithelia. Bulletin du Groupment International pour la Recherche Scientifique en Stomatologie et Odontologie 40: 4–22

Bosshardt DD, Lang NP 2005 The junctional epithelium: from health to disease. Journal of Dental Research 84: 9–20

Fiorellini JP, Kim DM, Ishikawa SO 2007 The gingival. In: Newman MG, Takei HH, Carranza FA (eds) Carranza's clinical periodontology, 10th edn. Saunders, London, pp 46–67

Gibbs S, Ponec M 2000 Intrinsic regulation of differentiation markers in human epidermis, hard palate and buccal mucosa. Archives of Oral Biology 45: 149–158

Mackenzie ICM, Rittman G, Gao Z et al 1991 Patterns of cytokeratin expression in human gingival epithelia. Journal of Periodontal Research 26: 468–478

Mayer J, Squier CA, Gerson SJ (eds) 1984 The structure and function of oral mucosa. Pergamon Press, Oxford

Newman HN 1990 The tooth–gingival interface: weak or strong? Journal of the Western Society of Periodontology 38: 5–9

Presland RB, Dale BA 2000 Epithelial structural proteins of the skin and oral cavity: function in health and disease. Critical Reviews in Oral Biology and Medicine 11: 383–408

Salonen JI 1986 Epithelial attachment of human gingiva. A descriptive and experimental study. Proceedings of the Finnish Dental Society 82: 1–92

Schroeder HE 1981 Differentiation of human and stratified epithelia. Karger, Basel

Schroeder HE 1986 The gingiva. In: Oksche A, Volrath L (eds) The periodontium. Handbook of microscopic anatomy, vol 5. Springer Verlag, Berlin, pp 233–323

Schroeder HE, Listgarten MA 1977 Fine structure of the developing epithelial attachment of human teeth. Monographs in Developmental Biology 2

Schroeder HE, Listgarten MA 1997 The gingival tissues: the architecture of periodontal protection. Periodontology 2000 13: 91–120

Schroeder HE, Listgarten MA 2002 The junctional epithelium: from strength to defence. Journal of Dental Research 82: 151–161

Seguier S, Godeau G, Brousse N 2000 Immunohistochemical and morphometric analysis of intra-epithelial lymphocyes and Langerhans cells in healthy and diseased human gingival tissues. Archives of Oral Biology 45: 441–452

Squier CA 1992 The permeability of oral mucosa. Critical Reviews in Oral Biology and Medicine 3: 13–32

Squier CA, Finklestein MW 1998 Oral mucosa. In: Ten Cate AR (ed) Oral histology: development, structure and function, 5th edn. Mosby, St Louis, pp 345–385

Tachibana T 1995 The Merkel cell: recent findings and unresolved problems. Archives of Histology and Cytology 58: 379–396

Thomson PT, Potten CS, Appleton DR 2001 In vitro labelling studies and the measurement of epithelial cell proliferative activity in the human oral cavity. Archives of Oral Biology 46: 1157–1164

## Temporomandibular joint

Berkovitz BKB 2000 Collagen crimping in the intra-articular disc and articular surfaces of the human temporomandibular joint. Archives of Oral Biology 45: 749–756

Berkovitz BKB, Becker D 2002 The detailed morphology and distribution of gap junction protein associated with cells from the intra-articular disc of the rat temporomandibular joint. Connective Tissue Research 203: 12–18

Berkovitz BKB, Pacy J 2000 Age changes in the cells of the intra-articular disc of the temporomandibular joints of rats and marmosets. Archives of Oral Biology 45: 987–995

Berkovitz BKB, Pacy J 2002 Ultrastructure of the human intra-articular disc of the temporomandibular joint. European Journal of Orthodontics 24: 151–158

Copray JCVM, Dibbets JMH, Kantomaa T 1988 The role of condylar cartilage in the development of the temporomandibular joint. Angle Orthodontist 58: 369–380

Detamore MS, Athanasiou KA 2003 Structure and function of the temporomandibular joint disc: implications for tissue engineering. Journal of Oral and Maxillofacial Surgery 61: 494–506

Detamore MS, Orfanos JG, Almarza AJ et al 2005 Quantitative analysis and comparative regional investigation of the extracellular matrix of the porcine temporomandibular joint disc. Matrix Biology 24: 45–57

Detamore MS, Hegde JN, Wagle RR et al 2006 Cell type and distribution in the porcine temporomandibular joint disc. Journal of Oral and Maxillofacial Surgery 64: 234–248

Gross A, Bumann A, Hoffmeister B 1999 Elastic fibres in the human temporomandibular joint disc. Journal of Oral and Maxillofacial Surgery 28: 464–468

Haskin CL, Milan SB, Cameron IL 1995 Pathogenesis of degenerative joint disease in the human temporomandibular joint. Critical Reviews in Oral Biology and Medicine 6: 248–277

Luder HU 1996 Postnatal development, aging and degeneration of the temporomandibular joint in humans, monkeys and rats. In: McNamara JA Jr (ed) Craniofacial growth series, vol 32. Center for Human Growth and Development, University of Michigan, Ann Arbor, MI, pp 133–168

Mills DK, Fiandaca DJ, Scapino RP 1994 Morphological, microscopic and immunohistochemical investigations into the function of the primate temporomandibular joint disc. Journal of Orofacial Pain 8: 136–154

Nakano T, Scott PG 1989 A quantitative chemical study of the glycosaminoglycans in the articular disc of the bovine temporomandibular joint. Archives of Oral Biology 34: 749–757

Nakano T, Scott PG 1989 Proteoglycans of the articular disc of the bovine temporomandibular joint. 1. High molecular weight chondroitin sulphate proteoglycan. Matrix 9: 277–283

Rabie A, Hagg U 2002 Factors regulating mandibular condylar growth. American Journal of Orthodontics and Dentofacial Orthopaedics 122: 401–409

Takisawa A, Ihara K, Jinji Y 1982 Fibro-architecture of human temporomandibular joint. Okajimas Folia Japonica 59: 141–166

Visnapuu V, Peltomaki T, Isotupa K et al 2000 Distribution and characterisation of proliferative cells in the rat mandibular condyle during growth. European Journal of Orthodontics 22: 631–638

Zarb GA, Carlsson GE, Sessle BJ, Mohl ND (eds) Temporomandibular joint and masticatory muscle disorders, 2nd edn. Munksgaard, Copenhagen

## Salivary glands

Azevedo LR, Dammante JH, Lara VS, Lauris JRP 2005 Age-related changes in human sublingual glands. Archives of Oral Biology 50: 565–574

Dale AC, Ten Cate AR 1998 In: Ten Cate AR (ed) Oral histology: development, structure and function. Mosby, St Louis, pp 386–407

Ellis GL, Auclair PL 1996 The normal salivary glands. In: Tumors of the salivary glands, 3rd series, fascicle 17. Armed Forces Institute of Pathology, Washington, DC, pp 1–26

Ferguson DB 1998 Oral biosciences, 2nd edn. Churchill Livingstone, Edinburgh, pp 117–157

Garrett JR 1998 Myoepithelial activity in salivary glands. In: Garrett JR, Ekstrom J, Anderson LC (eds) Glandular mechanisms of salivary secretion. Frontiers in oral biology 10. Karger, Basel, pp 132–152

Garrett JR 1999 Nerves in the main salivary glands. In: Garrett JR, Ekstrom J, Anderson LC (eds) Glandular mechanisms of salivary secretion. Frontiers in oral biology 10. Karger, Basel, pp 1–25

Garrett JR, Kidd A 1993 The innervation of salivary glands as revealed by morphological methods. Microscopy Research and Techniques 26: 75–91

Harrison JD 2005 Histology and pathology of sialolithiasis. In: Witt RL (ed) Salivary gland diseases: surgical and medical management. Thieme, Stuttgart, pp 71–78

Ihrler S, Blasenbreu-Vogt S, Sendelhofert A et al 2004 Regeneration in chronic sialadenitis: an analysis of proliferation and apoptosis based on double immunohistochemical labelling. Virchows Archiv 444: 356–361

Proctor GB 1998 Secretory protein synthesis and constitutive (vesicular) secretion by salivary glands. In: Garrett JR, Ekstrom J, Anderson LC (eds) Glandular mechanisms of salivary secretion. Frontiers in oral biology 10. Karger, Basel, pp 73–88

Scott J 1986 Structure and function in aging human salivary glands. Gerontology 5: 149–158

Scott J 1987 Structural age changes in salivary glands. In: Ferguson DB (ed) Frontiers of oral physiology 6. Karger, Basel, pp 40–62

Scott J, Flower EA, Burns J 1987 A quantitative study of histological changes in the human parotid gland occurring with adult age. Journal of Oral Pathology 16: 505–510

Tandler B 1993 Structure of mucous cells in salivary glands. Microscopical Research Techniques 26: 49–56

Tandler B 1993 Structure of serous cells in salivary glands. Microscopical Research Techniques 26: 32–48

Tandler B 1993 Structure of the duct system in mammalian major salivary glands. Microscopical Research Techniques 26: 57–74

Yamashina S, Tamaki H, Katsumata O 1999 The serous demilune of rat sublingual gland is an artificial structure produced by coventional fixation. Archives of Histology and Cytology 62: 347–354

## CHAPTERS 17–27

### Development of craniofacial region

Evans DJR, Francis-West P 2005 Craniofacial development: making faces. Journal of Anatomy 207 (Symposium issue): 435–683

Ferguson MWJ 1988 Palate development. In: Thorogood P, Tickle C (eds) Craniofacial development. Development 103(Suppl): 41–60

Fitchett JE, Hay ED 1989 Medial edge epithelium transforms to mesenchyme after embryonic palatal shelves fuse. Developmental Biology 131: 455–474

Graham A, Morriss-Kay G 2001 The evolution of developmental mechanisms. Journal of Anatomy 199 (Symposium issue): 1–229

Kerrigan JJ, Mansell JP, Sengupta A et al 2000 Palatogenesis and potential mechanisms for clefting. Journal of the Royal College of Surgeons of Edinburgh 45: 351–358

Meikle MC 2002 Craniofacial development, growth and evolution. Bateson Publishing, Norfolk

Singh GD, Moxham BJ, Langley MS, Embery G 1994 Changes in the composition of glycosaminoglycans during normal palatogenesis in the rat. Archives of Oral Biology 39: 401–407

Singh GD, Moxham BJ, Langley MS et al 1997 Glycosaminoglycan biosynthesis during 5-fluoro-2-deoxyuridine-induced palatal clefts in the rat. Archives of Oral Biology 42: 355–363

Slavkin HC, Diekwisch T 1996 Evolution in tooth developmental biology: of morphology and molecules. In: Nanci A, McKee MD, Smith CE (eds) The biology of dental tissues. Anatomical Record 245: 131–150

Sperber GH 2001 Craniofacial development, 4th edn. BC Decker, Hamilton, Ontario

Stricker M, van der Meulen J, Raphael B et al 1990 Craniofacial malformations. Churchill Livingstone, Edinburgh

Taya Y, O'Kane S, Ferguson MWJ 1999 Pathogenesis of cleft palate in TFG-β knockout mice. Development 126: 3869–3879

Thorogood P, Ferretti P 1998 Craniofacial development. In: Harris M, Edgar M, Meghji S (eds) Clinical oral science. Wright, Oxford, pp 38–48

Thorogood P, Tickle C (eds) 1988 Craniofacial development. Development 103(Suppl)

### Tooth development

Chen Y, Zhang Y, Jiang T-X et al 2000 Conservation of early odontogenic signaling pathways in Aves. Proceedings of the National Academy of Sciences of the United States of America 97: 10044–10049

Domingues MG, Jaeger MMM, Araujo VC, Araujo NS 2000 Expression of cytokeratins in human enamel organ. European Journal of Oral Science 108: 43–47

Duailibi SE, Duailibi MT, Vacanti JP, Yelick PC 2006 Prospects for tooth regeneration. Periodontology 2000 41: 177–187

Harris MP, Hasso SM, Ferguson MWJ, Fallon JF 2006 The development of Archosaurian first-generation teeth in a chicken mutant. Current Biology 16: 371–377

Jarvinen E, Salazar-Ciudad I, Birchmeier W et al 2006 Continuous tooth generation in mouse is induced by activated epithelial Wnt/β-catenin signaling. Proceedings of the National Academy of Sciences of the United States of America 103: 18627–18632

Linde A (ed) 1998 Odontogenesis and craniofacial development. European Journal of Oral Sciences 106(Suppl 1)

Lubbock MJ, Harrison VT, Lumsden AGS, Palmer RM 1996 Development and cell fate in interspecific (*Mus musculus/Mus caroli*) intraocular transplants of mouse molar tooth-germ tissues detected by in situ hybridization. Archives of Oral Biology 41: 77–84

Matalova E, Tucker, AS, Sharpe PT 2004 Death in the life of a tooth. Journal of Dental Research 83: 11–16

McCollum M, Sharpe PT 2001 Evolution and development of teeth. Journal of Anatomy 199: 153–160

McCollum MA, Sharpe PT 2001 Developmental genetics and early hominid craniodental evolution. Bioessays 23: 481–493

Mitsiadis TA, Caton J, Cobourne M 2006 Waking up the sleeping beauty: recovery of the ancestral bird odontogenic program. Journal of Experimental Zoology (Molecular and Developmental Evolution) 306B: 227–233

Schwabe GC, Opitz C, Tinschert S, Mundlos S, Sharpe PT 2005 Molecular mechanisms of tooth development and malformations. Oral Biology and Medicine 1: 77–91

Sharpe PT, Young CS 2005 Test tube teeth. Scientific American 295: 34–41

Smith M (ed) 2006 Vertebrate dentitions: genes, development and evolution. Journal of Experimental Zoology, Part B. (Molecular and Developmental Evolution) 306B: 177–316

Srisuwan T, Tilkorn DJ, Wilson JL et al 2006 Molecular aspects of tissue engineering in the dental field. Periodontology 2000 41: 88–108

Teaford MF, Meredith Smith M, Ferguson MWJ (eds) 2000 Development, function and evolution of teeth. Cambridge University Press, Cambridge

Thesleff I 2003 Developmental biology and building a tooth. Quintessence International 34: 613–620

Thesleff I, Vaahtokari A, Vaino S, Jowett A 1996 Molecular mechanisms of cell and tissue interactions during early tooth development. In: Nanci A, McKee MD, Smith CE (eds) The biology of dental tissues. Anatomical Record 245: 151–161

Trentini CJ, Proffit WR 1996 High resolution observations of human premolar eruption. Archives of Oral Biology 41: 63–68

Tucker AS, Sharpe PT 1999 Molecular genetics of tooth morphogenesis and patterning: the right shape in the right place. Journal of Dental Research 78: 826–834

Tucker AS, Sharpe PT 2004 The cutting edge of mammalian development: how the embryo makes teeth. Nature Reviews Genetics 5: 499–508

Tucker AS, Matthews KL, Sharpe PT 1998 Transformation of tooth type induced by inhibition of BMP signaling. Science 282: 1136–1138

### Amelogenesis

Aoba T 1996 Recent observations on enamel crystal formation during mammalian amelogenesis. Anatomical Record 245: 208–218

Bartlett JD, Simmer JP 1999 Proteinases in developing dental enamel. Critical Reviews in Oral Biology and Medicine 10: 425–441

Brookes SJ, Robinson C, Kirkham J, Bonass WA 1995 Biochemistry and molecular biology of amelogenin proteins of developing dental enamel. Archives of Oral Biology 40: 1–14

Den Besten PK 1999 Mechanism and timing of fluoride effects on developing enamel. Journal of Public Health Dentistry 59: 247–251

Deutsch D, Catalano-Sherman J, Dafni L et al 1995 Enamel matrix proteins and ameloblast biology. Connective Tissue Research 32: 97–107

Fincham AG, Simmer JP 1997 Amelogenin proteins of developing dental enamel. In: Chadwick D, Cardew G (eds) Ciba Foundation Symposium 205. Wiley, New York, pp 118–130

Fincham AG, Moradian-Oldak J, Simmer JP 1999 The structural biology of the developing dental enamel matrix. Journal of Structural Biology 126: 270–299

Fincham AG, Luo W, Moradian-Oldak J et al 2000 Enamel biomineralization: the assembly and disassembly of the protein extracellular organic matrix. In: Teaford MF, Meredith Smith M, Ferguson MWJ (eds) Development, function and evolution of teeth. Cambridge University Press, Cambridge, pp 37–61

Gibson CW, Collier PM, Yuan ZA, Chen E 1998 DNA sequences of amelogenin genes provide clues to regulation of expression. European Journal of Oral Sciences 106(Suppl 1): 292–298

Goldberg M, Septier D, Lecolle S et al 1995 Dental mineralization. International Journal of Developmental Biology 39: 93–110

Hu JC-C, Sun X, Zhang C, Simmer JP 2001 A comparison of enamelin and amelogenin expression in developing mouse molars. European Journal of Oral Sciences 109: 125–132

Robinson C, Brookes SJ, Bonass WA et al 1997 Enamel maturation. In: Chadwick D, Cardew G (eds) Ciba Foundation Symposium 205. Wiley, New York, pp 156–170

Robinson C, Brookes SJ, Shore RC, Kirkham J 1998 The developing enamel matrix: nature and function. European Journal of Oral Sciences 106(Suppl 1): 282–291

Sasaki T 1990 Cell biology of tooth enamel formation. Monographs in Oral Science 14. Karger, Basel

Sasaki T, Takagi M, Yanagisawa T 1997 Structure and function of secretory ameloblasts in enamel formation. In: Chadwick D, Cardew G (eds) Ciba Foundation Symposium 205. Wiley, New York, pp 2–46

Simmer JP, Fincham AG 1995 Molecular mechanisms of dental enamel formation. Critical Reviews in Oral Biology and Medicine 6: 84–108

Simmer JP, Hu JC 2001 Dental enamel formation and its impact on clinical dentistry. Journal of Dental Education 65: 896–905

Slavkin HC 1990 Molecular determinants of tooth development: a review. Critical Reviews in Oral Biology and Medicine 1: 1–16

Smith CE 1998 Cellular and chemical events during enamel maturation. Critical Reviews in Oral Biology and Medicine 9: 128–161

Smith CE, Nanci A 1995 Overview of morphological changes in enamel organ cells associated with major events in amelogenesis. International Journal of Developmental Biology 39: 153–161

Takano Y 1995 Enamel mineralization and the role of ameloblasts in calcium transport. Connective Tissue Research 33: 127–137

Uchida T, Murakami C, Wakida K et al 1998 Sheath proteins: synthesis, secretion, degradation and fate in forming enamel. European Journal of Oral Sciences 106(Suppl 1): 308–314

Woltgens JH, Lyaruu DM, Bronckers AL et al 1995 Biomineralization during early stages of the developing tooth in vitro with special reference to secretory stage of amelogenesis. International Journal of Developmental Biology 39: 203–212

## Dentinogenesis and pulp development

Boskey AL 1995 Osteopontin and related phosphorylated sialoproteins: effects on mineralization. Annals of the New York Academy of Sciences 760: 249–256

Chiego DJ 1995 The early distribution and possible role of nerves during odontogenesis. International Journal of Developmental Biology 39: 191–194

Embery G, Hall R, Waddington R et al 2001 Proteoglycans in dentinogenesis. Critical Reviews in Oral Biology and Medicine 12: 331–349

Frank RM, Nalbandian J 1989 Development of dentine and pulp. In: Oksche A, Volrath L (eds) Teeth. Handbook of microscopic anatomy, vol 6. Springer Verlag, Berlin, pp 73–171

Fried K, Nosrat C, Lillesaar C, Hildebrand C 2000 Molecular signaling and pulpal nerve development. Critical Reviews in Oral Biology and Medicine 11: 318–332

Goldberg M, Septier D, Lecolle S et al 1995 Dental mineralization. International Journal of Developmental Biology 39: 93–110

Linde A 1995 Dentin mineralization and the role of odontoblasts in calcium transport. Connective Tissue Research 33: 163–170

Linde A, Goldberg M 1993 Dentinogenesis. Critical Reviews in Oral Biology and Medicine 4: 679–728

Nosrat CA, Fried K, Ebendal T, Olson L 1998 NGF, BDNF, NT3, NT4 and GDNF in tooth development. European Journal of Oral Sciences 106(Suppl 1): 94–99

Ruch JV 1998 Odontoblast commitment and differentiation. Biochemistry and Cell Biology 76: 923–938

Smith AJ, Lesot H 2001 Induction and regulation of crown dentinogenesis. Embryonic events as a template for dental tissue repair. Critical Reviews in Oral Biology and Medicine 12: 425–437

Thomas HF 1995 Root formation. International Journal of Developmental Biology 39: 231–237

Tziafas D 1994 Mechanisms controlling secondary initiation of dentinogenesis: a review. International Endodontic Journal 27: 61–74

Weiner S, Veis A, Beniash E et al 1999 Peritubular dentin formation: crystal organization and the macromolecular constituents in human teeth. Journal of Structural Biology 126: 27–41

## Development of root

Bosshardt DD, Nanci A 2004 Hertwig's epithelial root sheath, enamel matrix proteins, and initiation of cementogenesis in porcine teeth. Journal of Clinical Periodontology 31: 184–192

Bosshardt DB, Schroeder HE 1996 Cementogenesis reviewed: a comparison between human premolars and rodent molars. Anatomical Record 245: 267–292

Crzesik WJ, Narayanan AS 2002 Cementum and periodontal wound healing and regeneration. Critical Reviews in Oral Biology and Medicine 13: 474–484

D'Errico JA, MacNeil RL, Strayhorn CL et al 1995 Models for the study of cementogenesis. Connective Tissue Research 33: 9–17

Diekwisch TGH 2001 Developmental biology of cementum. International Journal of Developmental Biology 45: 695–706

Hammarstrom L 1997 Enamel matrix, cementum development and regeneration. Journal of Clinical Periodontology 24: 658–668

Hammarstrom L, Alatli I, Fong CD 1996 Origins of cementum. Oral Diseases 2: 63–69

Karring T, Linde J, Cortellini P 1998 Regenerative periodontal therapy. In: Linde J, Lang NP (eds) Clinical periodontology and implant dentistry, 3rd edn. Munksgaard, Copenhagen, pp 597–646

King GN 2001 New regenerative technologies: rationale and potential for periodontal regeneration. 2. Growth factors. Dental Update 28: 60–65

Moxham BJ, Grant DA 1995 Development of the periodontal ligament. In: Berkovitz BKB, Moxham BJ, Newman HN (eds) The periodontal ligament in health and disease. Mosby-Wolfe, London, pp 161–181

Rippamonti U, Renton L 2006 Bone morphogenetic proteins and the induction of periodontal tissue regeneration. Periodontology 2000 41: 73–87

Venezia E, Goldstein M, Bouan BD, Schwartz Z 2004 The use of enamel matrix derivative in the treatment of periodontal defects: a literature review and meta-analysis. Critical Reviews in Oral Biology and Medicine 15: 382–402

Wikesjo UME, Selvig KA (eds) 2000 Periodontal wound healing and regeneration. Periodontology 2000 19: 7–172

Yamamoto H, Cho SW, Kim E-J et al 2004 Developmental properties of the Hertwig's epithelial root sheath in mice. Journal of Dental Research 83: 688–692

Yamamoto TT, Domon T, Takahashi S, Arambawatta AKS, Wakita M 2004 Immunolocalization of proteoglycans and bone-related non-collagenous glycoproteins in developing acellular cementum of rat molars. Cell and Tissue Research 317: 299–312

Yamashiro T, Tummers M, Thesleff I 2002 Expression of bone morphogenetic proteins and Msx genes during root formation. Journal of Dental Research 82: 172–176

Zeichner-David M 2006 Regeneration of periodontal tissues: cementogenesis revisited. Periodontology 2000 41: 196–217

Zeichner-David M, Chen LS, Hsu Z et al 2006 Amelogenin and ameloblastin show growth-factor like activity in periodontal cells. European Journal of Oral Science 114: 244–253

## Development of the dentitions

Berkovitz BKB, Moxham BJ 1989 Tissue changes during eruption. In: Oksche A, Volrath L (eds) Teeth. Handbook of microscopic anatomy, vol 6. Springer Verlag, Berlin, pp 21–71

Jones SJ, Boyde A 1988 The resorption of dentine and cementum in vivo and in vitro. In: Davidovitch Z (ed) Mechanisms of tooth eruption, resorption and replacement by implants. EBSCO Media, Birmingham, AL, pp 335–354

Krarup S, Darvann TA, Larsen P, Marsh JL, Kreiborg S 2005 Three-dimensional analysis of mandibular growth and tooth eruption. Journal of Anatomy 207: 669–682

McDonald F, Ireland AJ 1998 Diagnosis of the orthodontic patient. Oxford University Press, Oxford

Moxham BJ 1994 What the structure and the biochemistry of the periodontal ligament tell us about the mechanisms of tooth eruption. In: Davidovitch Z (ed) Mechanisms of tooth eruption, resorption and replacement by implants. EBSCO Media, Birmingham, AL, pp 437–450

Moxham BJ, Berkovitz BKB 1995 The periodontal ligament and physiological tooth movements. In: Berkovitz BKB, Moxham BJ, Newman HN (eds) The periodontal ligament in health and disease. Mosby-Wolfe, London, pp 183–214

Moxham BJ, Pycroft JM, Hann A 1998 The role of the cells of the periodontal connective tissues in tooth eruption. In: Davidovitch Z, Mah J (eds) Biological mechanisms of tooth eruption, resorption and replacement by implants. Harvard Society for the Advancement of Orthodontics, Cambridge, MA, pp 79–88

Van der Linden FPGM 1983 Development of the dentition. Quintessence, Chicago

Wise GE, Frazier-Bowers S, D'Souza RN 2002 Cellular, molecular, and genetic determinants of tooth eruption. Critical Reviews in Oral Biology and Medicine 13: 323–334

## Ageing and archaeological and dental anthropological applications of tooth structure

Bentley RA 2006 Strontium isotopes from the earth to the archaeological skeleton: a review. Journal of Archaeological Method and Theory 13: 135–187

Bentley RA, Wahl J, Price TD, Atkinson TC 2008 Isotopic signatures and hereditary traits: snapshot of a Neolithic community in Germany. Antiquity 82: 290–304

Budd P, Montgomery J, Barreiro B, Thomas RG 2000 Differential diagenesis of strontium in archaeological human dental tissue. Applied Geochemistry 15: 687–694

Burke FM, Samarawickrama DY 1995 Progressive changes in the pulpodentinal complex and their clinical consequences. Gerodontology 12: 57–66

Buzon MR, Simonetti A, Creaser RA 2007 Migration in the Nile Valley during the New Kingdom period. A preliminary strontium isotope study. Journal of Archaeological Science 34: 1391–1401

Cho MI, Garant PR 1984 Formation of multinuclear fibroblasts in the periodontal ligaments of old mice. Anatomical Record 208: 185–196

Cowpe JG, Longmore RB, Green MW 1985 Quantitative exfoliative cytology of normal oral squames: an age, site and sex-related survey. Journal of the Royal Society of Medicine 78: 995–1004

Gogly B, Godeau G, Gilbert S et al 1997 Morphometric analysis of collagen and elastic fibres in normal skin and gingival in relation to age. Clinical Oral Investigations 1: 147–152

Kingsmill VJ, Boyde A 1998 Mineralisation density of human mandibular bone: quantitative backscattered electron images analysis. Journal of Anatomy 192: 245–256

Kingsmill VJ, Gray CM, Moles DR, Boyde A 2007 Cortical vascular canals in human mandible and other bones. Journal of Dental Research 86: 368–372

Kvaal SI, Solheim T 2008 Incremental lines in human dental cementum in relation to age. European Journal of Oral Sciences 103: 225–230

Lipsinic FE, Paunovich E, Houston GD, Robison MF 1986 Correlation of age and incremental lines in the cementum of human teeth. Journal of Forensic Sciences 31: 982–989

Miller CS, Dove SB, Cottone JA 1988 Failure of use of cementum annulations in teeth to determine the age of humans. Journal of Forensic Sciences 33: 137–143

Morse DR, Esposito JV, Schoor RS, Williams FL, Furst ML 1991 A review of aging of dental components and a retrospective radiographic study of aging of the dental pulp and dentin in normal teeth. Quintessence International 22: 495–501

Muller W, Fricke H, Halliday AN, McCulloch MT, Wartho J-A 2003 Origin and migration of the alpine iceman. Science 302: 862–866

Needleman I 2007 Aging and the periodontium. In: Newman MG, Takei HH, Carranza FA (eds) Carranza's clinical periodontology, 10th edn. Saunders, London pp 93–98

Ohtani S, Ito R, Arany S, Yamamoto T 2005 Racemization in enamel among different types of teeth from the same individual. International Journal of Legal Medicine 119: 66–69

Price TD, Manzanilla L, Middleton WD 2000 Immigration and the ancient city of Teotihuacan in Mexico: a study using strontium isotope ratios in human bone and teeth. Journal of Archaeological Science 27: 903–913

Richards MP, Maays S, Fuller BT 2002 Stable carbon and nitrogen isotope values of bone and teeth reflect weaning age at the medieval Wharram Percy site, Yorkshire, UK. American Journal of Physical Anthropology 119: 205–210

Richards MP, Pettitt PB, Trinkhaus E et al 2000 Neanderthal diet at Vindija and Neanderthal predation: the evidence from stable isotopes. Proceedings of the National Academy of Sciences of the United States of America 97: 7633–7666

Richards MP, Taylor G, Steele T et al 2008 Isotopic dietary analysis of a Neanderthal and associated fauna from the site of Jonzac (Charente-Maritime), France. Journal of Human Evolution 55: 179–185

Scott J 1987 Structural age changes in salivary glands. In: Ferguson DB (ed) Frontiers of oral physiology, 6. Karger, Basel, pp 40–62

Scott J, Valentine JA, Balasooriya BA 1983 A quantitative histological analysis of the effects of age and sex on human lingual epithelium. Journal de Biologie Buccale 11: 305–315

Slavkin HC 1997 Sex, enamel and forensic dentistry. Journal of the American Dental Association 128: 1021–1025

Sinibaldi M, Goodfriend GA, Barkay G et al 1999 Aspartic acid racemization in teeth from Ketef Hinnom, a late Holocene burial cave in Jerusalem: evidence for reuse. Geoarchaeology 14: 441–454

Wang Y, Cerling TE, Quade J et al 1993 Stable isotopes of paleosol carbonates and fossil teeth as paleoecology and paleoclimate indicators: an example from the St. David Formation, Arizona. Climate Change in Continental Isotopic Records. Geophysical Monographs 78: 241–248

Whittaker DK 2000 Ageing from the dentition. In: Cox M, Mays S (eds) Human osteology in archaeology and forensic sciences. Cambridge University Press, Cambridge, pp 83–99

Whittaker DK 2000 Historical and forensic aspects of tooth wear. In: Addy M, Embury G, Edgar WM, Orchardson R (eds) Tooth wear and sensitivity. Martin Dunitz, London, pp 77–85

# Index

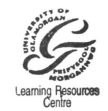